Perfume Bottles for Purse and Dresser

From Czechoslovakia, 1920s-1930s

Perfume Bottles for Purse and Dresser

From Czechoslovakia, 1920s-1930s

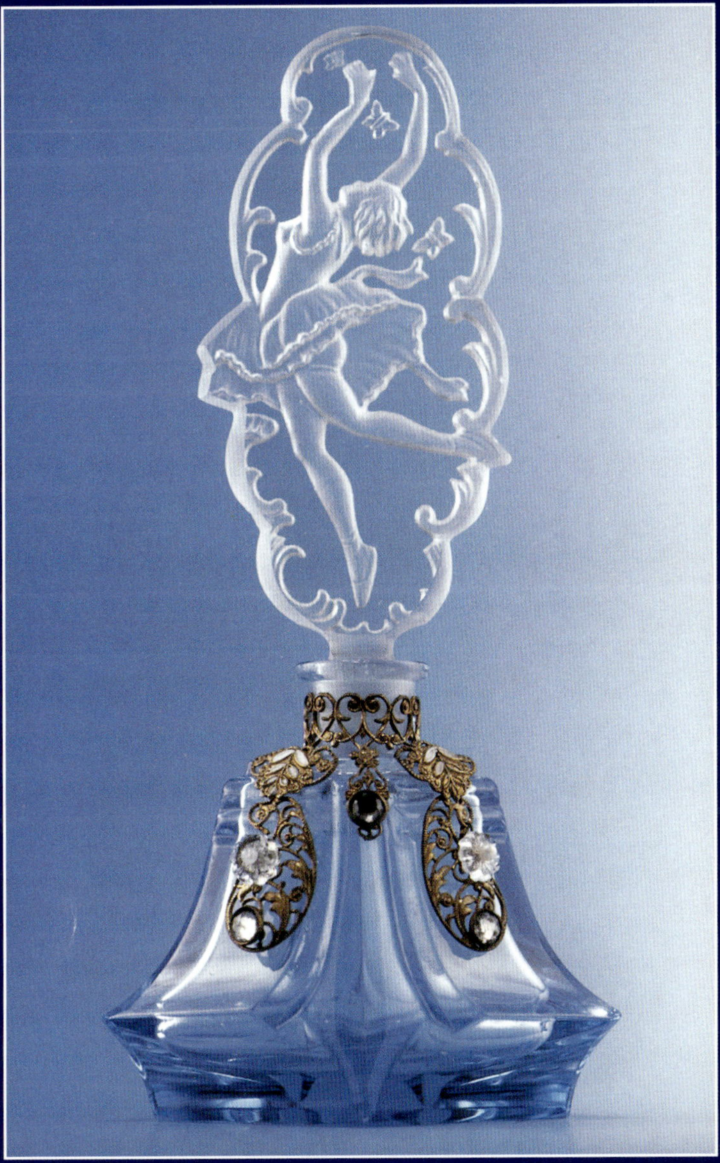

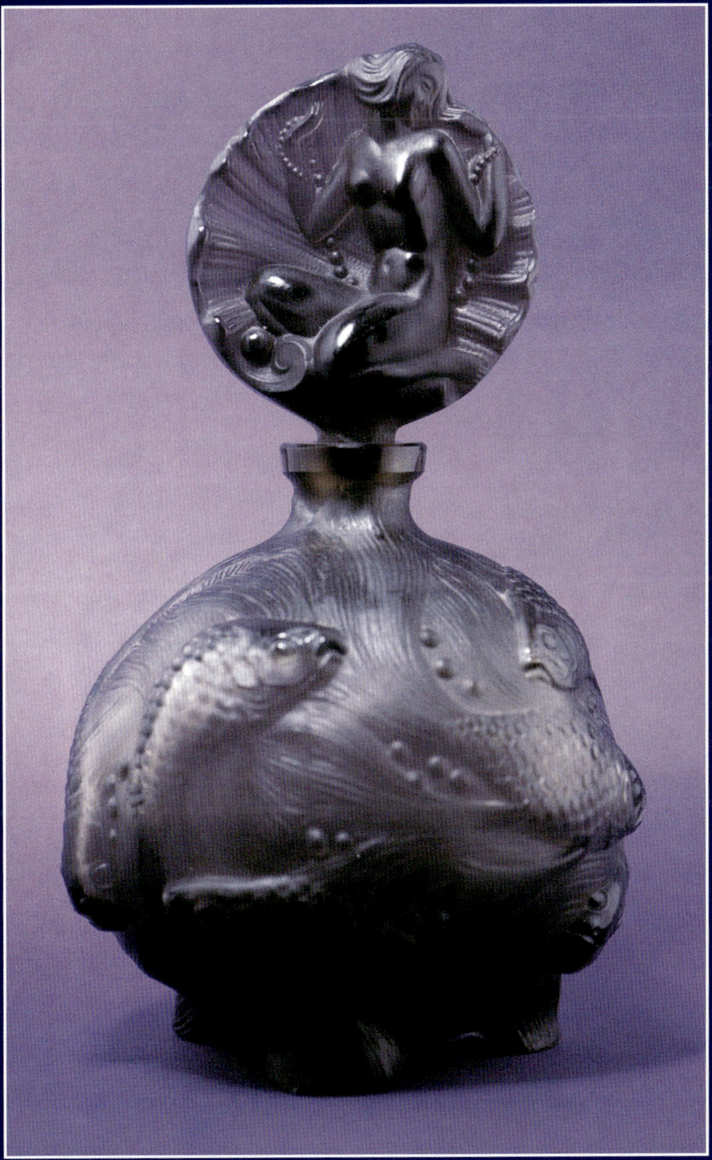

Verna J. Kocken

Schiffer Publishing Ltd®

4880 Lower Valley Road, Atglen, PA 19310 USA

Dedication

To my mother, Edith Wildish Pattee, who has always believed that I could do anything (as long as it is not mechanical—that is my sister, Jan.); and to my grandsons, Brandon, Noah, and Jacob, who bring their own kind of joy.

Library of Congress Control Number: 2005936397

Designed by John P. Cheek
Type set in Lydian BT

ISBN: 0-7643-2412-8
Printed in China
1 2 3 4

Published by Schiffer Publishing Ltd.
4880 Lower Valley Road
Atglen, PA 19310
Phone: (610) 593-1777; Fax: (610) 593-2002
E-mail: Info@schifferbooks.com

For the largest selection of fine reference books on this and related subjects, please visit our web site at
www.schifferbooks.com
We are always looking for people to write books on new and related subjects. If you have an idea for a book please contact us at the above address.

This book may be purchased from the publisher.
Include $3.95 for shipping.
Please try your bookstore first.
You may write for a free catalog.

In Europe, Schiffer books are distributed by
Bushwood Books
6 Marksbury Ave.
Kew Gardens
Surrey TW9 4JF England
Phone: 44 (0) 20 8392-8585; Fax: 44 (0) 20 8392-9876
E-mail: info@bushwoodbooks.co.uk
Free postage in the U.K., Europe; air mail at cost.

Contents

Acknowledgments

The preparation for writing this book started four years prior to its completion, and during that time I have encountered amazing support. Though it would be impossible to name everyone who has been helpful, the encouragement of friends, family, and acquaintances throughout the process has been a key factor.

That said, I am indebted to some individuals for specific help they have provided. To Ruth Forsyth, not only for the inspiration of her courageous pioneer work on the topic of Czechoslovakian ware, but also for taking the time to point me in some productive directions. Ruth, you are the epitome of graciousness.

Special thanks to Earline and Tom Kopriva, Nancy and Frank Dooley, Donna Everitt, Michael Genger, Don Orban, and David Kirk of Kirk Photography, Ft. Wayne, Indiana, who enhanced the scope of this book by providing some of pictured pieces, printed matter, or formal expertise—in some cases, all three.

Thank you, Tom Brennan and Henry Basch, for information on Irice and Petr Vondrich of Jablonex.

Thanks to Paula Walker, Diane Goldfarb, Donna Sims, Rocky and Marilyn Rockholt, Steve and Terry Blumrich, Ken Leach, Sandy Bilsky, and other friends from the International Perfume Bottle Association who have shared stories, expertise, pictures, and enthusiasm with me.

Thanks to dealer friends who make collecting and learning a special joy: Chloe and Jim McKinney, Jacqueline and Robert Johnson, Liz and Mark Thompson, and Suzy and Claude Prince.

Thanks also to the folks at Dotson's camera shop, who gave me photographic advice, assistance, and the senior discount.

To my partner, Don Baldwin, and all my family—DJ, Jan, Bob, Charles, Jeff, Tina, and Richard—I could not have done it without you.

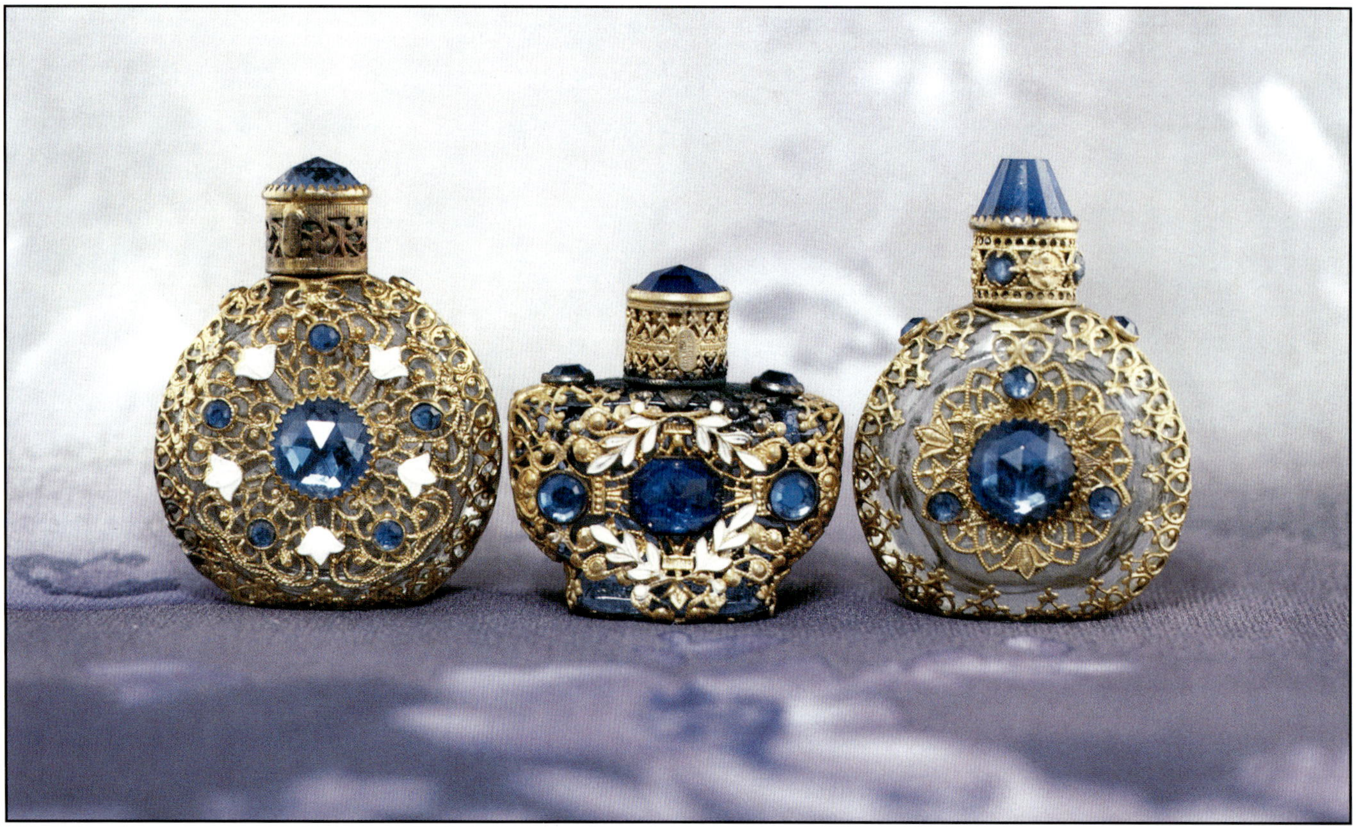

Introduction

Students of human behavior probably have sophisticated answers as to why people collect and could perhaps shed light on why they fixate on a particular category of items to collect. I collect perfume bottles, preferably the tiny ones, and the older, the better.

I have always been fascinated by miniaturization. My earliest childhood memories include playing with a metal dollhouse and enjoying the tiny plastic dolls, furniture, and accessories. Child-sized tea sets and dishes were also favorite toys. But when the Watkins™ man came to our house with helpful items to sell to Mom, he sometimes left a tiny sample bottle of perfume for the "young lady" of the house. That would be me. The sample would be a treasure, one to be placed in a position of importance in my young world. None of these special toys or items survived my childhood, however—after all, there were three younger siblings and no space for storing things that were not being used.

In the late 1980s, a good friend took me to my first huge antique and collectible show. It was a trip into yesteryear. I saw items connected with events, people, and places that were long gone. A tablecloth printed with brightly colored cherries, a glass milk bottle with a cardboard cap, a tatting shuttle, a particular gaudy vase, a letter opener commemorating the Seattle World's Fair, an "I Like Ike" button, a gas station calendar from 1951, a Dick and Jane reader, a cup and saucer in Grandma's good china pattern, a lamp, a jar full of marbles—all were items that tugged at memories, items that connected with my personal and shared history, items that told the times.

At the end of my day's adventure, my "new" old finds included a boxed set of wooden-headed bottles labeled "Floral Quintuplets" (commemorating the Dionne Quintuplets), a miscellany of small, old commercial bottles, and a tiny cut crystal bottle with a flat green cut crystal stopper, complete with a dauber. It was acid-marked Czechoslovakia on the bottom, a two-inch tall work of art. I showed my treasures to my friend; I was hooked!

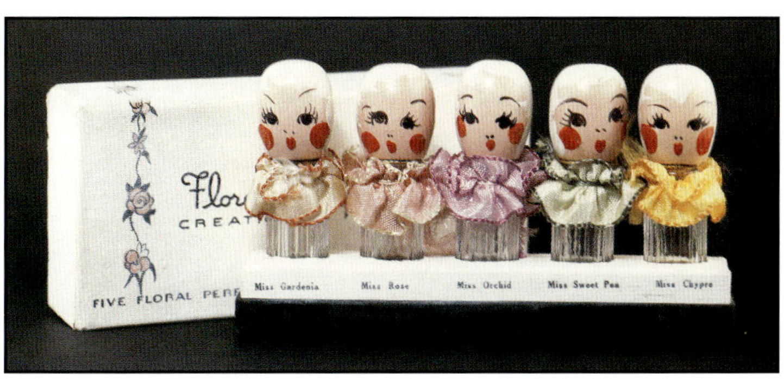

Stuart Products, "Floral Quintuplets, Creation by Karoff, Five Floral Perfumes for Milady's Every Mood." This presentation appeared in 1935 and commemorated the Dionne quintuplets.

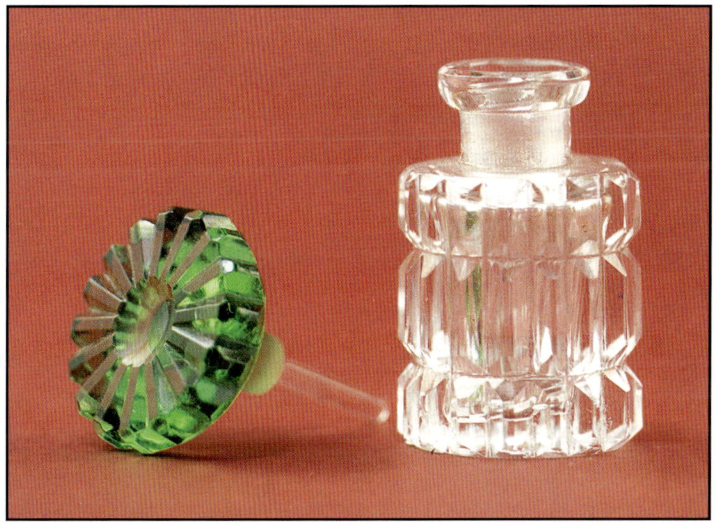

A perfect Czech bottle, later discovered to be one of an original twin set, this 1.875" charmer was the start of the author's love affair with Czech perfume bottles.

Choosing perfume bottles to collect has had certain advantages. I already had my own special bottles, saved from high school and college days. I was soon to discover that a vast number and variety were available. Women get perfume as tokens of love, as promotions, as advertising giveaways, even as plate-side favors at ladies' luncheons or fashion shows. Miniatures come as samples or as "purse bottles" in sets. Too appealing to throw away, they stick around long after the perfume has evaporated or grown rancid with age, gathering in lingerie drawers, dressing tables, even in sewing baskets. Victims of household downsizing or the detritus of estate closings, they end up at garage sales, resale outlets, or flea markets, So, the supply is readily available. And often cheap!

At first, I was not terribly discriminating. If it was cute, did not cost too much, and I did not already have it, I bought it. As time went by, however, I acquired reference books that told me more about what I had in my growing collection. At this point, collecting became "treasure hunting." I bought a 1 dram bottle, still in its tiny sample box, of California Perfume Company/Avon's™ "Gardenia," and was able to date it from the graphics on the box as a 1936 piece. Later, when I found an identical bottle with a similar label but the totally unfamiliar name of "Lucy Hays," I knew to look in the Avon reference. I discovered that this perfume, only available with another purchase, originally sold for twenty cents and only from March 3 to March 23, 1936. Another time, I picked up several bottles at a sale and among them were two Faberge™ purse bottles in original boxes. Much later, I noticed that both boxes were printed on the side with the words, "Buy defense bonds." The word "defense" was struck through with a single line and "War" printed above it. My reference confirmed that both fragrances came out in 1938. Another treasure, which I obtained from a second hand shop for a trade, turned out to be a rare round black Lanvin™ mini-bottle. By this time, I had learned what all collectors and dealers learn—that you simply cannot know everything about everything, but you *can* learn enough to be savvy about a more limited subject. You just hope, for the sake of bargaining, that the particular dealer does not share your particular passion.

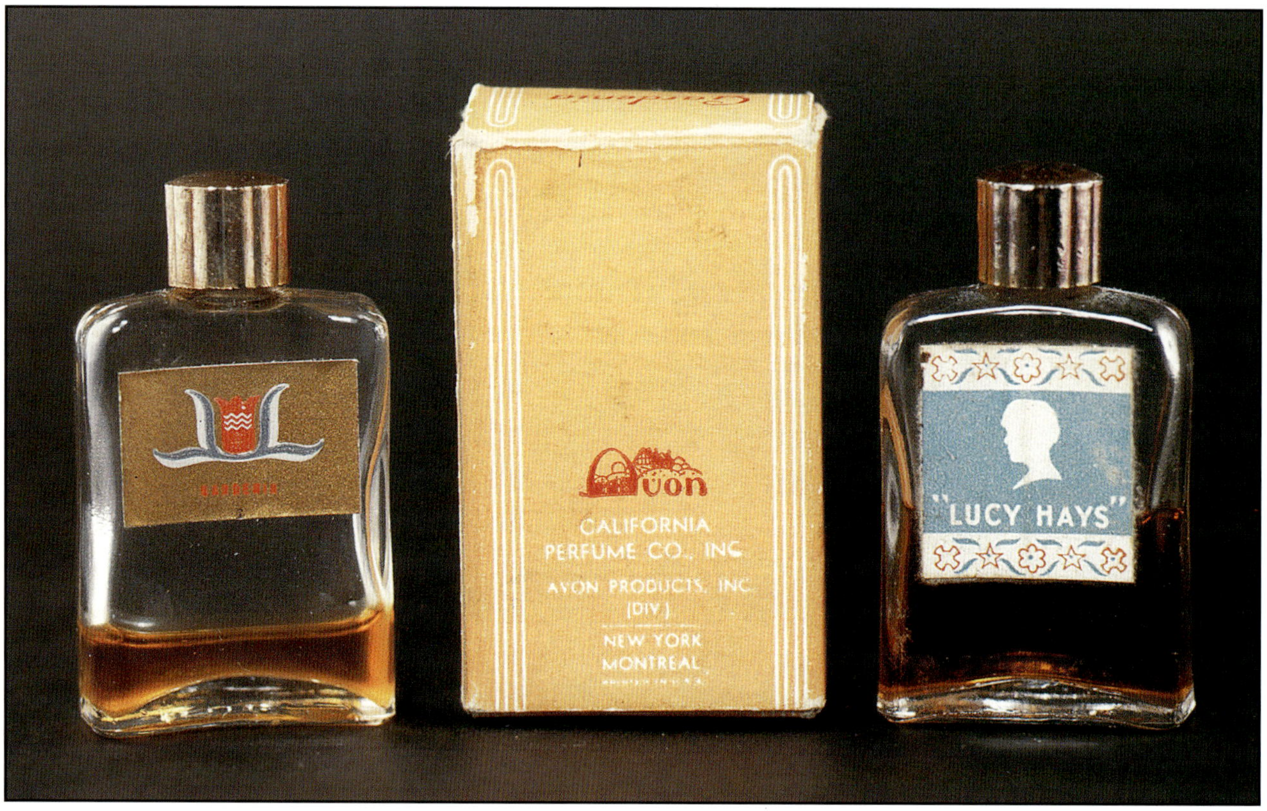

Left: Avon's Gardenia, 1936, with its box. Right: Avon's Lucy Hays, sold March 3-23, 1936. Both 2".

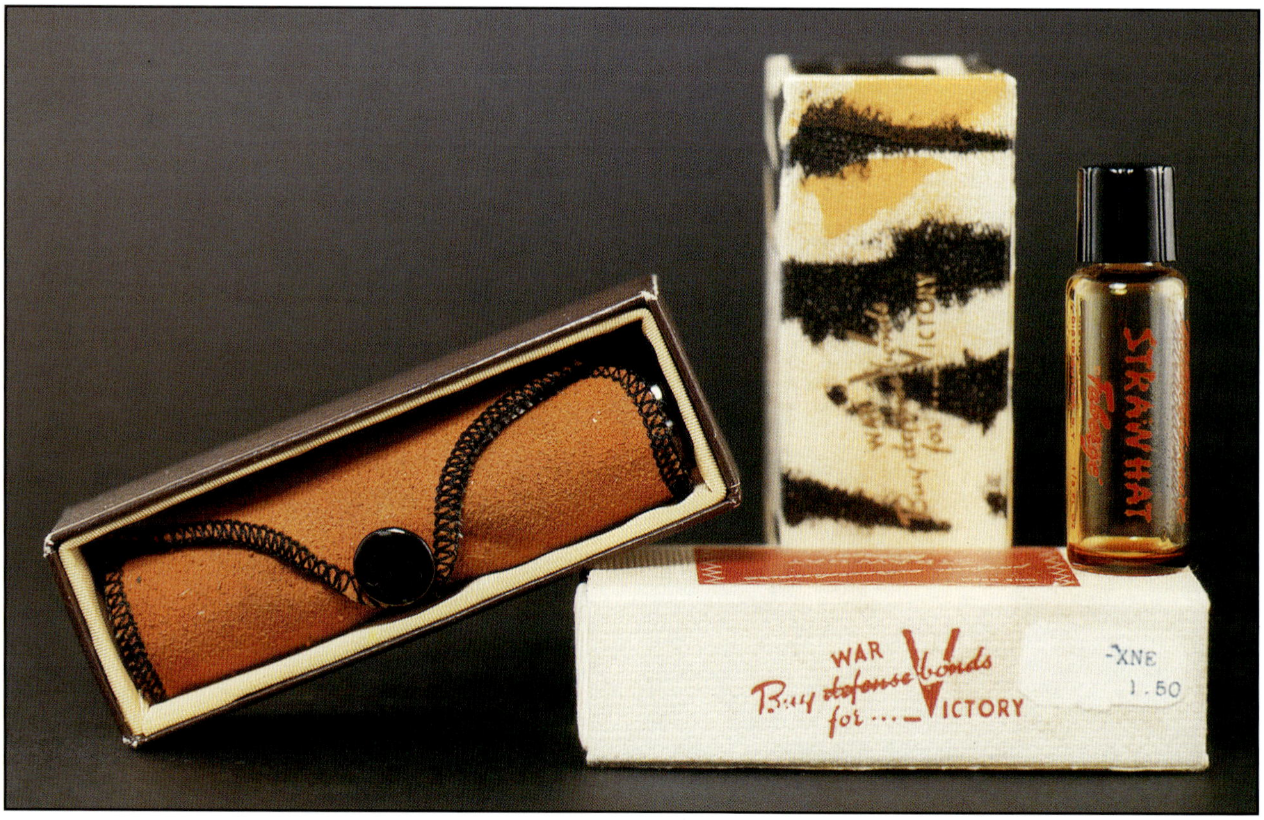

Faberge bottles from 1938: Tigress in the suede roll up and tiger box; Straw Hat in a small, black-capped bottle with box and felt sleeve. Note the pre WWII captions on the boxes.

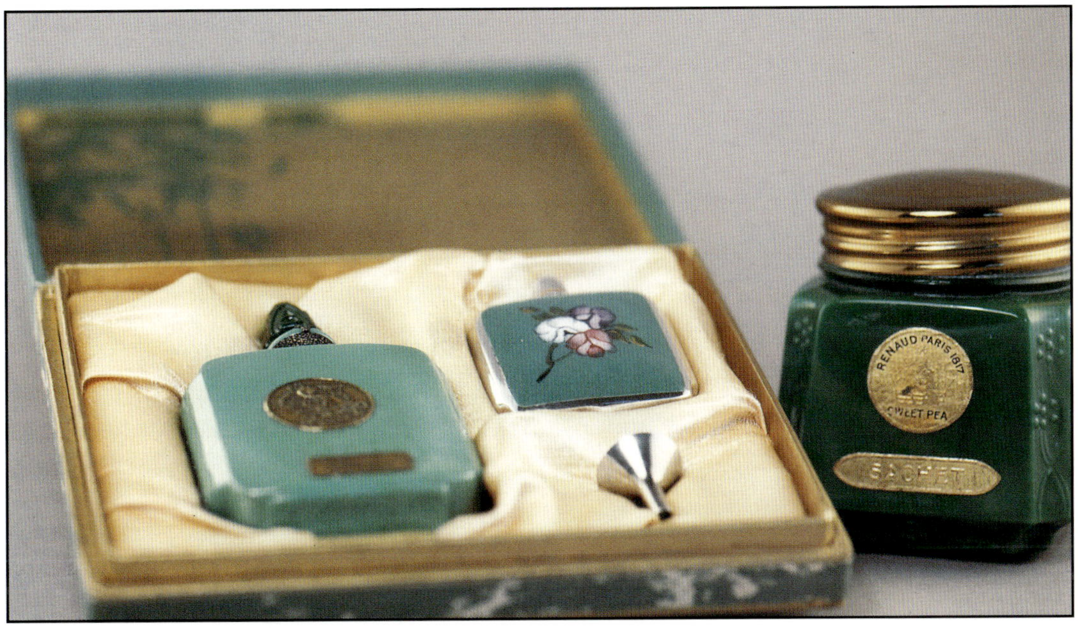

Renaud's Sweet Pea in its box, along with sterling and enamel purse bottle and funnel. On the right, a green slag bottle of Sweet Pea sachet.

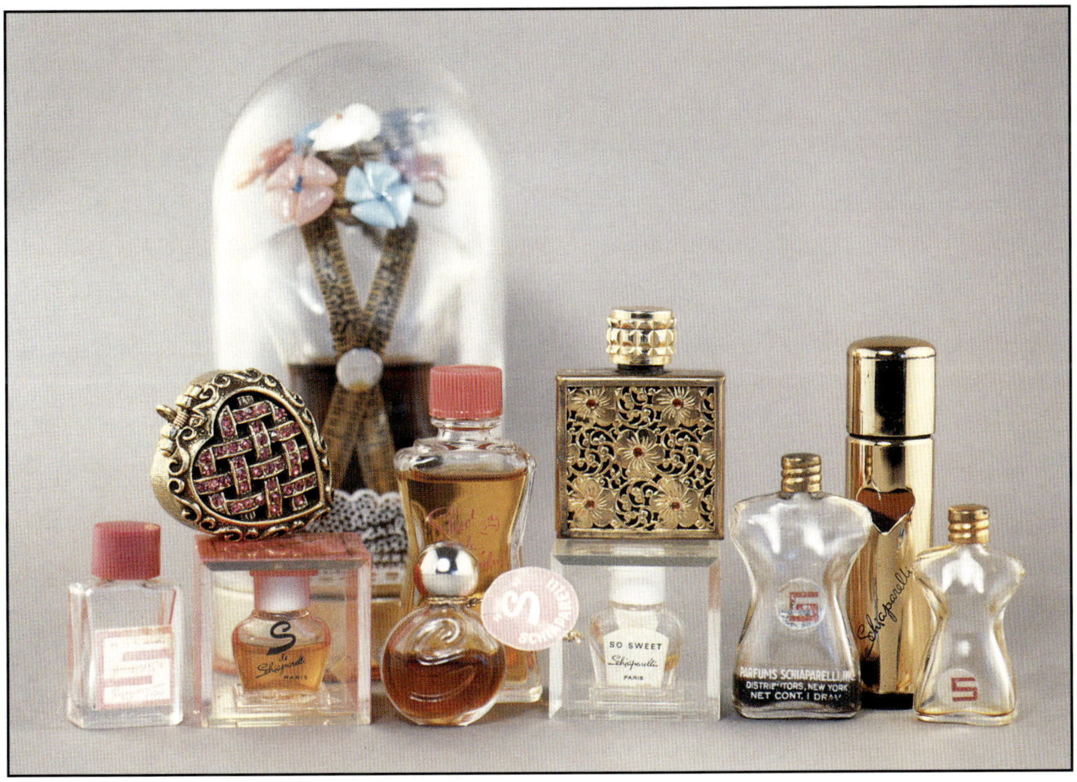

A variety of Schiaparelli bottles for Shocking, "S," and So Sweet. The dressmaker bottle's crystal cover was made in Czechoslovakia. This is an older bottle with a glass stopper. The small bottle on the far left was produced with an upside-down label.

Perfume bottles are great artifacts! They reflect the attitudes and the economics of their time. In the late nineteenth and early twentieth centuries, perfume was presented as a practical commodity. Thus, the title for the perfume was often descriptive of its floral component. It would not be unusual to find Tuberrose, Carnation, Narcisse, Chypre, Lilac, Muget or Lily of the Valley, Trailing Arbitus, Violet, and Heliotrope presented, sometimes by more than one manufacturer. Bottles tended to be apothecary style, practical and relatively unimaginative, certainly unadorned. The druggist or shopkeeper sometimes carried perfumes in bulk and provided, filled, and labeled the bottle for a customer. Sometimes the perfumer provided empty bottles to be filled on site.

By the 1920s and '30s, the whole package began to change. Apparel designers added fragrance and cosmetic lines, and perfumes were marketed to sophisticated women. Elizabeth Arden™, who created Arden Jasmin and Arden Rose in 1922, produced "Black Lace" in 1938. Lanvin came out with "My Sin" in 1923 and "Scandal" in '31. Schiaparelli™, with her dressmaker form shaped bottle, marketed "Shocking" in 1936. D'Orsay's™ "Intoxication" appeared in 1942; Evyan's™ classic, "White Shoulders" in '43. Perfumes were named "Jockey Club," "Opening Night," "Evening in Paris," "Twenty Carats," "White Satin," and "Chantilly." The marketing appeal was similar to that of romance novels, capitalizing on the image evoked—be it of youth and innocence, extravagance and luxury, intrigue, the exotic, the regal, the idolized, the naughty, the provocative, or mostly, the fantastical. Women were invited to use scent as a personal statement—a different statement, perhaps, for daytime use than for evening wear. A woman could choose different perfume to suit her every mood, her choice of fabric or color, her purpose. Packaging, labels, and the bottles themselves had become pieces of art, and the art portrayed something much bigger than the scent alone. It became a woman's entree to her image or her dream.

Acquiring several scents in addition to her "signature" scent, a woman might also adorn her dressing table with special receptacles for the scents. A market thus emerged for dresser sets, which often included hand mirrors, trinket boxes, and dresser jars. These were accompanied by atomizer and drop-stoppered bottles, and sometimes by a fancy mirrored tray to hold and display them on the dressing table. Personal flacons were sold as well, designed to carry a supply for travel or to keep in the reticule for refreshing the toilette. Jewelry stores and upscale shops carried crafted bottles of precious metals or crystal. A wide range of bottles was produced and sold to please a variety of tastes, décor, and pocketbooks. Among these were bottles made in Czechoslovakia in the 1920s and '30s. With their stunning diversity of color, style, and composition, these Czechoslovakian bottles are artistic treasures to find and display today.

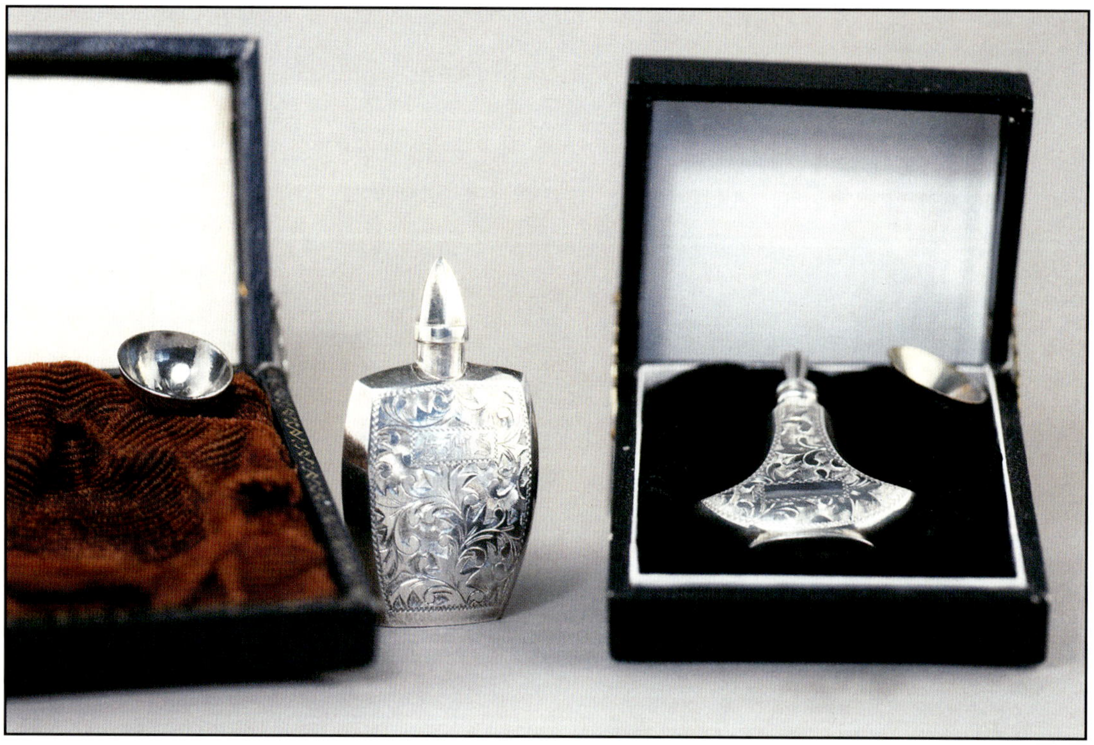

Two silver monogrammed purse bottles with boxes and sterling funnels.

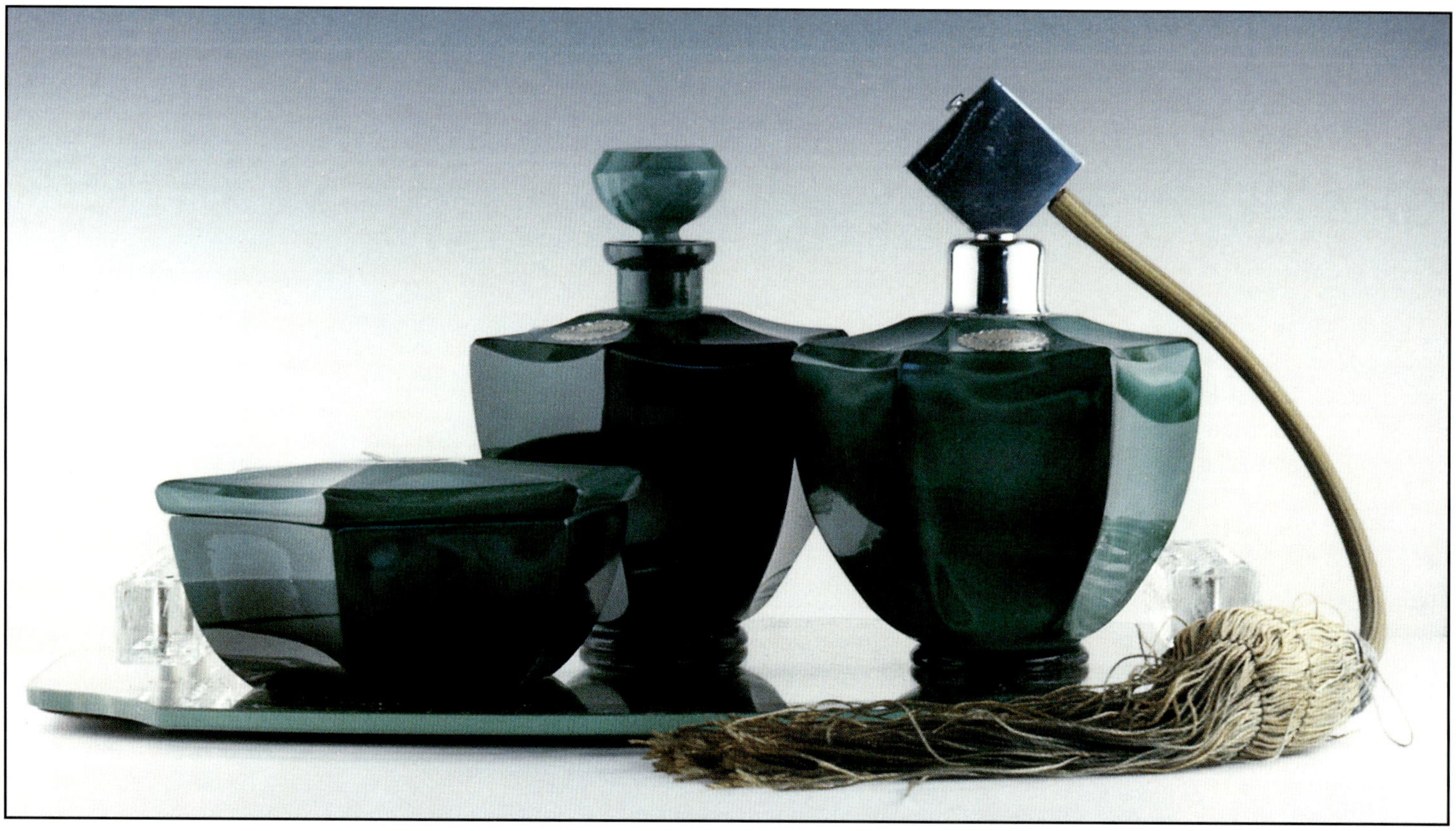

An Ingrid malachite dresser set with paper labels. This set includes a powder box, perfume bottle, and atomizer and is displayed on an unmarked mirrored tray.

Czechoslovakia: Historical Perspective

Czechoslovakia was a unique place in the 1920s and '30s. Created after the defeat of Austria-Hungry at the end of World War I, the country's newly-formed government attempted to bring together and represent several diverse ethnic groups already occupying the area. These groups had quite different cultures, histories, economic statuses, and even languages. The three largest were the Czechs, who were primarily entrepreneurs and landowners; the Suden Germans, generally workers; and the Slavs, who were agrarian. Tradition, family ties, skills handed down from parent to child, and social mores kept each group separate.

Many makers of the Czechoslovakian scent bottles of the 1920s and 1930s were Suden Germans—descendents of German speaking peasants who emigrated to the Bohemian area after the Thirty Years War (1618-1648). The mountainous, forested area was already steeped in a tradition of glass making. These people settled in clusters around the glass factories and applied their skills in producing or refining the rough glass to products ready for use or trade. For many generations, landlords profited from glass making and exported products from Bohemia that included glass fittings for chandeliers, buttons, beads, crystal, and jewelry.

A rapidly changing world, post World War I Europe was busy repairing war damage. The industrial revolution was impacting jobs, creating goods faster and in greater numbers, as well as creating a working populace that could better afford to buy such goods. Machine produced items competed in the marketplace with hand crafted items, forcing prices down on labor-intensive goods. The market demanded a quality product, but wanted it at a lower cost. Cutting production costs via efficient use of materials or cutting down on labor-intensive processes was necessary for market survival. Even so, many glass houses faced bankruptcy. Workers labored long hours for less pay. Just when the economy appeared to be leveling out, the stock market crashed, people stopped buying luxury items, and workers were made idle.

The Suden Germans, looking for economic relief that was not forthcoming from the Czechoslovakian government, were vulnerable to overtures from Germany. In 1938, the Bohemian area was annexed to Germany as a result of the Munich agreement. Hopes of better times were soon dashed as both their currency and their goods were devalued. German alliances and impending war further evaporated export avenues. Many factories were altered to produce war related items. When World War II ended with Germany's defeat, Suden Germans were, by order of the then reinstated Benès government, expatriated from their homes and land. Many settled in Neu Gablonz and other towns in West Germany. All industry became nationalized over the span of 1945-48.

Though many of the skilled workers and designers were gone, glass was continuously produced in northern Bohemia. Some pieces were still made from the old molds but in general, the style and the finished quality were different. With the removal of the Communist government in 1993, the glass industry was once again privatized and began producing art glass in the old style. New bottles in a variety of sizes, colors, and shapes are currently on the market. They are identified as Bohemian glass from the Czech Republic. Many of the exquisite old molds have been restored to use.

Spectacular designs from Hoffman, Schlevogt, and other masters have long been collectors' items. Drawing less attention through the years have been the Czech purse bottles and minis. These tinier bottles were press molded in large quantities and went through the hands of many refiners, whose only signature outside of an acid mark or metal tag declaring "Czechoslovakia" was the beauty or unique aspects of the bottle itself. Anonymous workers cut, polished, etched, enameled, formed or stamped metal bits, caged, and jeweled these bottles in various combinations of refinements as dictated by fashion. They were then ordered by exporters, who found a ready market in the US, England, and other countries. The bottles have survived through the years because they are unique and beautiful art pieces.

Originally selling for from twenty-five cents to a couple of dollars, these colorful prizes now sell for a great deal more—from twenty-five dollars to several hundred. The price often depends less on the hand labor involved and more on the rarity of the item and the fancy of the collector.

The fact that some purse bottles continue to be produced in northern Czechoslovakia makes it important for collectors to be as familiar as possible with features unique to the bottles of the 1920s and '30s. The indicators of age for purse bottles are the styles of the caps, the component parts of the metal caging filigree, and the metal cover of the bottles' necks that receive the threads of the cap. Markings were important, too, but many, especially later bottles, were marked with paper labels that were vulnerable to age and wear or were removed by the buyer.

Setting Values

Part of the benefit of a reference on collectibles is the placing of an economic value on the pieces pictured. While I have attempted to do that, I need to tell a family story in order to put the whole pricing issue into perspective. My grandmother's heritage is Irish and she collected in her lifetime some lovely pieces of Beleek china. Eventually, my own mother acquired a few pieces as well. Several years ago, when I first began attending antique and collectible shows, I found an exquisite Beleek teapot and paid dearly for it. I presented it to my mother as a Mothers' Day gift. When shown the teapot, my younger brother turned it over in his hands. He saw the tag on the bottom and his eyes got big. He carefully placed it back on the table and with arched brows and soft voice asked, "What kind of tea do you use in a teapot like this?" The answer, of course, is that no tea will brew or taste any better made in Beleek than in crockery, but acquiring and displaying a fine piece of bone china—or a fine antique perfume bottle—is simply a pure pleasure.

Setting a market value on perfume and scent bottles, especially on these Czech and other bottles from the '20s and '30s is difficult. These items were originally sold in shops between sixty-eight and eight-five years ago. It is safe to say that few, if any, are currently in the hands of the individuals who originally purchased them. By their nature, these bottles are fragile and the decorative elements or attachments were subject to damage or loss through the years. Sometimes metalwork has been discolored by perfume contact. Vulnerable drop stoppers, which were affixed to the shaped and polished dowel, are often broken off or missing. "Flea bites" and tiny chips are common. Most collectors look at the overall appearance of the bottle. The patina of age and wear marks from use are likely to add interest and authentication rather than detract from the value. Finding a dauber intact is often seen as a bonus, while very few lovely bottles are rejected because of a missing dauber rod.

With each passing year, the number of available bottles diminishes. A prudent collector will pick up stray parts to combine and complete bottles when possible. The good "marriage" will increase the value of the separate parts; the stopper or cap should be a match for the bottle in style, balance, fit, and in origin.

Market trends fluctuate constantly; the overall value of a collection can shift as easily as the stock market. The value of an individual bottle is only what a buyer will pay for it, and in a declining market, buyers may well hold on to their discretionary money. Part of the joy of collecting, it seems, should be an appreciation of each item for its own sake. Financial security attained through collecting as investment lies in the ability to keep and enjoy the collection until an optimum time for sale.

In recent years, Internet auctions have moved the collectible supply within easy reach of individual buyers and have expanded the consumer base from weekend antique mall explorers to the whole online world. Serious collectors give careful thought to value and bidding strategies and become wise to the identities and practices of others vying for the same types of items. Keep in mind, too, that a collector might pay top price in a contested auction for a bottle that he or she wants for the collection, but once that piece is obtained, the position is filled and identical bottles at a quarter of the price are subsequently ignored.

Some observations can be safely made from watching the bidding and the end prices over time. Expect to pay more for colored bottles than for clear. Colored stoppers are less common than clear crystal. Except for black bottles, which often had different colored tops, most colored tops matched the base. Colored daubers are also unusual. Expect to pay more for figural bottles and tops. Figural or floral intaglio bottles and stoppers are more highly desired than geometric cuts. Cut glass bottles with jeweled filigree are harder to find and are popular among collectors. Pressed bottles with no hand cuts are of lesser value. Check for authentication marks—acid marks on the cut glass base or metal tags on caps or filigree. These help verify the age and origin. Unusual dangles are harder to find. They should be suspended on the characteristic delicate brass chain, and affixed by standard methods of joining parts and hanging the dangles. Heavier chains or unusual couplings could mean that a repair or alteration has been made.

The word among collectors is that some of the dangle bottles are being reproduced. Look for authentication in the form of a "Czecho-Slovakia" metal tag, which appeared on the coin and bangle (with gems) and the bold flower caps. Tags did not appear on the railroad track cap or on the plain coin and bangle caps. Look for signs of age. The cap and dangle that are too shiny and perfect may be too good to be true.

Examine the item carefully, checking for stopper fit. When the stopper is twisted firmly in place, it should be snug enough to support the weight of the bottle. Examining the item personally is far better than buying from a picture. Catalog or e-mail pictures are simply not as good. Color is often not "true," and the size can be hard to determine when shown in isolation. Holding a ruler up to the picture and noting the dimensions given can prevent mistaking the size.

In summary, placing a market value on an item should include many factors: the actual price paid for the item in today's money; reference values, taking into consideration the publication date of the reference; and current demand and the availability of that particular item or similar items. It should consider the appearance and condition of the item overall. It should also consider the craftsmanship of the item and its rarity, keeping in mind that, especially with dangles, the craftsmanship sometimes takes a back seat to the appeal of the item's uniqueness and charm. Taking all of the above into consideration, values given in this book are not absolute, but are in an "expect to pay" range.

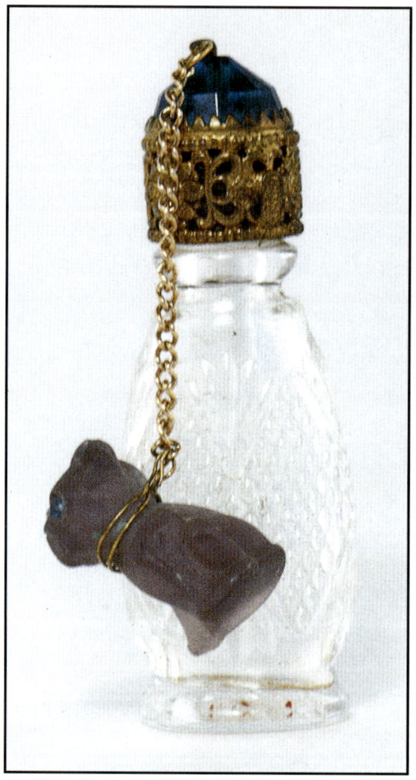

This "restored" dog dangle appears as purchased on the Internet. The chain is heavier than is normally found. The dog's collar is missing and has been replaced by a thin doubled wire around his neck. Usually, the dangle is a match to the color of the capstone.

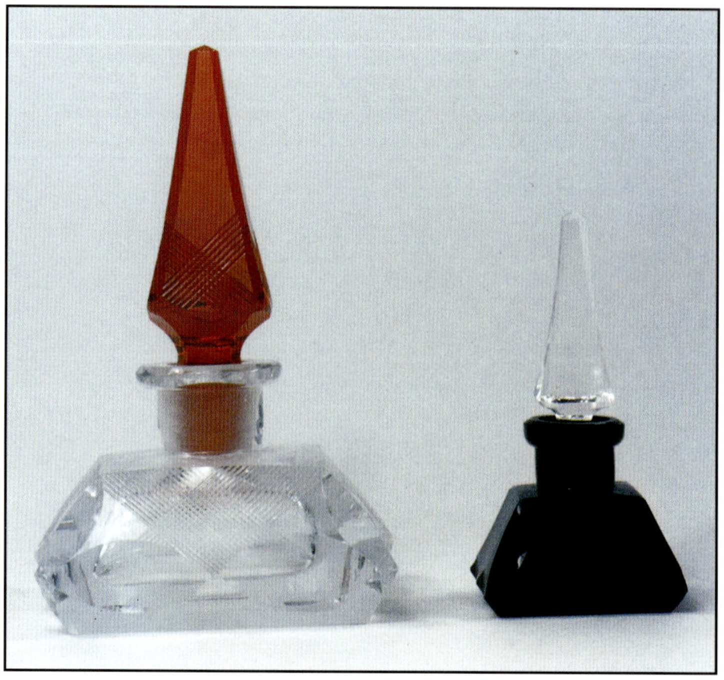

Little or big? These two bottles are very different in size, but similar in shape. It is wise to pay careful attention to dimensions given when purchasing from an online auction or from a picture. Holding a 6" ruler up to the picture helps give a more accurate perception. Left: 4"; Right: 2.75".

Part I

Purse Bottles

A purse bottle is a flask or vial designed to hold a small amount of perfume. The bottle itself, therefore, is usually small and made with a secured closing, typically a screw cap, in order to be carried easily and without spillage in a lady's handbag. The precursor of the purse bottle was the vinaigrette or scent box, both of which were used earlier to hold smelling salts or herbal restoratives.

Through the years, purse bottles have been made of a variety of materials, including precious metals and precious or semi-precious gems, which were only accessible to the wealthy.

The Czechoslovakian purse bottles included here were formed of mold-blown glass and, unless otherwise noted, were decorated with base metal and glass gems. Some, like the dangle bottles, had little refining, while others were finished with extensive hand labor. These bottles were affordable and were a popular export item.

In each type of purse bottle, the detail is important to the collector as a means of identification and of placing a value on the piece. The caps in particular provide evidence about the order in which certain styles and details appeared.

Items that are acid marked or marked with a metal tag in the cap or filigree with the word "Czechoslovakia" are products of the years between the world wars. The name "Czechoslovakia" for this area did not exist prior to that time and after World War II, different forms of identification were used, usually paper tags. The absence of a mark makes exact identification and time placement more difficult.

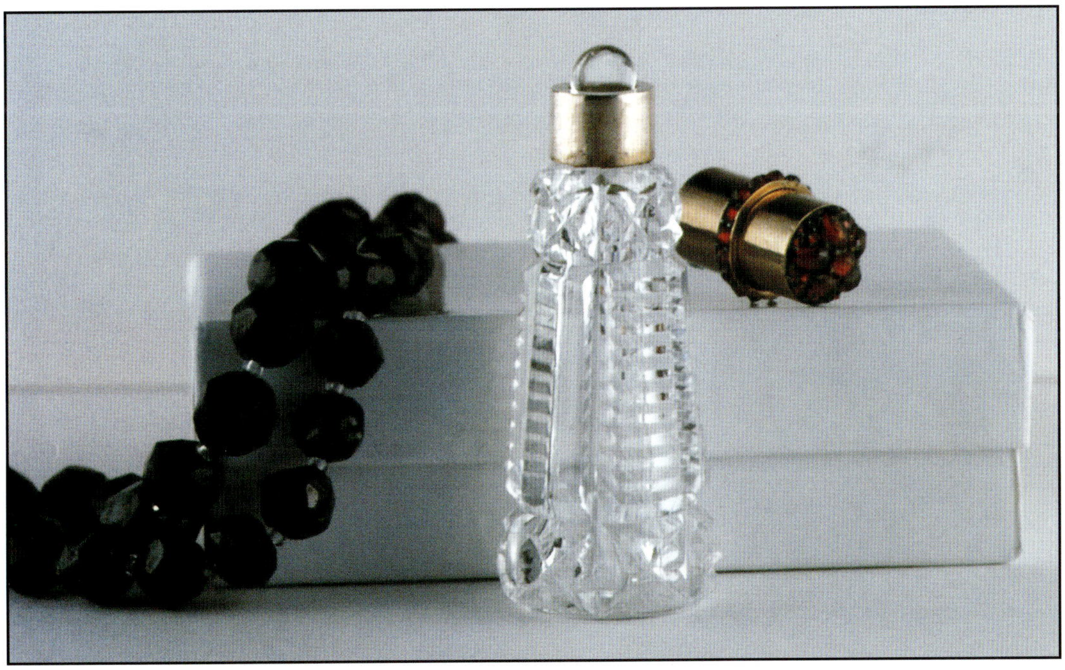

This bottle has a hand cut base and a 10 carat gold neck piece and cap. The stones are garnets, for which the Bohemian area has long been known. The bottle is unmarked and is attributed to the late 1800s. $700-800. Shown with faceted garnet beads. $50.

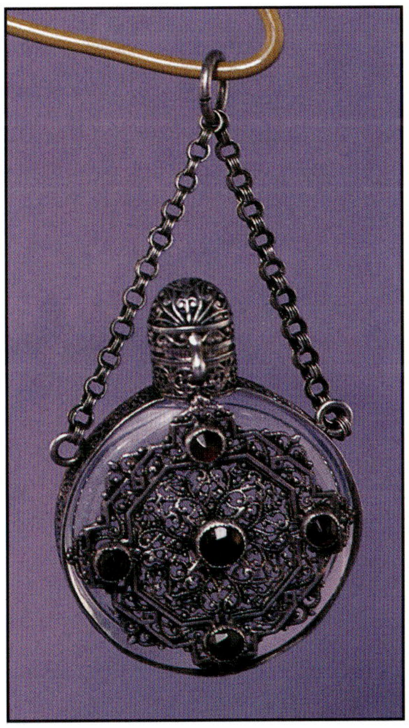

Crystal pendant bottle with beveled edges, silver wire filigree, and garnet stones. It has a hinged top and glass stopper with dauber. It dates from the late 1800s. 1.75". $550- 600.

Several distinctive types of purse bottles are included in this section. First are the Irice dangles and dangle style bottles. These are easily identified because they have only a few standard shapes and because the importer's name "Irice" appears in the base of the bottle. Sold as novelty items, their appeal is in the cap detailing and the frequently present dangling charms.

If Irice dangles fit into a novelty category, cut glass purse bottles are clearly "a cut above." Though they are considered purse bottles because of the screw cap closure, they have the fine appearance and hand finish work of a dresser bottle. Indeed, some identical bases can be found with both a screw cap and a glass stopper. While some cut glass purse bottles are relatively plain, many have the additional adornment of filigree and jewels.

Created by Curt Schlevogt and named for his young daughter, the Ingrid line included several purse bottle styles. They are in a category of their own because of their distinctive molded opaque glass. Most commonly found in green, black, and blue, these bottles appeared in 1934 and became quite popular. The molds of these bottles are currently in use in the Czech Republic and clear, colored, and frosted versions are available in quantity today.

From the early 1950s until 1961, a company known as Jablonex or Jaco, Czechoslovak Export Company Ltd., exported both purse and dresser bottles in the miniature size. Photographs of some of the bottles shown in the sales brochure, as well as the brochure itself, are shown here.

Victorian style purse bottles are more reminiscent of the chatelaine, evoking images of the lady of the house who was literally the "keeper of the keys." Though chatelaines were originally worn at the waist, many of these have a finger ring, a pendant loop and chain, or a brooch pin, and have become functional pieces of jewelry.

The Victorian bottles were much smaller than most of the purse bottles, often not much more than an inch square. These were popular and were produced in France and Germany at the same time. Since only a few were marked, attribution is difficult to establish with certainty. The groupings here are intended to give a feel for what was usually credited to each country. Where an item is marked, it will be noted.

Irice, The Import Company

The Irving W. Rice and Company of New York (Irice) was probably the best known of several importers of Czech bottles from the 1920s and '30s. According to current company spokesman Tom Brennan, Irving Rice started the company in 1908. He traveled in Europe seeking items to re-sell in the United States. Along with other products, he imported crystal perfume bottles, atomizers, and other vanity items from Czechoslovakia. The company sold these items to department stores, gift shops, and drug stores. During World War II, when Czechoslovakia was occupied by Germany, Irice bought from Imperial Glass, a US company. After the war, Irice continued to buy from glass manufacturers, many of them Suden Germans who had been expatriated from Czechoslovakia and settled in West Germany.

When Irving Rice died in the 1950s, he left the company to his sales manager and his top buyer, who ran it successfully for about ten years. They ultimately sold the company to a successful conglomerate, Avnet. In the mid '60s, a young man by the name of Henry Basch was hired. He worked as a buyer, eventually becoming company president and serving in that capacity for about twenty years. During that time, the company continued to specialize in perfume bottles, atomizers, purse atomizers, mirrors, compacts, trays, and vanity items.

In an interview with the author, Mr. Basch told of buying excursions to Europe where he would visit showrooms to contract goods, which were then shipped to the company warehouse in New Jersey. The search for quality at affordable prices led him to focus less on West Germany and more on the Orient, where growing commerce gave the buyer more control and merchants were anxious to please.

In the late 1980s, many department stores in the US were closing as the economy struggled. In 1993, the company was sold again, this time to John Craddock, whose specialty was manufacturing and cosmetic products. Perfume bottles were no longer a featured item. In 1997, Craddock's daughter, Kathleen, took over the company and is its present owner.

It is possible to see reprints of original Irice advertisements in Jacqueline Jones-North's book, *Czechoslovakian Perfume Bottles and Boudoir Accessories* (Antique Publications, 1990 original copyright; 1999 revised edition). The ads date from 1932 to 1940 and include a variety of perfume bottles and vanity items sold to retailers. These items may have the acid-etched word "Czechoslovakia" on the bottom, and some still wear the black and silver Irice paper and foil sticker.

Mr. Basch spoke of Irice's quest for "quality first." While Irice products span the range from pressed glass dangle bottles to the finest cut crystal, there is no doubt of the enduring popularity of these products—then or now. The Irice Company is now located in Holmdel, New Jersey.

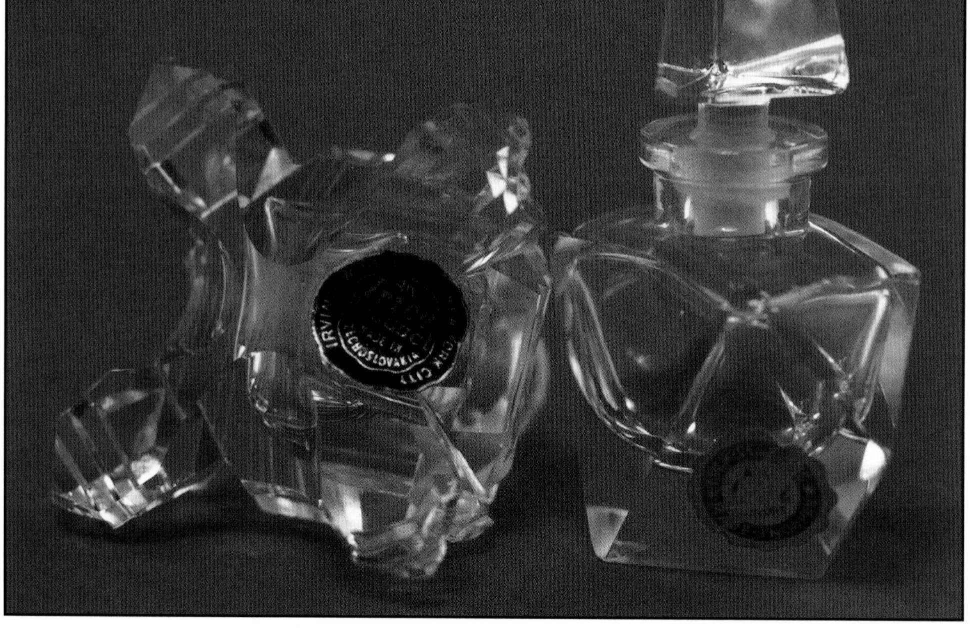

Irice labels. Left: black and silver, seen on the bottom of a cut glass Czechoslovakian dresser bottle. Right, on the back of a crystal dresser bottle, probably from the late 1940s or early '50s, marked Japan.

Irice Dangle Bottles

The most common of the Irice dangle bottles is cone-shaped, slightly wider at the base than at the shoulders. The pressed pattern forms a series of "X's" and "O's". This bottle appears most frequently in 2.25" height, measuring without the cap. It is also found, though less commonly, in a 2.5" (bottle only) height. Shorter, stubby bottles have a bulb-shaped base with a hobnail-like pattern in the glass and a thinner, plain neck that comprises about half of the bottle height of 1.75". The words, "Irice" and Stubby" are embossed in the bottom. The bottles are topped with metal screw caps in a variety of cap styles and have a glass dauber. Some caps have an affixed small metal tag reading "Czechoslovakia," some do not. Note: measurements given in the captions include the cap unless otherwise specified.

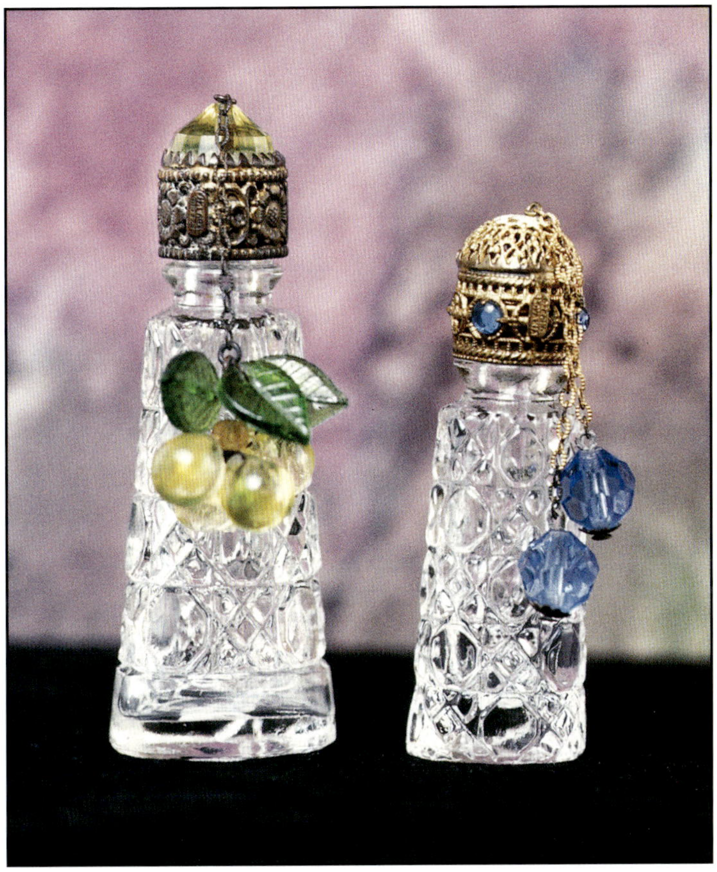

Two sizes of the typical Irice dangle bottles, including caps. On the left, 3"; on the right, 2.5".

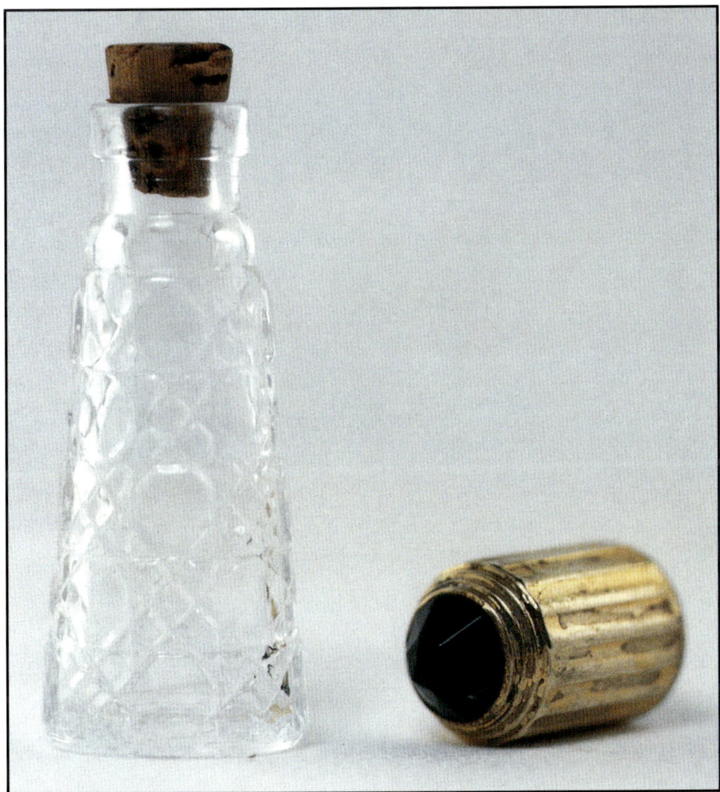

A rough beginning? This unmarked bottle with its cork stopper and green jeweled cover is possibly an early version of the typical Irice dangle base. The unthreaded corked bottle is the same height as a standard Irice dangle bottle. $50- $100.

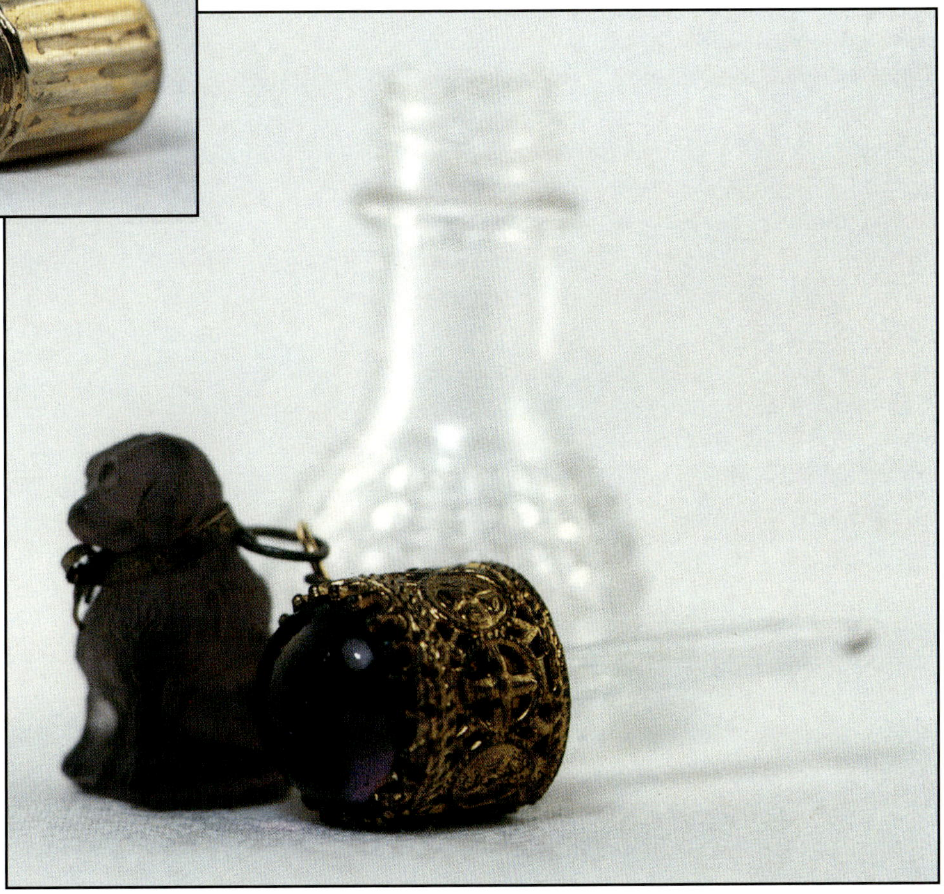

The words "Irice" and "Stubby" are embossed in the glass in the bottom of the bulb-shaped bottles. 2.125".

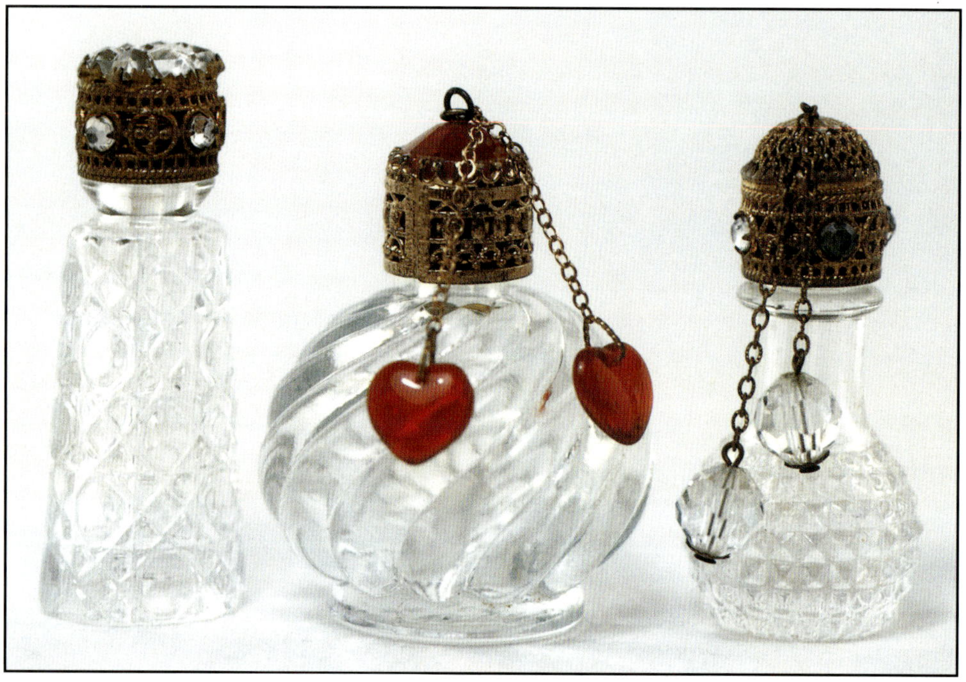

On the left, a clear, star flower capstone on a coin and bangle cap, and right, a Stubby with clear bead dangles. Both are marked with a metal tag on the cap. $75-$150 each. Center, an unusual Irice base with unmarked railroad track cap and red heart dangles. $150-$250.

As the base in these bottles is clear and molded in one or two consistent patterns, it is the caps that provide the color, decoration, and unique designs that draw collectors. The caps are made of stamped metal overlaying a utilitarian metal screw cap base. They are usually brass colored, but occasionally one can be found in silver colored metal. Often caps are fitted with colored glass jewels, either faceted or cabochon, and are literally the crowning glory to the bottle.

A collection of Czech minis and purse bottles would surely contain a variety of these Irice "dangle" bottles, so called because beads or other charms were often suspended from the cap by a single or double chain. The anchor loop for the chain was at the peak of the crown of the bottle or, in a few bottles, affixed to the filigree on the upper side of the cap.

Charms on the dangle bottles take many forms, but most are made of glass. Some charms are simple faceted beads and others are clusters or groupings of beads that resemble dolls, flowers, or clusters of fruit and leaves. Animal and bird dangles were popular, as well as hearts, stars, dice, and geometric shapes. The dangles are sometimes further decorated with gems set in; examples include the sets in toes of the Dutch shoes and the eyes of the animal pets.

All of the dangle bottles were designed to be appealing and to sell. The suggested retail price on dangle style bottles in the mid to late 1930s was a quarter. (The Helen Farnsworth CD shows a McKesson & Robbins Inc. advertisement from 1938, with a box of heart and dice dangles and the suggested retail price of $.25.)

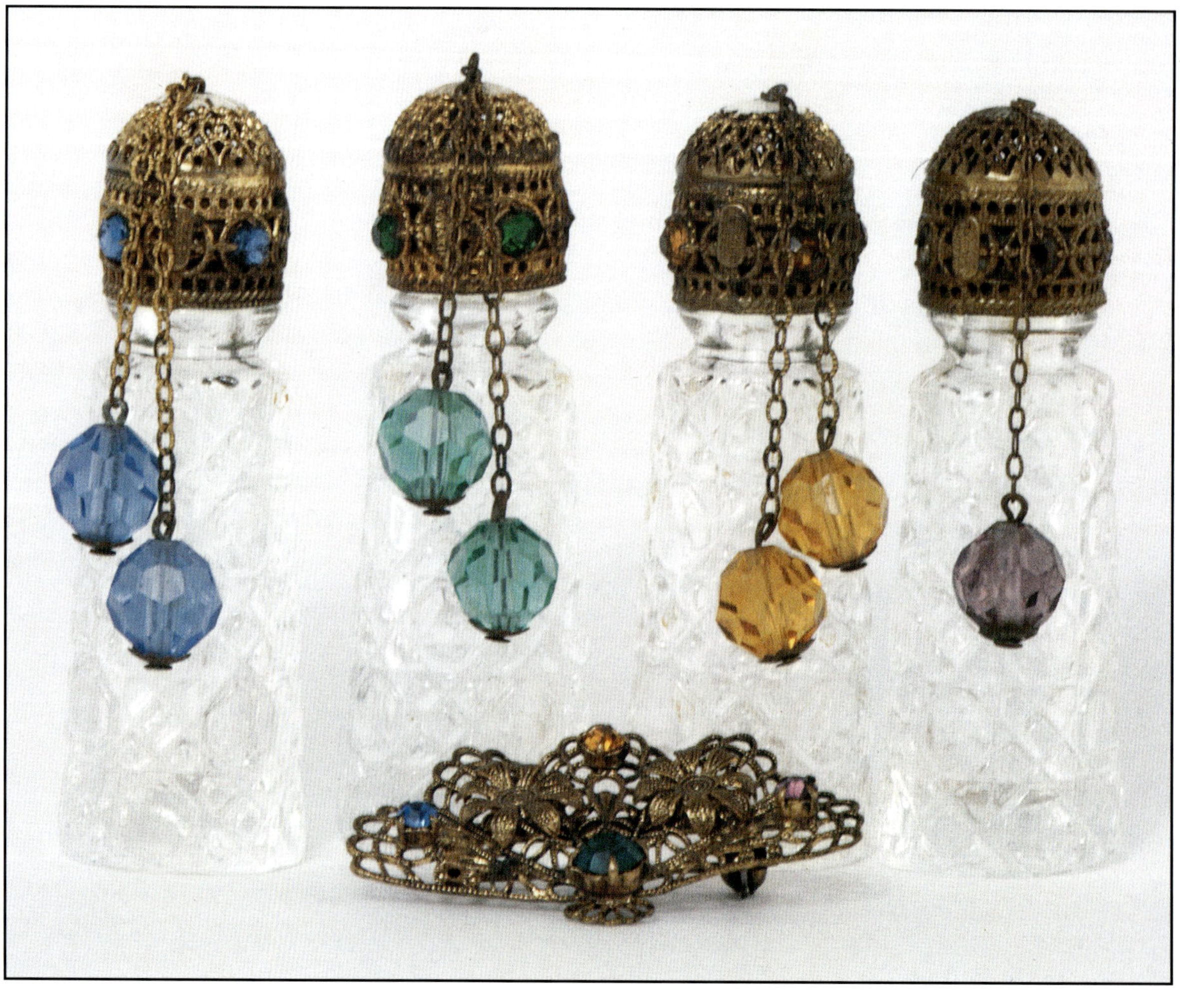

Single and double bead dangles, $75-150 each. Unmarked filigree fan pin, $40.

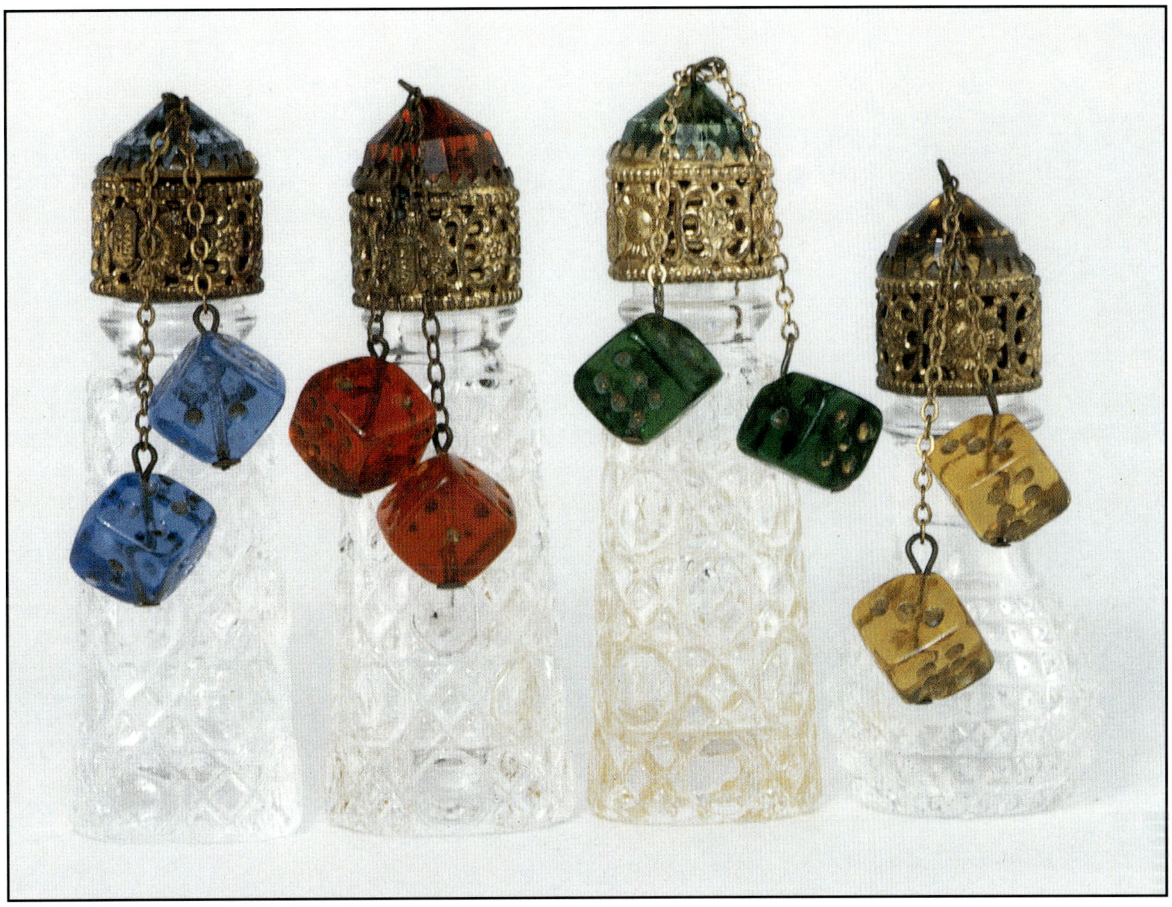

Dice dangles in primary colors with matching colored capstones. Note that the bottle with the green dice is light yellow, which is unusual. 1938. $200-300 each.

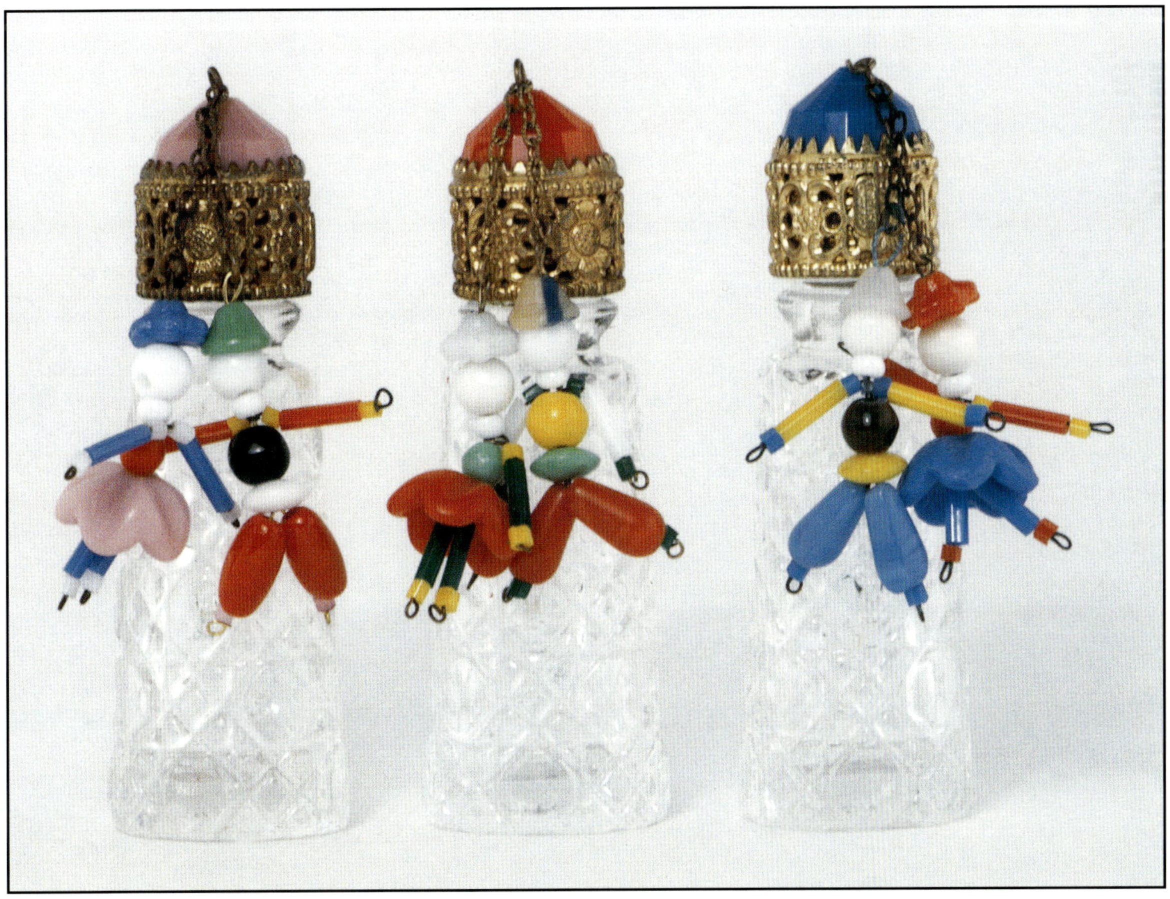

Doll or "Raggedy Dangles." The capstones are colored, faceted opaque glass. $150-250 each.

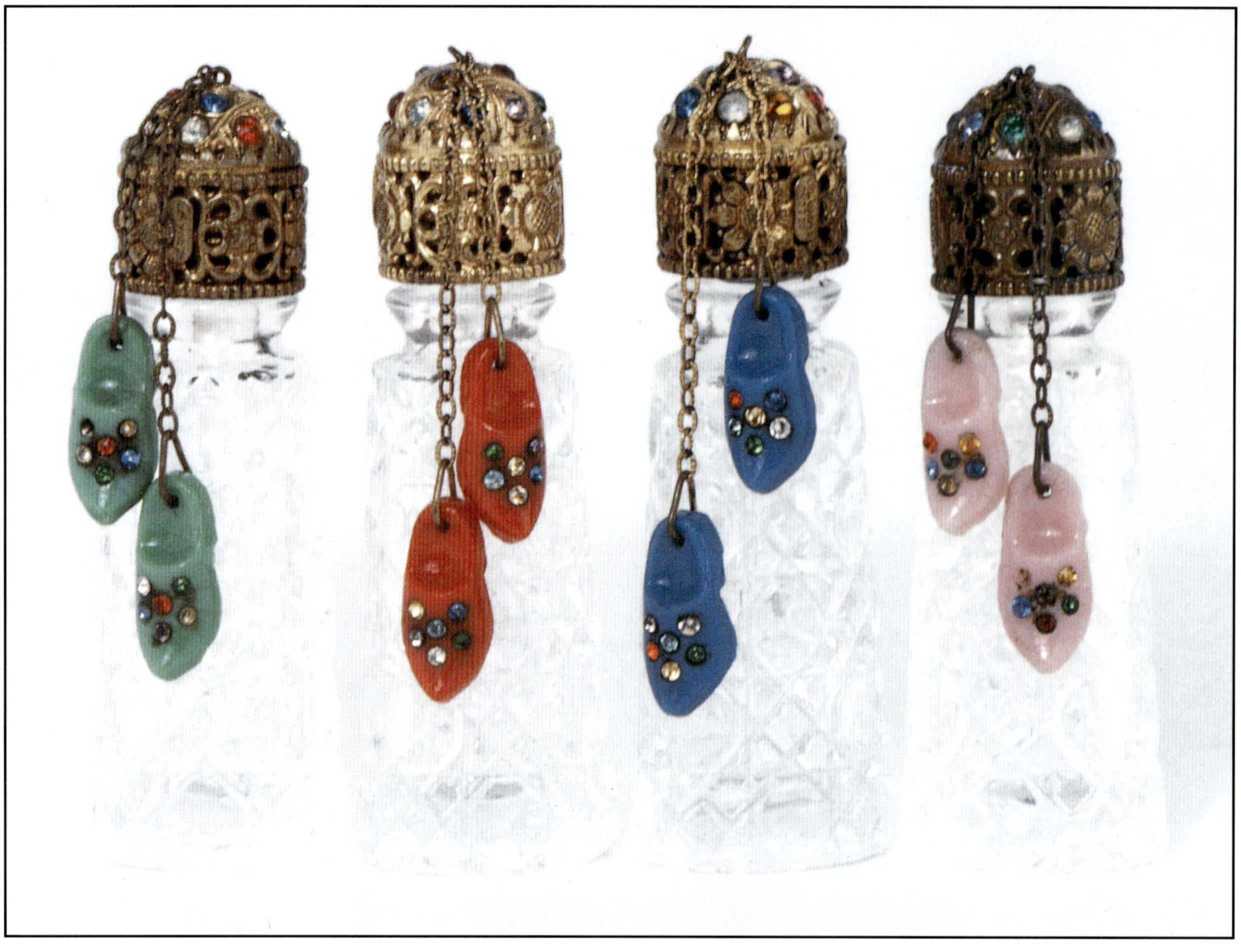

Dutch shoe dangles. Multi-colored gems are sprinkled in the crowns of the caps and sparkle in the toes of the shoes. $300-400 each.

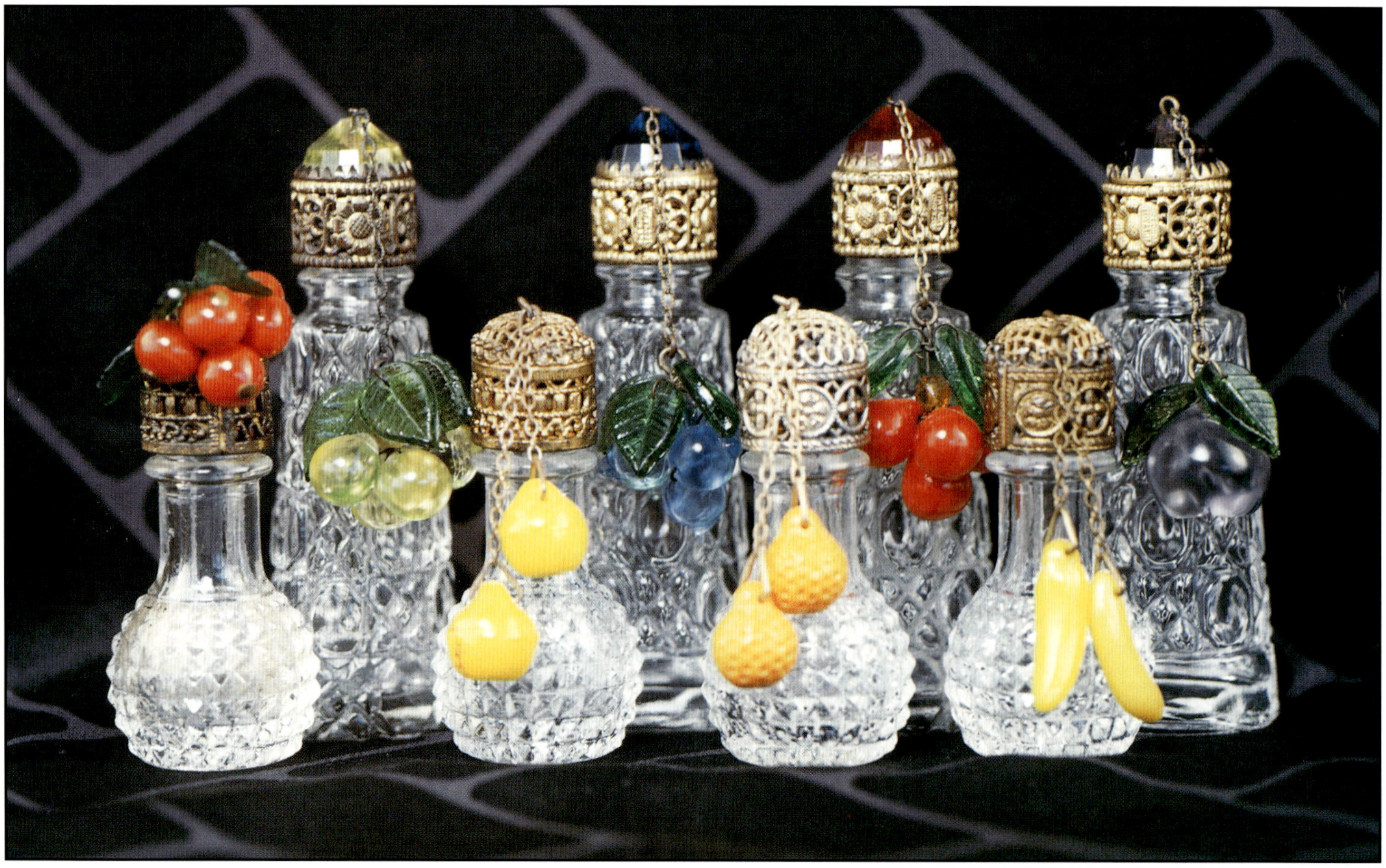

Fruit salad mix. Back row: gooseberries, blueberries, cherries, and a plum, all caps marked. $200-400 each.
Front row: currents, pears, oranges, and bananas. $100-200 each.

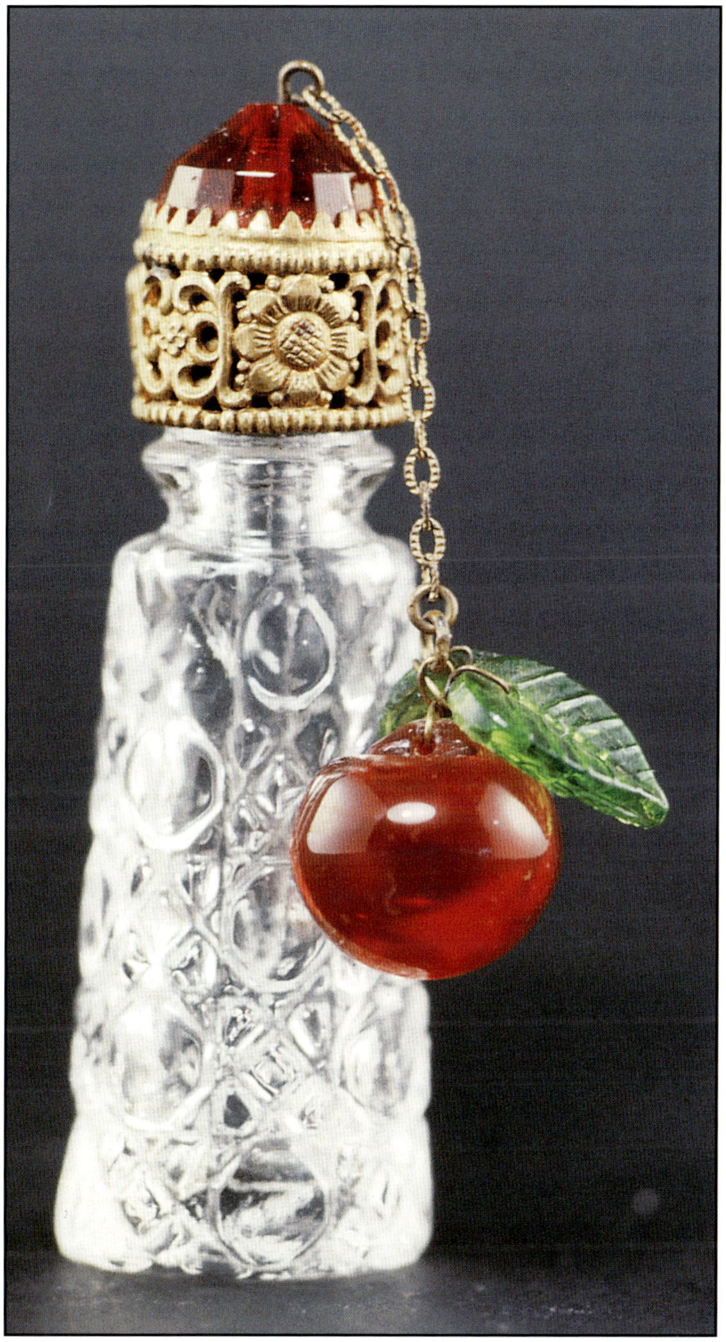

Apple dangle. $200-400.

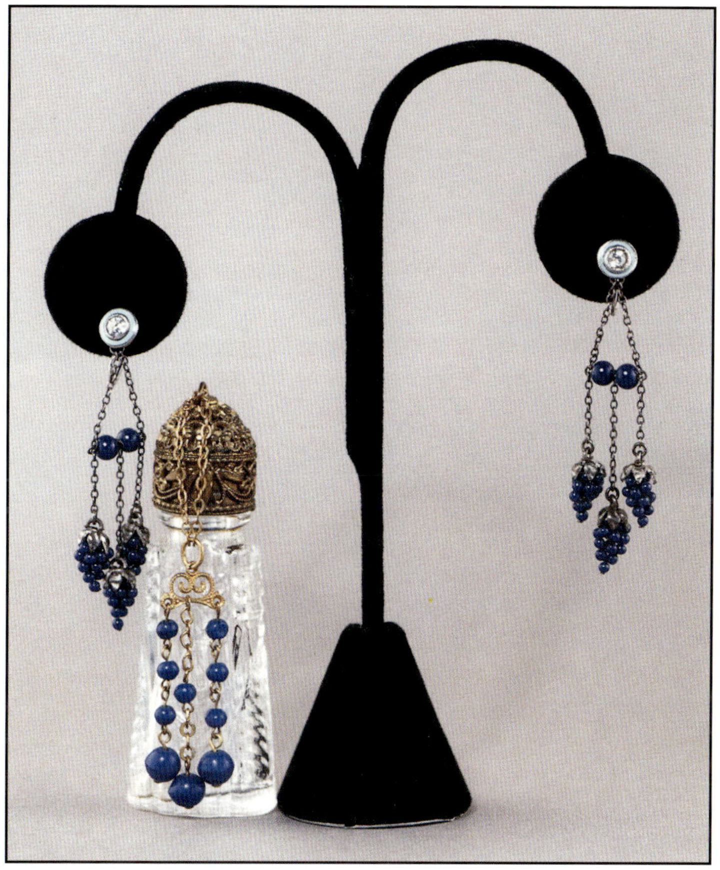

A dangle of lapis colored beads and filigree shown with sterling and lapis grape cluster earrings. Bottle, $150-200; earrings, $150.

Happy Holidays assortment. Opaque red glass Valentine heart with silver colored cap, $125-200; Easter chick, $150-250; and St. Pat's shamrock dangles, $125-200.

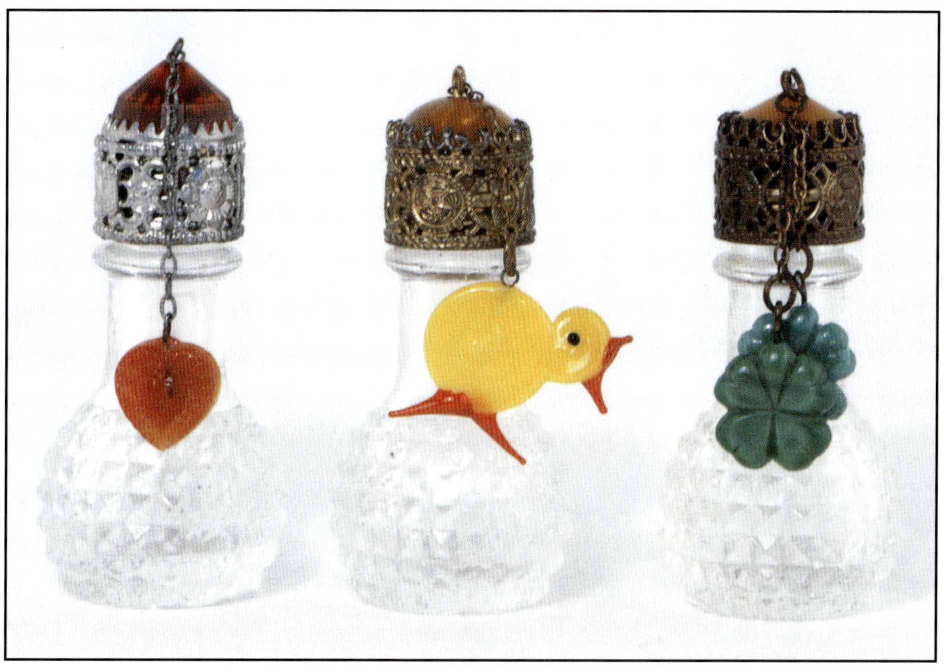

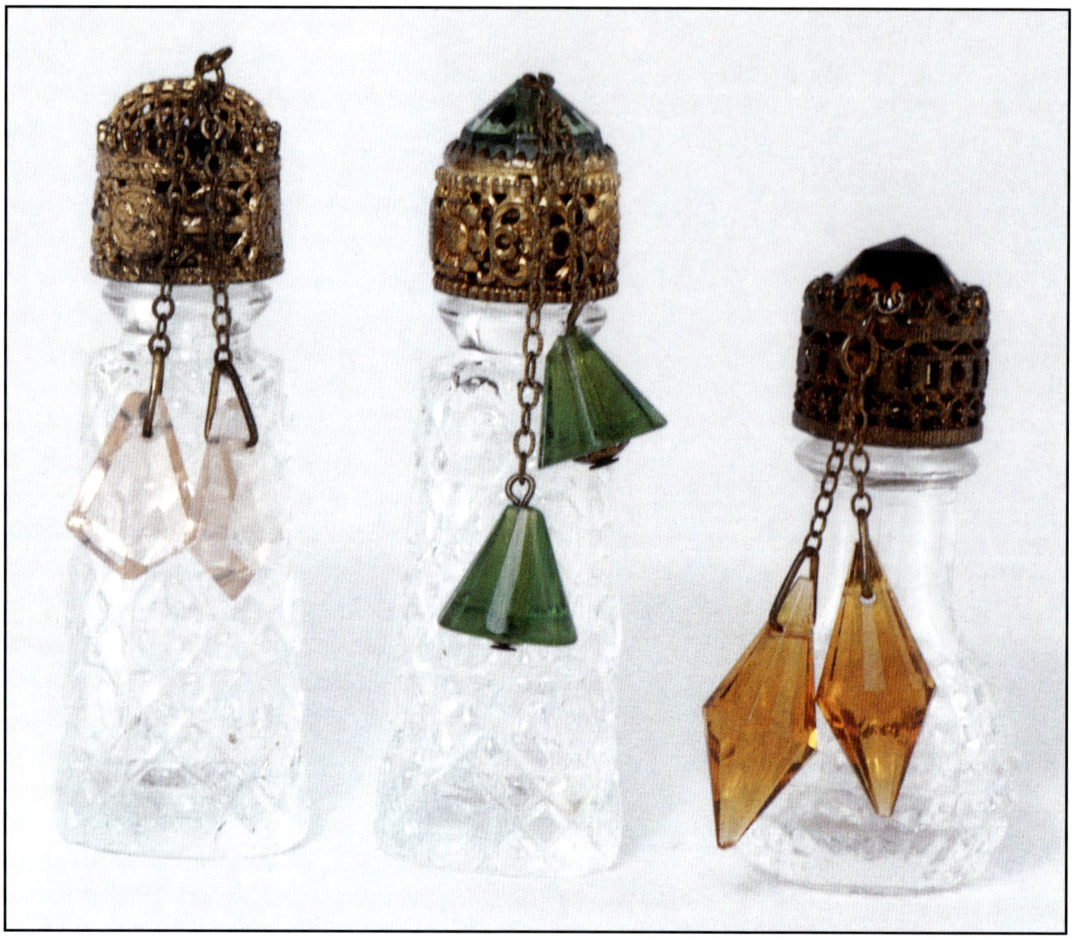

Geometric shapes. Pink prisms and green cones, $150-200 each. Amber prisms, $100-200.

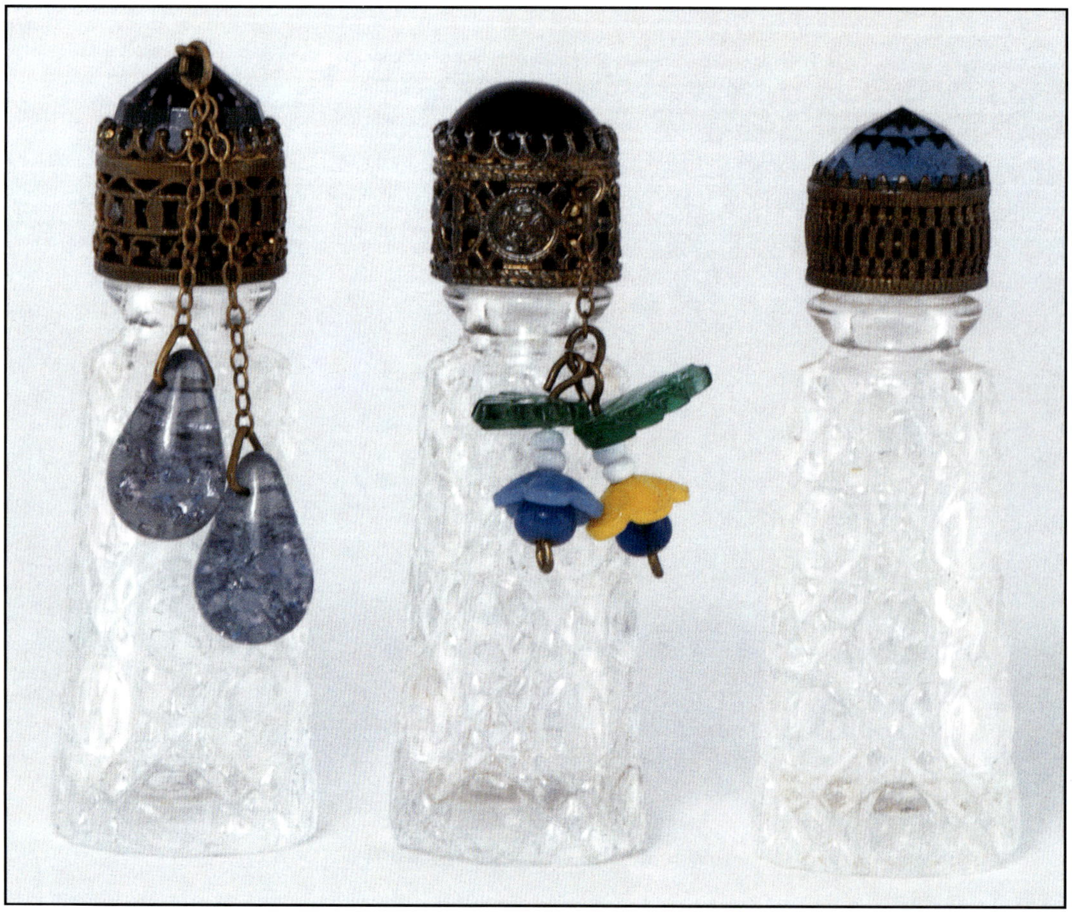

Purple crackle drop beads, $50-100; bead flowers on a split chain, $100-200; blue faceted capstone in a plain, mesh, marked cap, 1935, $50-100.

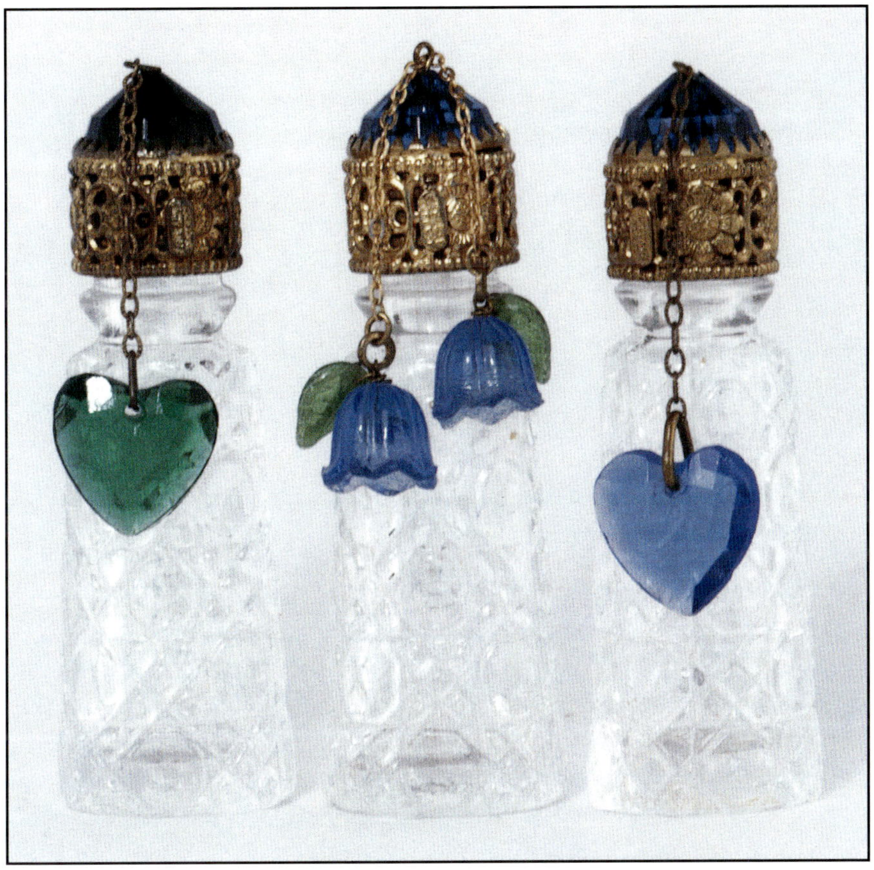

Hearts and flowers. Green and blue hearts, dating to 1938; bluebells, date unknown. $150-250 each.

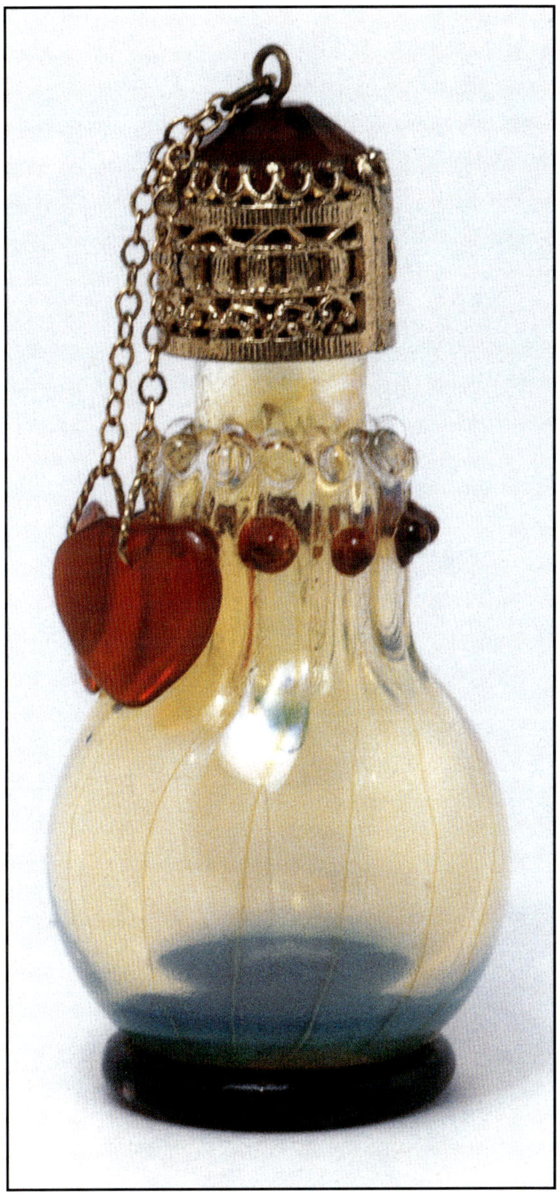

This unique, unmarked bottle looks like it is drawn up in a uranium glass bag. The red glass base and the red dot decorations are applied glass. The double red heart dangles fall from the crest of a railroad track cap. $250-400.

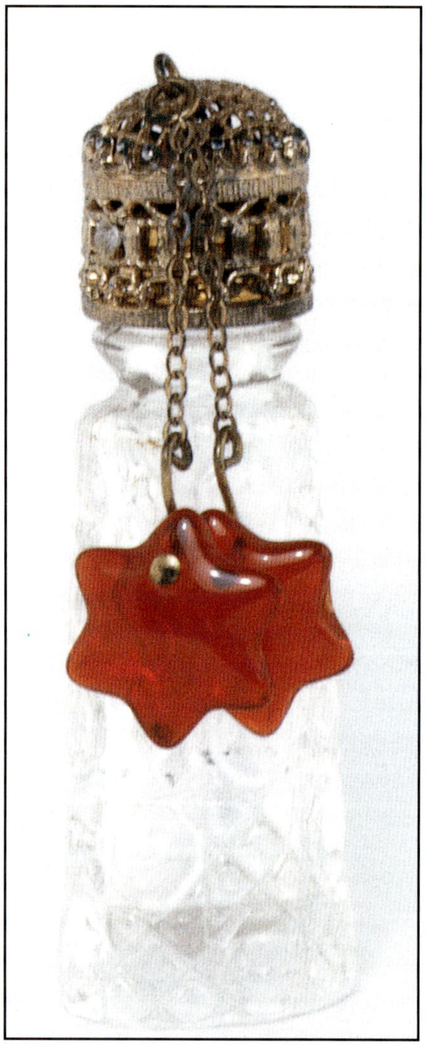

Six pointed red stars. $150-300.

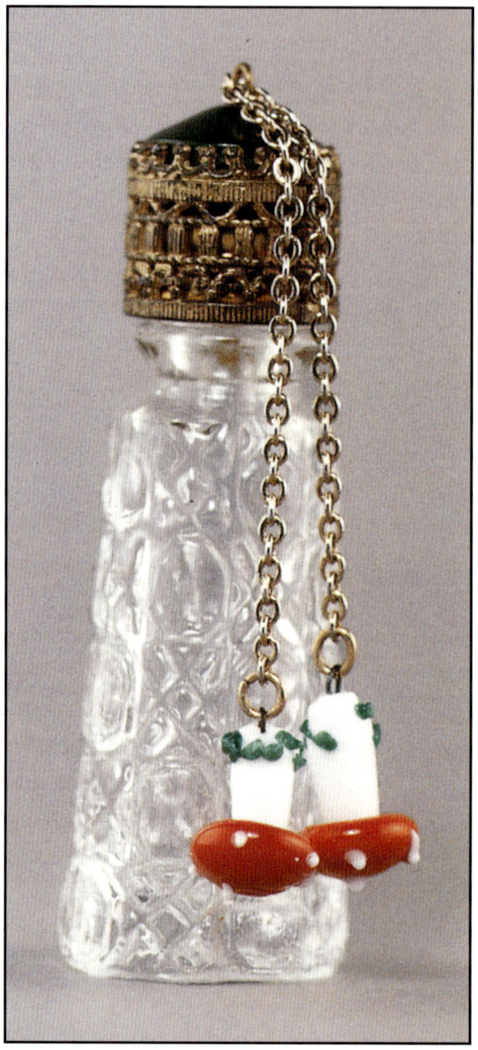

Mushroom dangles from a green Bakelite capstone. This dangle has unusually long chains. Note the applied dots and trailings on the lampworked mushroom beads. $150-250.

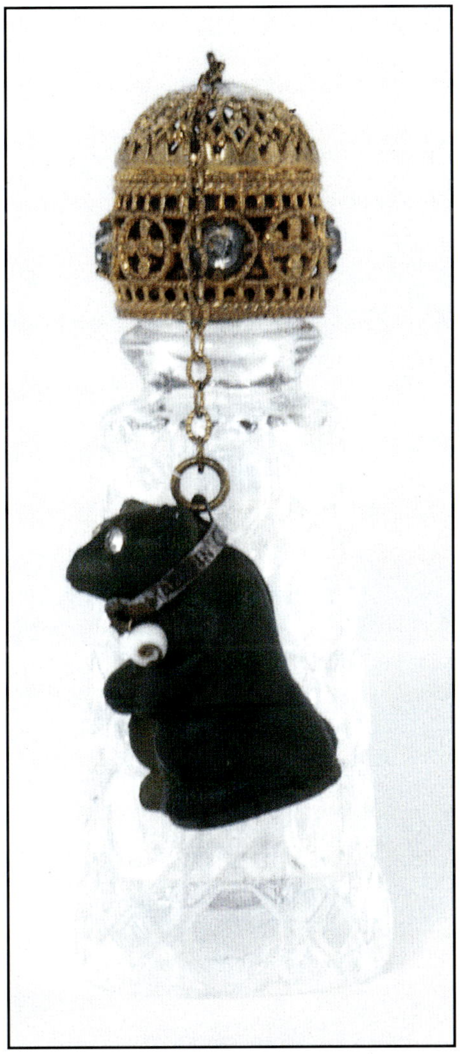

This rare black bear has "Czechoslovakia" marked in his collar; the cap is also marked with a metal tag. The bear shows dark, olive green through the light. $250-350.

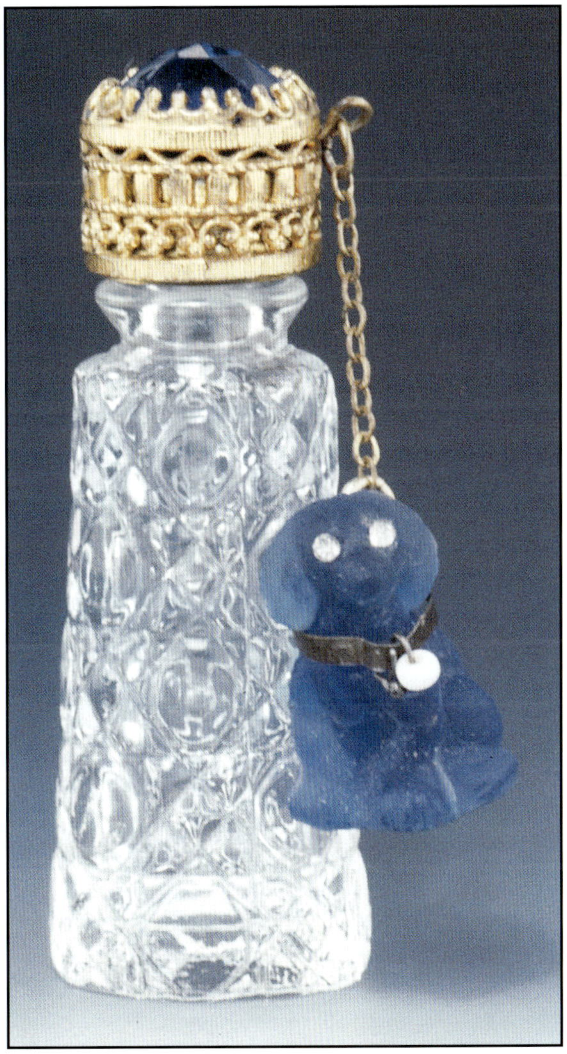

The blue dachshund is supported by a chain on the side of the cap. He is the same intense blue as the capstone. $250-350.

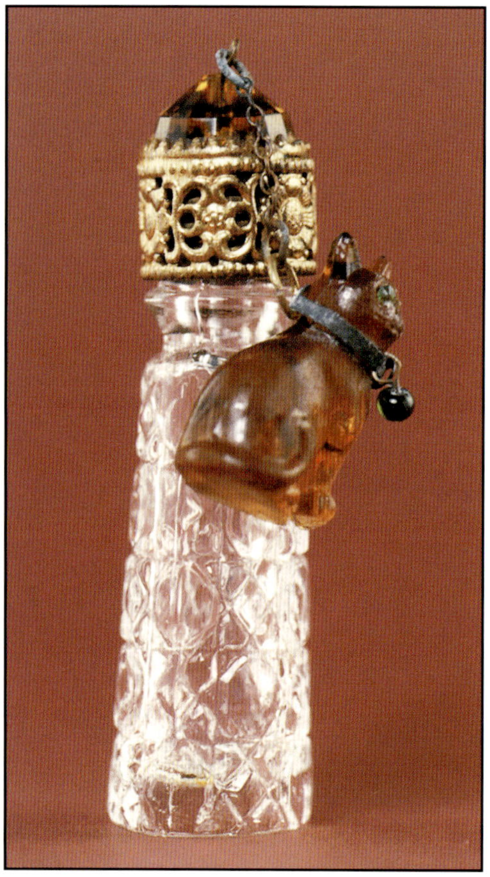

The amber cat is attached to a matching amber capstone. $175-250.

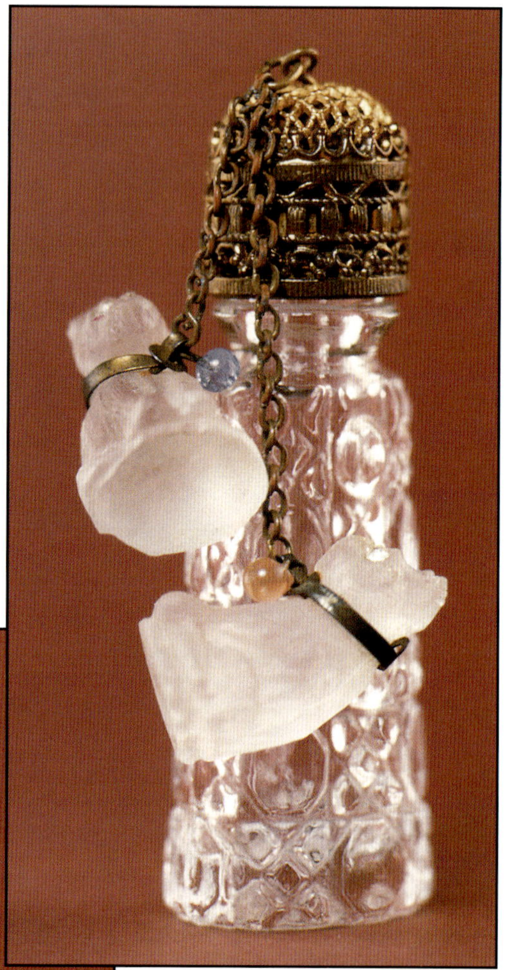

Unusual double pet dangles are attached from the front of their collars. These show off pink and blue beads. $300-400.

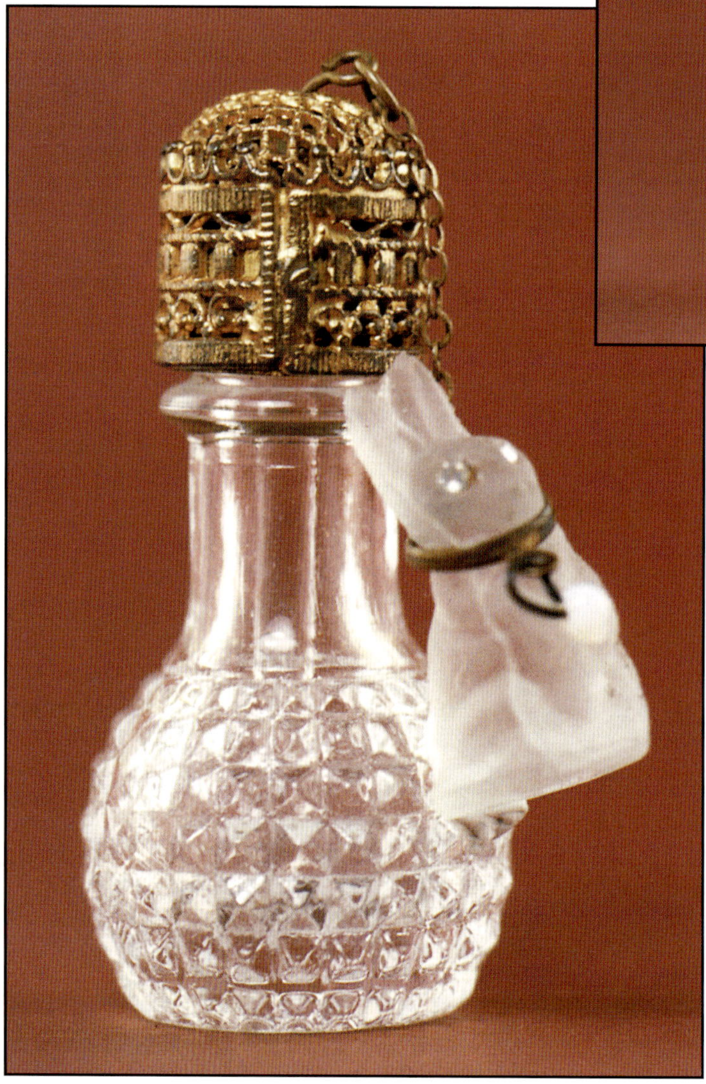

A hard-to-find rabbit charm is suspended from a railroad track cap on a Stubby bottle. $175-250.

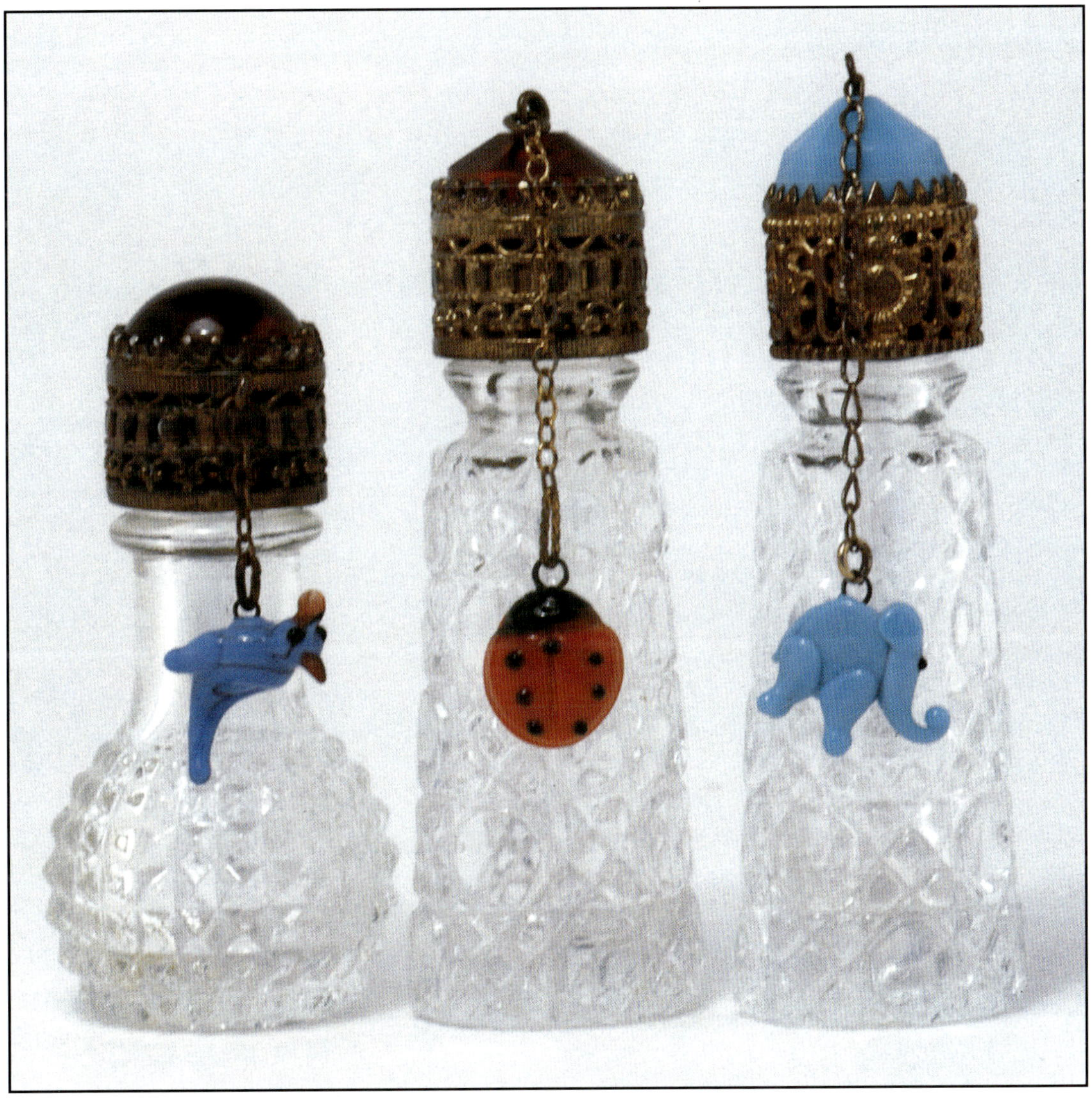

More from the menagerie: a bluebird, ladybugs, and a blue elephant. The dangles are lamp worked with sculpting or features added. The elephants can also be found in doubles. $150-200 each.

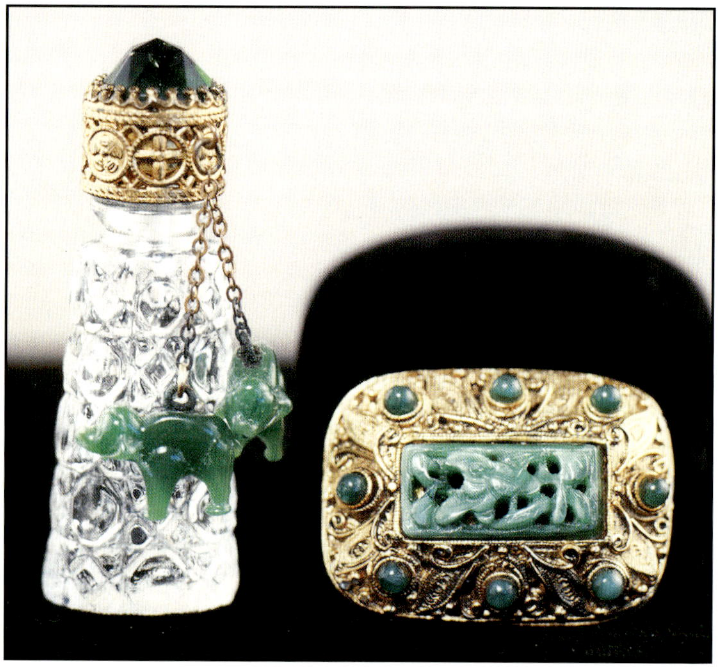

Twin green elephants that have lost the tips of their trunks and now resemble piglets are attached to the cap from the side. They are shown with an unmarked pin with a "carved" floral medallion. Bottle, $100-150; pin, $45.

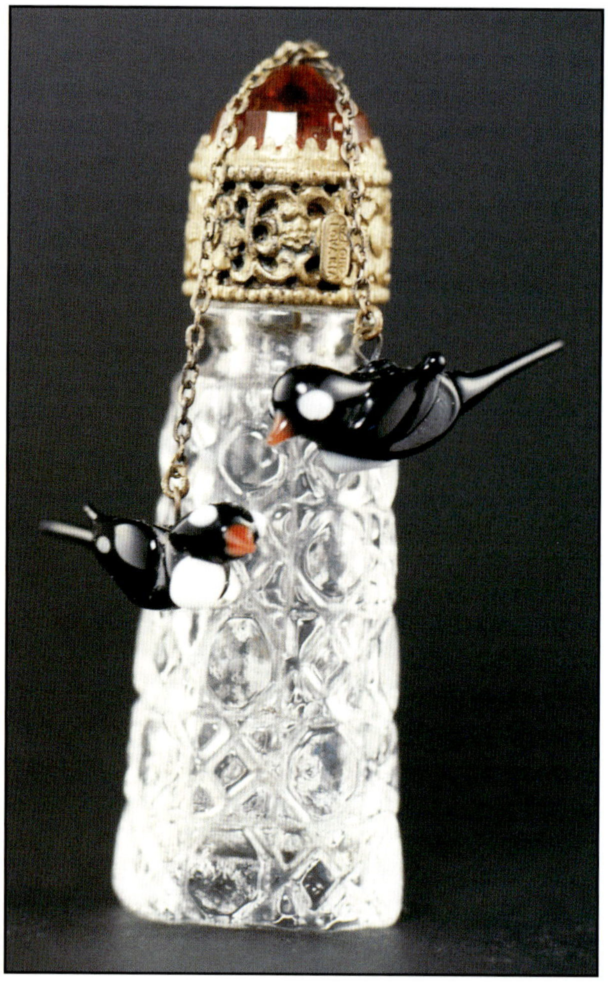

The magpies are suspended in flight. Red and white detailing was applied to the black birds. $150-200.

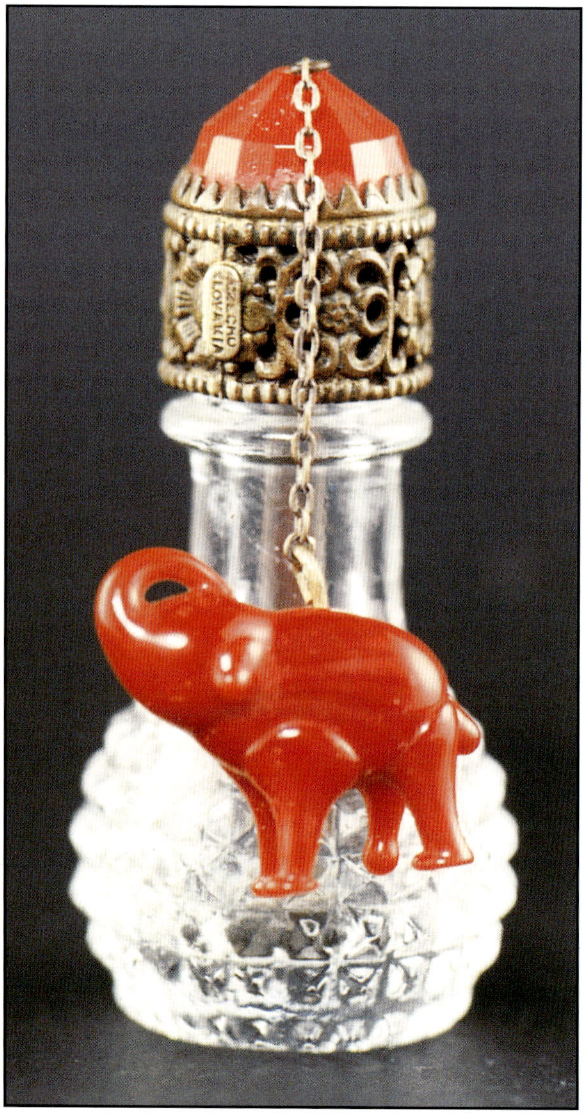

This spectacular elephant in molded opaque glass is an obvious match for the bottle's capstone. Note the style and mark on the cap. $200-300.

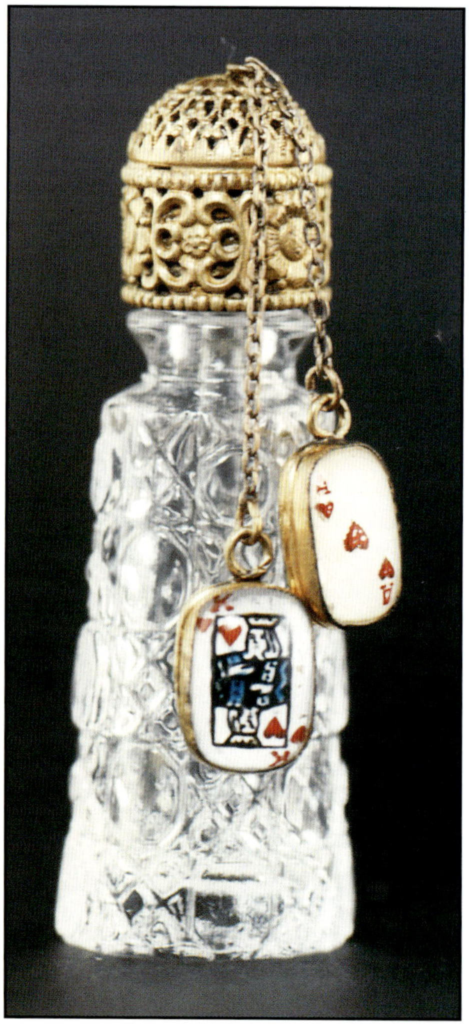

Unique and too rare to assign a value, this is truly "a winning hand."

Other Iríce Purse Bottles

Some bottles have no dangles, obtaining their interest from the detail of the cap instead. A sparkling initial embedded in a flat "onyx" surface or bright "star flowers" form some capstones, for example, while pearls surround faceted stones in others. Molded animal heads sometimes perched above the cap while other animals were molded in the base of a clear glass bubble then painted from underneath and mounted in the cap. Pictured with examples of this style bottle is a bracelet made of similar "bubble buttons," featuring a horse's head and scene of a horse and rider jumping a rail.

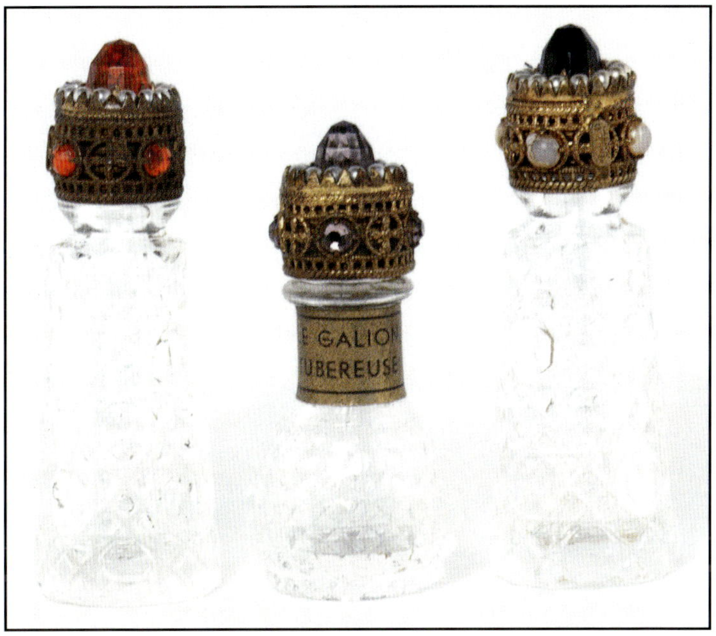

The gems atop these bottles are wreathed in pearls. The caps are marked. Note that the middle bottle was used commercially and still bears its "Le Galion, Tubereuse" label. The bottle on the right has an unusual opaque black faceted stone. $75-150 each.

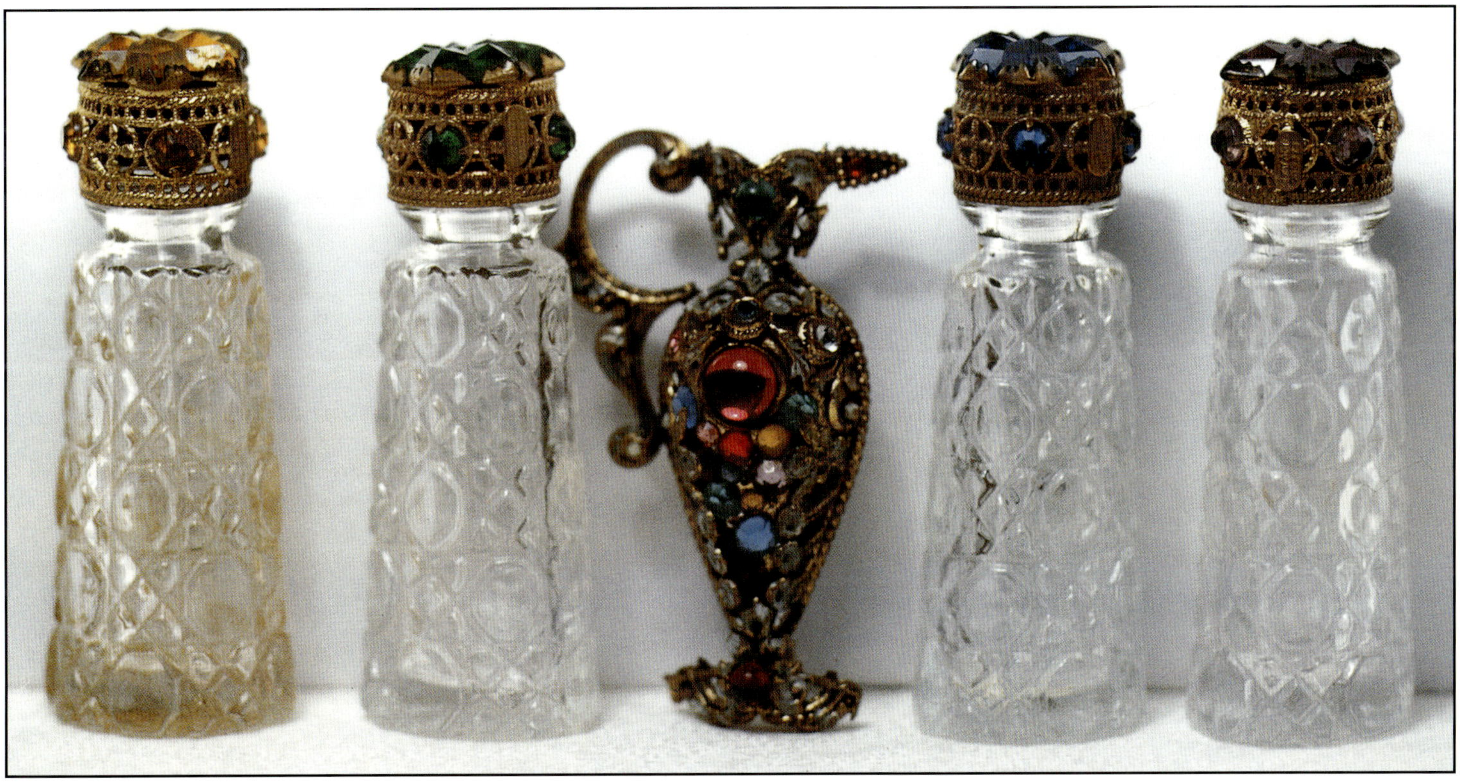

Flat star flowers form the tops of these bottles. Found in clear and a variety of colors, the gems around the caps match the tops. The yellow cap sits on an unusual yellow tinted base. The pitcher pin is marked "Czecho." Pin and bottles, $50-125 each.

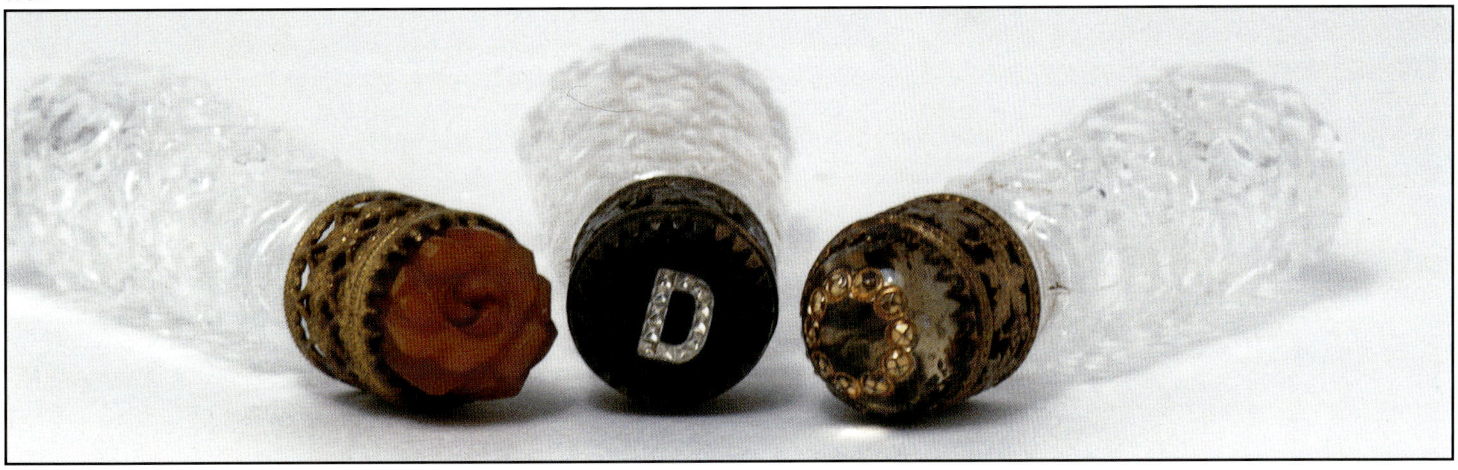

Three bottles with fancy capstones. From left: Carved "coral" rose, monogram or initial cap, and soft yellow cap with molded, gold painted "beads" in a circle. $100-200 each.

Czech portrait bracelet in similar style as the dog portrait bottles shown below. These picture a horse head and a jumping horse and rider. $100.

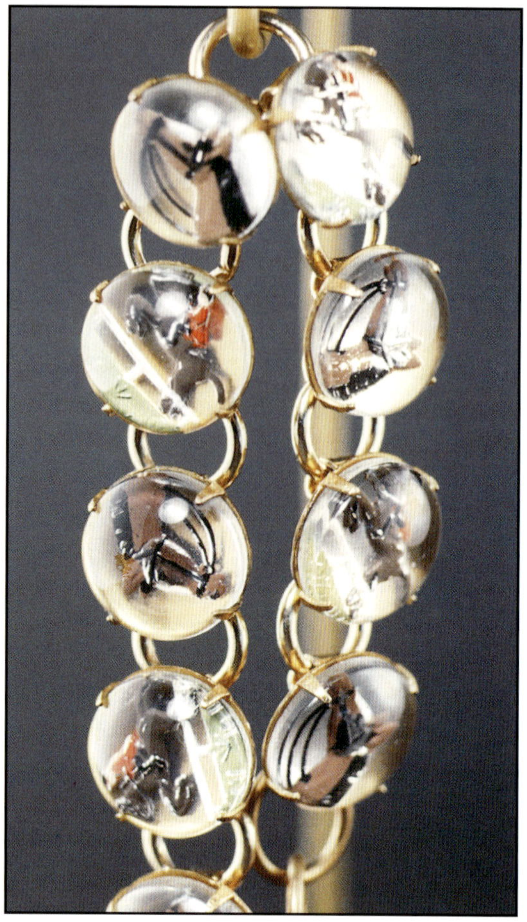

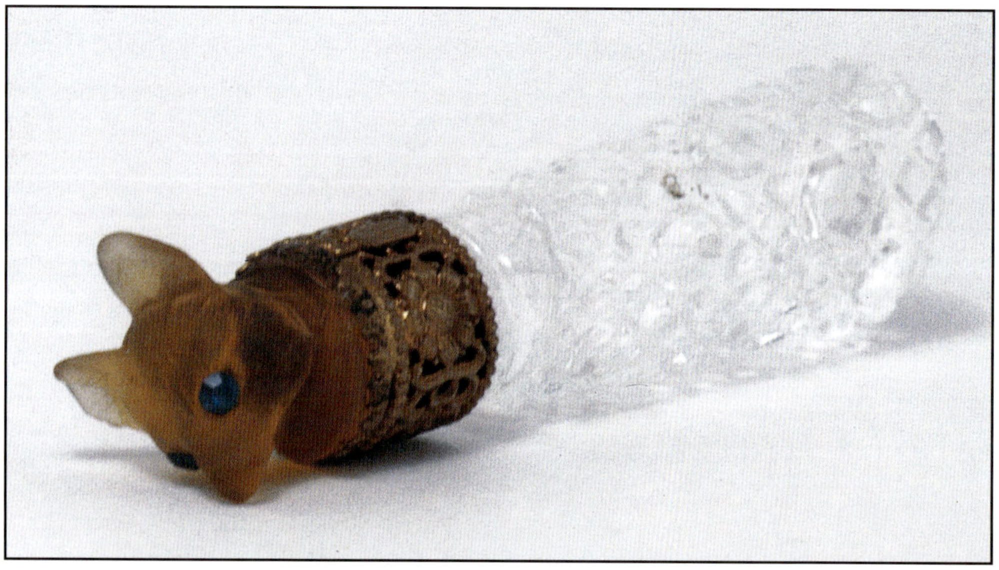

The fox. Several animals were depicted in this manner, most commonly, a dog or fox. These are seldom seen on the market. $300-500.

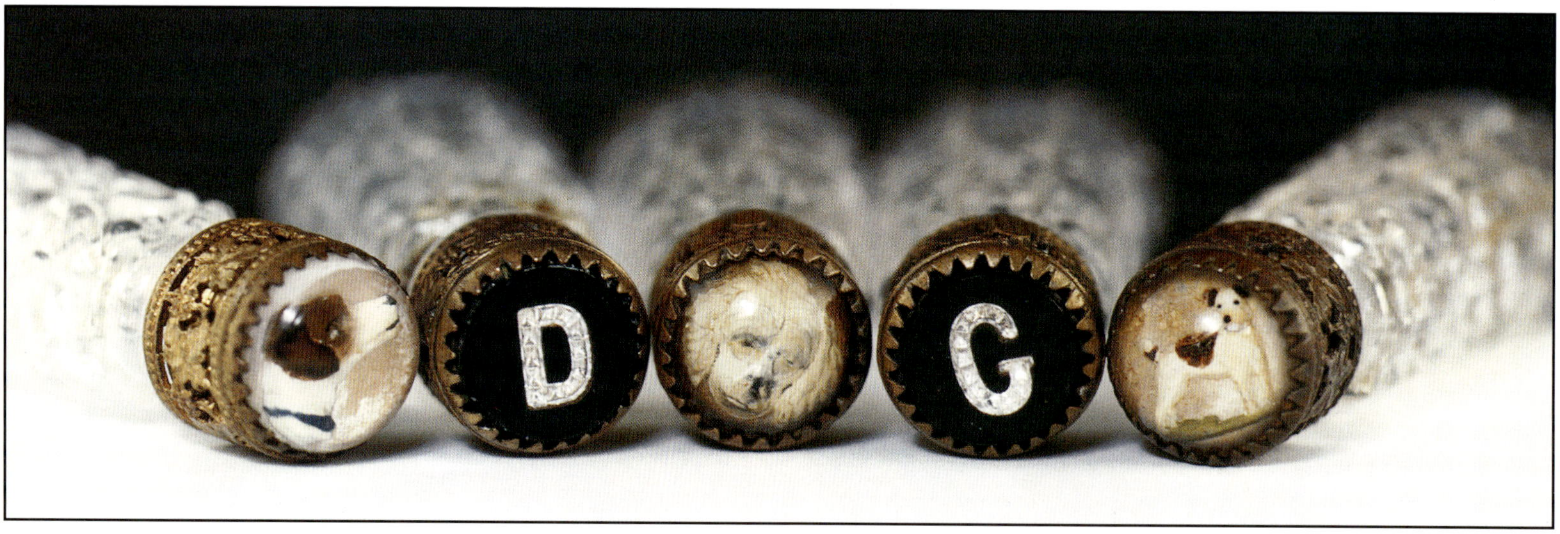

Going to the dogs. These dogs intaglio and reverse side painted are rarely, if ever seen. Monogram bottles and dog portrait bottles *courtesy of Nancy and Frank Dooley*. No price available.

Mystery Bottles

Pictured in this section along with some Irice bottles are unmarked bottles that most likely competed for the same buyers as the Irice dangles. "Snowman" bottles appeared with a variety of cap styles. Most of these bottles have no identifying mark, but some are marked USA. The bell and pinch bottles (round bottles with three indented or "pinched" sides) are cold painted and have survived the years in surprisingly good condition. They have a slightly different picture on each of the three sides. The metal caged bottles are adorned with the same style of caps (double bow) and are marked Irice in the molding in the metal of the base. The bottle with the pointed plastic cap and the orange bead dangles is completely unmarked, as are the trio with dangles and brass ball caps. These are the mystery bottles that are sometimes seen advertised as Czech—and whether they are or not, they certainly come from the same era and have the same appeal.

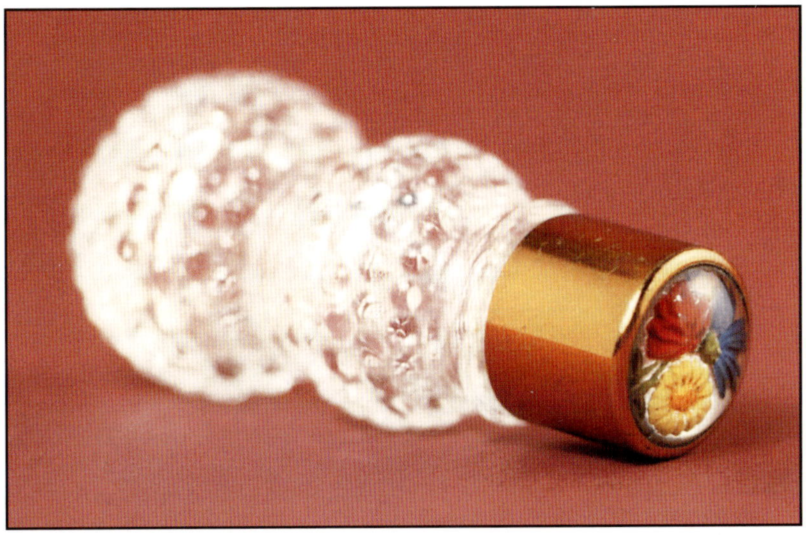

A cap feature similar to the previously shown dog portraits is this reverse painted intaglio floral trio. The "snowman" bottle is unmarked and of undetermined origin. $50.

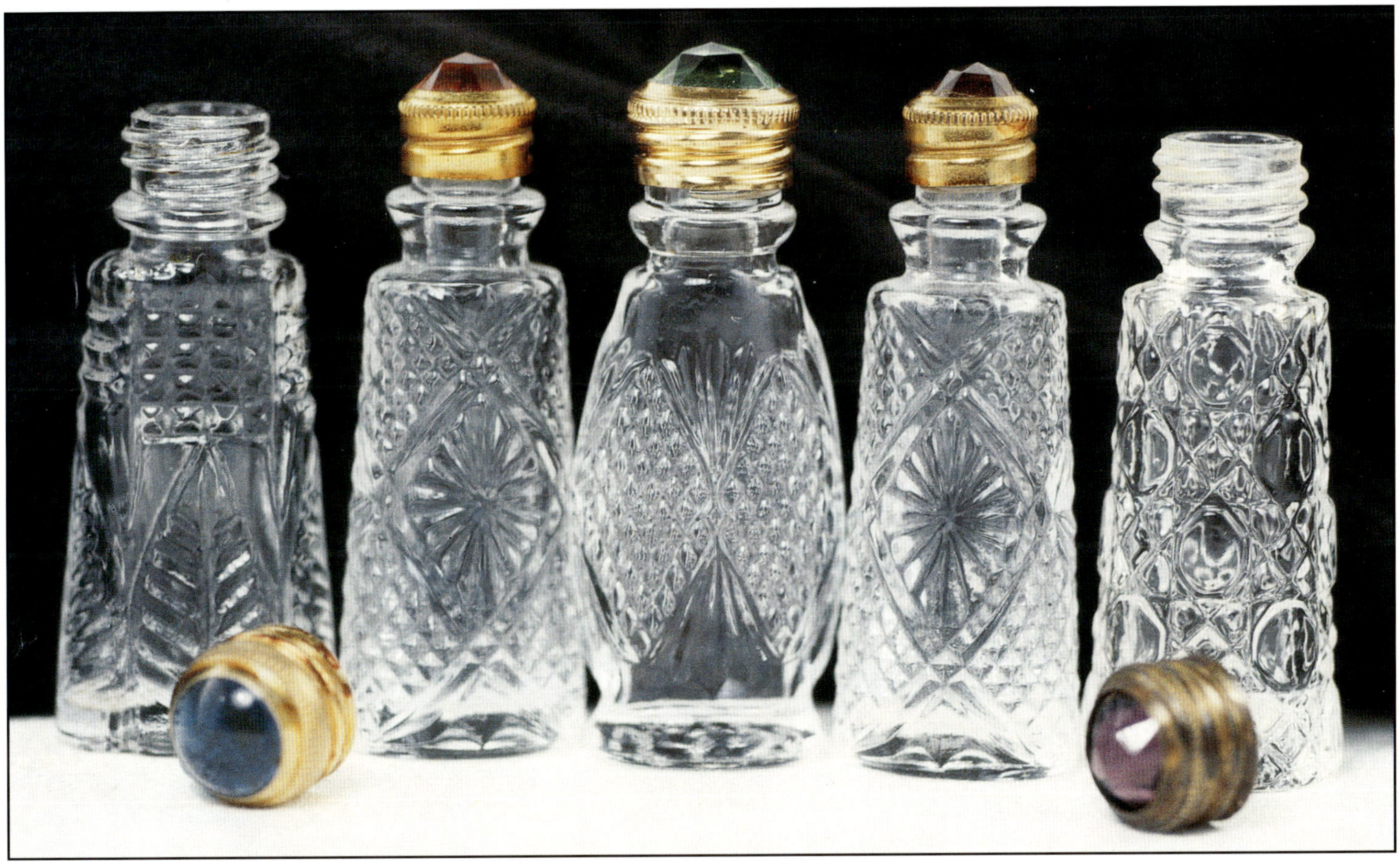

A medley of bottle base styles with plain caps. $50.

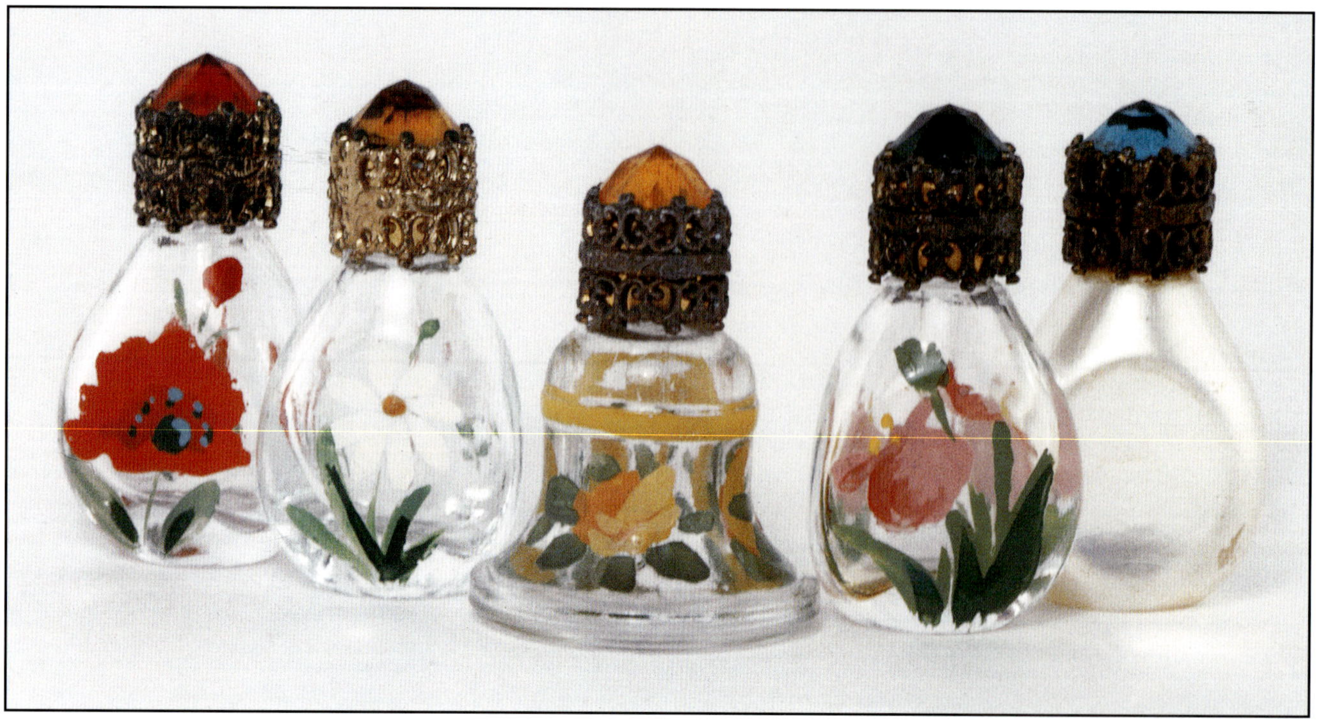

A center bell is flanked by pinch bottles, all less than 2" in height. The pinch bottles have different cold painted flowers on each of their three sides. The pinch bottle on the right has no flowers, but has been painted with a pearl-like gloss. These bottles are unmarked. $35-95 each.

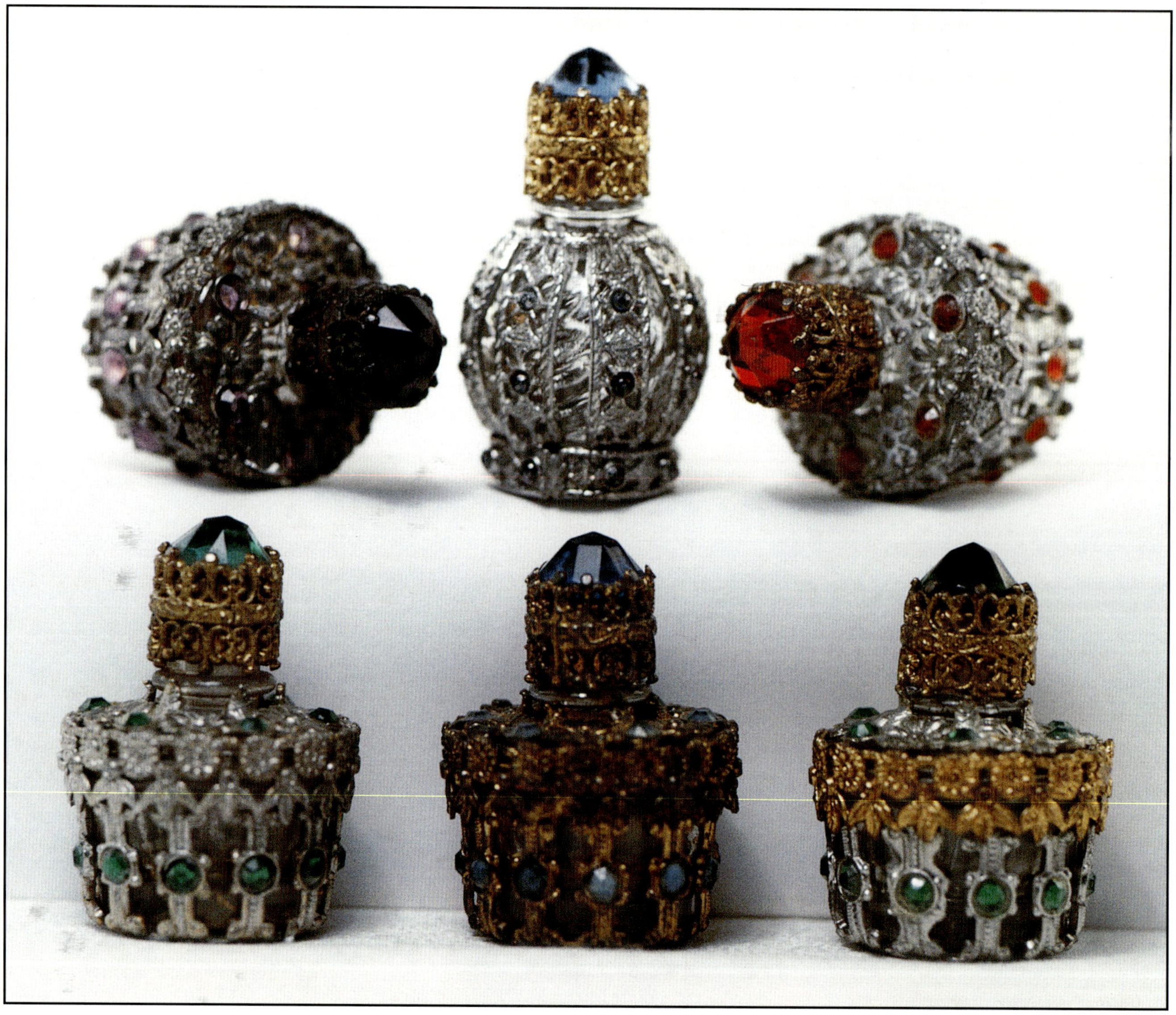

These diminutive, jewel-studded caged bottles are all marked Irice in the metal in the base. The cap style is identical to those in the previous grouping. $50-125 each.

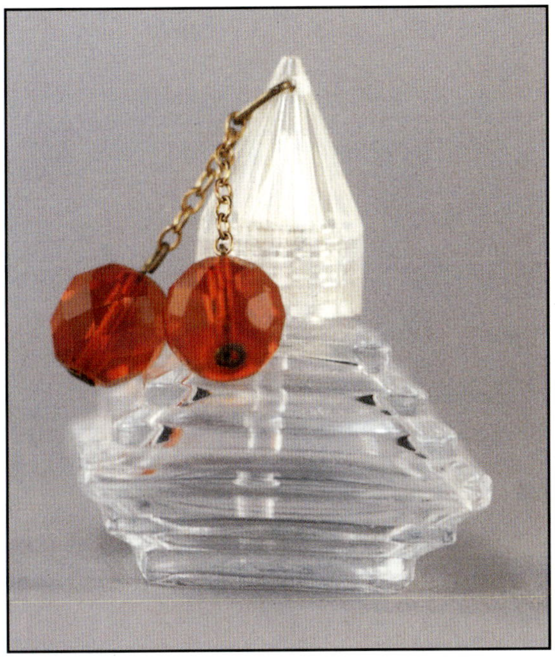

This bottle is unmarked. It has a plastic lid, but a glass dauber. The beads are heavy crystal and clean cut, but in a bright orange that is not common to Czech perfume bottles. I have seen similar bottles listed as Czech. $50-100.

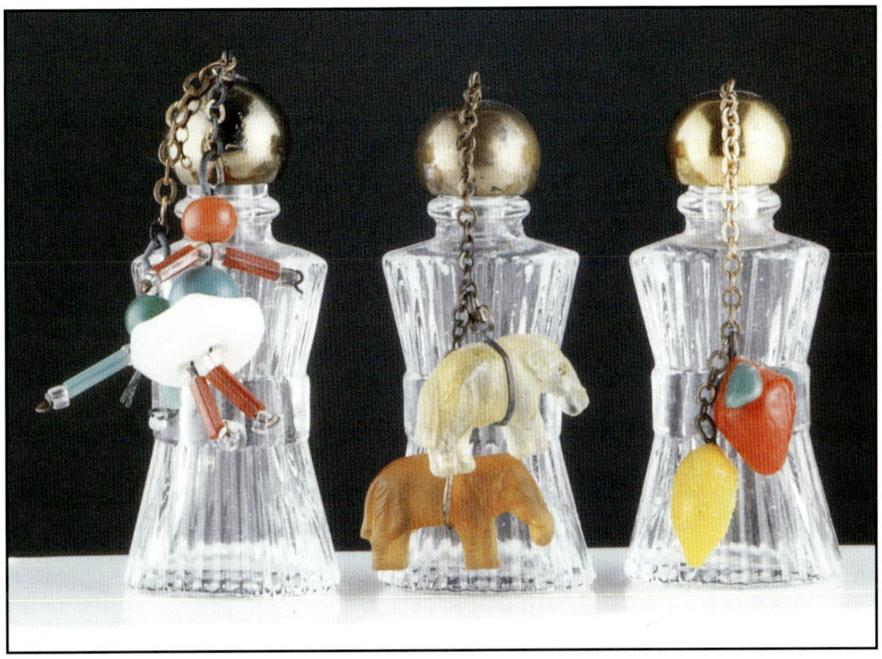

A trio of mystery bottles. These bottles all have glass stoppers, heavy brass ball caps. All are unmarked. If not Czech, they were surely targeting the same market. $50-$100 each.

Cut Glass Purse Bottles

In a separate class from the Irice dangles are the miniatures with cut and polished glass bases and screw tops. Most of these are acid etched in the base and many also have the "Czechoslovakia" metal tag on the cap. Although most have glass daubers attached to the inside of the cap, some have glass stoppers with daubers, which seat inside the bottle opening. The screw cap serves as a stopper cover.

Cut glass purse bottles come in various sizes and shapes. What draws them together in a category of their own is their elegance. The caged purse bottle compared in this photo with a cut glass bottle of similar height looks chunky and busy. Its companion, with strips of filigree down each side, has clean lines, bevel-cut edges and corners, and a cap with gem-studded crown piece.

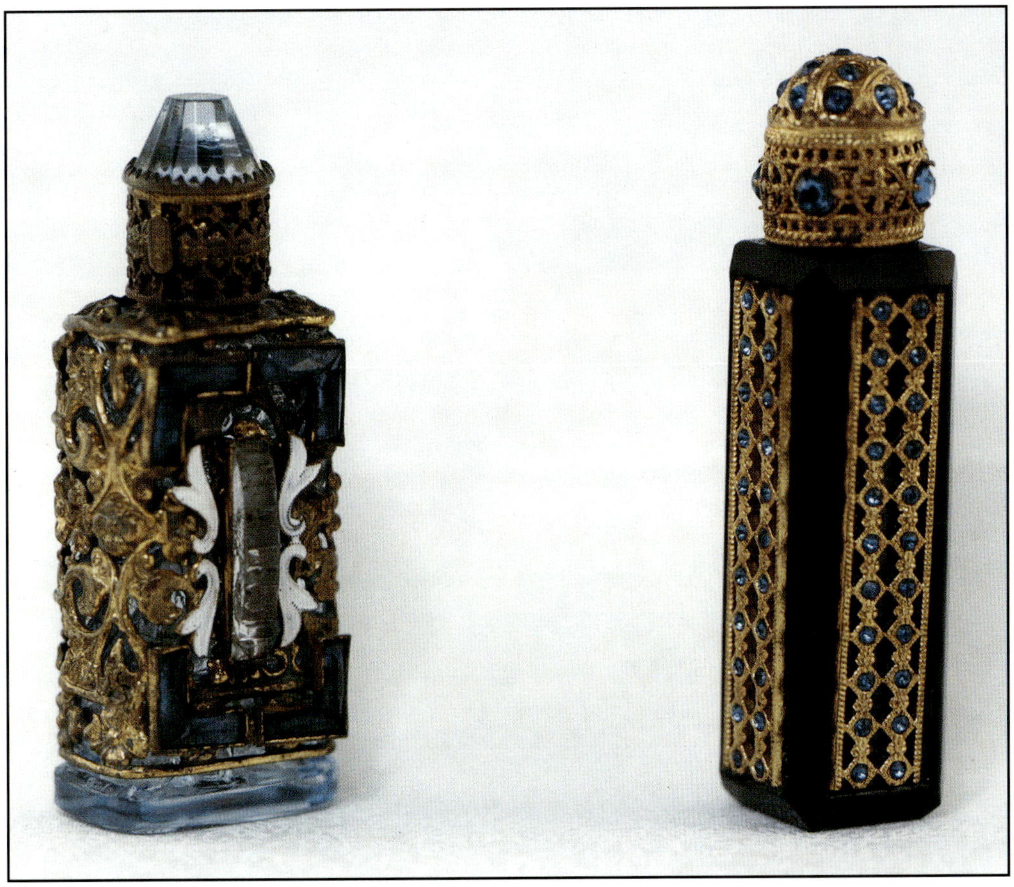

Left: Caged purse bottle, metal tag. 2.5". $150-200. Right: Black cut glass purse bottle, side panels of filigree, blue stones. 2.75". $250-300.

The bottles shown in the second of these two photos have openings the same size as the Irice dangle bottles. Some of the openings are glass only and some have metal threaded pieces over the glass. The metal threads are accepted as evidence of earlier productions, but the Irice dangle bottles, which had only glass threads, were advertised in the mid-1930s.

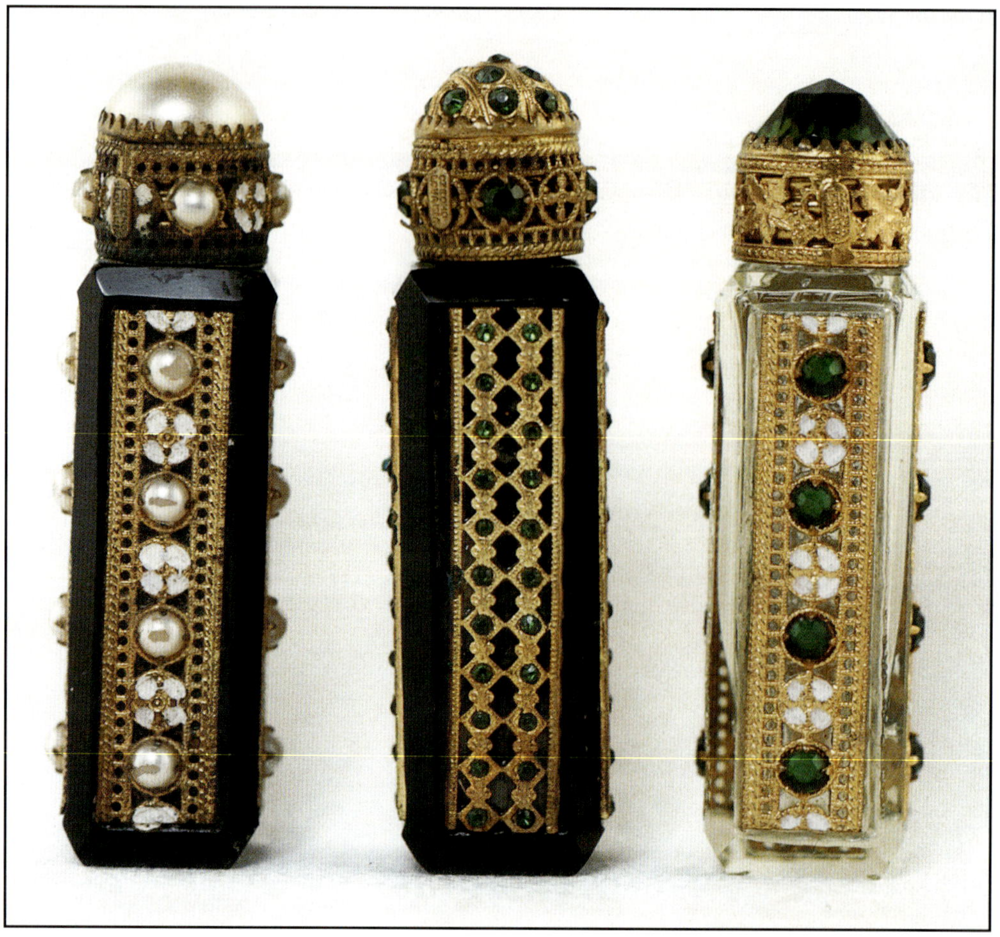

Left: Black cut glass purse bottle with side strips of enameled filigree and pearls. Center: Black cut glass with side strips of filigree and green jewels. Right: Light yellow cut glass with side panels of filigree and green stones. All marked. 2.75". $250-300.

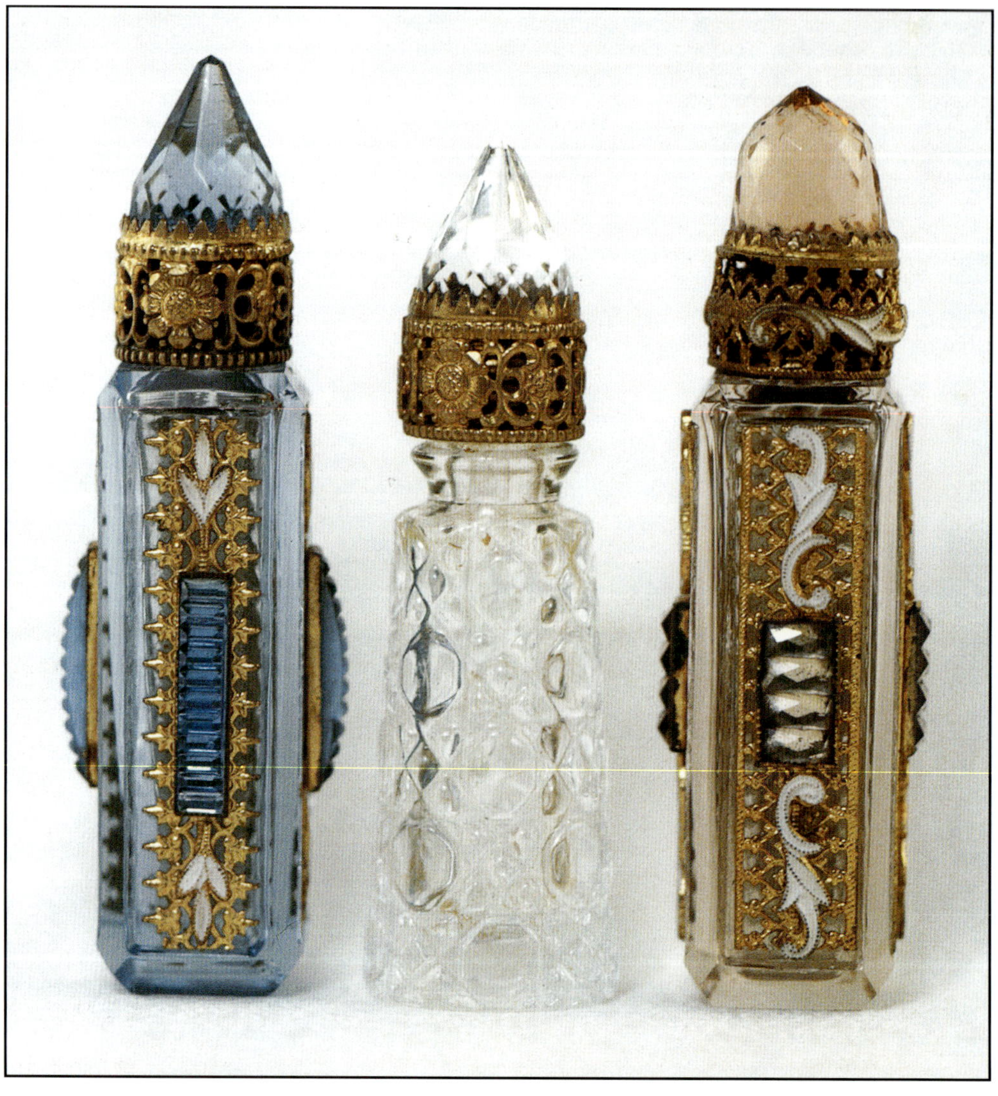

Left: Blue cut glass, enameled filigree, pointed, faceted top. 3.125". $300-400. Center: Irice base with elaborate cap. 3". $100-150. Right: Pink cut glass, applied filigree on sides and cap, elaborate faceted capstone. 3.125". $300-400.

Smaller and daintier, with metal inner threads, these bottles have caps that are the same size as caged purse bottles (that is, smaller than the Irice dangles). The metal inner rim, the detailing of the cuts and intaglio, and the styles and markings of the caps all indicate that these bottles were produced before the mid-1930s. The caps with the clover-leaves are not marked with metal tags, but in each example, the base is acid etched.

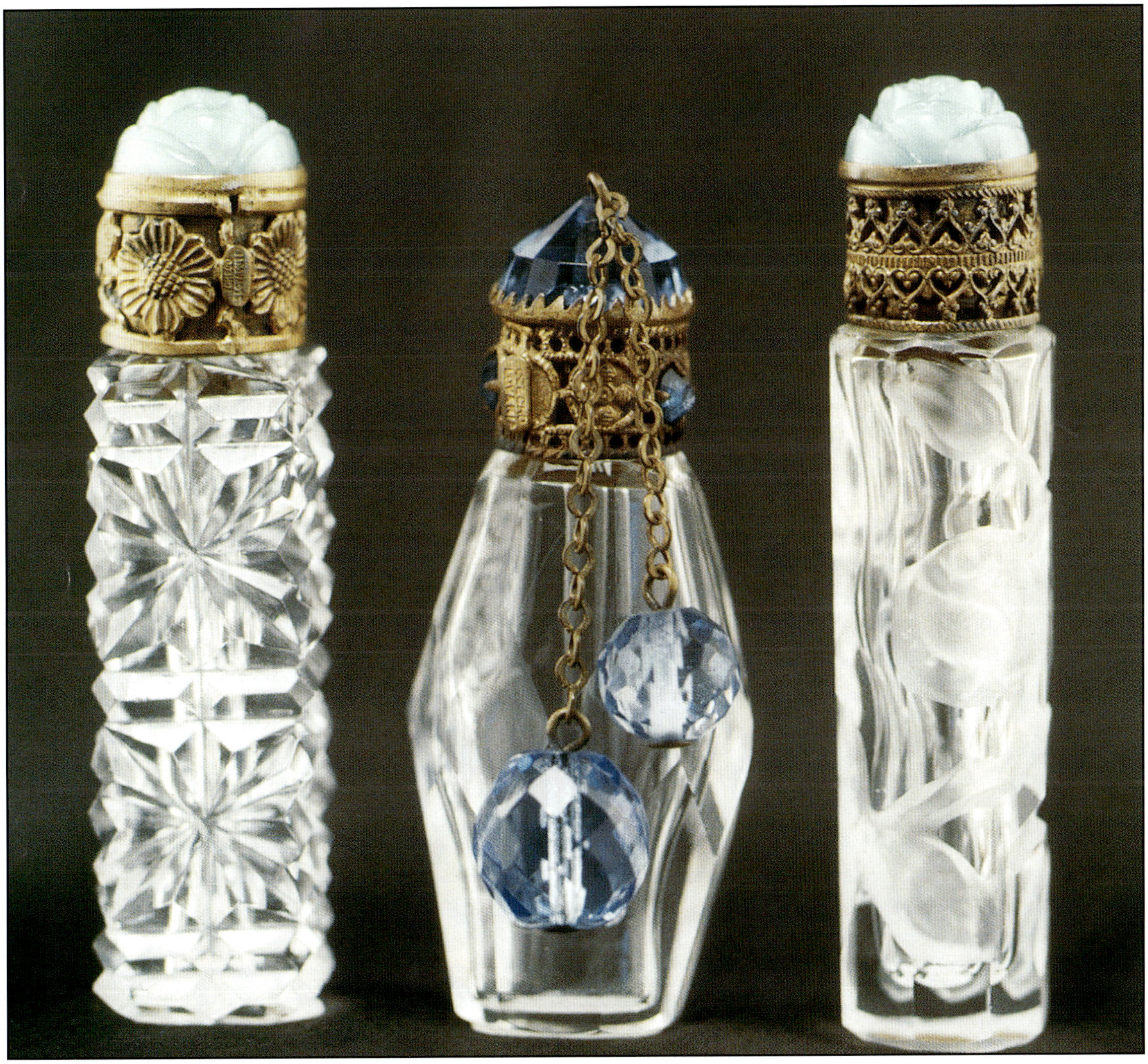

Left: Geometric cut, clover top with "jade" carved rose. 2.375". $200-250. Center: Facet cut bottle with blue crystal top and two sizes of cut beads dangles. 2.25". $150-200. Right: Eight-sided cut glass bottle, frosted, intaglio roses, jade carved rose top. 2.725". $250-300.

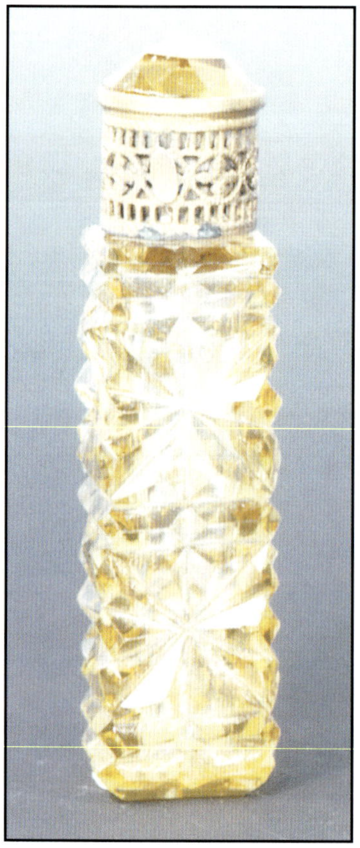

Amber geometric cut glass bottle, faint acid mark in base. 2.25". $200-250.

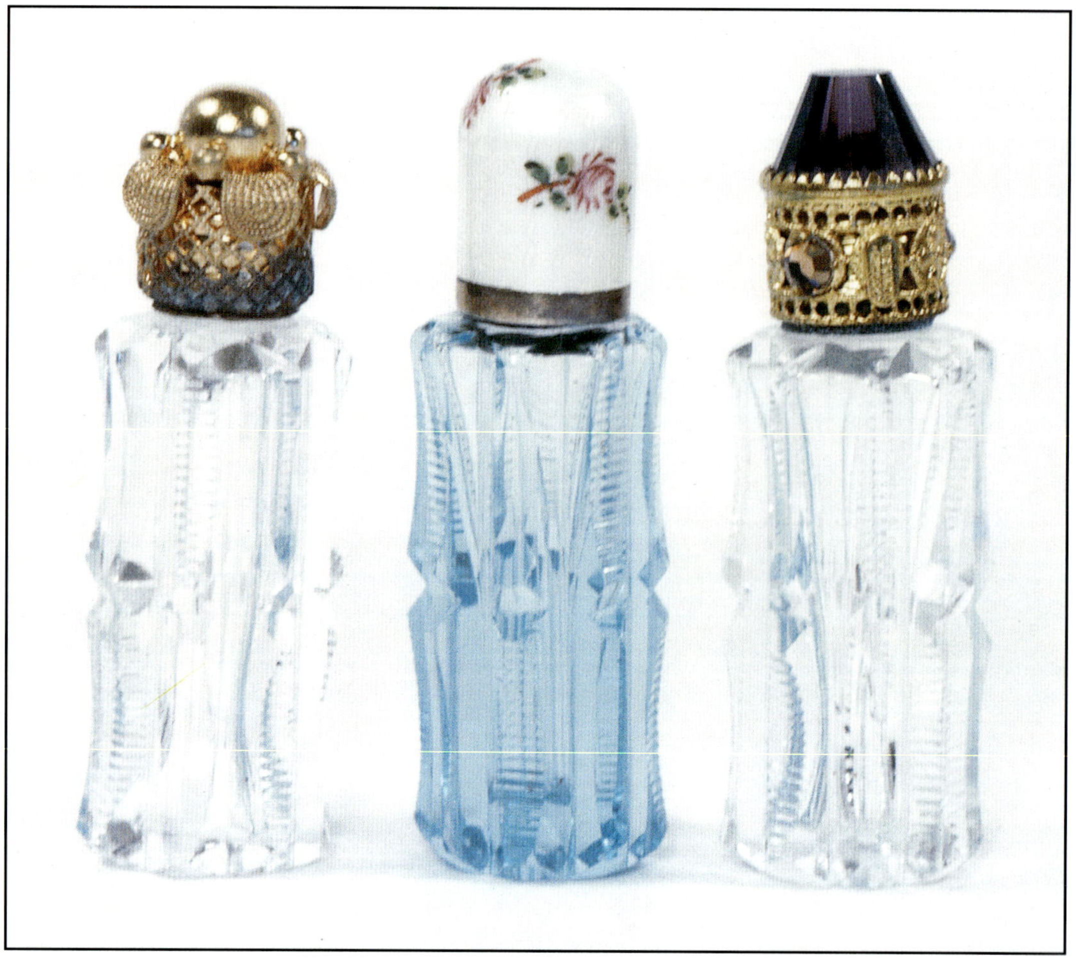

Left: Clear cut base, ornate brass flower on a mesh cap. $100-200. Center: The same base in rare, teal color, the cap (stopper cover) is fine enameling over sterling, marked Germany. The stopper is silver and cork. $250-300. Right: Same base design with amethyst stones in cap. $150-200.

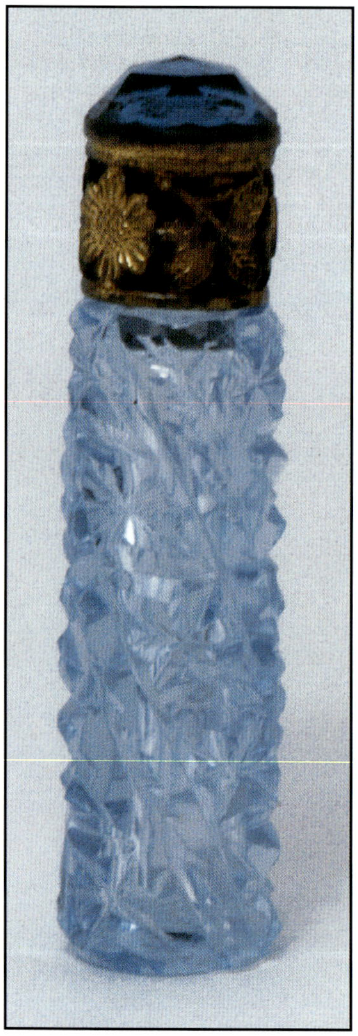

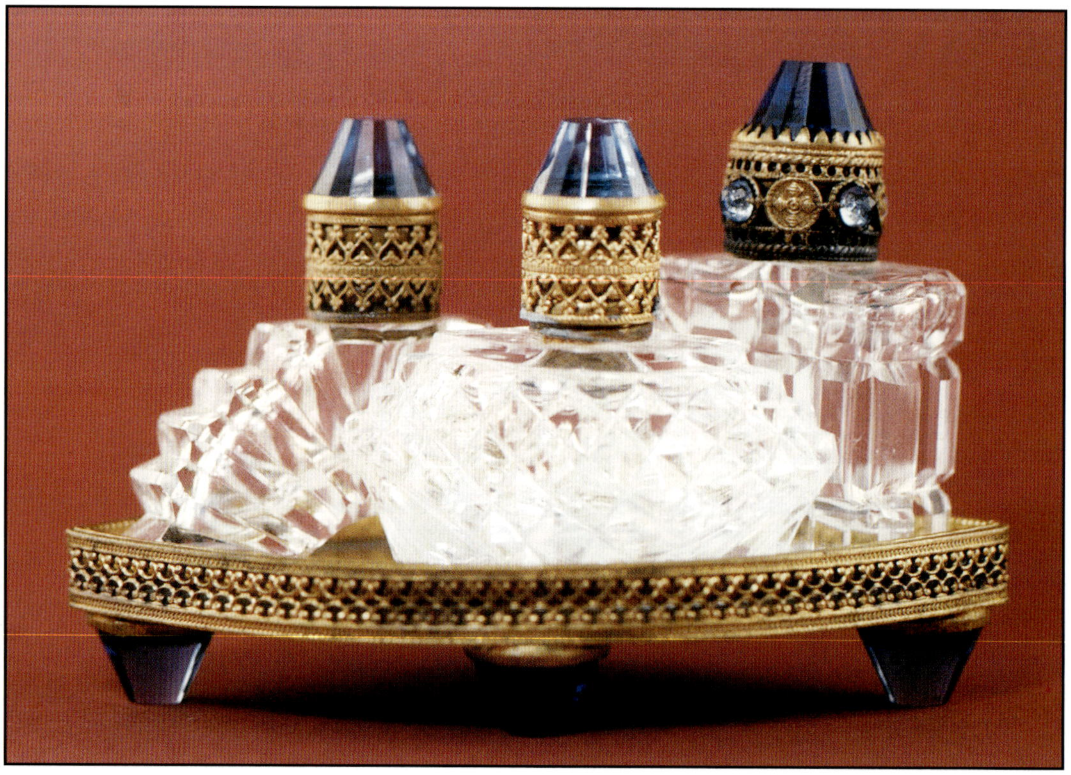

Trio of cut glass purse bottles on oval Czech tray.

Blue spiral-cut purse bottle. 2.5" $200-250.

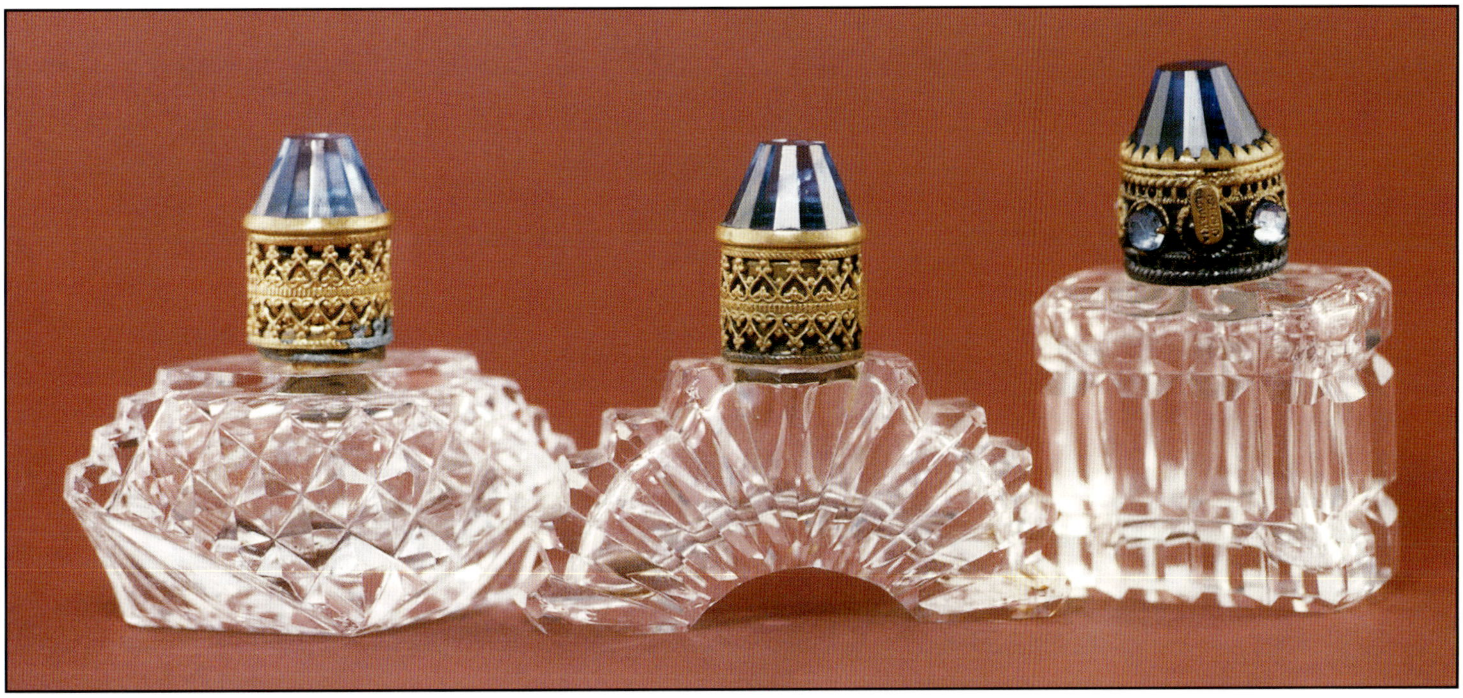

Left: 1.725", diamond geometric cuts, blue capstone. Center: "Bridge" bottle. These "zipper" caps are actually stopper covers. Right: "Ice block" bottle base, blue "coin and bangle" cap has attached dauber. The center and right bases can be found with a variety of finish detail. $100-150 each.

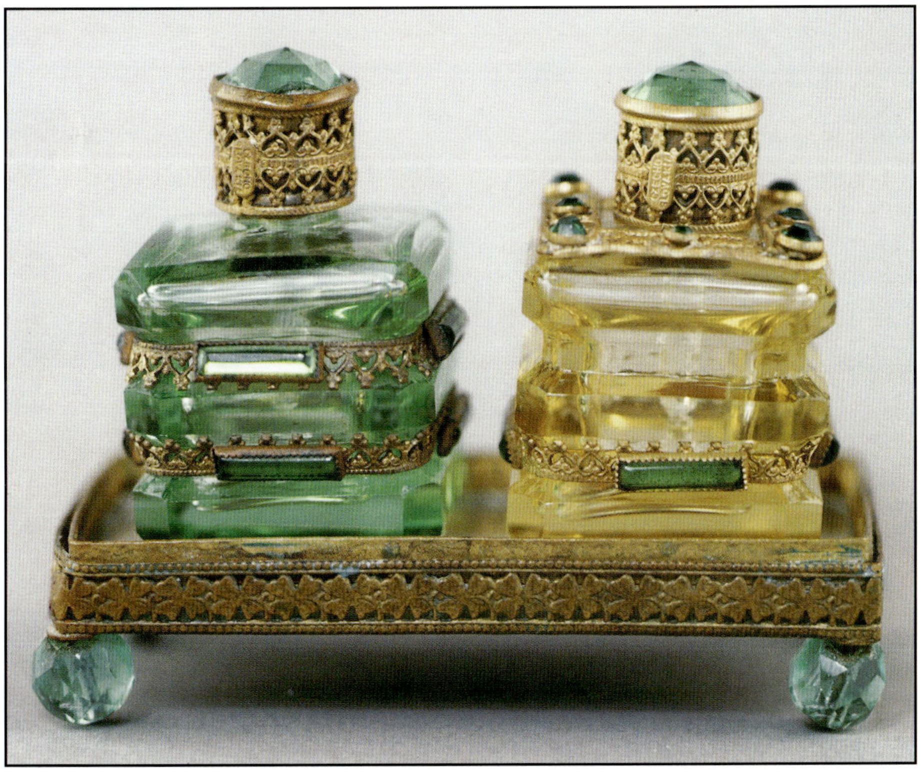

Complementary cut glass bottles on a rectangular Czech tray. The metal and jewel work is different on the two bottles. Because these were hand decorated, the difference was likely intentional. Bottles, 2.75", $200 each. Tray, $100. Bottles and tray are marked.

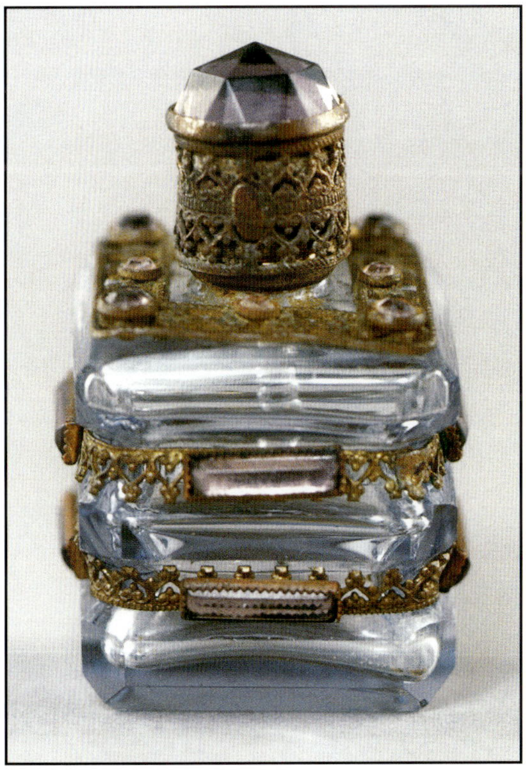

Same bottle with maximum decoration in amethyst. Metal tag reads, "Tcecho Slovacuie."

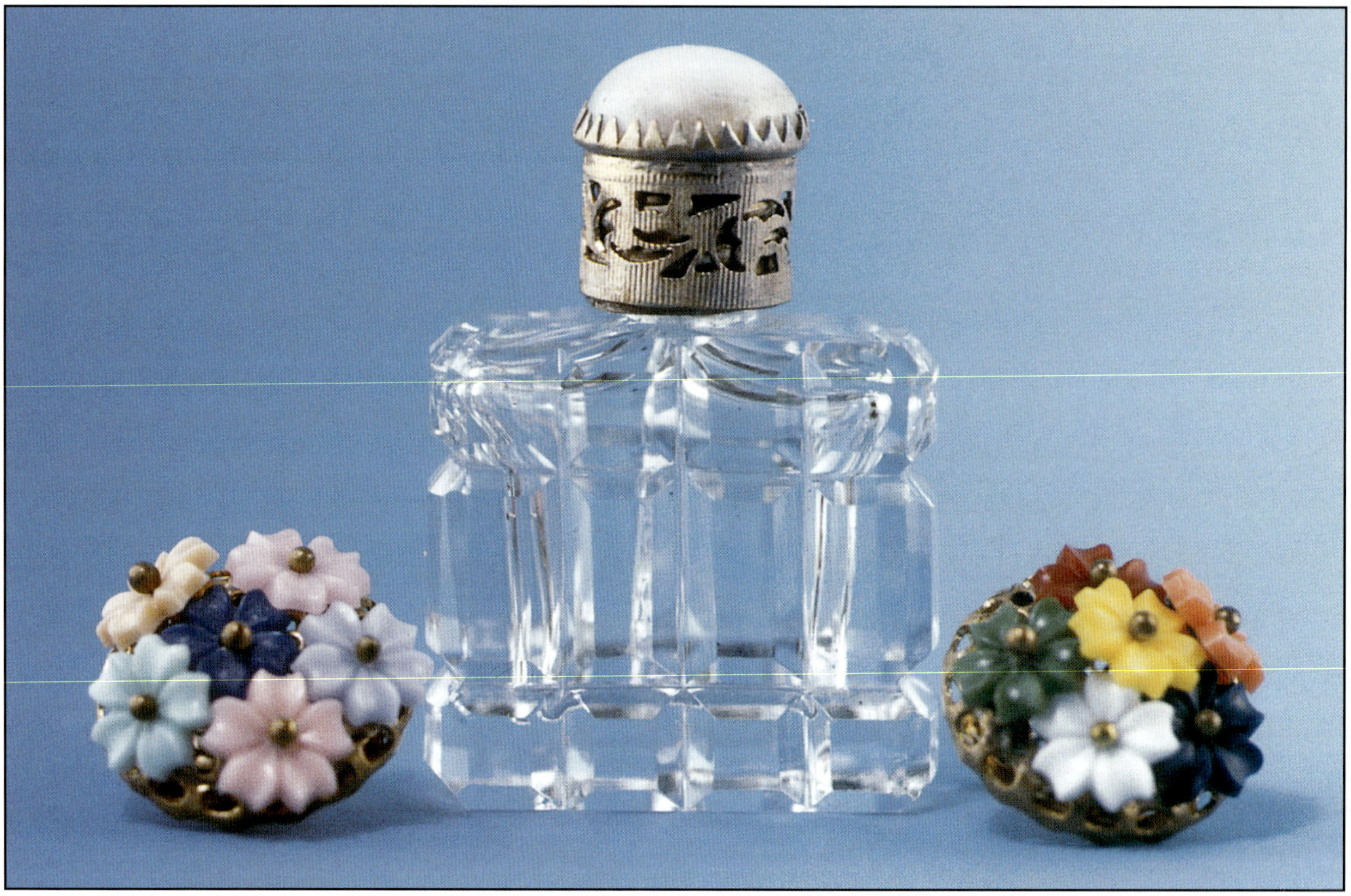

"Ice block" bottle with white cap, no marks. 1.75". $50-100. Shown with bead glass flower earrings. $20.

Some cut glass mini purse bottles have bouquets of bead flowers sprouting from the top of the caps. Under the beads in each cap top is a clear rose. A loop in the center of the rose serves as the anchor for the bead arrangement.

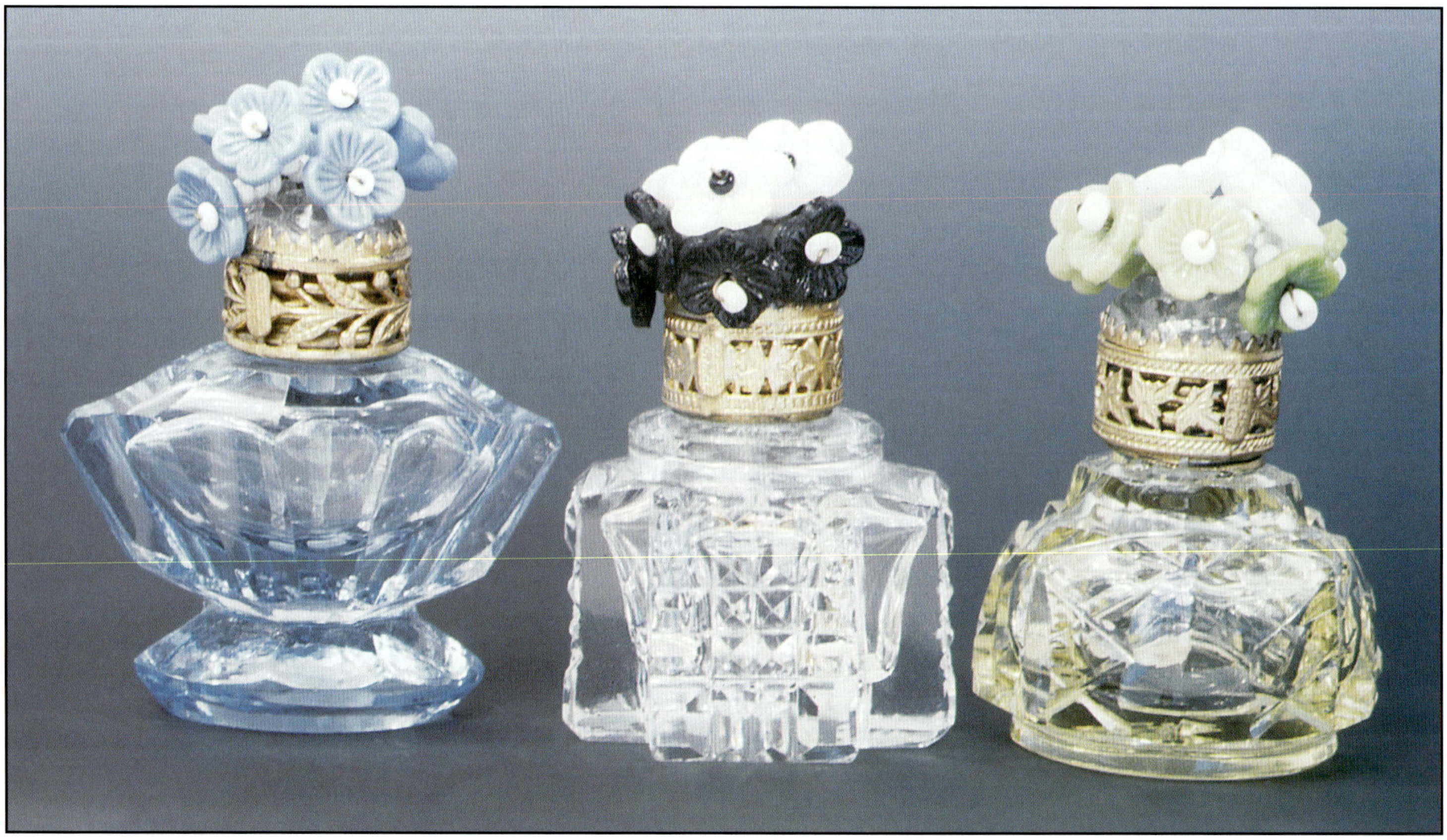

Bead bouquets. Left: Blue cut glass base, blue and white bead flowers. Center: Clear base, black and white flowers. Right: Yellow base, green and white bead flowers. All marked in the caps, all about 2", all $150-200.

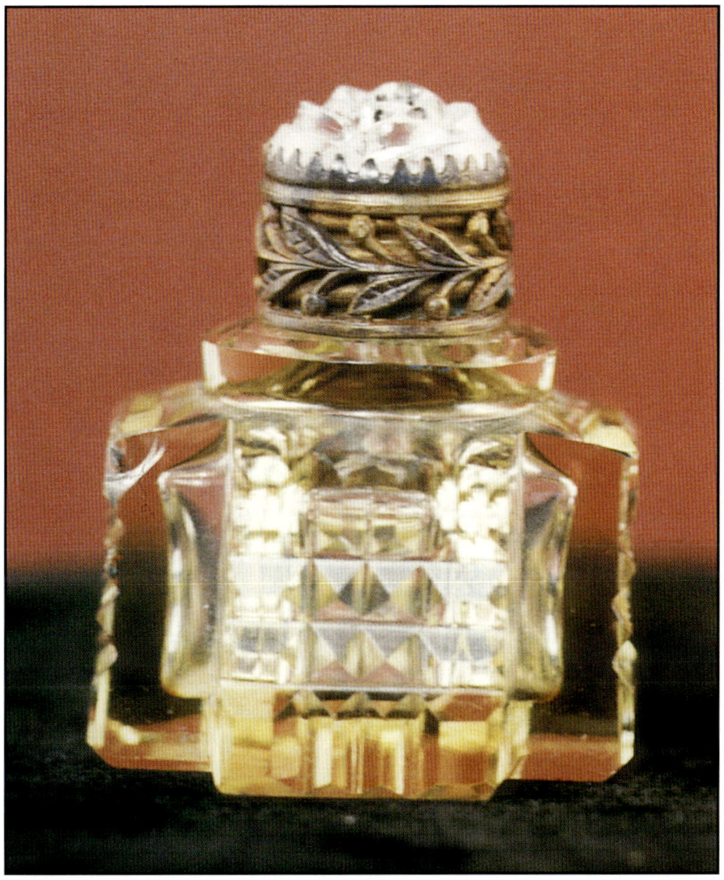

Yellow cut glass base, clear carved rose in cap, 1.725". A loop at the center top once anchored beaded flowers. $150-200.

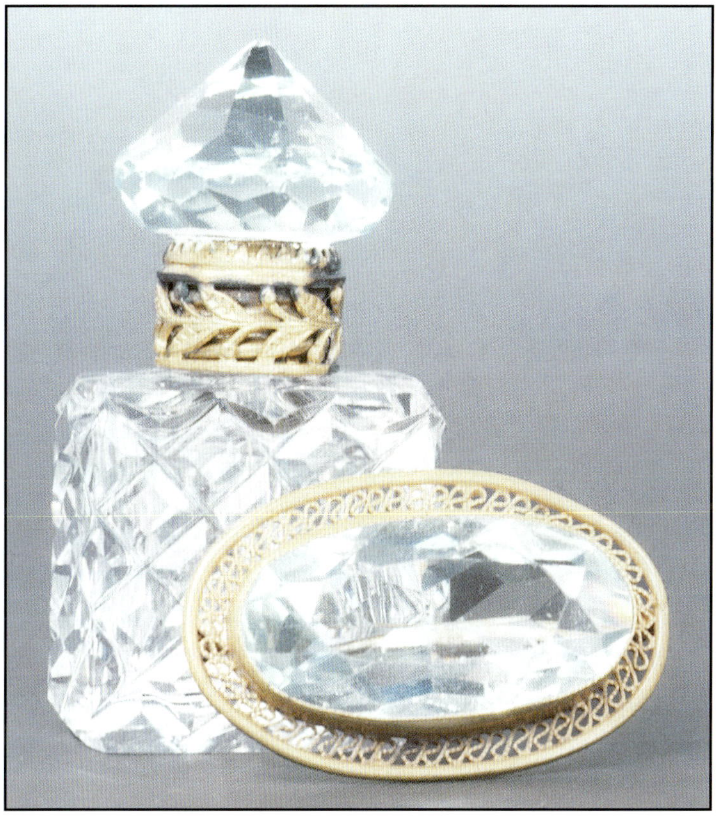

The same blank as the ice block, but cut in a diamond pattern with a bodacious aqua faceted capstone. The cap is marked and the base has an acid mark. 2.25". $150-200. Unmarked, cut glass aqua oval pin with filigree. $50.

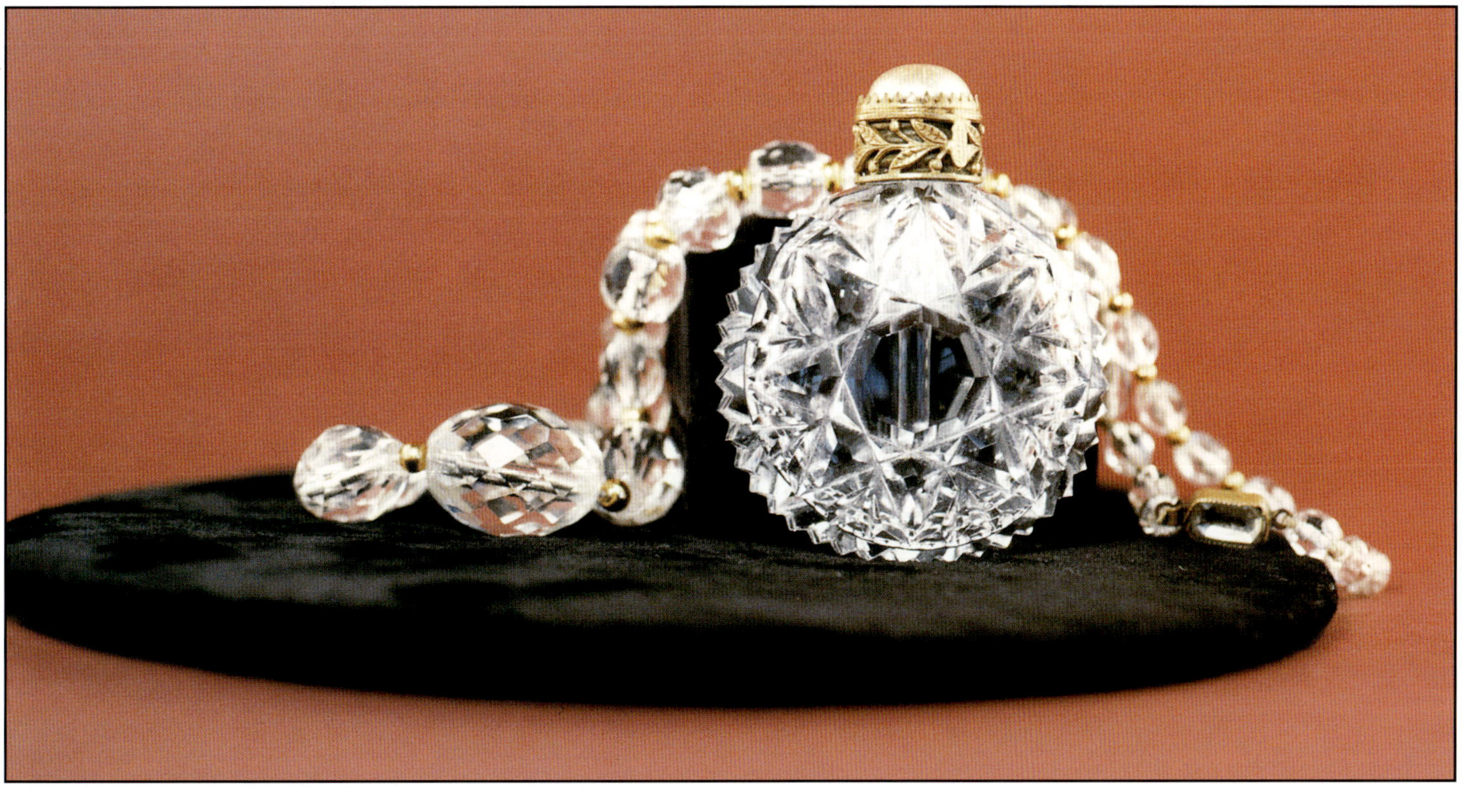

Star cut crystal laydown bottle with pearl set is shown with marked crystal beads. Bottle, $200-300; beads, $50.

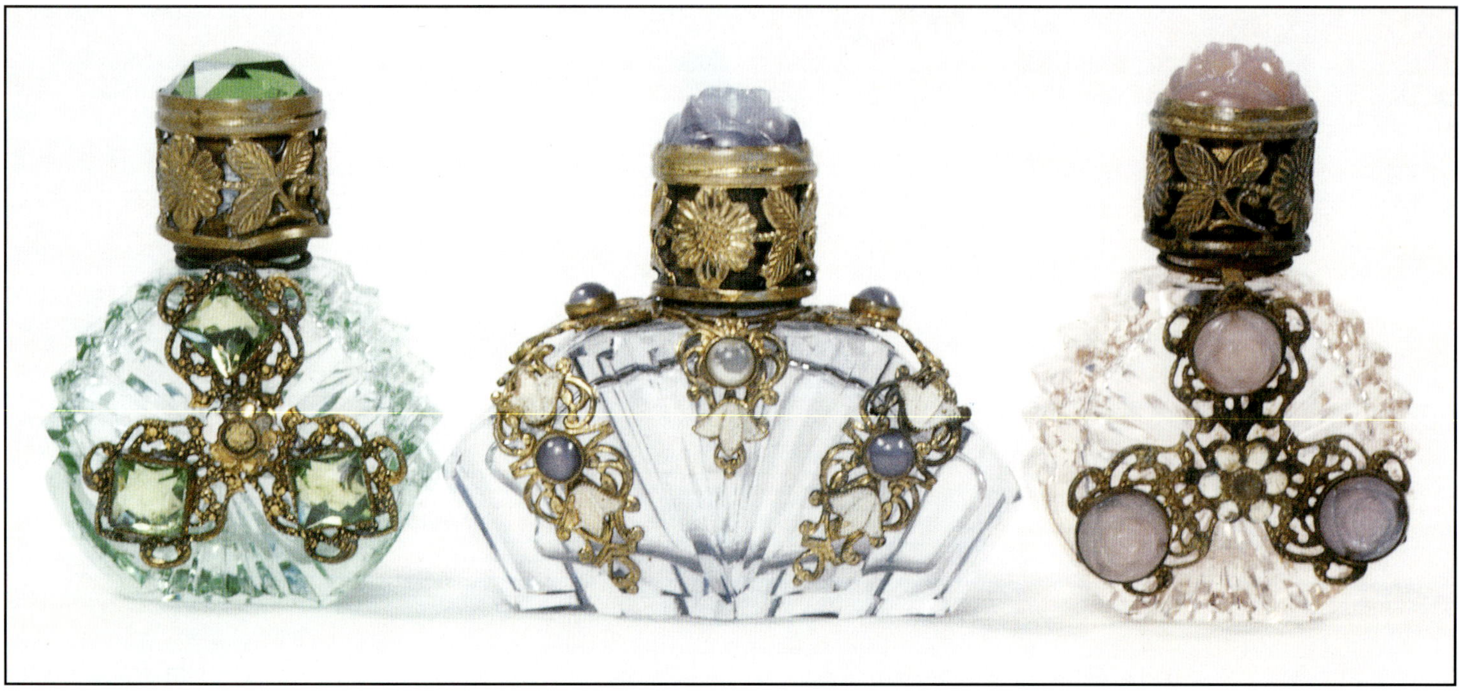

Easter pastels. Left: Green cut glass with green square-cut stones. Acid marked, 2.75". $150-200. Center: Amethyst with pearl, pearlized amethyst cabochons and an amethyst carved rose in the cap. 1.725". $250-300. Right: Round pink cut glass with enamel work and carved pink roses. 1.785". $250-300.

These pictures show the separate stopper/dauber from the left hand bottle in the previous photo, and how it is seated in the bottle. Note: the word "Czechoslovakia" appears on the top metal rim of the opening.

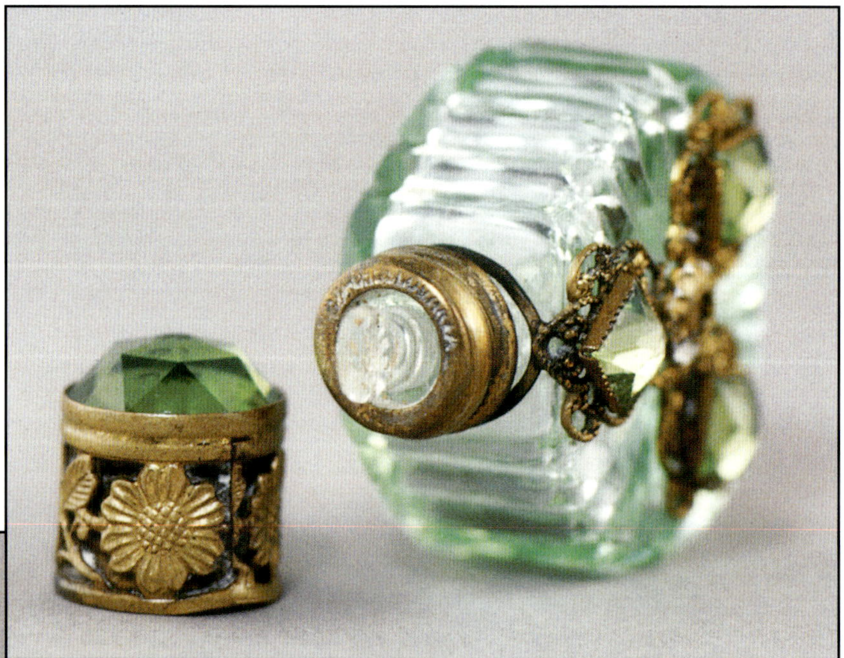

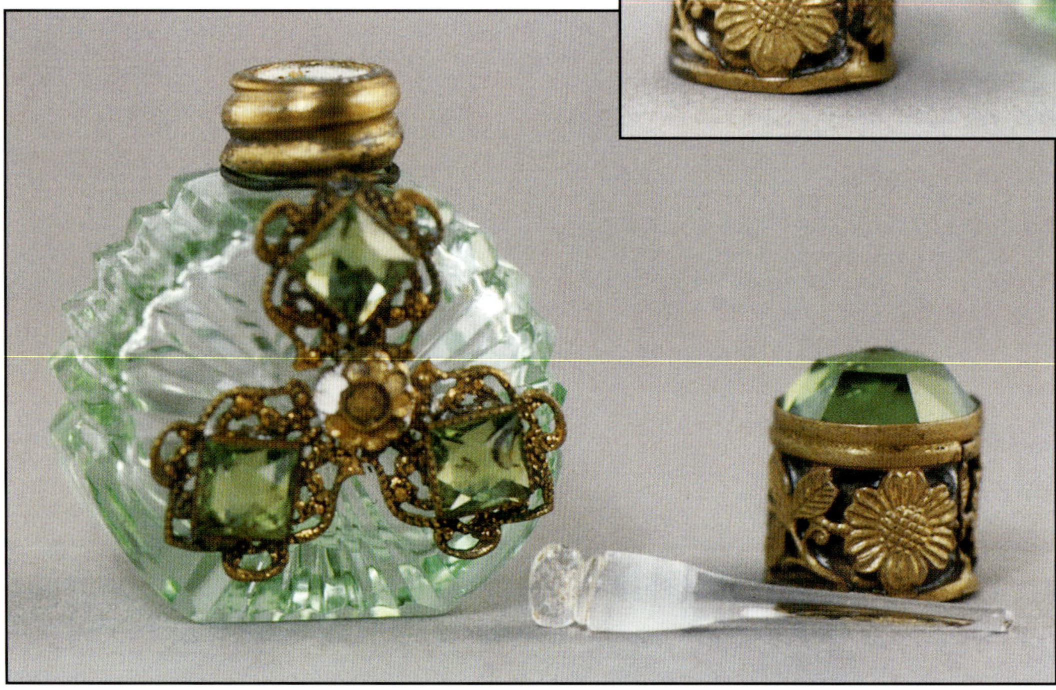

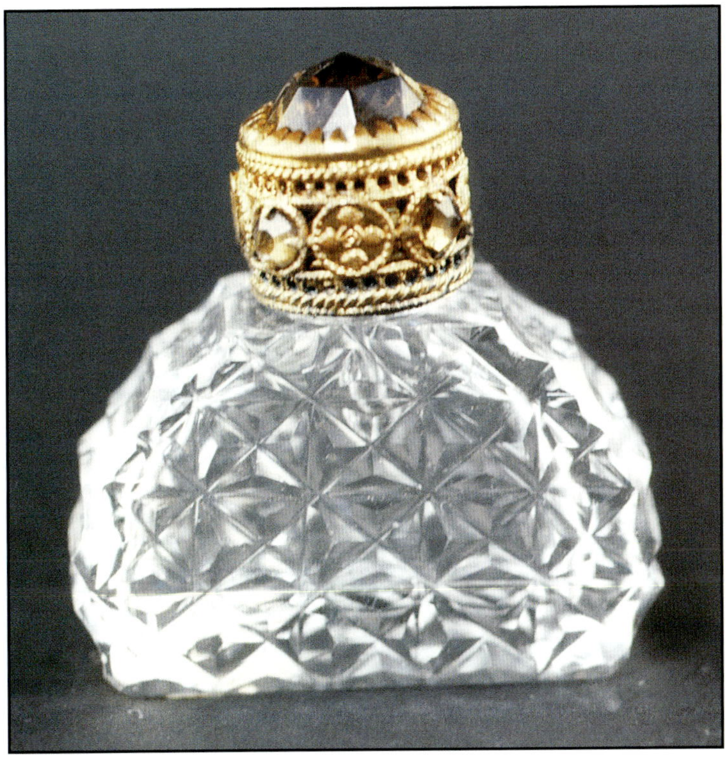

Half circle cut glass bottle with an amber capstone. Acid etched in base as well as a paper label, "Morlee." 1.725". $75-125.

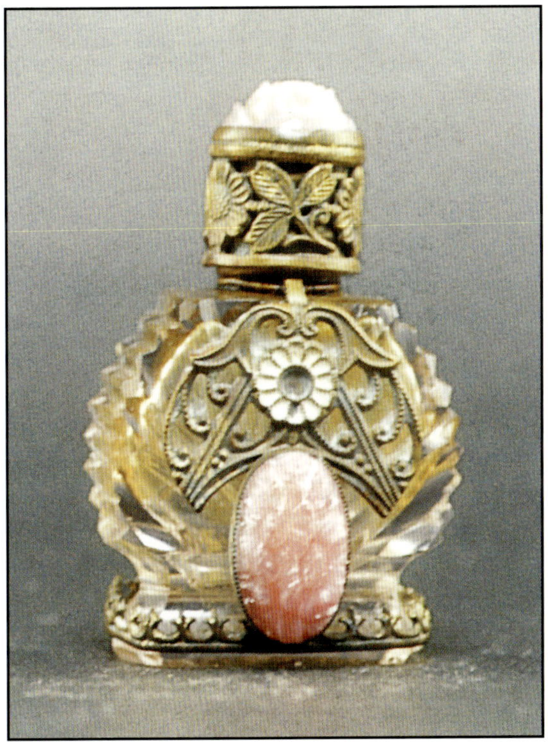

Clear cut glass, caged in filigree with enameled accents and a carved pink glass medallion and carved pink rose capstone. 2". *Courtesy of Earline Kopriva.* $300-350.

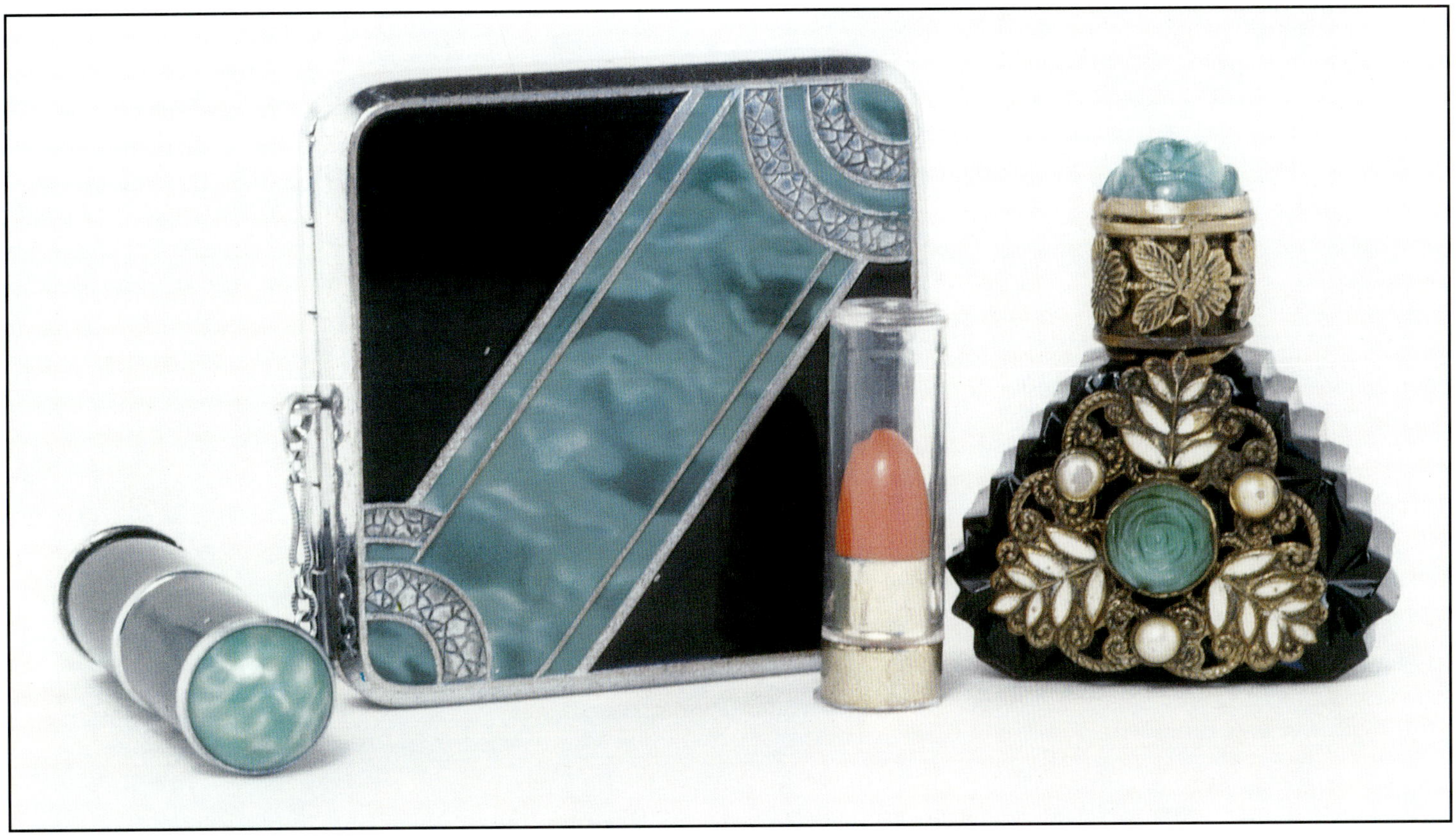

Black cut glass with enamel, filigree, and jade carved roses and pearls. Acid etched. The cap is a stopper cover. 1.875". $200-300. Shown with an art deco Evans vintage compact and chain-attached lipstick holder with its original lipstick filler. $150-200.

It is interesting to see how different finish work makes bottles with essentially the same base appear very different. Adding filigree to the bottom third and accenting with gems makes strangers out of these siblings.

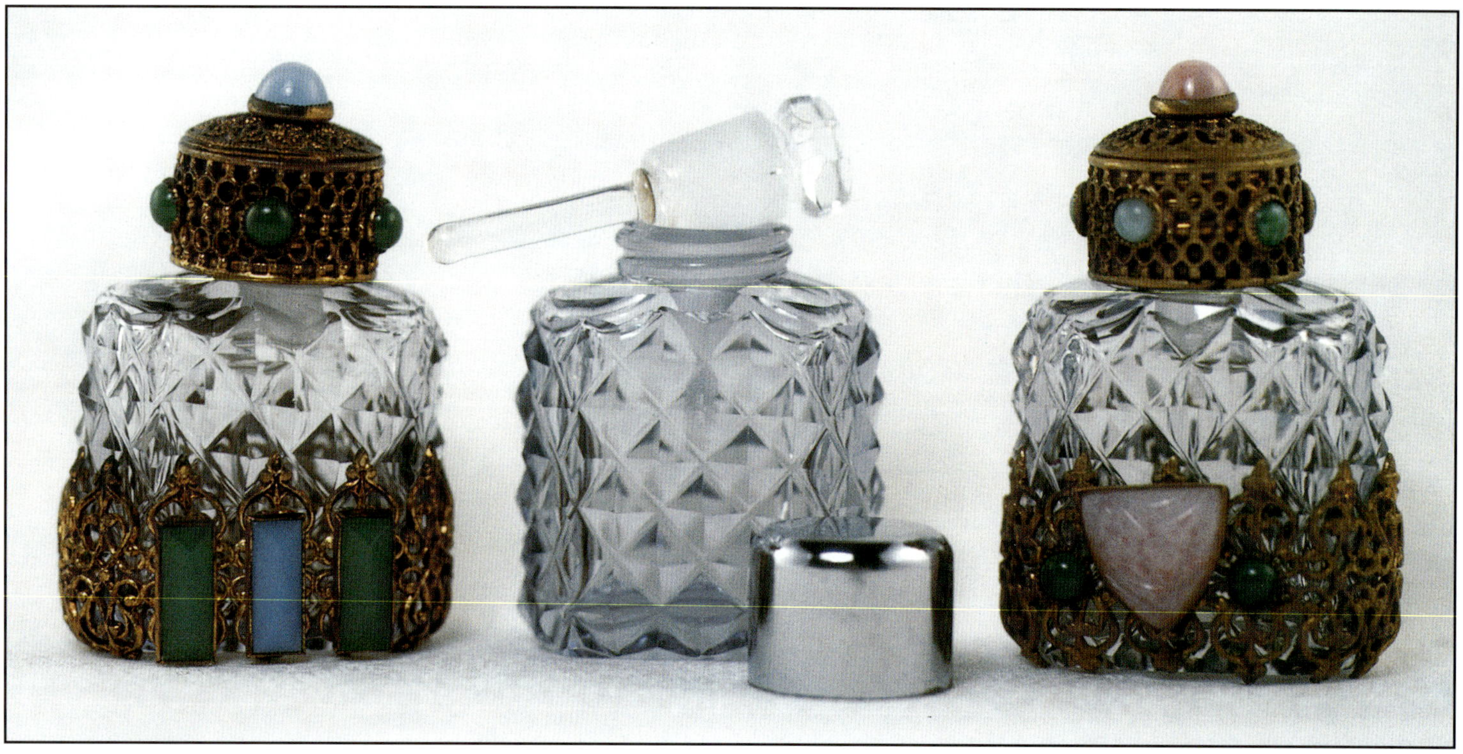

Left: Amethyst cut glass with filigree, green and blue stones. 2". $150-200. Center: Identical base shown with stopper and silver colored cover. $50-100. Right: Same base, but with different gems including a pink glass medallion. 2". $150-200.

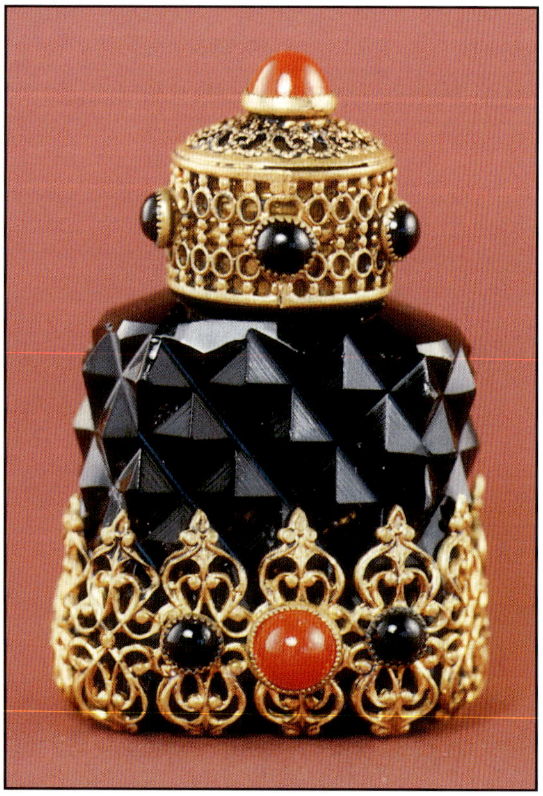

The same base again, in opaque black glass with filigree and red and black cabochons. Acid mark, inner stopper. 2". $250-300.

The photo below is of a cut glass base and dainty filigree bottle with a metal cap. Though this bottle, with its medallion and matching colored capstone, is in the Czech style, the cap is tag-marked "Austria."

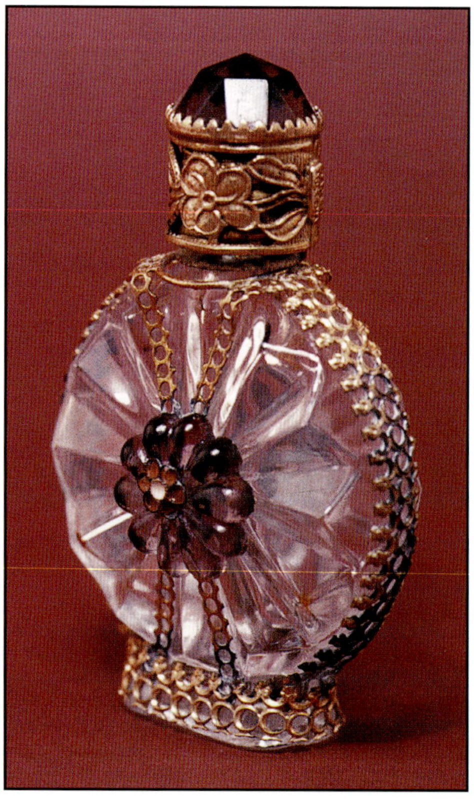

This dainty cut glass filigree purse bottle with amethyst colored accents is marked "Austria" on a tag affixed to the cap. 2.375". $75-125.

Many horn bottles were fitted with glass stoppers, but some were also produced with screw caps. The bottles shown have metal threads. Their "cousins," the tasseled laydowns, were often found in cut-to-clear in several colors similar to the black cut-to-clear pictured. The Vaseline green is more unusual. The marking on both is in the metal. The top piece in each unscrews, revealing a dauber of hard plastic. This hardware and dauber appear on other bottles as shown.

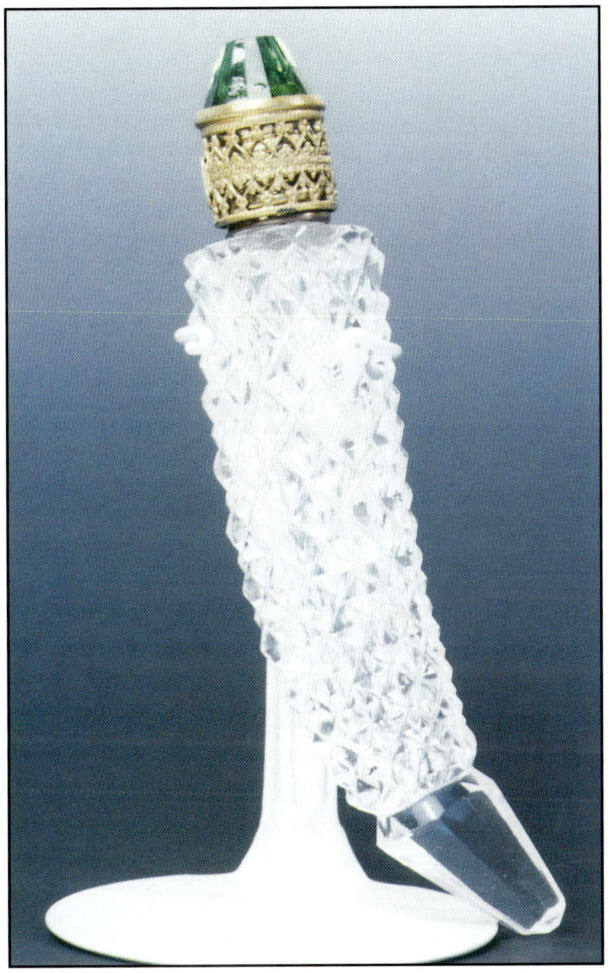

Cut glass laydown horn bottle with screw cap and green capstone. Marked with a tag. 3.5". $200-250.

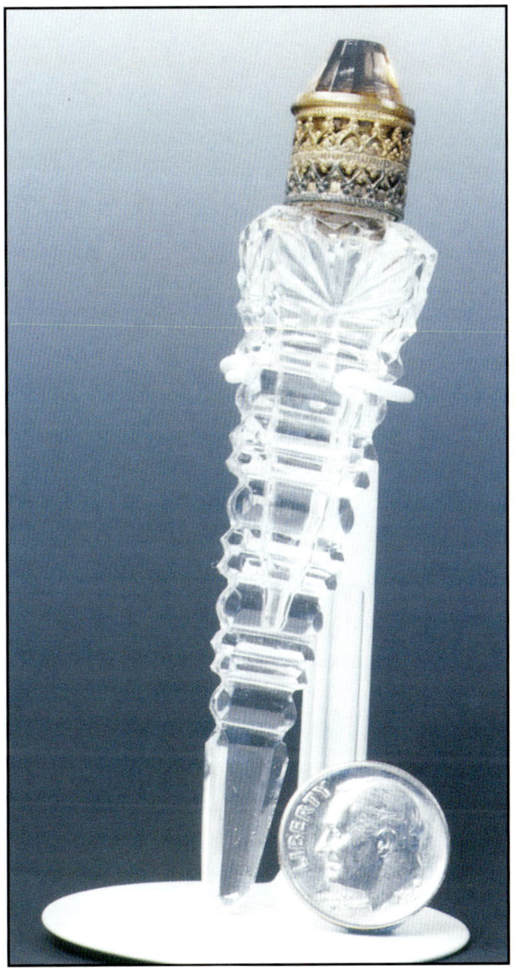

Cut glass laydown with a pink top, marked. 3.75". $200-250.

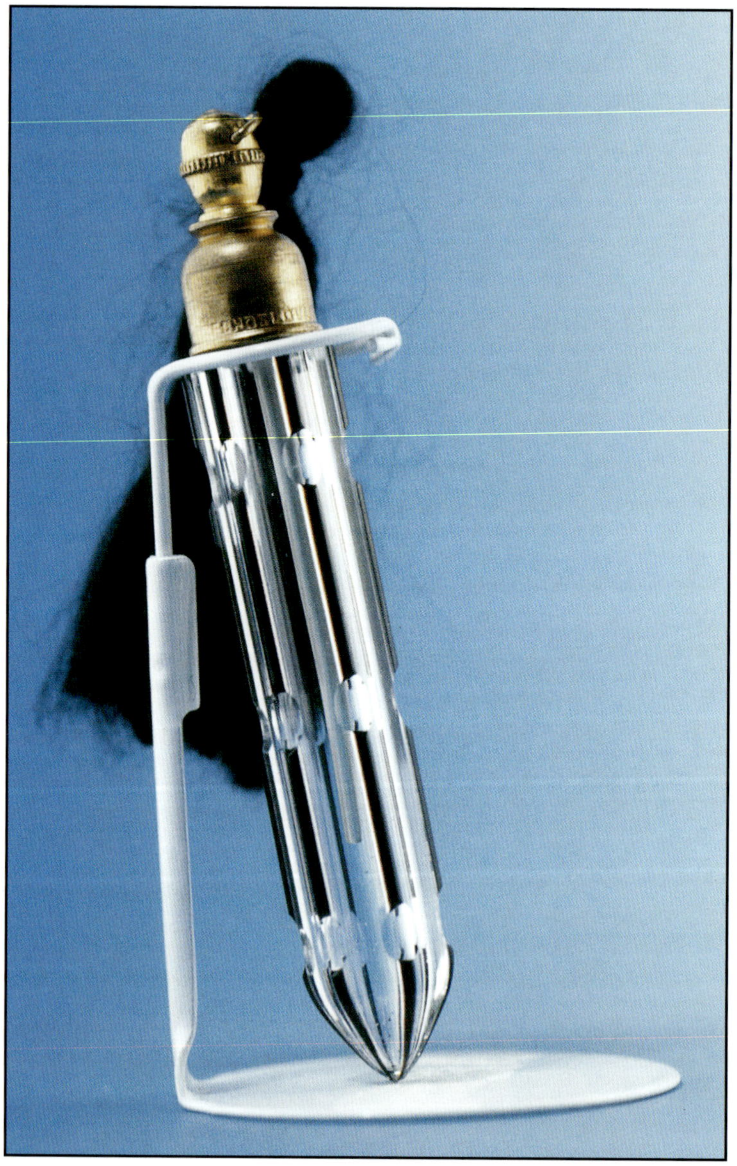

Black cut-to-clear laydown with a tassel. Marked in the metal. 3.5". $150- 200.

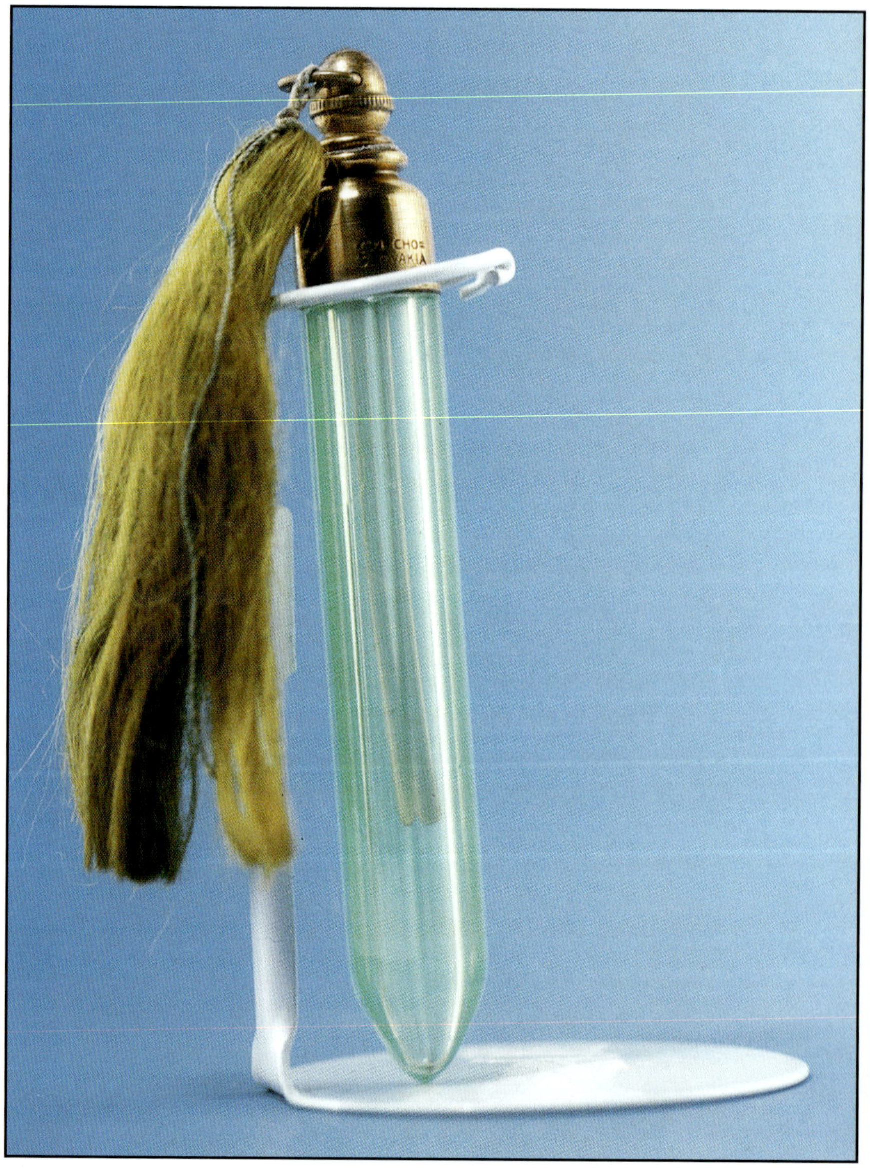

Vaseline glass, six-sided cut, laydown with tassel. 3.25". $150-200.

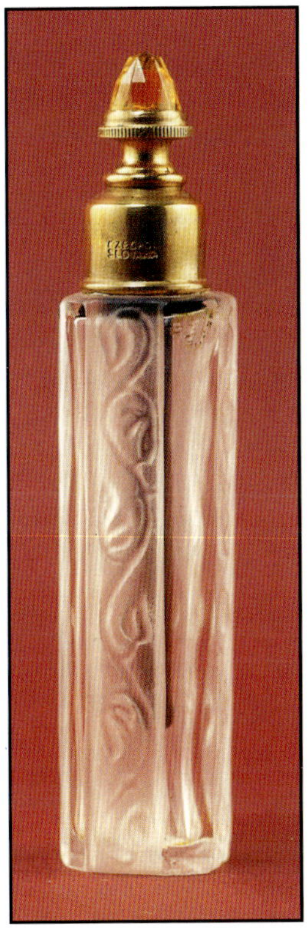

These three bottles share hardware that was probably from the mid-twenties. Each has a hard plastic dauber, which has discolored from time and contact with the perfume. The purple bottle has a subtle, but lovely frosted center motif. 3.5", 3", and 2.875". $125-175 each.

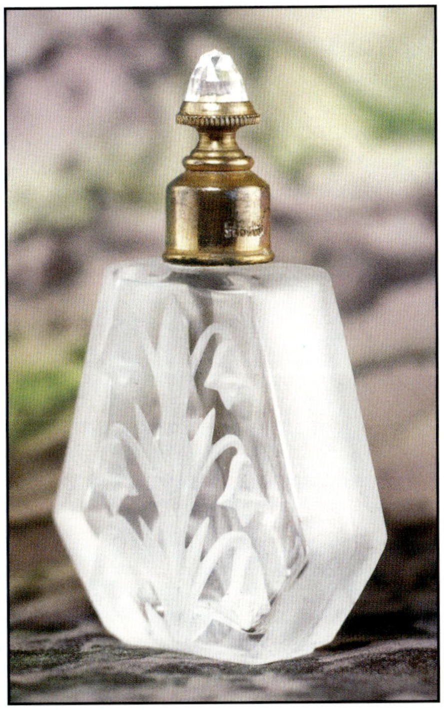

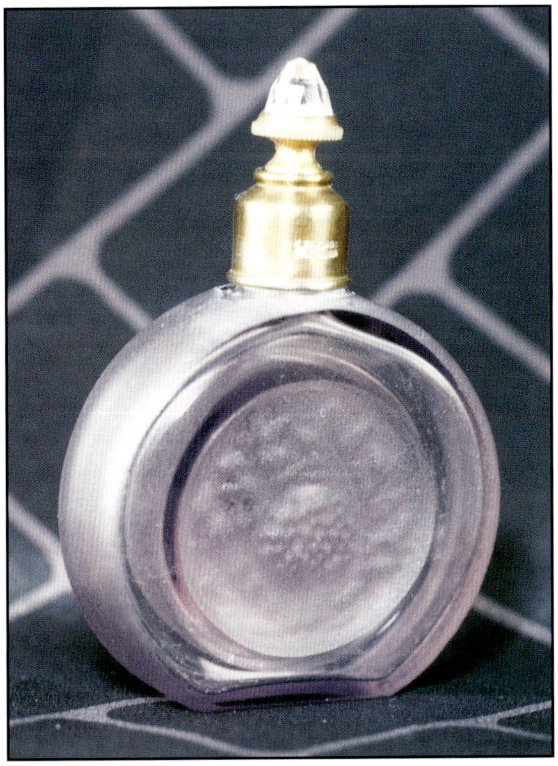

This photo of three laydown bottles shows a cut glass bottle and two mercury glass bottles. Bottles in this style often have a metallic look and a ball-topped dauber that slides into a metal-covered cork surround. Bottles in this style were also made in Germany, in which case, the marking can often be found in the metal lip edge.

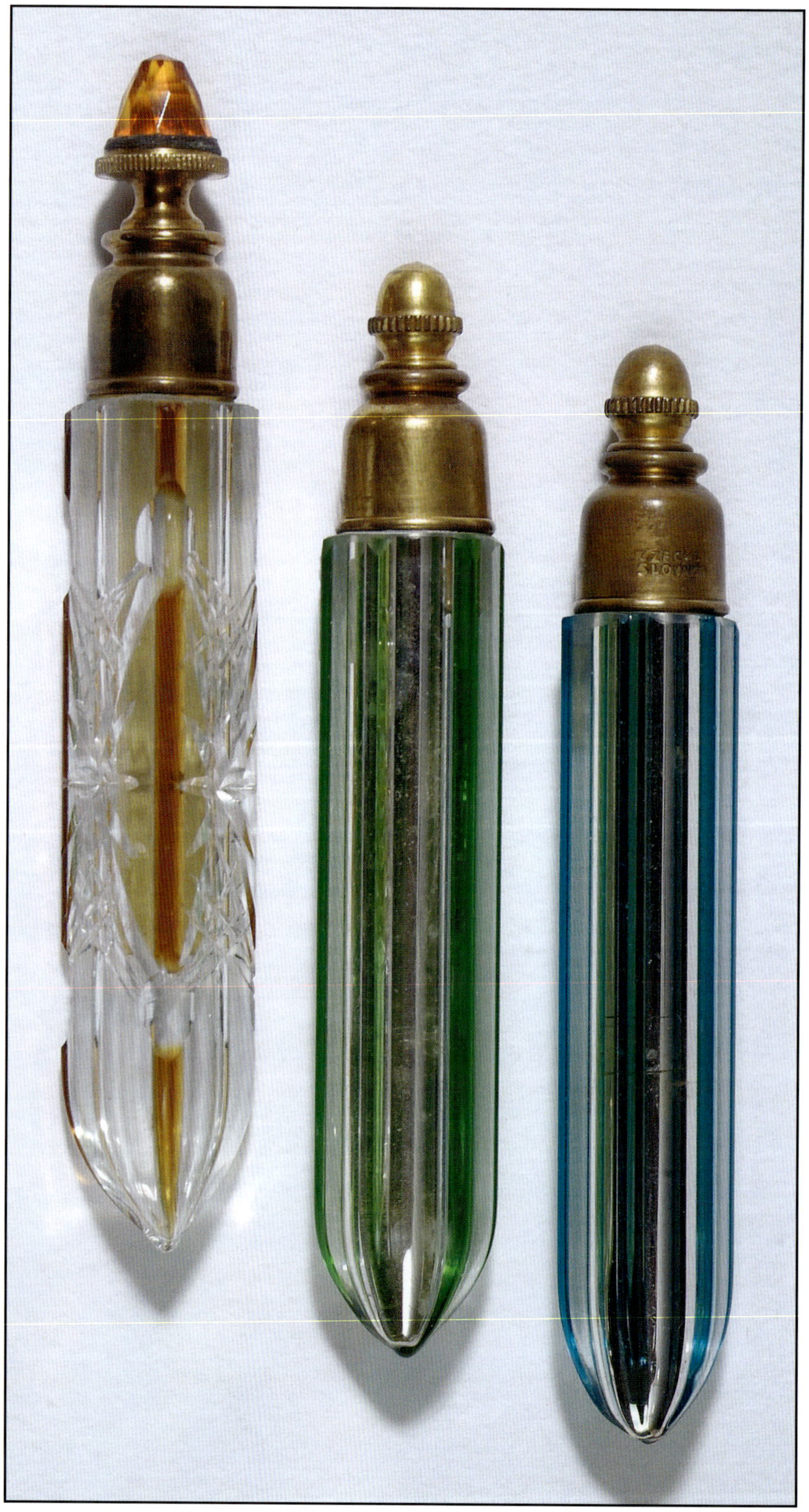

Three laydown bottles. Left: Long triangular shaped clear, cut bottle with amber edges. Cap topped by amber jewel. 3.5". $160. Center: Hexagonal mercury glass bottle with light green edges. 3.25". Right: Hexagonal mercury glass bottle with bright blue edges. 3.25". *Courtesy of Don Orban. Photo by David Kirk of Kirk Photography.* $125.

Ingrid Purse Bottles

The Petr Nový (2002, page 164) and Truitt, V.I. (1995, page 129) references both show pictures of mid-1930s advertising copy of Schlevogt's Ingrid glass product line. Shown among the vanity items is a grouping of several Ingrid purse bottles. The designs are mostly floral: iris, daisy, rose (footed), and chrysanthemum, along with the Oriental snuff bottle style. Nový also shows an elephant purse bottle. The early purse bottles shown have Bakelite tops and a few have filigree metal caps.

The most common production color was opaque green, or malachite glass. Less common, but somewhat available to collectors, were opaque blue (lapis glass) and opaque black. Rare examples can be found in aqua or turquoise. Though Donna Sims, in her article featured in Monson and Baer's *The Beauty of Perfume* ("Czechoslovakian Perfume Bottles: The Stunning Opaques," May, 1996, pp. 95-105) shows classic opaque Schlevogt and Hoffman bottles in fourteen colors and color combinations, the bottles featured are dresser bottles and atomizers, not purse bottles.

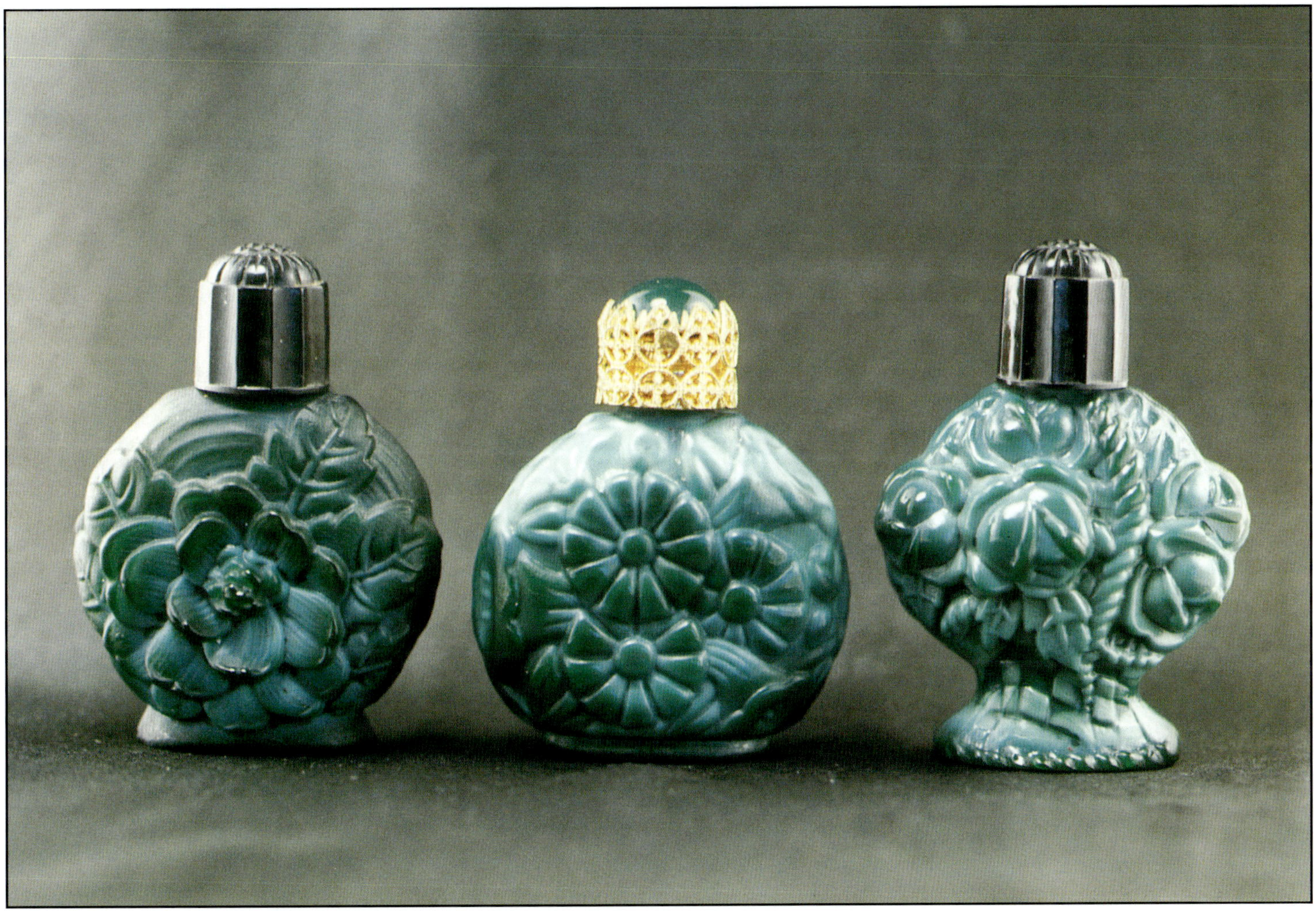

Three malachite glass bottles. Left: Opened rose surrounded by leaves on a footed base. Frosted, but with buffed glass on the petal edges. Black Bakelite cap, late 1930s. Unmarked. 2.25". $250-300. Center: Daisy design. This bottle is marked on the back (Ingrid) and on the base (Czechoslovakia) with paper labels. Possibly 1950s production. Reduced sized opening, no dauber. 2.125". $100-150. Right: Basket of cabbage roses; the handle reaches up one side and down the other. Black Bakelite cap, late 1930s. Unmarked. 2.25". $250-300.

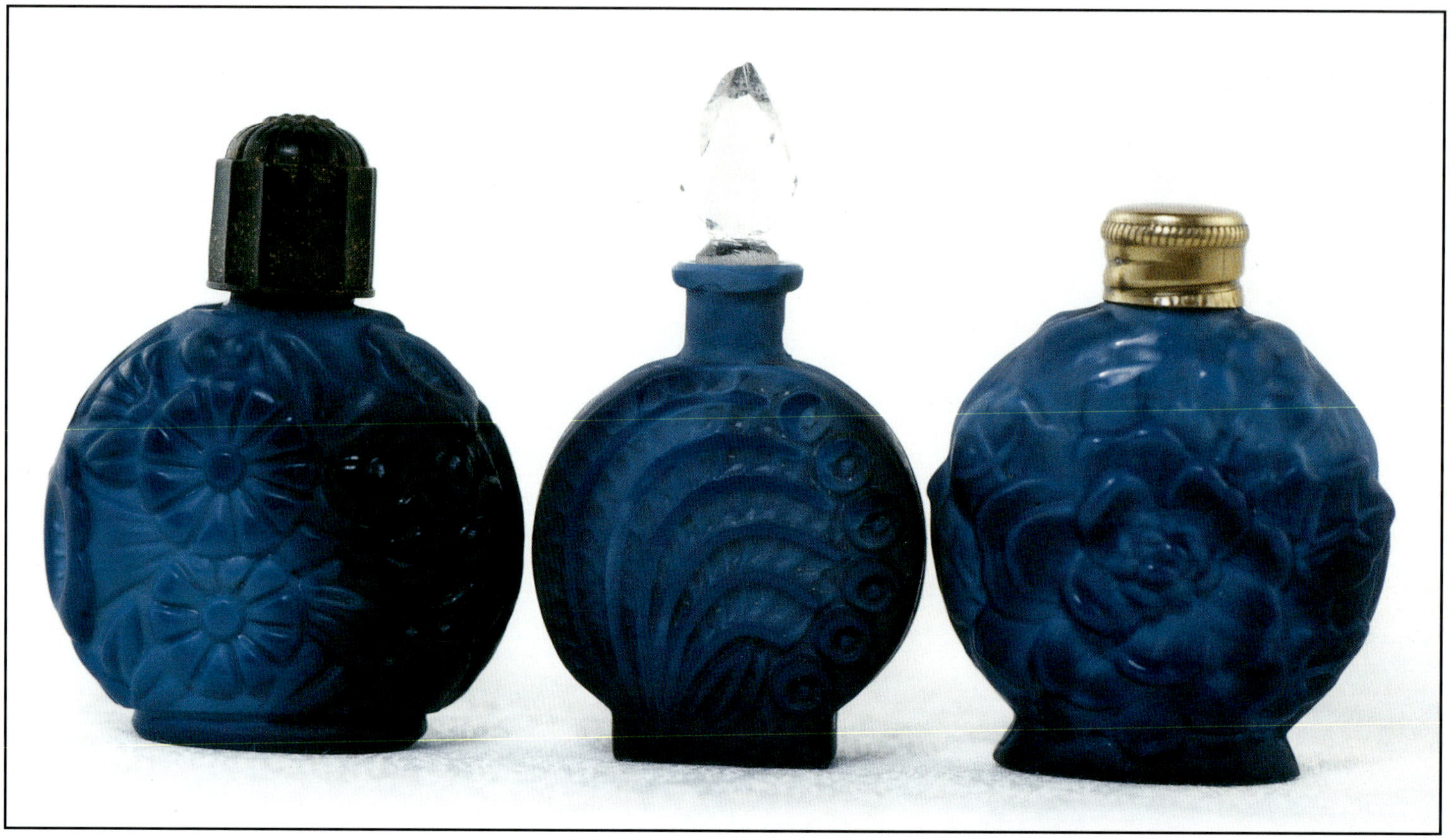

Three lapis glass bottles. Left: Daisy design with a Bakelite cap, late 1930s. 2.125". $250-300. Center: Art deco arrangement of flowers; stem and flower outlines are polished to contrast with the frosted background. Actually a dresser bottle, the stopper shown is not original. 2.5". As shown, $100-150. Right: A blue version of the opened rose design. This bottle has a plain cap and a reduced sized dome opening with no dauber. 2". $200-300.

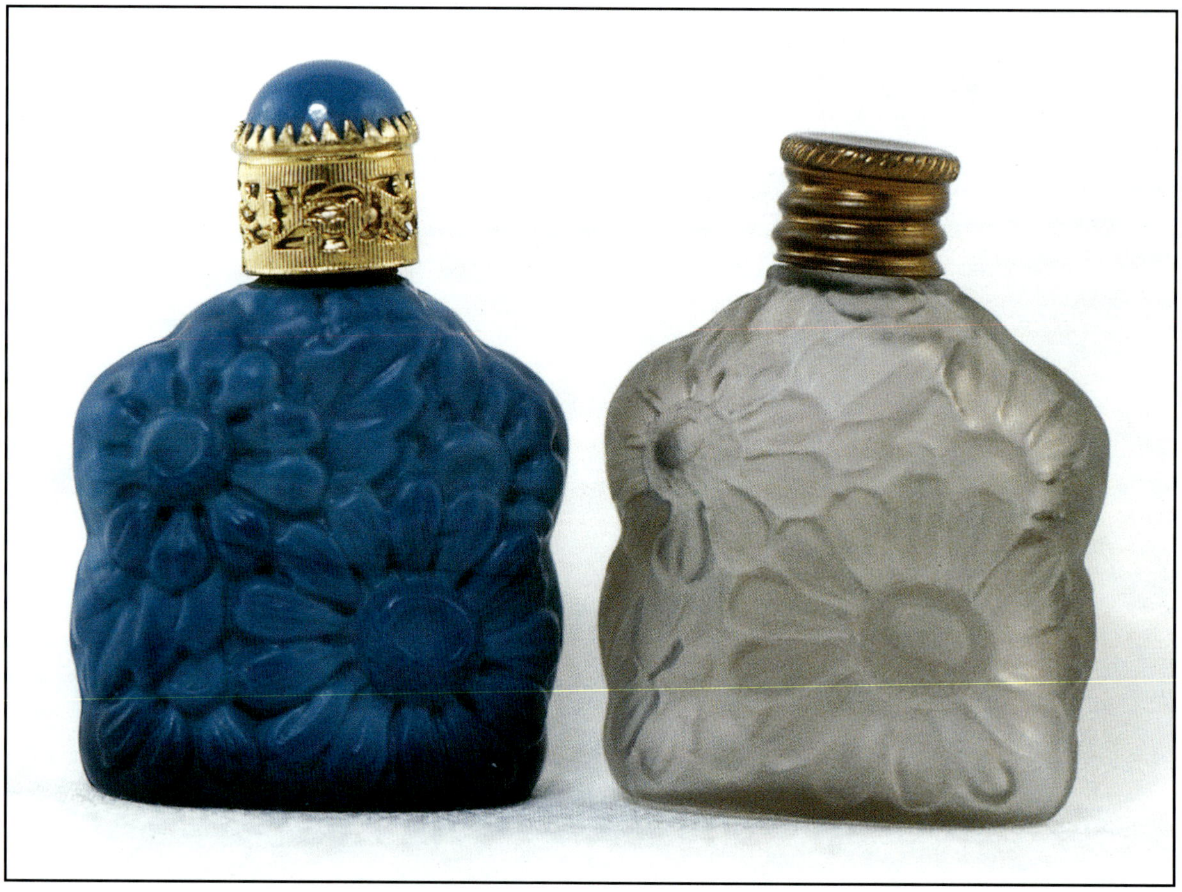

Chrysanthemums. Left: Lapis bottle with opaque blue capstone. This bottle has a metal neck fitting and a dauber. Unmarked. Late 1930s. 2.375". $250-300. Right: Smoky frosted, satin-finished bottle with plain cap. 2". $75-125.

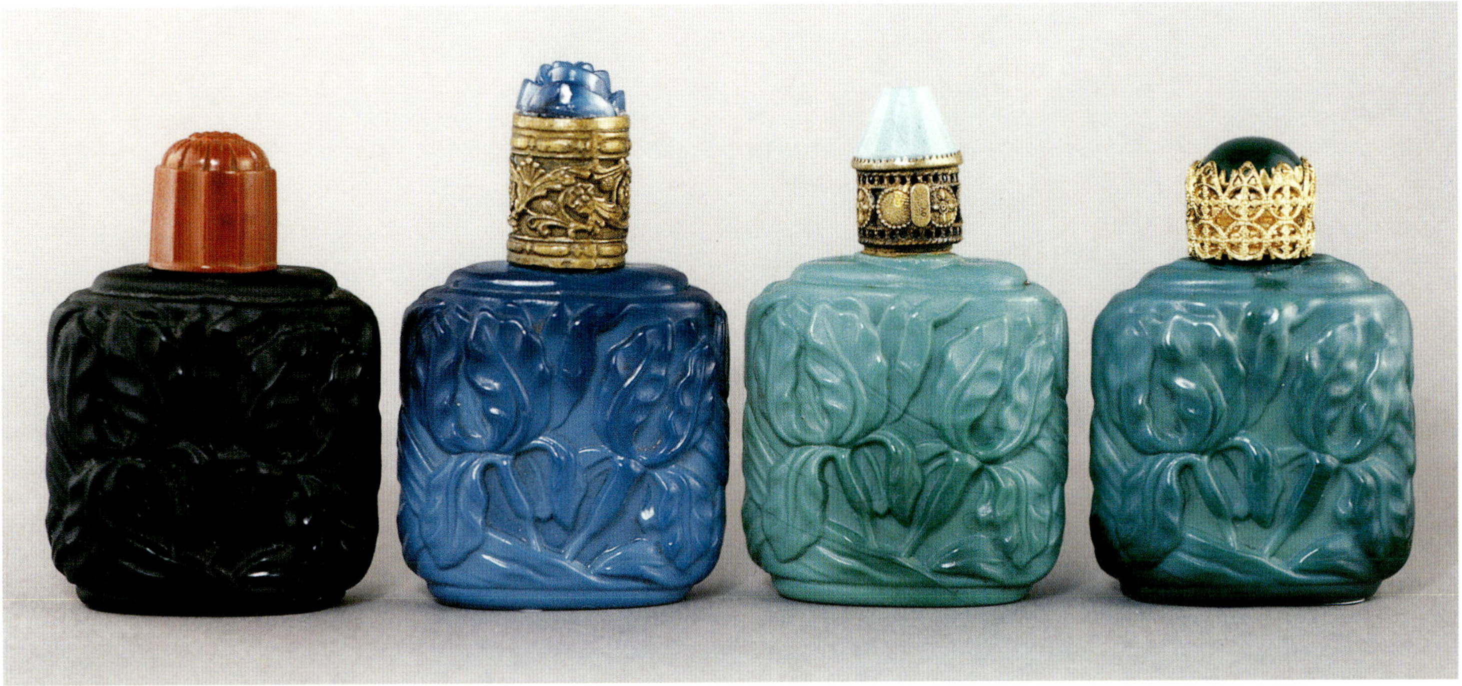

Four Iris bottles. From left: Black iris with a red Bakelite cap, acid marked "Ingrid Czechoslovakia" in the base. 2.25". $300-350. Lapis iris, also acid marked. This bottle has a metal covered opening, which is also marked on the lip. Note the elaborate, elongated cap with the lapis carved rose. 2.725". $300-400. Jade green iris bottle with metal neck fitting and metal tag on the cap. The cap may have originally had stones. 2.5". $300-400. Malachite Iris bottle. This bottle is marked with paper labels, probably 1950s. It has a small domed opening and no dauber. 2.25". $100-150.

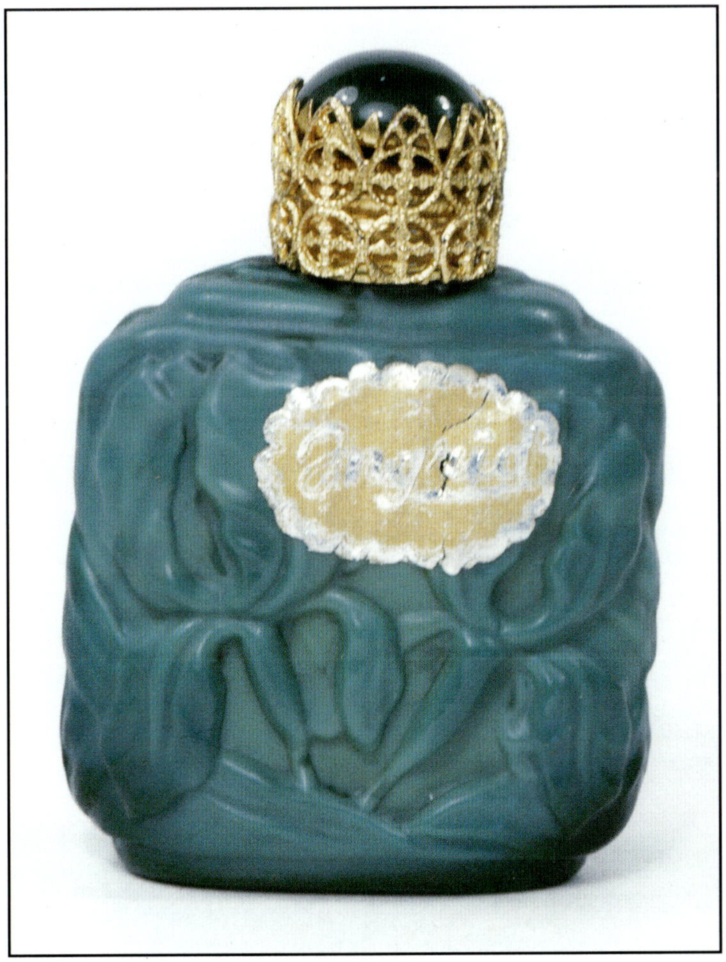

Back view of the malachite iris bottle, showing the Ingrid paper label.

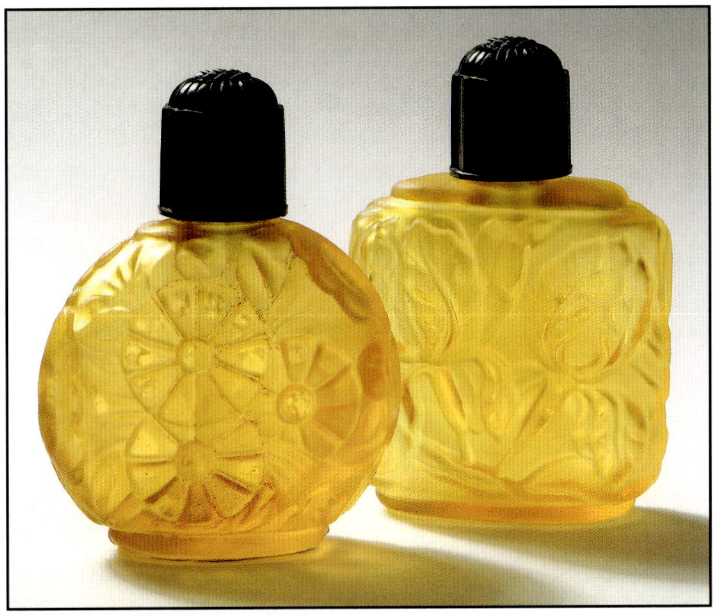

Ingrid purse bottles in frosted amber glass. Circular bottle on left has molded daisies and trumpet shaped flowers. Ingrid label on bottom. 2.125". Right hand bottle has molded iris blossoms. 2.25". Both bottles have black Bakelite caps with glass daubers. *Courtesy of Don Orban. Photo by David Kirk of Kirk Photography.* $125 each.

Indicators of earlier bottles (mid to late '30s) include an acid mark in the base, "Ingrid" in script and "Czechoslovakia," Bakelite caps of either black or red, and caps that are marked with a metal tag. Some bottles had plain metal (unmarked) caps and are also thought to be an earlier production as are any of the lapis purse bottles. Some bottles with metal-over-glass openings have the word "Czechoslovakia" printed in the lip.

It is tempting to attribute all opaque purse bottles to Schlevogt's Ingrid line, however, the white bottle pictured here is an unusual glazed ceramic composition. It is marked with red ink in the base. The pink bottle on the right is more likely an Ingrid, as it has the characteristic Bakelite top and the acid mark in the base is formed in an outline similar to other Ingrid bottles.

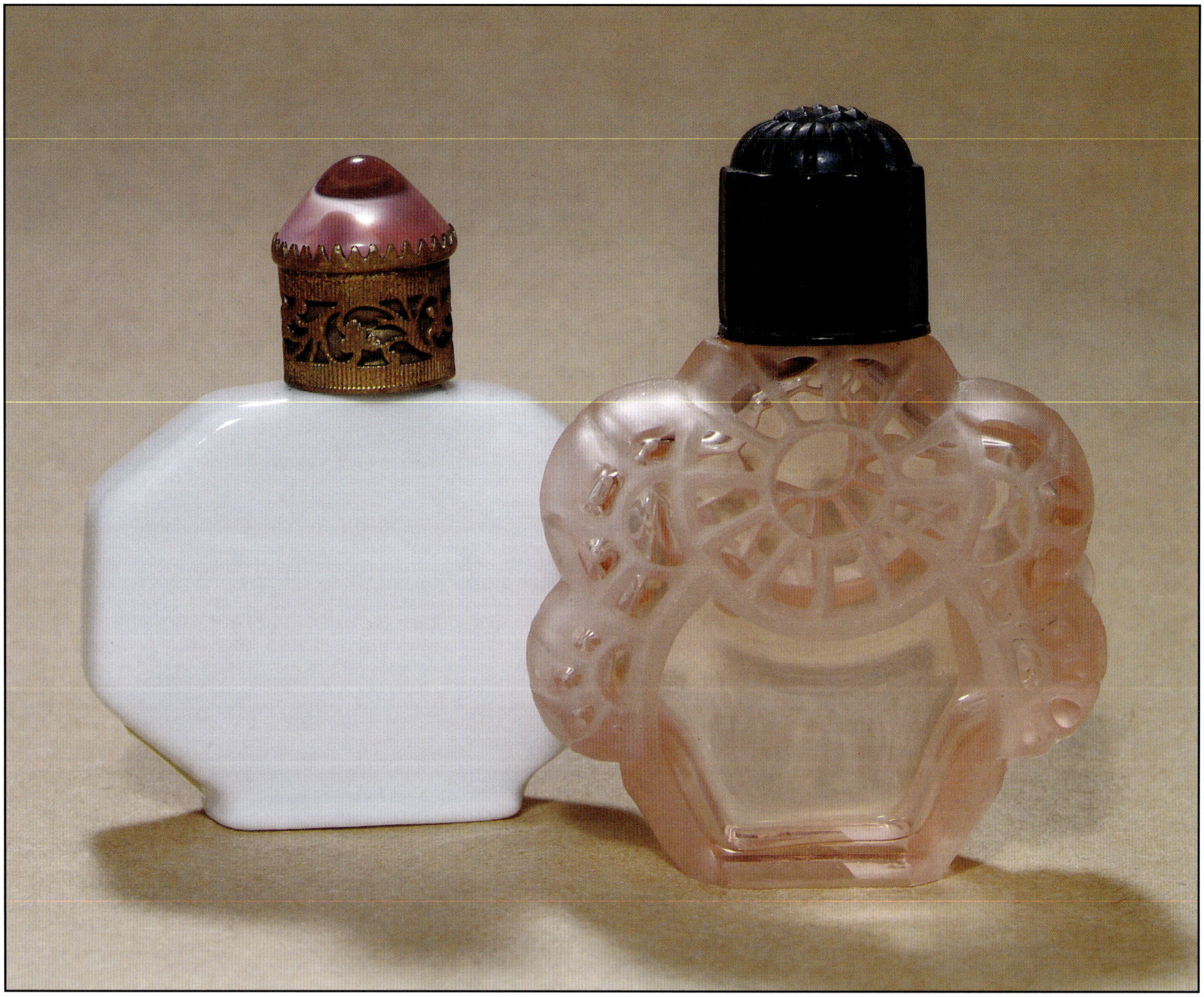

Left: White ceramic purse bottle with gold filigree screw cap topped by domed opalescent pink jewel. 1.875". Right: Clear and frosted pink glass purse bottle shaped like Deco flower basket with black Bakelite cap. 2.125".*Courtesy of Don Orban. Photo by David Kirk of Kirk Photography.* $125.

Jones-North includes in her book (1999, p. 86), advertising copy that includes Ingrid designs produced in the 1950s. The pictured grouping features all the bottles shown in Truitt and four additional designs. These all have metal caps and, according to the author, only appeared in opaque green glass. These bottles were identified with paper labels.

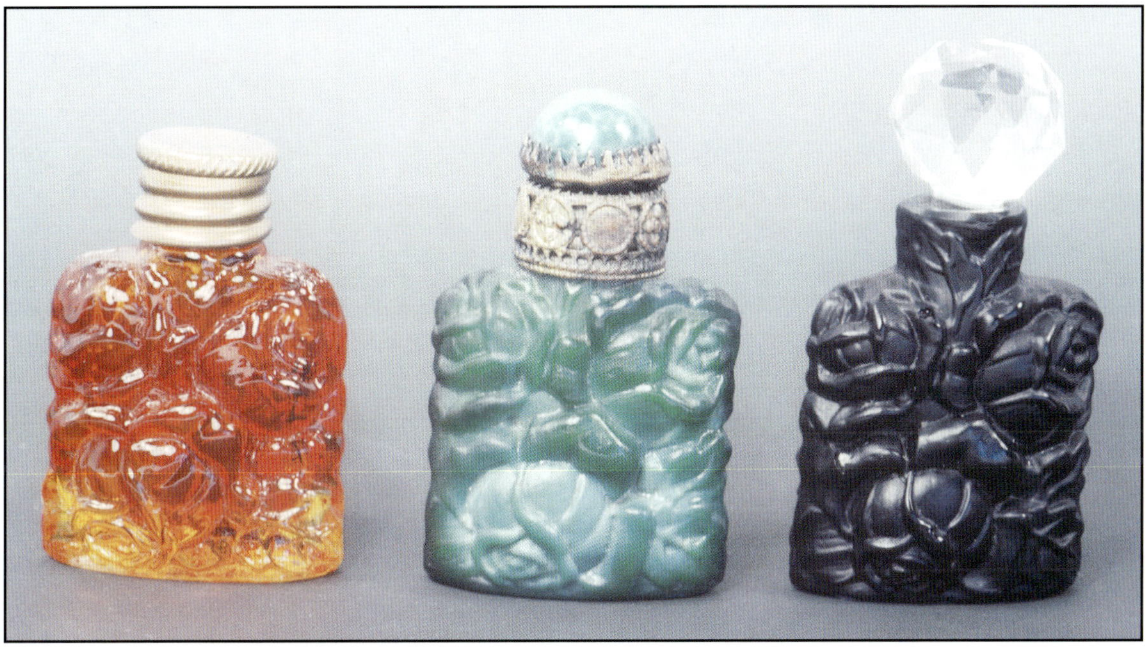

Three different cabbage rose treatments from the same mold. Left: Amberina, yellow to orange, with a plain cap. 2.725". Value unknown. Center: Malachite glass, with a metal neck fitting. The cap is damaged, dauber missing, unmarked. $100-125. Right: A dresser bottle with a stopper rather than a cap, this opaque black bottle is acid marked. Purchased without a stopper. 2.375". $100-150.

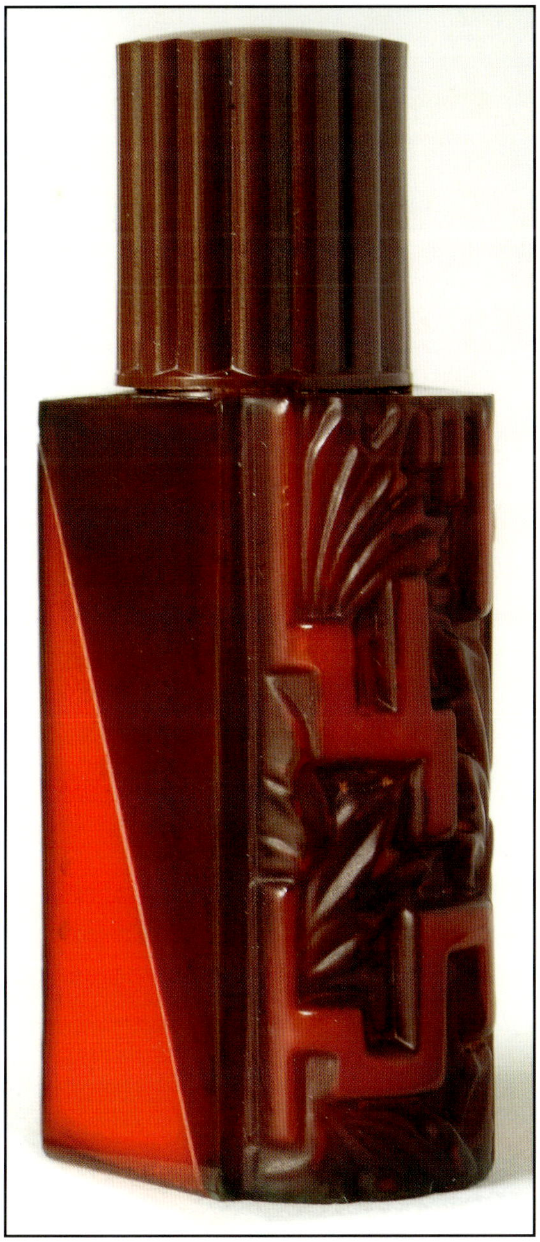

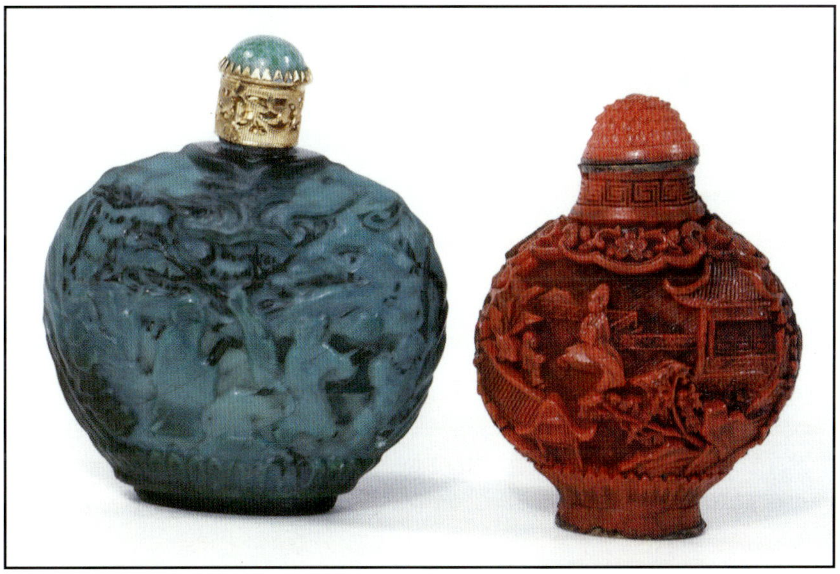

Malachite bottle with an oriental theme. Paper label in the base. 2.875". $100-150. Shown with an Oriental cinnabar snuff bottle. $50.

Extremely rare two-tone purse bottle in dark cinnabar and cherry red opaque glass. Oriental inspired design on end panels. Cinnabar colored Bakelite cap with glass dauber. 2.375". *Courtesy of Don Orban. Photo by David Kirk of Kirk Photography.* $400-450.

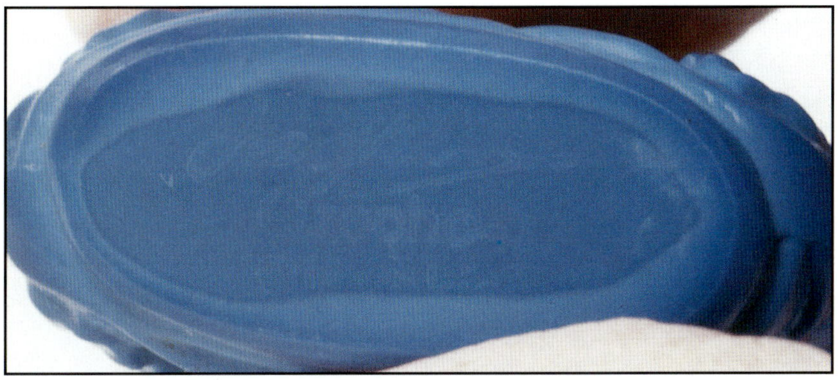

Although it is difficult to see, the acid mark from the base of the lapis iris bottle is shown in this picture.

The classic Ingrid purse bottle styles, however, re-appeared in the 1990s in clear and colored frosted bottles. They have a variety of modern styled caps and sell for about $10.

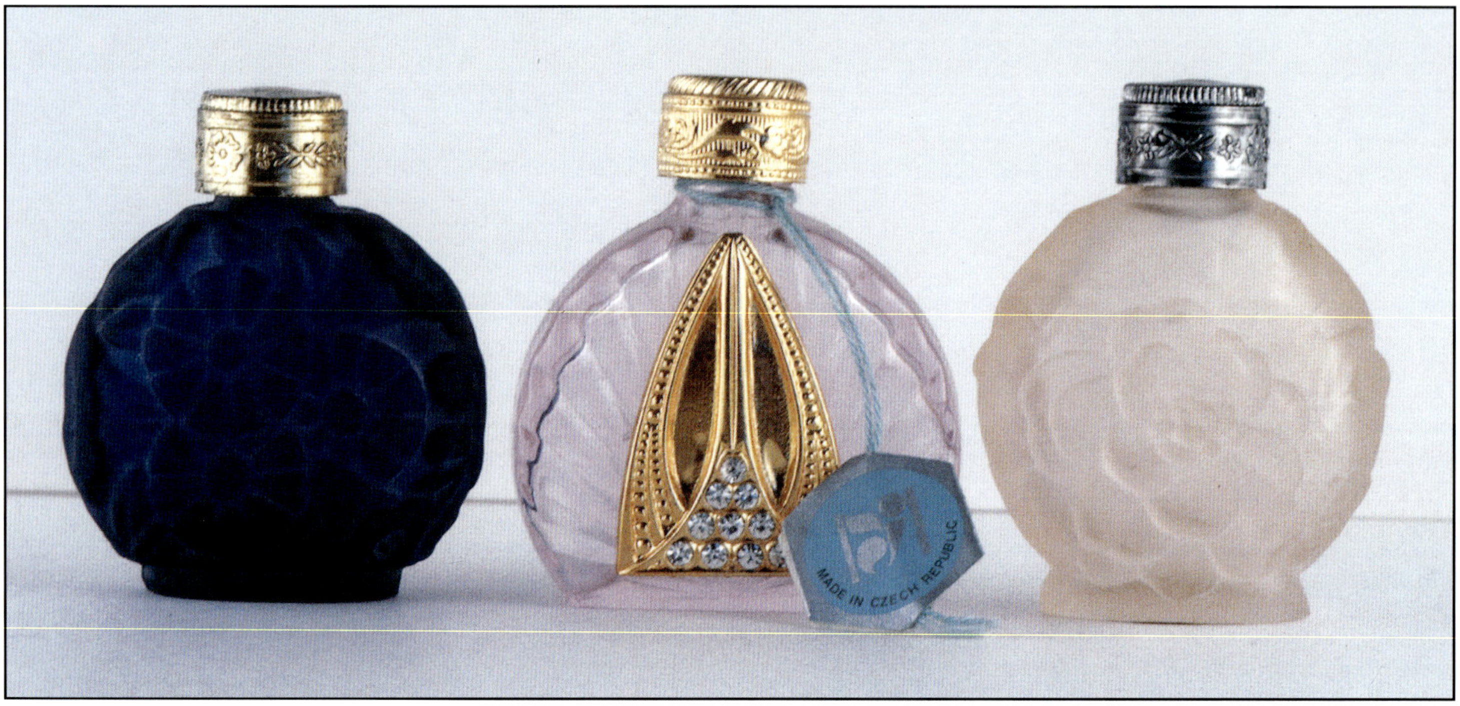

Left and right: modern productions from Ingrid molds. These bottles are marked with paper labels reading, "HAND MADE GLASS BOHEMIA CZECH REPUBLIC"; they were purchased in 2001 for less than $10 each. Center: purse bottle from Czech Republic, 1990s.

Caged Purse Bottles

Surrounded by "silver" or "gold," tombac or brass filigree and adorned in the manner of the colorful costume jewelry that was also produced by Bohemian cottage workers of the time, these press-molded, small glass scent bottles were consistently popular. Exporters set the style, production standards, and the laborers' pay, then merchandized the bottles to an eager market, with thirty percent or more going to the United States.

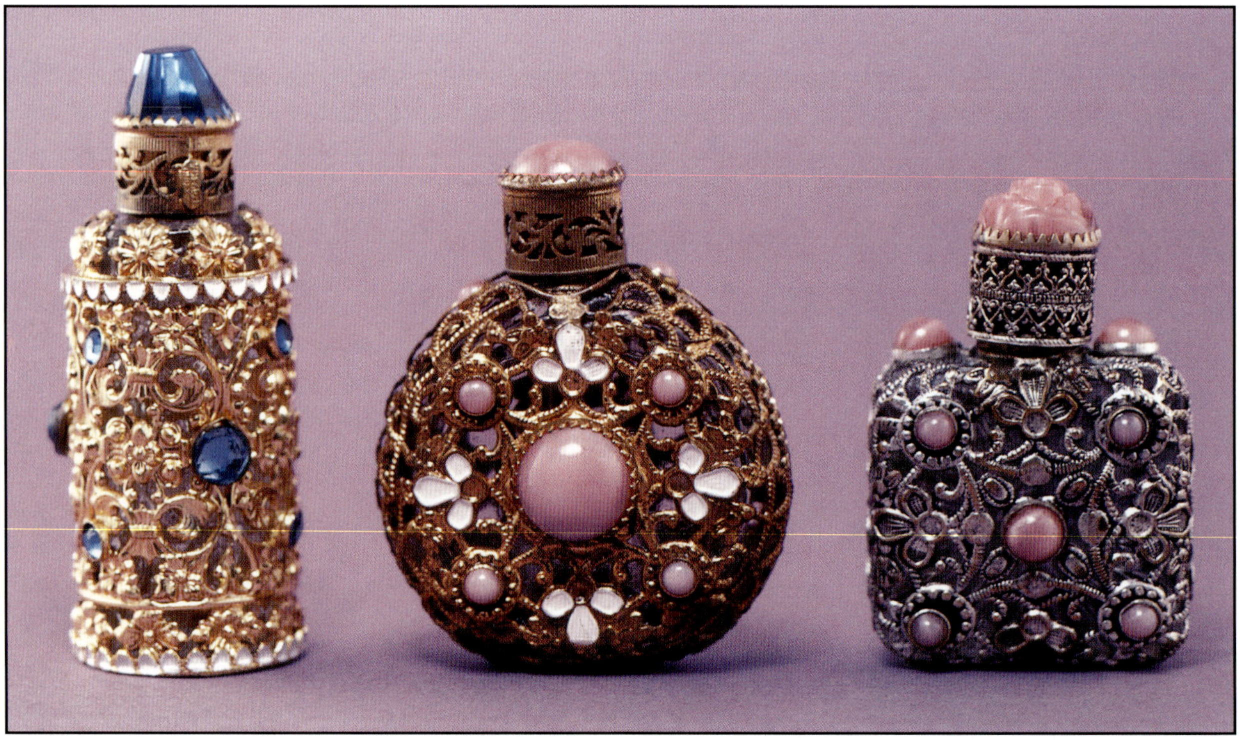

Caged purse bottles in three colors of metal. Left: in gold, a "lipstick" bottle with blue faceted stones. 2.5". $125-175. Center: Pink stone with enameling in copper color. 2.125". $150-200. Right: Unusual silver colored caging. 2" $150-200. Note that the stamped pattern in the metal is the same on the center and right bottles. This is a frequently used pattern.

The bottles embody the work of many northern Bohemian skilled craftsmen and women: the glass makers, producers of the metal fittings, and the finish workers, who added "gems" and final embellishments. The glass blanks were produced from the furnaces of the glasshouses to fill orders for the exporters, who hired refiners for the various decorative processes. Metal formers, called gürtlers, used molds to press and shape base metal. They produced a multitude of elements used in the manufacturing of costume jewelry, buttons, and chandelier fittings, as well as creating the thin, decorative caging components for the scent bottles. The metal filigree for the purse bottles is similar to the foundation pieces of a necklace pendant, dress clip, or brooch.

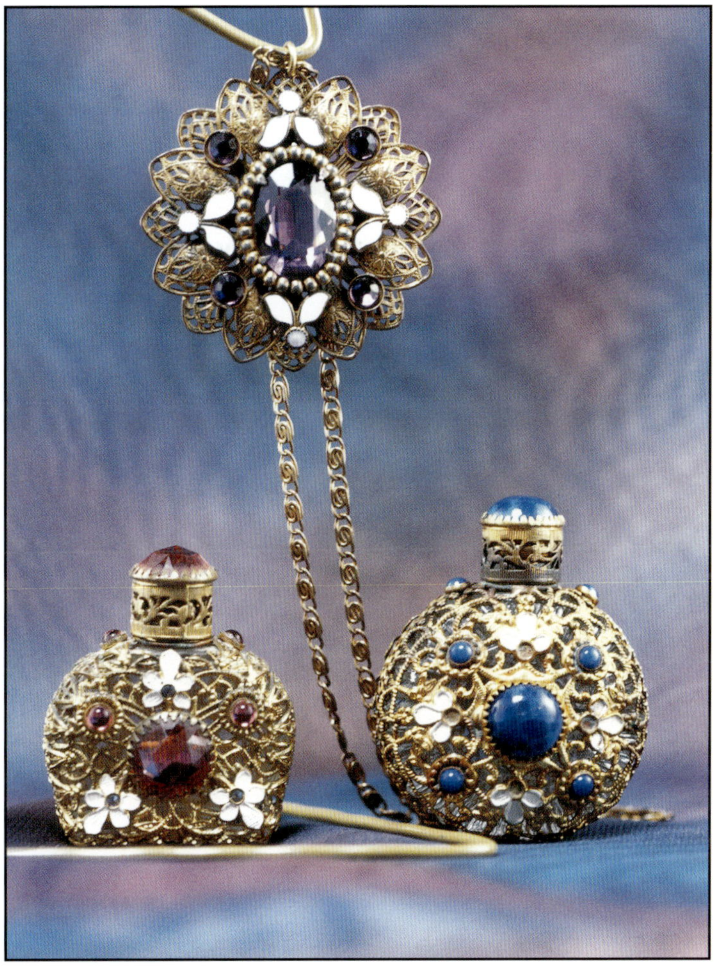

Shows the similarity of workmanship in a pendant necklace and caged purse bottles. All three have white enamel accents and faceted glass stones set in. Details of these bottles follow.

The bottles are finished or refined in similar fashion. Though the vast majority of caged purse bottles have a rough blank as a base, a few were cut and polished prior to being fitted with metal work.

Refiners, many of whom worked out of their homes, finished the scent bottles by forming and fixing the filigree, enameling and detailing the metal, and setting the stones. Careful examination and comparison of bottles shows repeated and clever use of some of the same stock components to cover and finish a variety of bottles of different sizes and shapes.

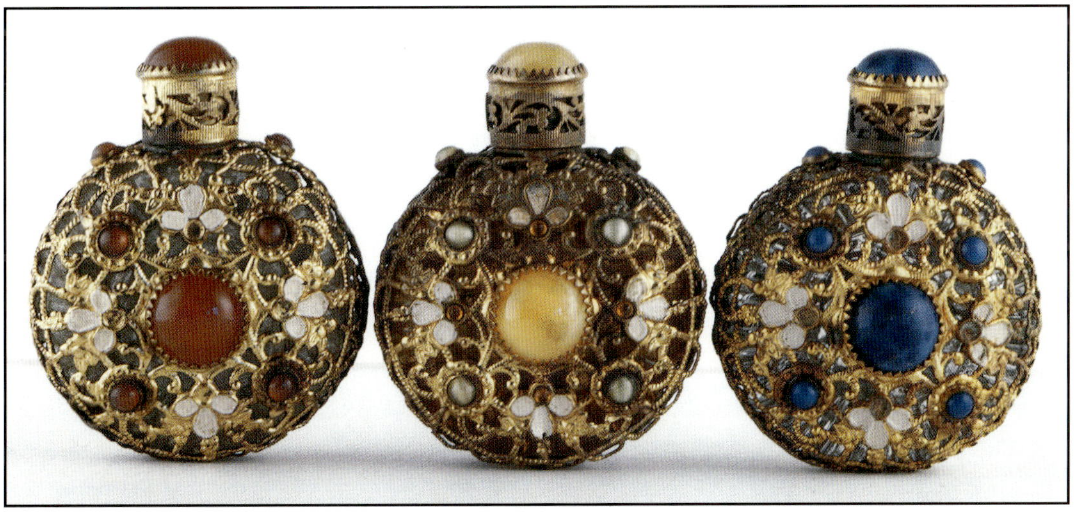

Front view of three laydown bottles. Left: Carnelian colored stones. Center: Yellow "moonstone." Right: Lapis, variegated. All are 2.25", $150-200.

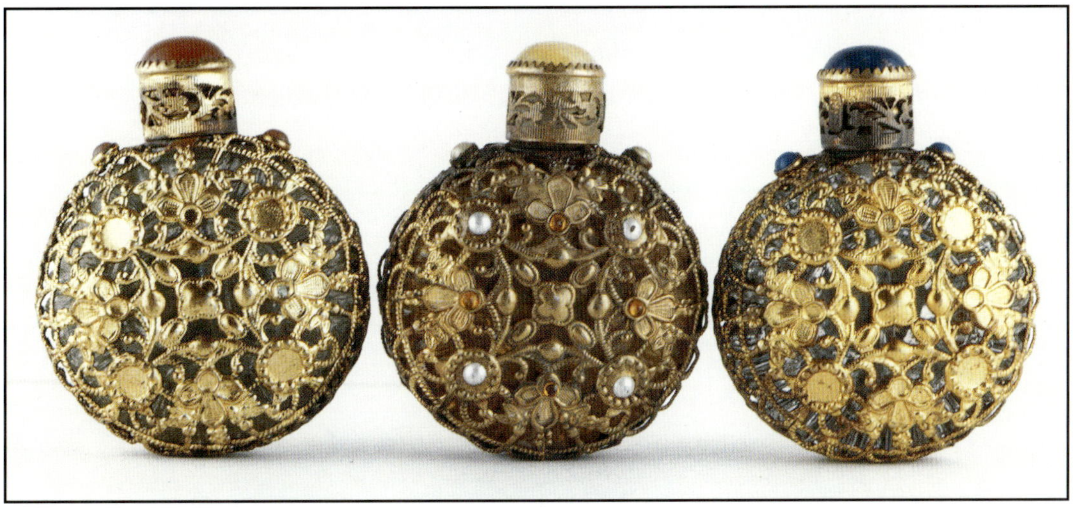

Back view. Note that the center bottle has yellow brilliants set in the back, as well as in the center of the enameled leaves in the front. This probably indicates an earlier bottle.

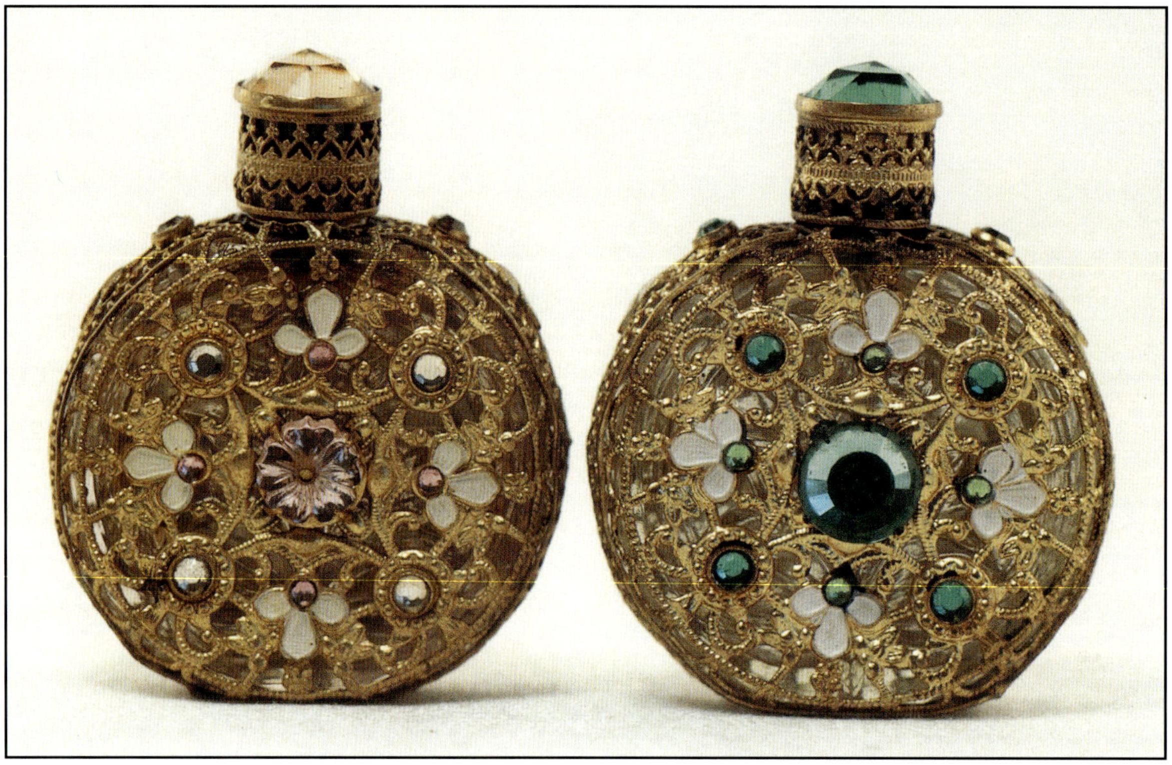

Front view of two additional bottles. These use the same stamped plates front and back as the preceding set. Both are 2.375", $150-200.

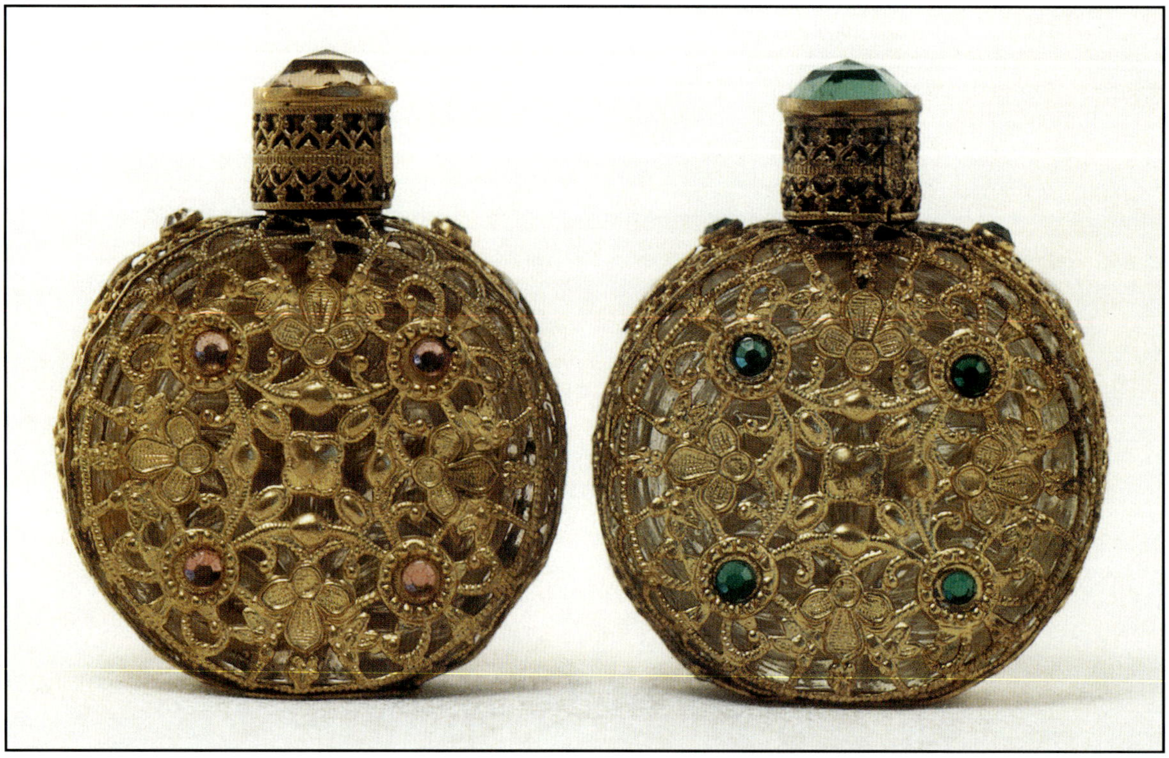

Back view. Shown in the Premier ad in Jones-North (1999, p. 112), these are dated at 1937. Stones are prong and bezel set, with some stones in the back.

It is interesting to note the different methods for placing and fixing the filigree on the various bottles. For many bottles, separate, identical circular "medallions" or plates of delicate filigree are placed to cover the front and the back and are anchored to a ring at the neck of the bottle. A strip of mesh-like metal filigree encircles the sides and base, connects to the front and back pieces at contact points, and anchors to the neck ring.

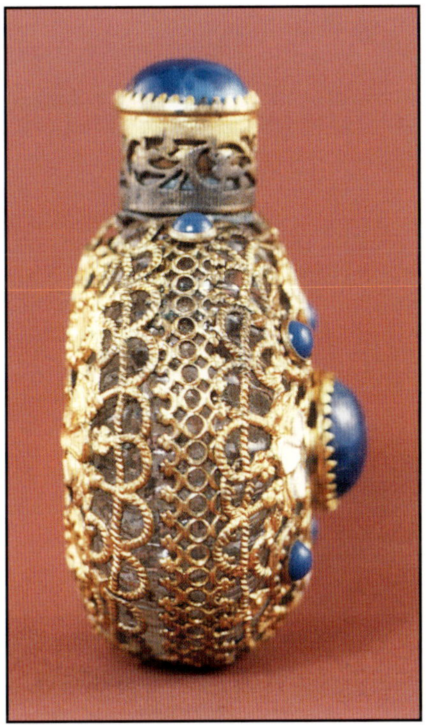

Side view of caged bottle, showing the slight overlap of front and back plates to the side strip.

Bucket shaped bottles are enclosed from the bottom. The bottle is placed on a thin solid round base piece from which radiate segments of filigree. These segments fold up the sides, encasing the bottle. Over the neck, a round flat collar piece is added, the edges of which crimp in place over the sides.

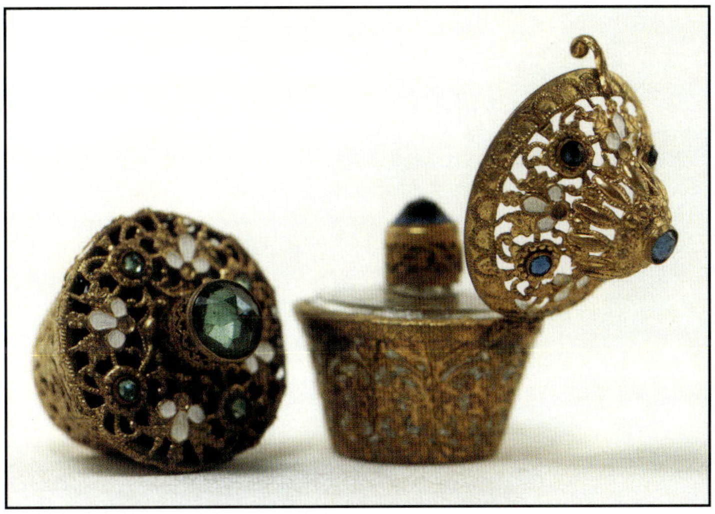

Left: Bucket shaped bottle. 1.75". $150-200. Right: Hinged bottle. 2". The top plates and the basket top repeat the filigree pattern shown previously. $275-325.

"Offset" bottles are unusual and eye-catching. A strip of filigree goes around the bottle from the angled opening, dividing the front and back of the bottle in two parts. The rest of the front plate is formed from one medallion, cut in half, and joined to opposite sides of the center strip. Overlapping plates from the front and back are joined at the sides. Enameled pieces and jeweled sets finish off the center strip and the rest of the front, giving it a balanced look.

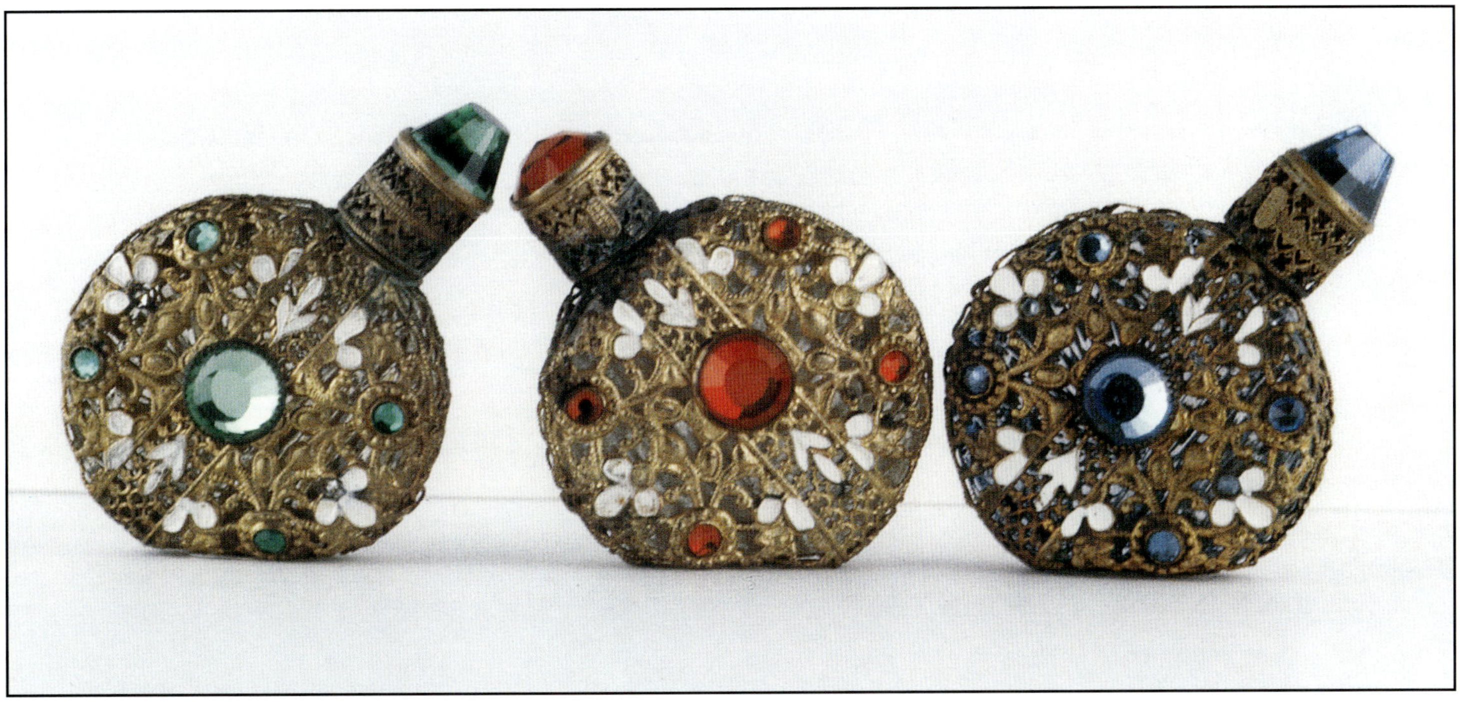

Offset bottles, all marked, all 2.25". Note that the blue bottle has extra gems and the base bottle is of blue, not clear glass. $150-200 each.

Some lipstick shaped bottles are caged by slipping the glass inside a tube of filigree formed around a solid or mesh base. The decorative top edges are then folded over the shoulders of the bottle. Others are enclosed by a tube that fits down over body and shoulders of the bottle, resting on a glass flange at the base.

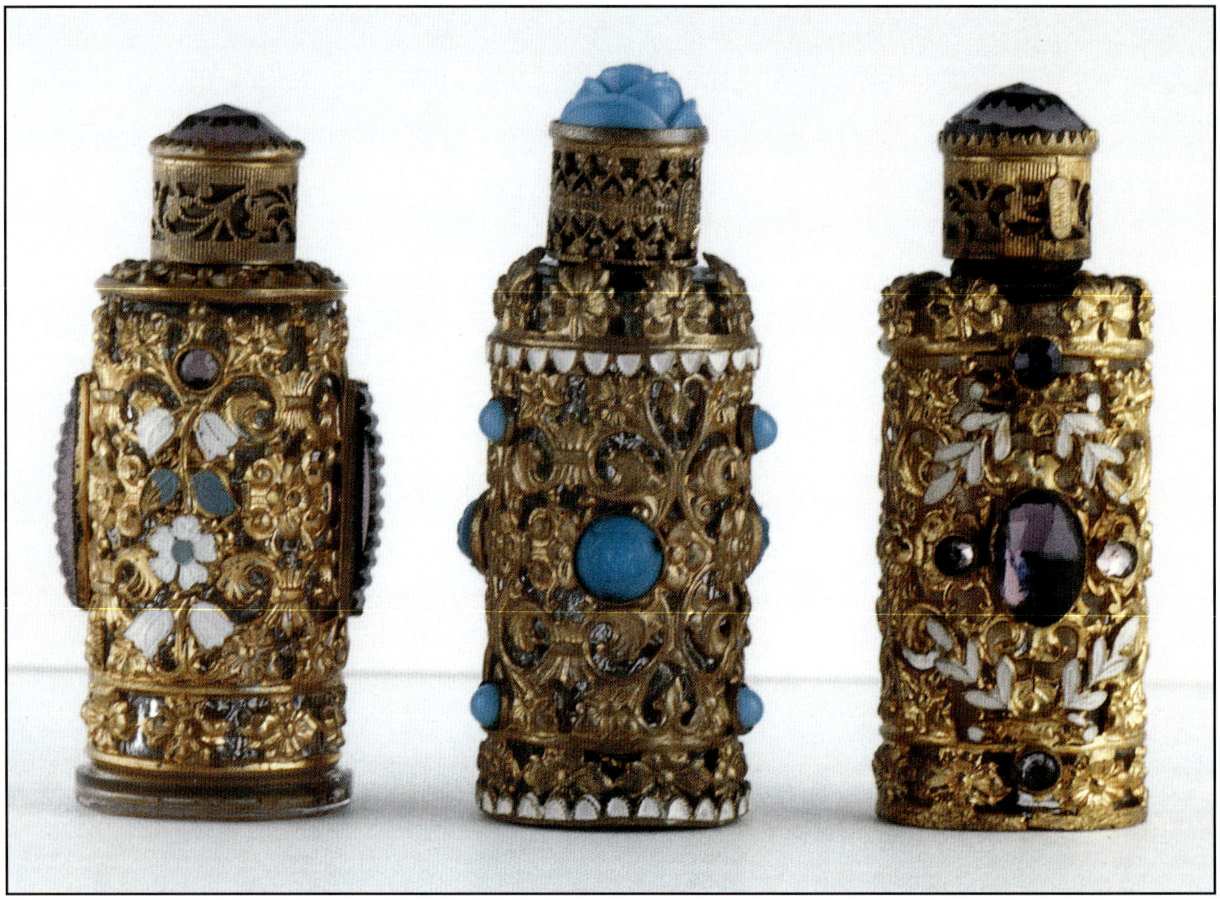

Lipstick caged bottles. Left: Purple glass, caging rests on the bottom flange. The polished base has an acid mark. 2.375". Center: Turquoise carved roses. 2.5". Right: Faceted amethyst brilliants. 2.375". $175-225 each.

On some bottles, enameling appears to have been added directly to the original front plate piece. On others, detailed pieces have been fixed to the top of the surface of the filigree, giving it added character and depth. Most of the enameling was done in white, perhaps to keep from competing with the jewel sets, but sometimes the detailing has additional color, usually green or red to add to a flower motif. Fittings for the sets were also added to the filigree and the glass stones set carefully in place. It is a tribute to the workmanship that the vast majority of the stones have remained in place over time. Except for a very few bottles, stones were not set in the back. This was most likely a necessary cost saving measure.

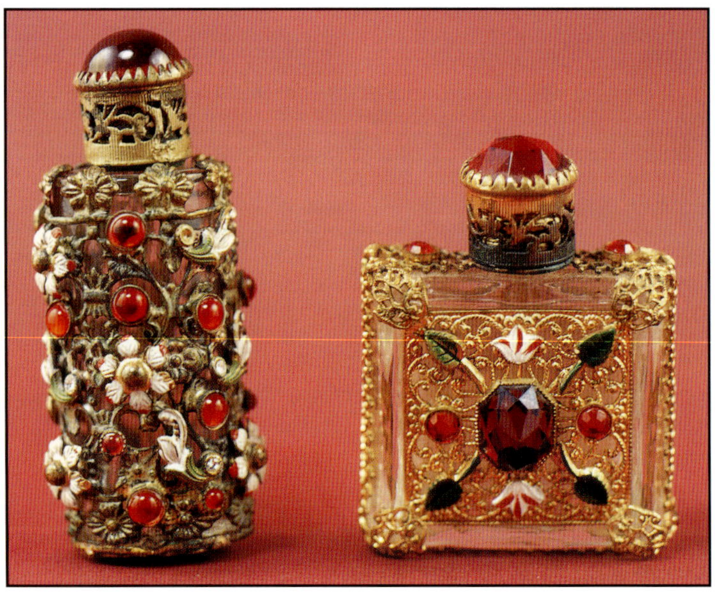

Left: Square bottle with colorful enamel work. 2". $100-200. Right: Applied enamel pieces. 2.375". $150-200.

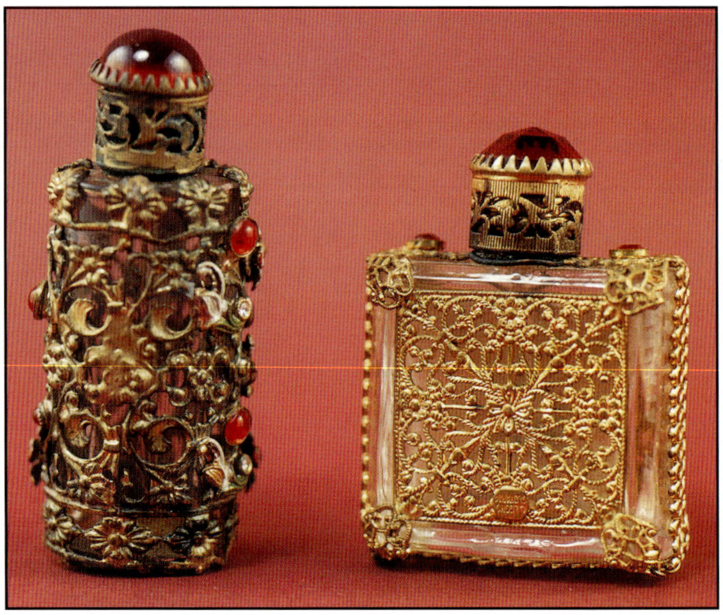

Back view.

Caged purse bottles have a variety of "gemstone" and capstones. Usually a central stone is matched by color and type in the capstone. Most stones are clear, faceted, or cabochon stones. Less common, but no less lovely, are the opaque lapis, malachite, turquoise, carnelian, or opaque red stones. A smaller number of bottles were decorated with carved roses in a surprising variety of colors. Most are made to resemble rose quartz, lapis, turquoise, jade, or coral. Press molded medallions were featured on some of these bottles and also appeared on some of the popular jewelry produced at the same time.

Many of the caged purse bottles from between the world wars were made with a metal fitting over the glass neck of the bottle. Caged purse bottles that were made and sold in the 1960s were finished in similar filigree, enamel work, and gems, and can be identified by the glass bottle neck and the distinctive, solid cap. These caps were not marked.

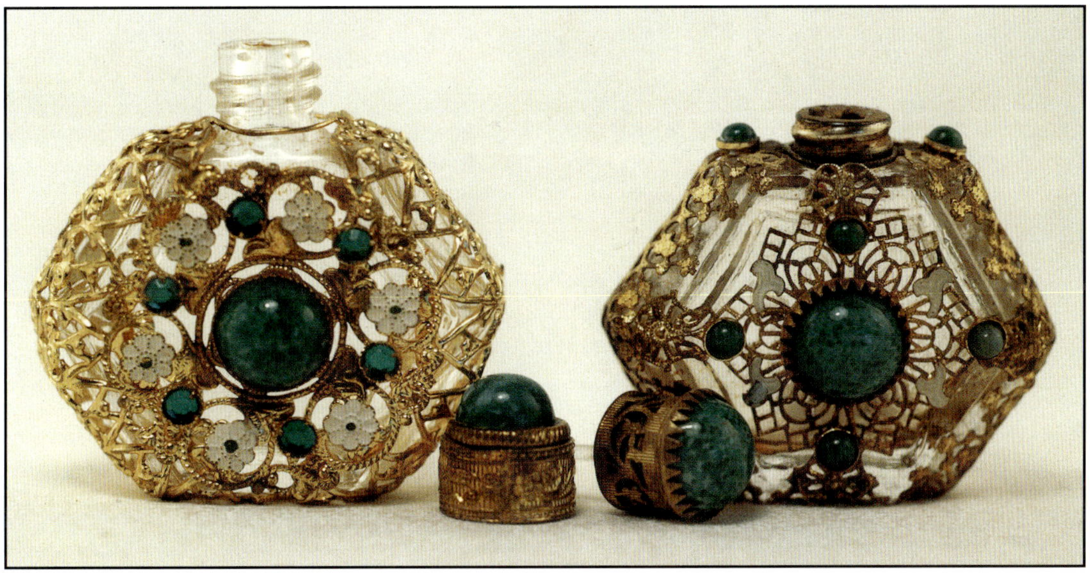

Left: A caged, jeweled, and enameled bottle from the 1960s. Note the solid cap and glass bottle neck. $50-100. Right: A bottle of the same mold shape, also with filigree, enamel work, and jewels, but with a metal neck and a cutaway cap. This bottle dates from the 1920s or '30s. $150-175.

Front view. Left: Lapis floral medallion. 2.25". Center: Opaque red floral medallion. 2". Right: Amethyst carved rose; the bottle base is yellow glass. 2". $175-$225 each.

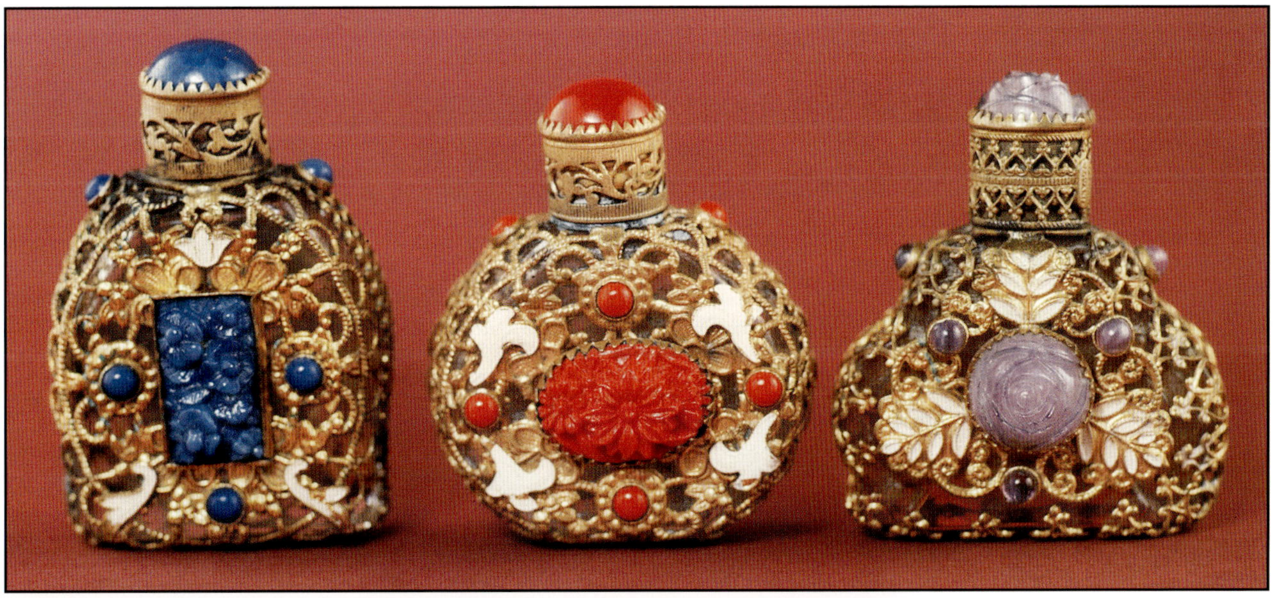

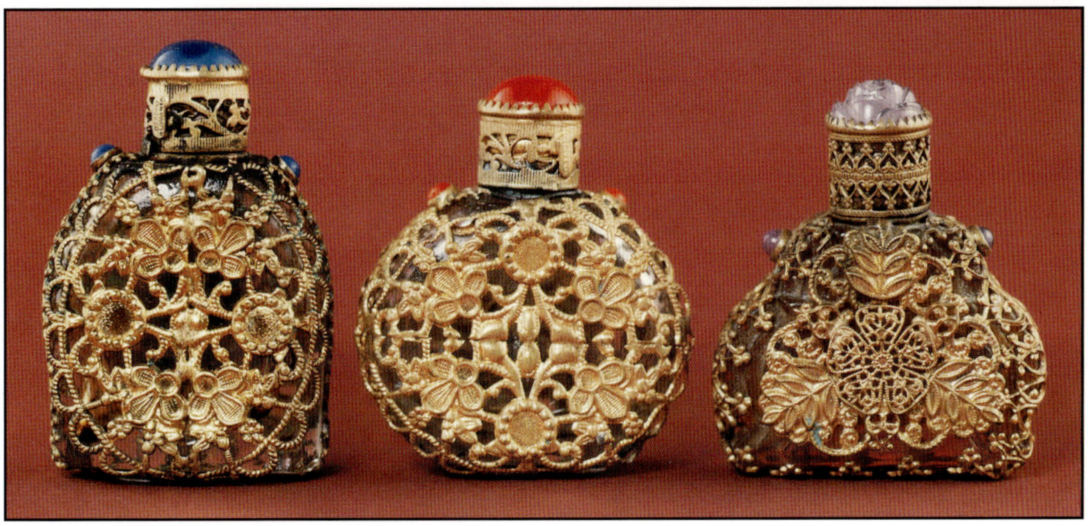

Back view. Note the layers of filigree on the amethyst topped bottle.

Purse bottle with green medallion. 1.875". $175-225. Shown with unmarked necklace with pink glass and tombac beads, about $50.

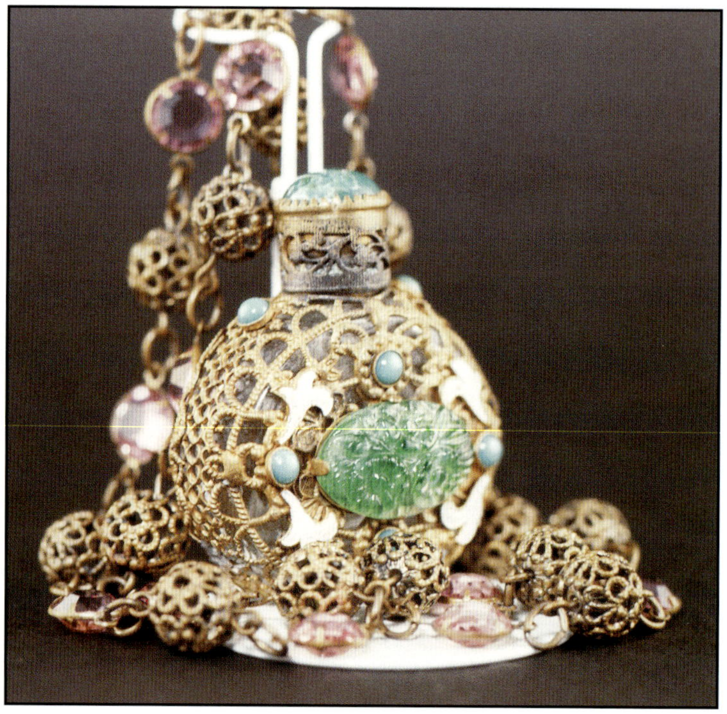

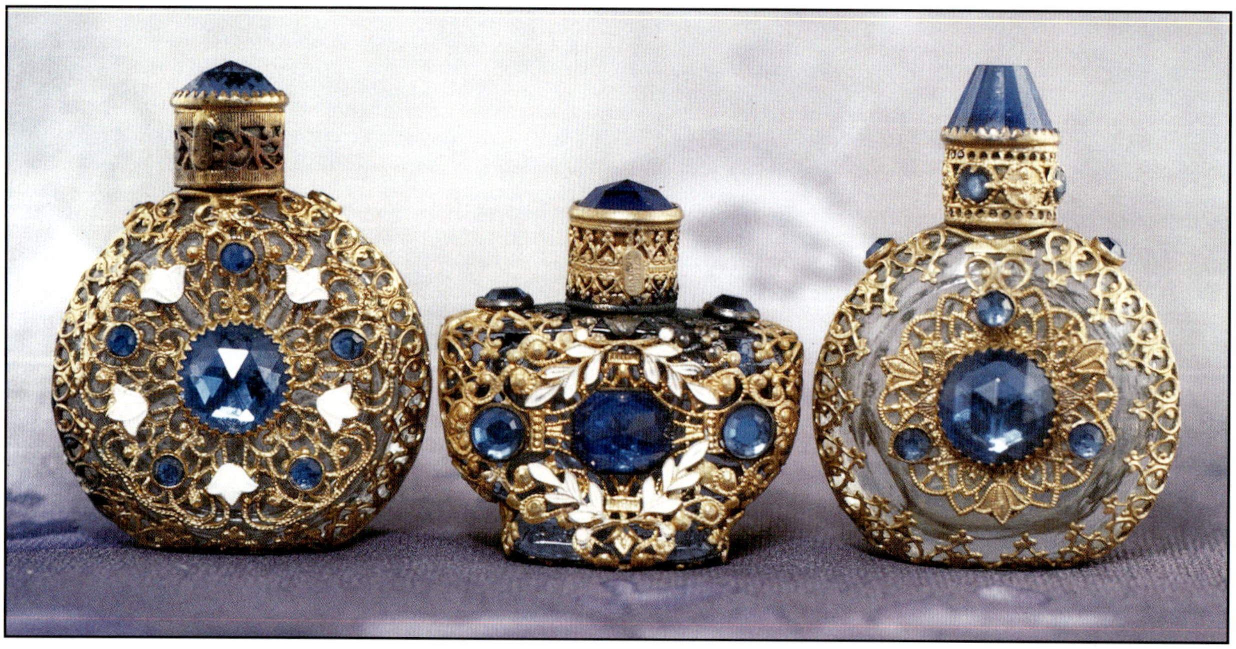

Three styles of filigree with blue stones. Left: Dainty filigree and enamel. 2.125". Center: Heavily jeweled, blue glass base. 1.725". Right: Lacy filigree and applied plain metal pieces. 2.25". $175-225 each.

The same bottle mold with pink, aqua, and green stones. 2". $150-200 each.

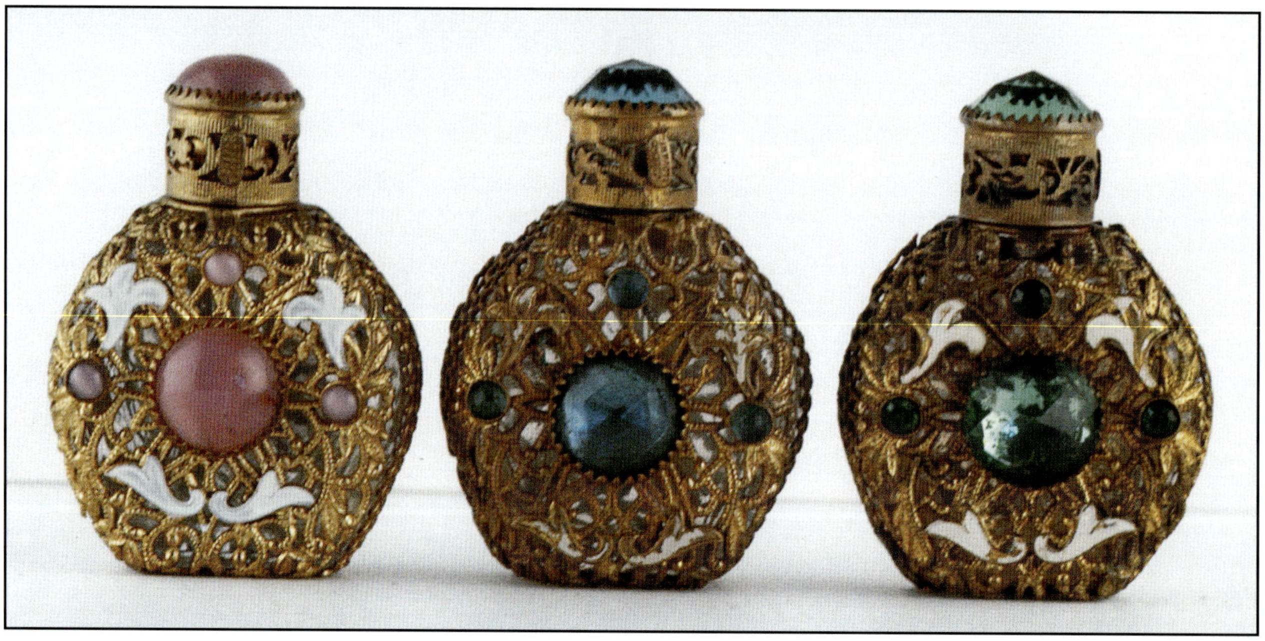

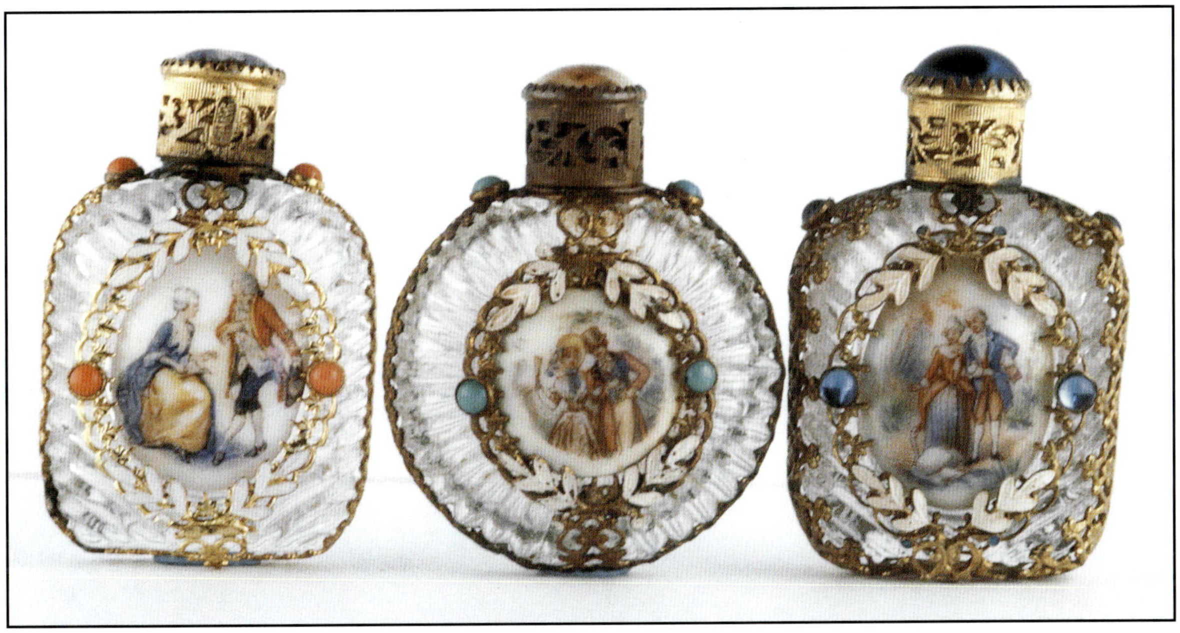

Three cameo bottles, each with Victorian couples. Left: Coral colored cabochons. 2.125". Center: Round bottle with green or turquoise cabochons. 2.25". Right: Clear blue cabochons 2.25". $175-225 each.

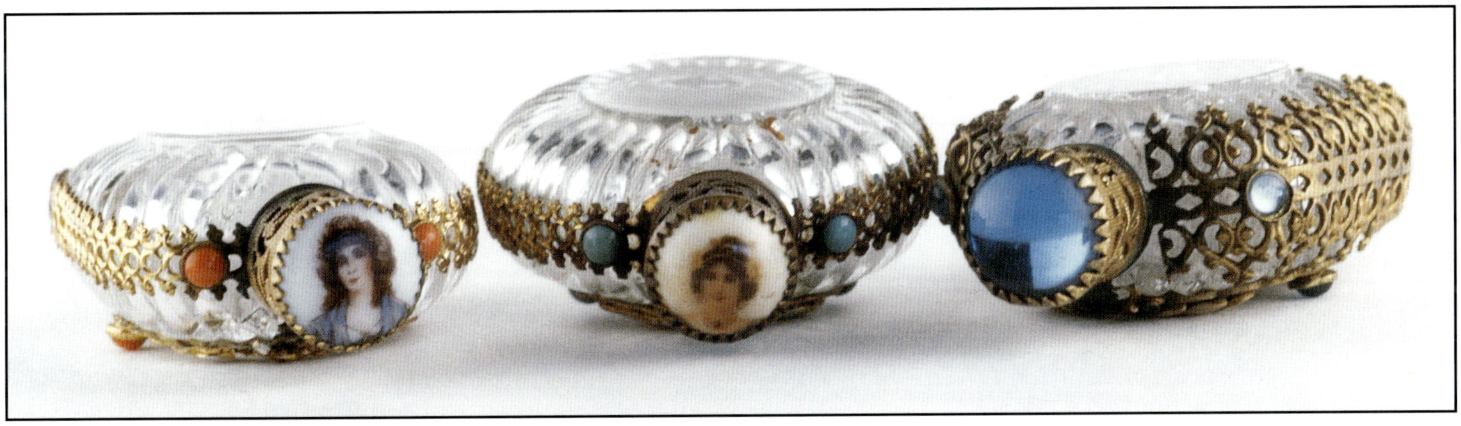

Caps on the cameo bottles.

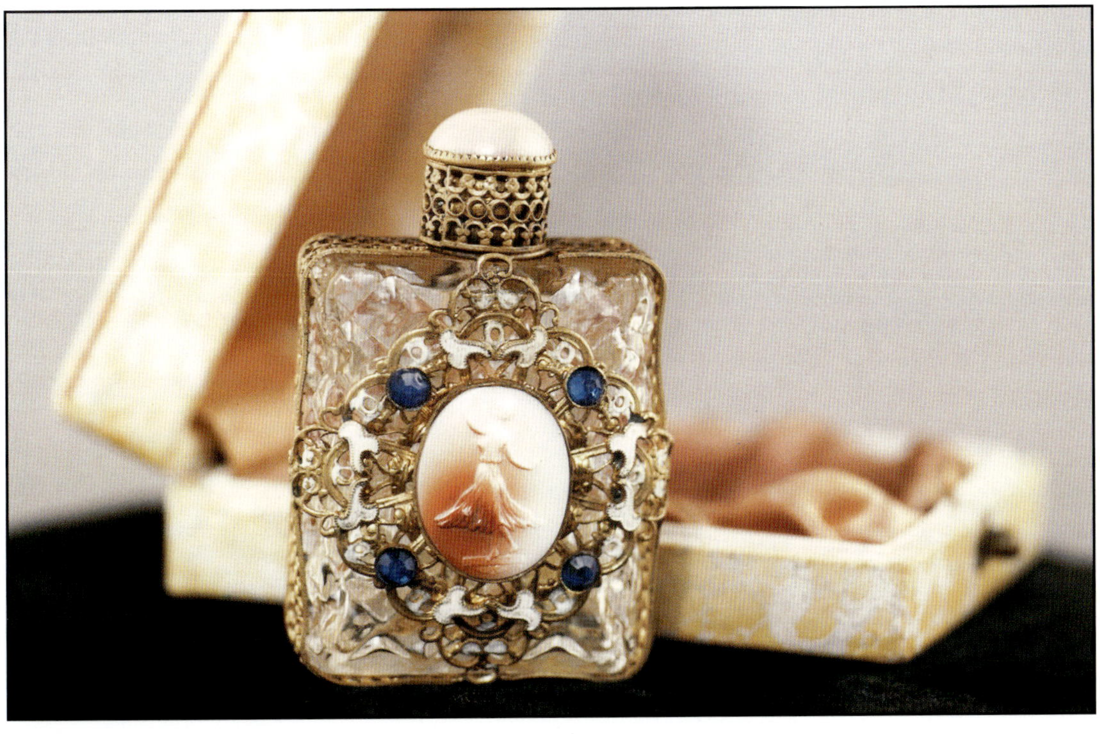

Another style of cameo, this full-skirted, swirling woman is surrounded by blue brilliants and enamel work. The tag is found in the bottom band. Original box marked Dralle. 2.25". $200-250.

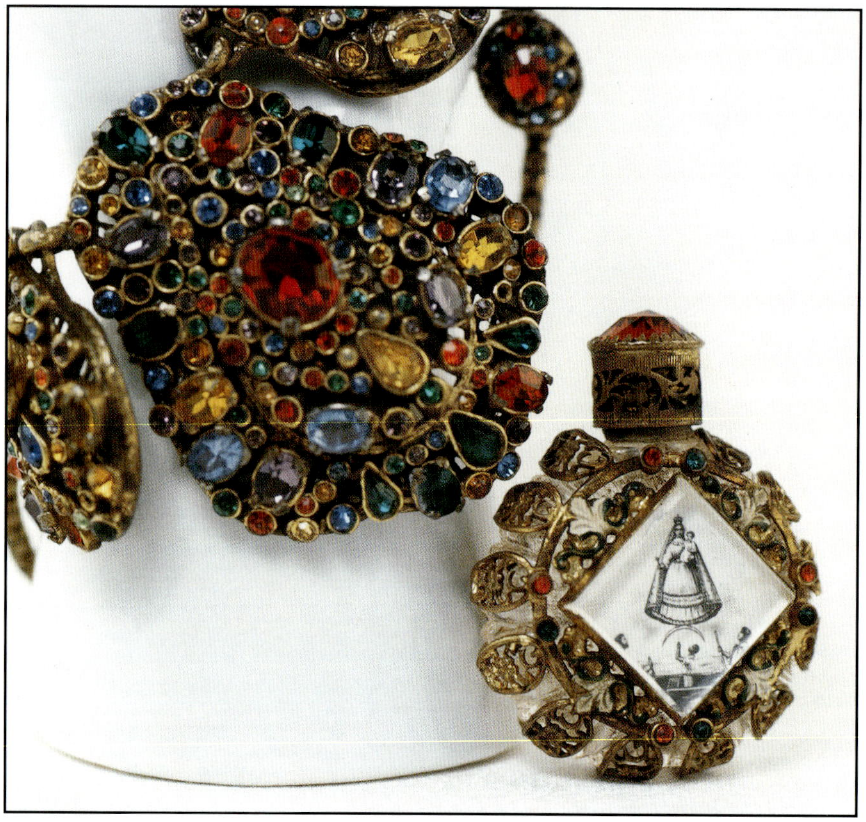

This unusual bottle features a crowned Madonna holding her child and a cross. The three figures below appear to be standing in a boat. The bottle has a red faceted cap, red and green stones, and detailed filigree and enamel work. 2.125". $200-250. It is shown with a three lobed necklace with multi-colored gems, about $150.

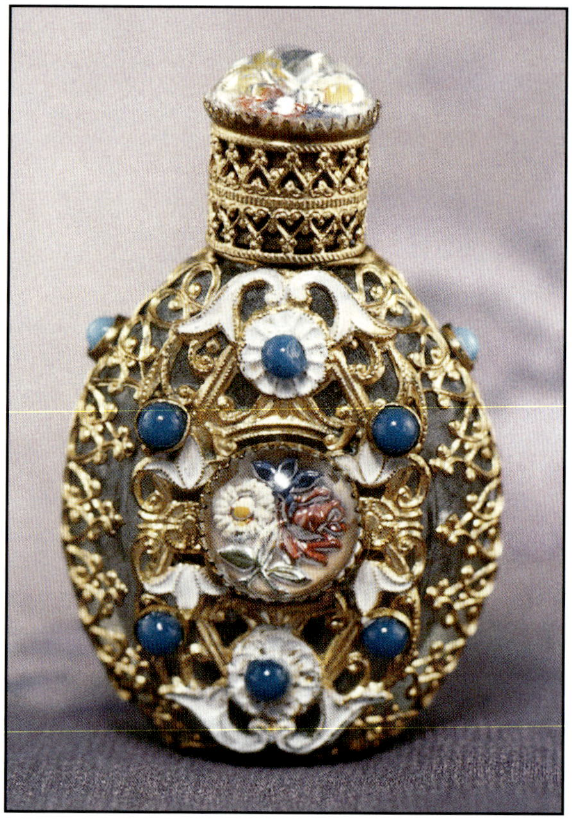

This bottle features reverse molded flower bouquets painted from the underside as a central medallion and as a capstone. It is embellished with filigree, lapis, and lighter blue cabochons. 2.5". $175-225.

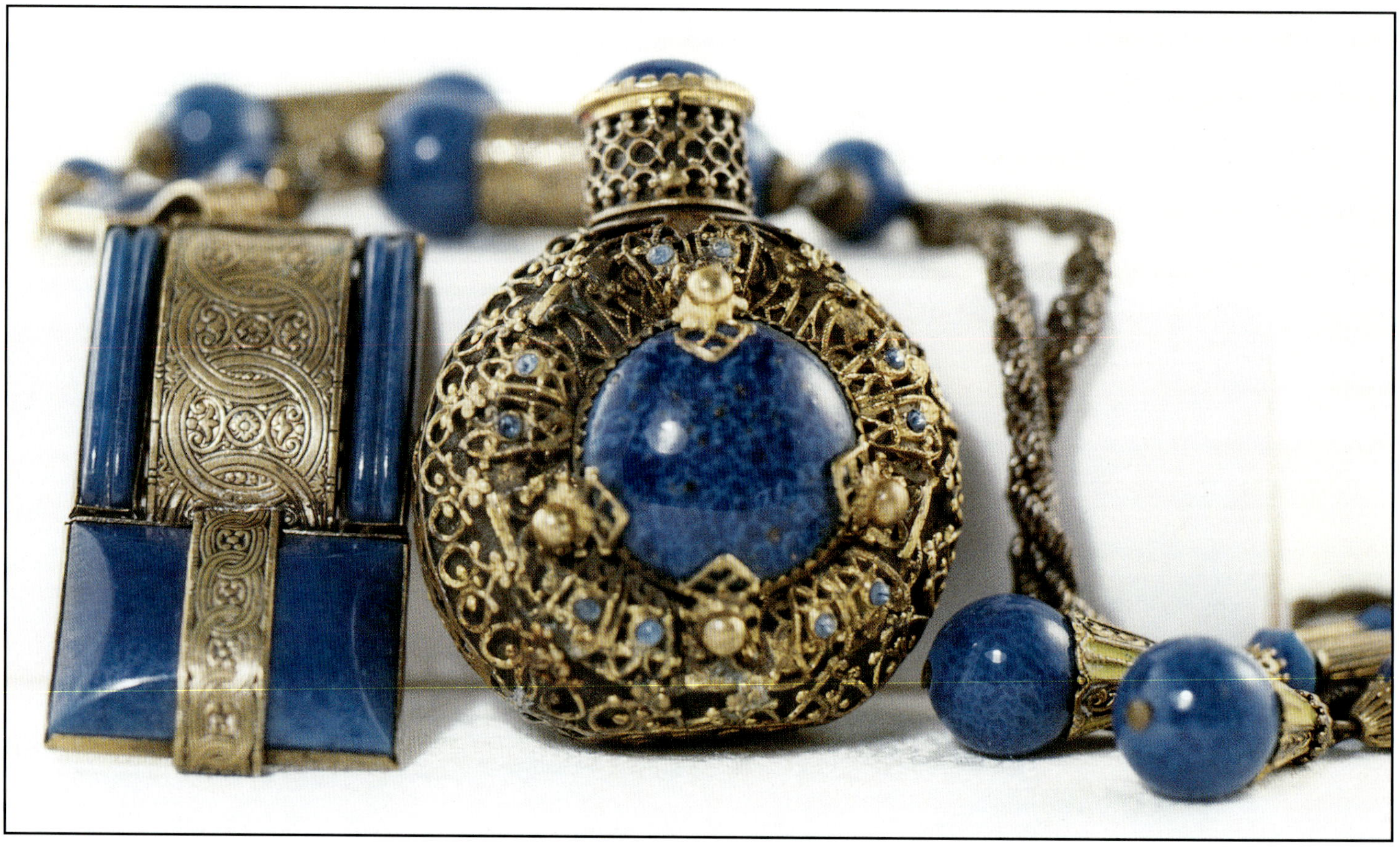

Beautifully elaborate filigree and tiny blue brilliants frame this mottled lapis stone that is flecked with gold. This unmarked bottle was purchased from Germany. 2". $200-250. Shown with a marked lapis necklace and earrings. $150-200.

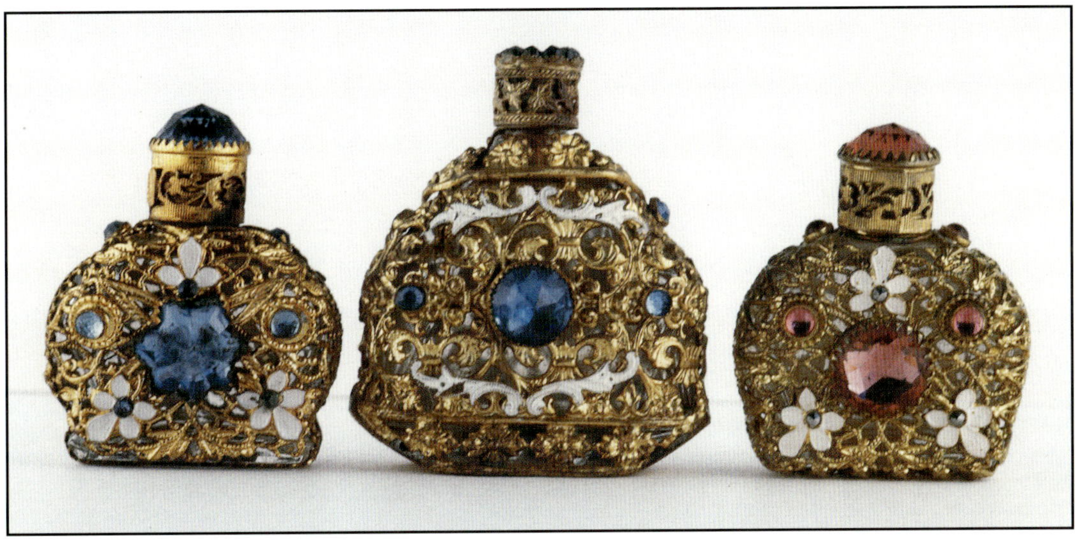

Left: The blue star flower in the center is the same as found in the caps of some Irice purse bottles. The top enameled flower is smaller than on the bottle on the right to accommodate the shape of the center flower. 2". Center: This bottle also has a glass flower of a more regular shape as a capstone. Note that although the bottle is larger (2.25"), the cap is undersized. Right: Nearly identical to the left bottle. Mark in the bottle filigree. 1.875". $150-200 each.

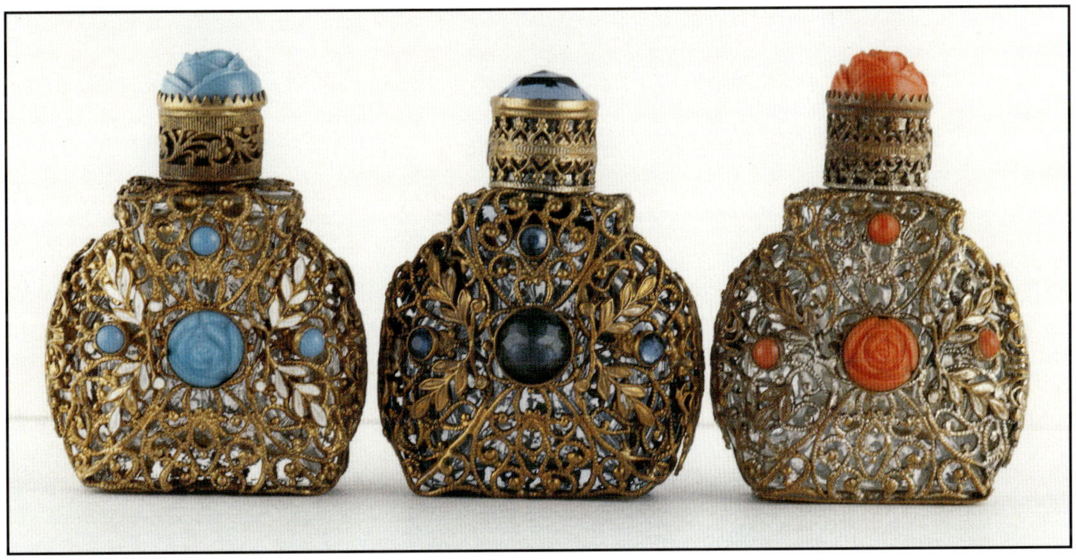

The same bottle with minor variations. All have marked caps. The center bottle has a blue glass base. All 2.375", $150-200.

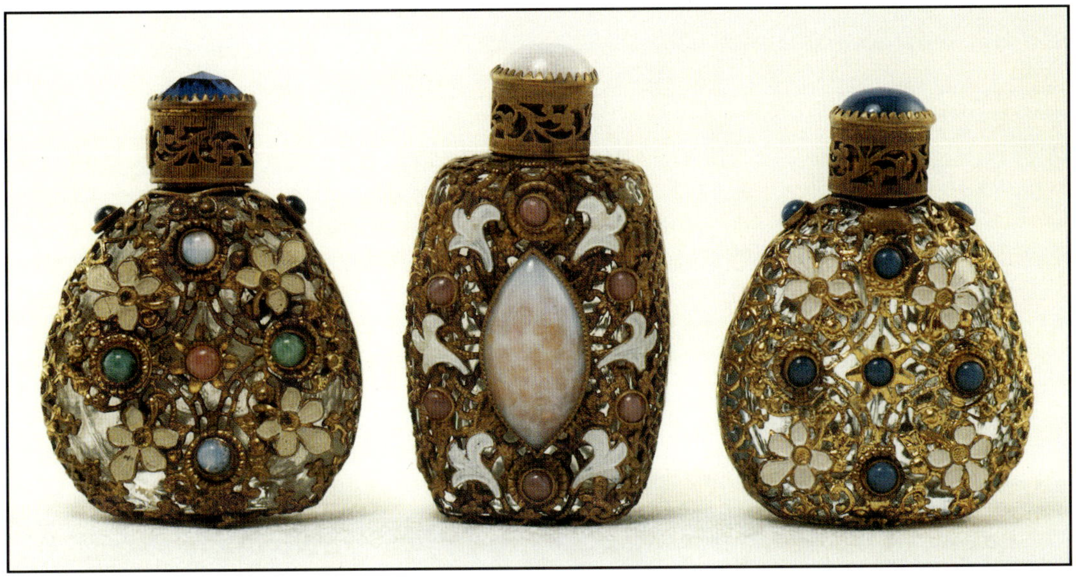

The left and right bottles are similar, but with different colored stones. The bottle on the left is made with light blue glass. 2.125". Center: Pink, 2.375". $150-200 each.

Left: Aqua green stones with marked mesh caging and applied filigree. Right: Lipstick shaped caged filigree with dark red faceted stones. 2.5". $175-225 each.

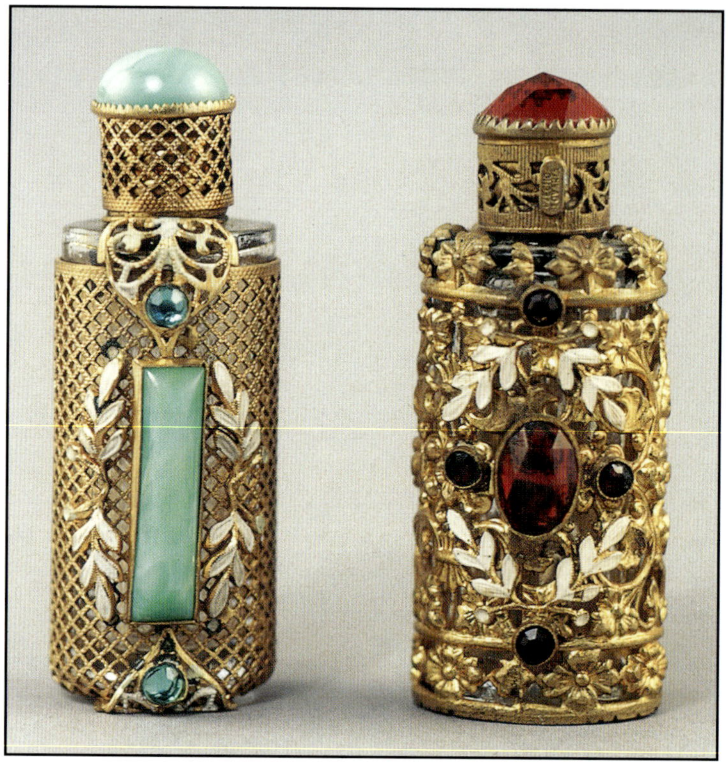

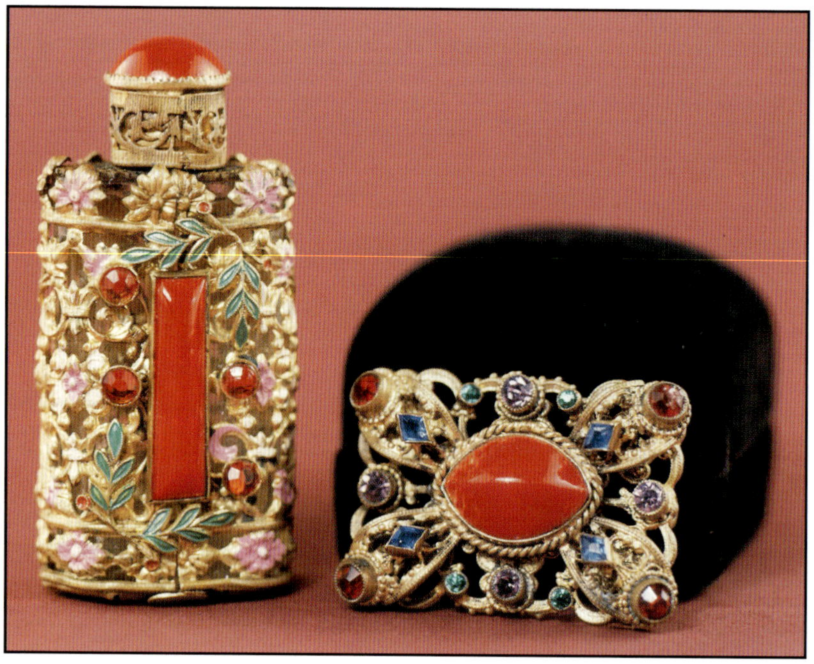

Purse bottle with a long red opaque center stone and red capstone, plus pink, red, white, and yellow enameling. Marked with a tag in the base. 2.375". $200-250 Shown with vintage pin, unmarked, about $50.

This pair of similar bottles have cut and polished glass bases. Bottles like these were sometimes used commercially for the Dralle perfume company. Both marked. 1.75". Left: Aqua mirrored sets. Right: Oblong cut lapis glass sets. $150-200 each.

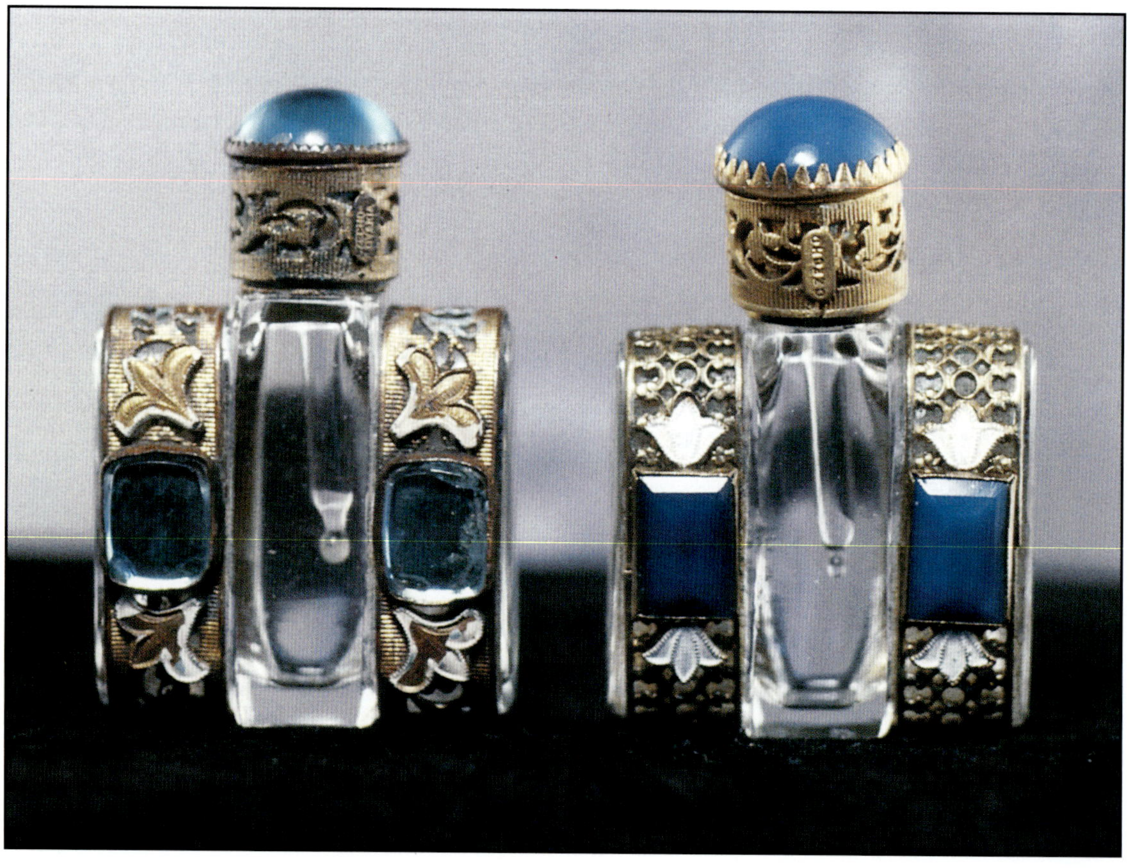

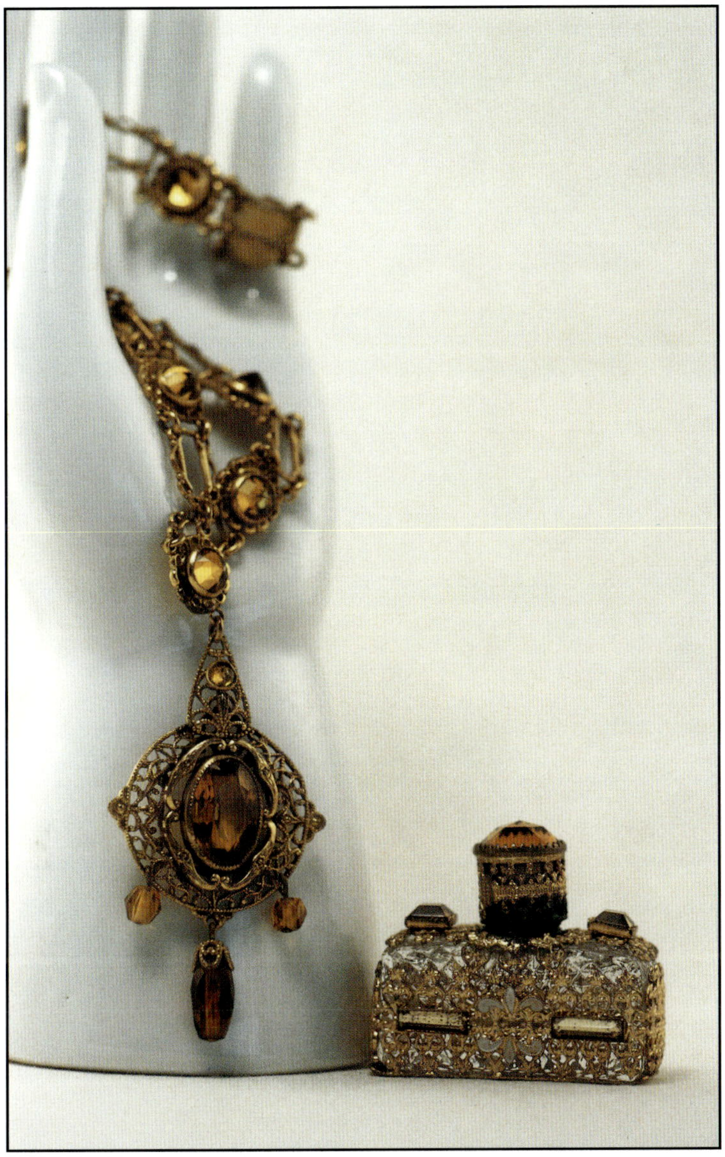

Short at 1.25", this purse bottle has enamel work and yellow stones. $150-200. Shown with an unmarked necklace, about $75.

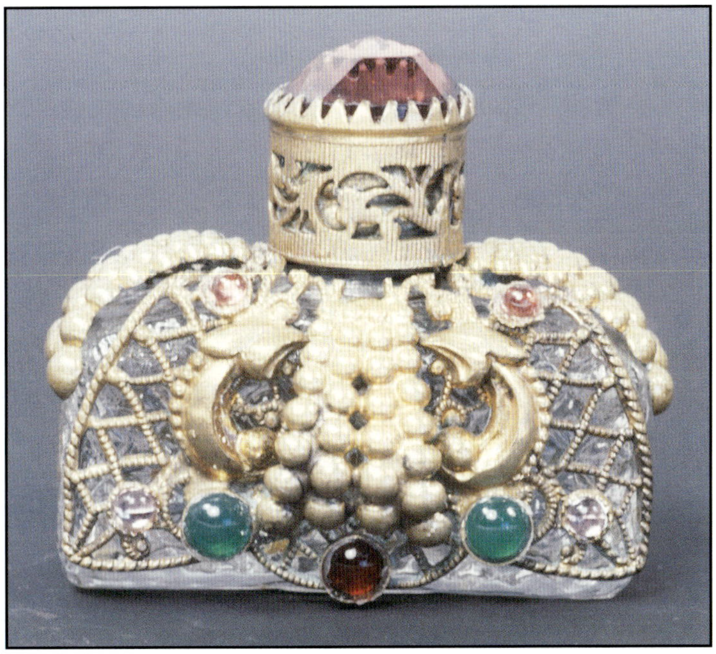

Also measuring 1.25", this unmarked bottle was purchased from Israel. The bead "waterfall" flows down all four sides. Beautiful cabochon stones. $150-200.

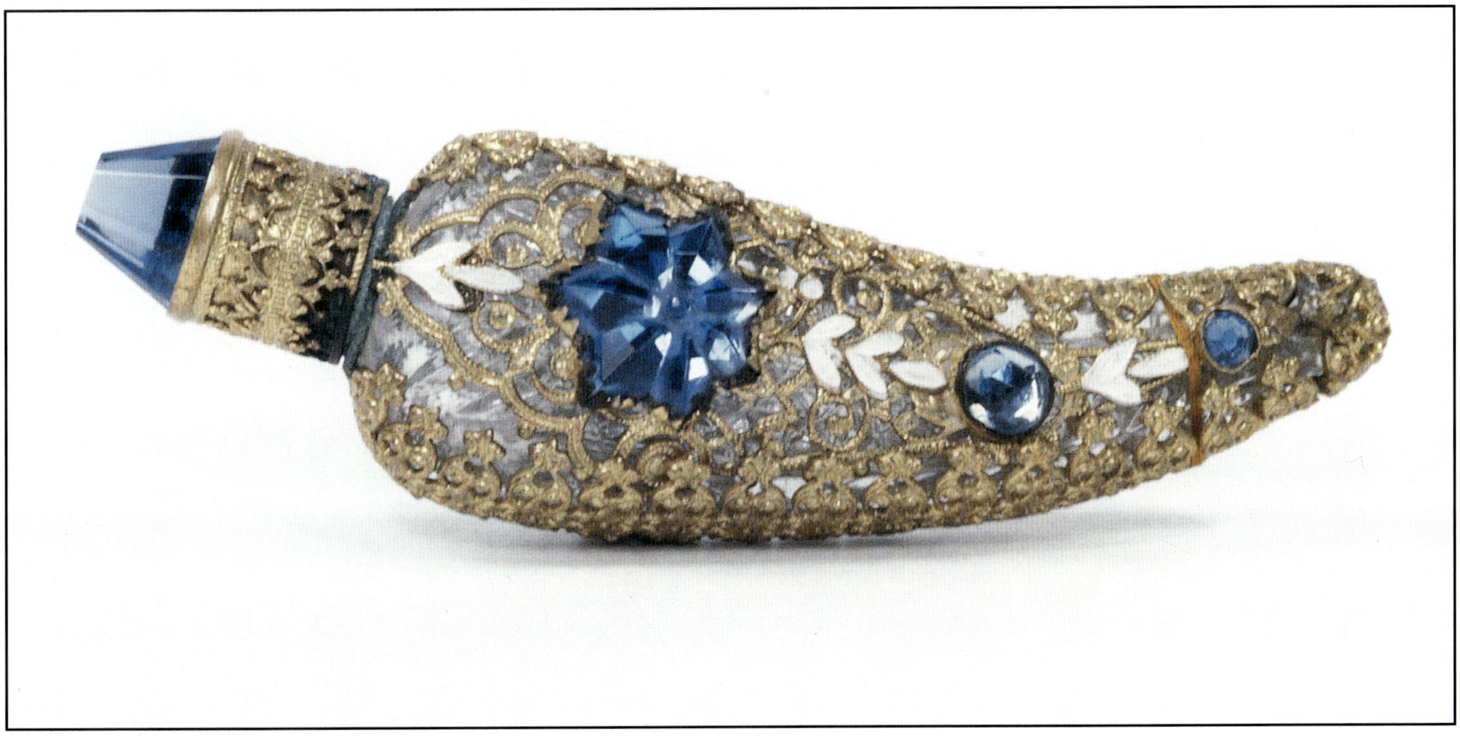

An unusual caged laydown with a star flower set and blue stones. 3.25". $200-300.

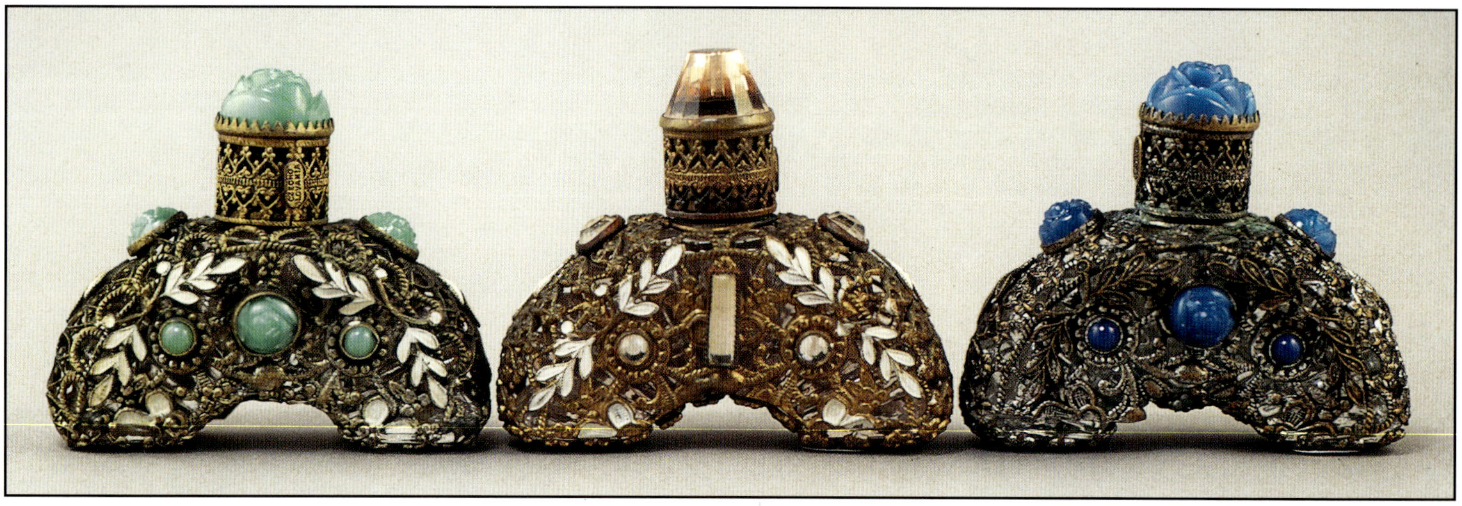

Three caged bridge bottles. Left: Silver colored metal with enamel work, green carved roses. Center: Gold colored metal on a pink glass base, enamel work. Right: Blue carved roses, silver metal, no enamel work. All 1.75", $250-300.

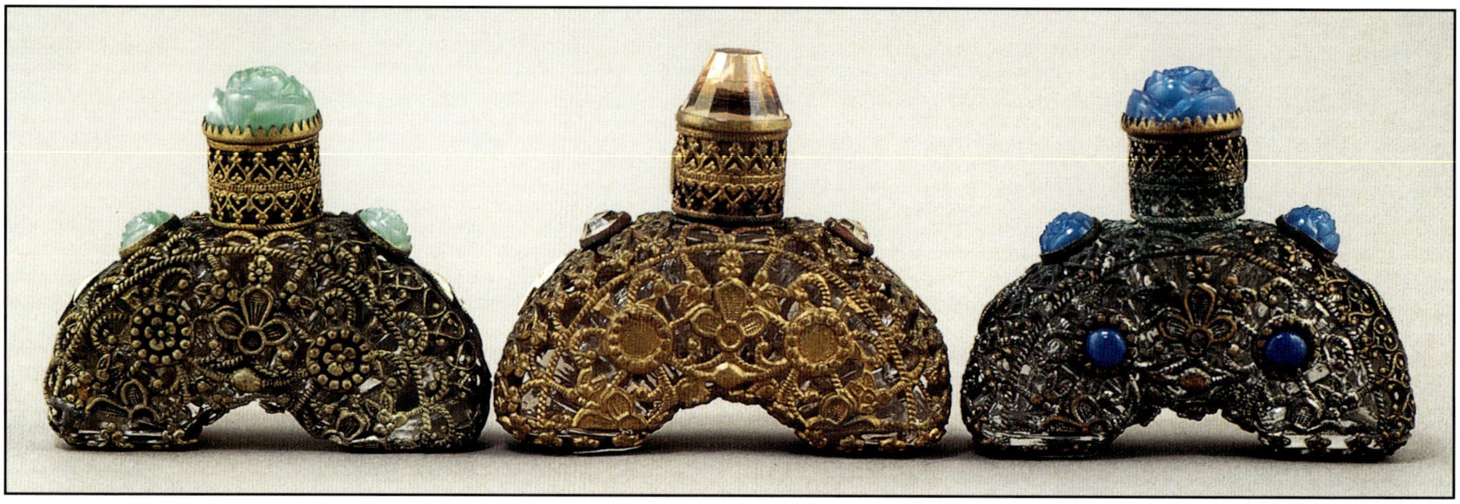

Bridge bottles' back view. Note that the blue bottle has sets in the back. The metal pattern is similar, but the green bottle back has more detailing.

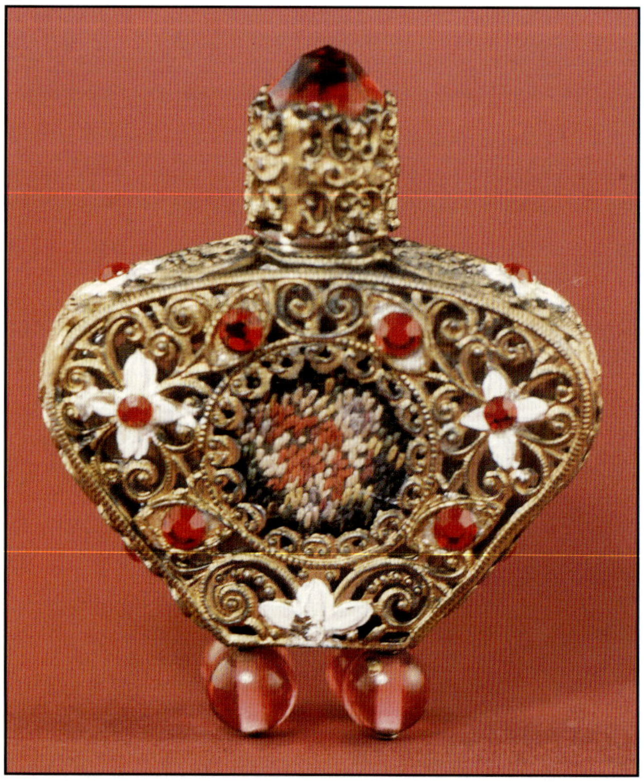

Bead-footed bottle with needlework center medallion is marked Irice in the base. It has complete decoration front and back. 2.25". $150-200.

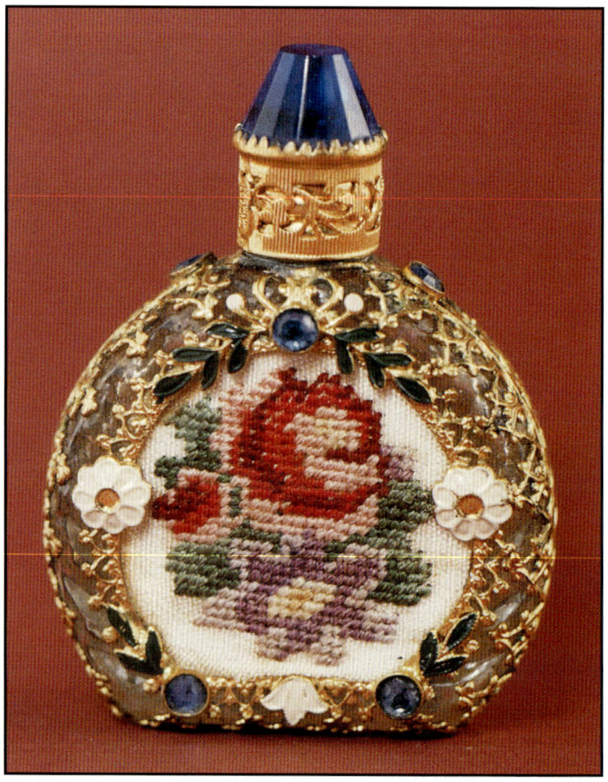

Beautiful detailing in the petit point bouquet as well as the enamel work. Cap is marked Czechoslovakia. Needlework is often an indicator of Austria and this part might have been produced there. 2.375". $150-200.

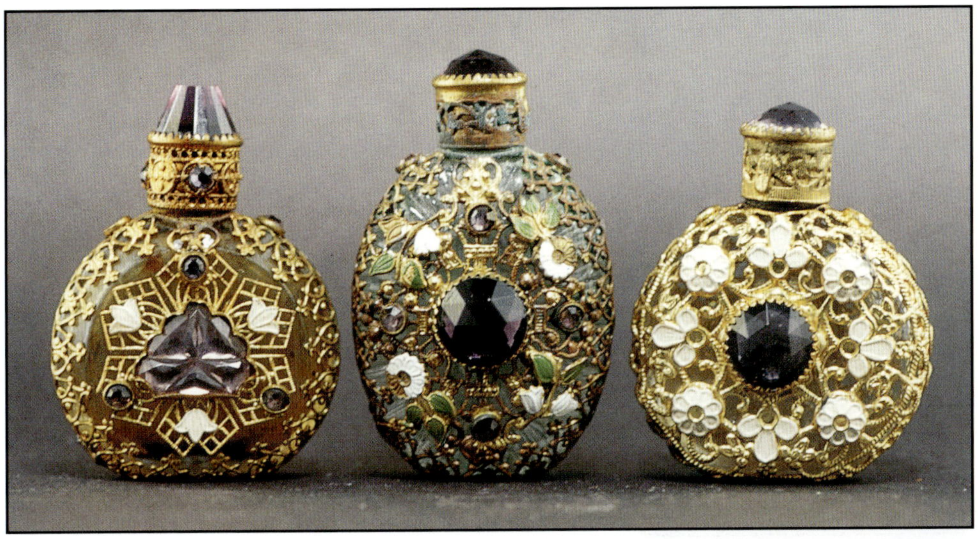

Left: Wispy filigree pattern with amethyst medallion, added amethyst stones, and white enameled detail. 2.5". Center: Blue base bottle with elaborate green and white enamel work, amethyst central, capstone, and incidental stones. 2.25". Right: Two enameled flowers are applied to the face plate with its flat enameled flowers. Center and capstone are amethyst faceted glass. 2.25". *Courtesy Earline Kopriva.* $175-225 each.

A boxed purse bottle used for Dralle perfumes is shown with a boxed micro mini for contrast. The purse bottle has an opaque red cabochon center and capstone and contrasting colored faceted stones. 2.25". $175-225. Micro mini: $100-150.

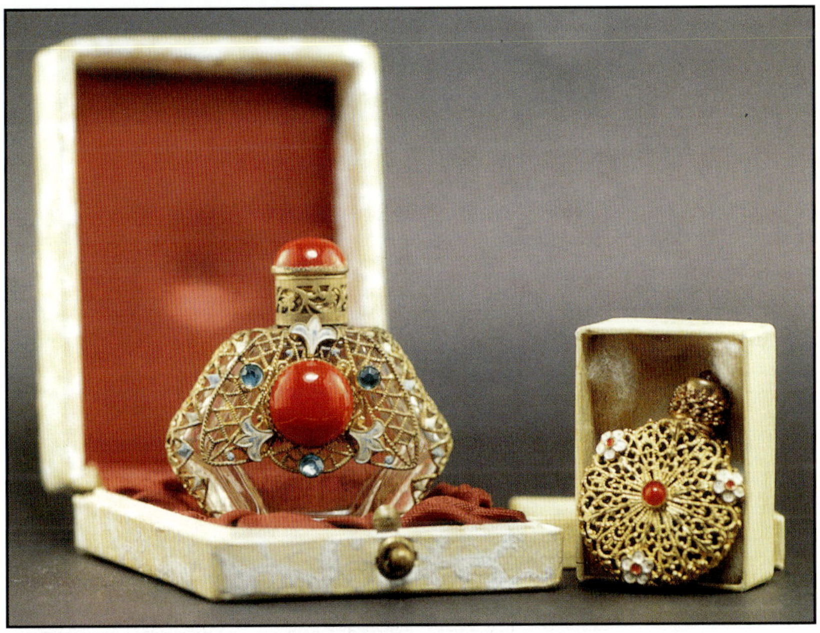

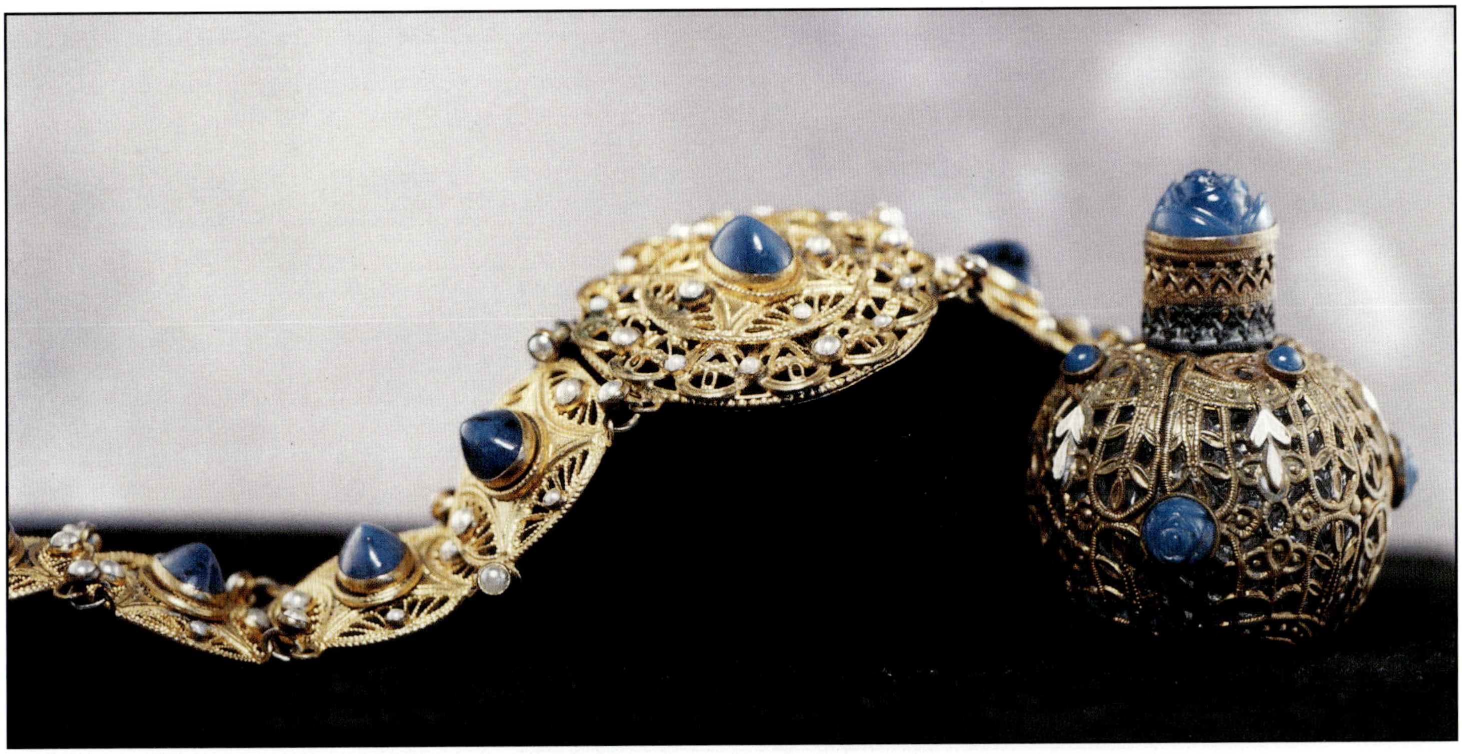

Round blue bottle is surrounded by six metal segments folded up and attached at the neck. It has three lapis carved roses and three lapis cabs. Marked in the bottle lip. 2". $150-200. Shown with a filigreed lapis and pearl bracelet marked "Austria." $125-150.

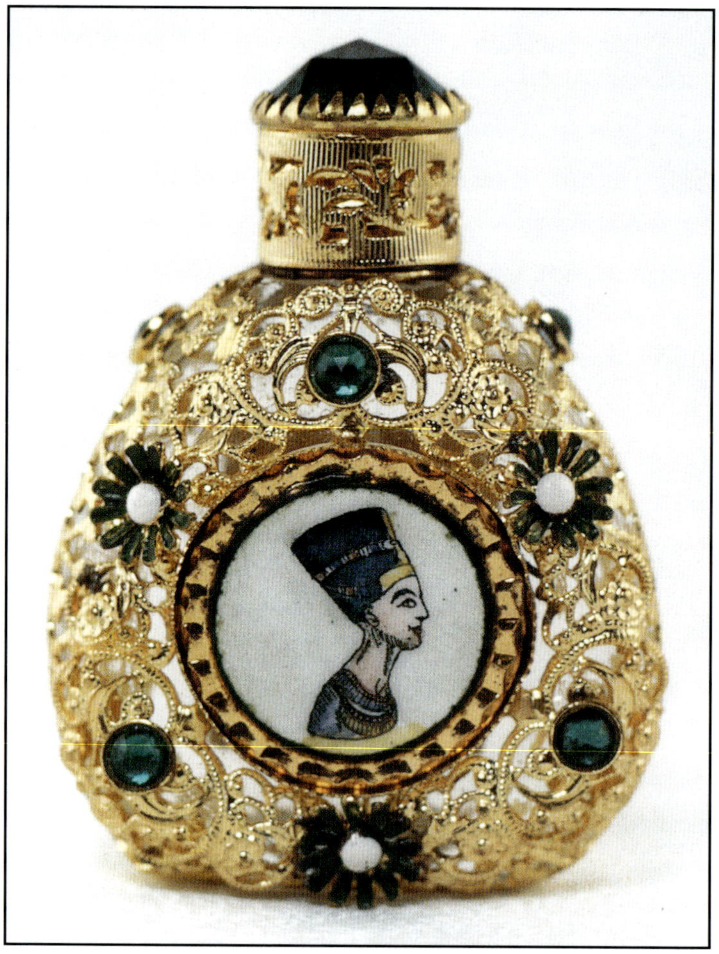

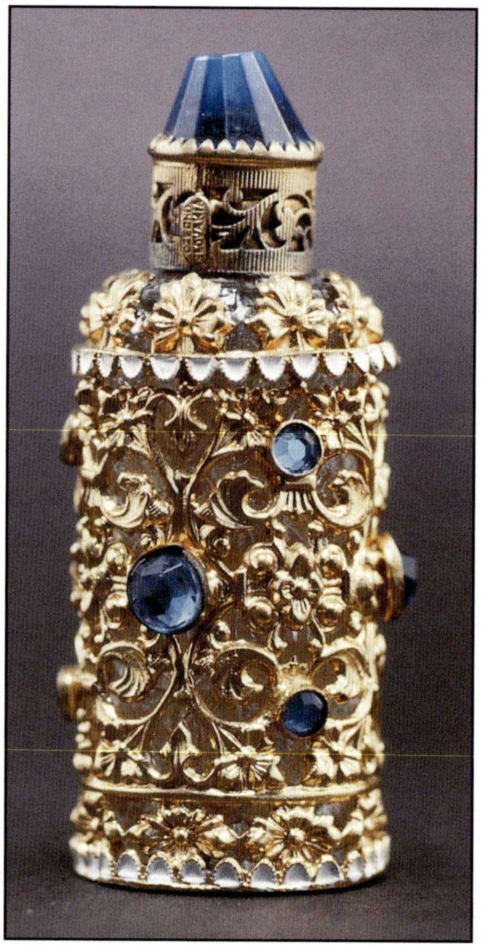

Gold filigree with blue faceted stones and white enameled rings at the shoulders and base. Cut-away cap with a faceted truncated blue capstone. 2.5". $150-175.

Another portrait bottle, of Nefertiti. This bottle with blue stones is pictured in the *Perfume Bottle Quarterly* for Spring, 2002. It is from the collection of Helen Farnsworth and dated as 1935. 2.375". $150-200.

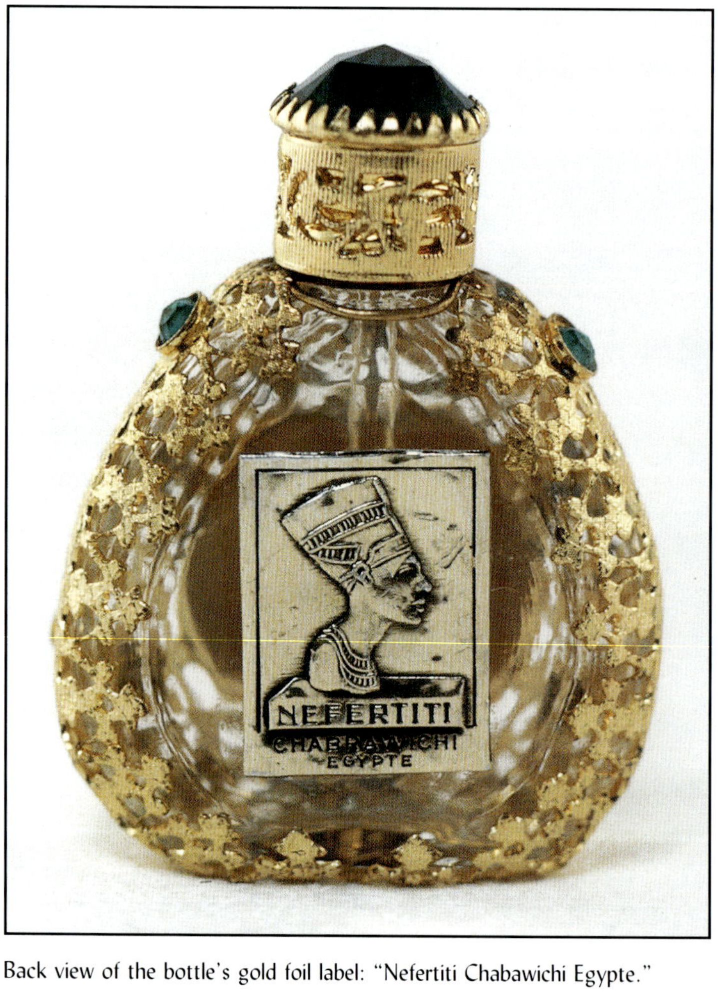

Back view of the bottle's gold foil label: "Nefertiti Chabawichi Egypte."

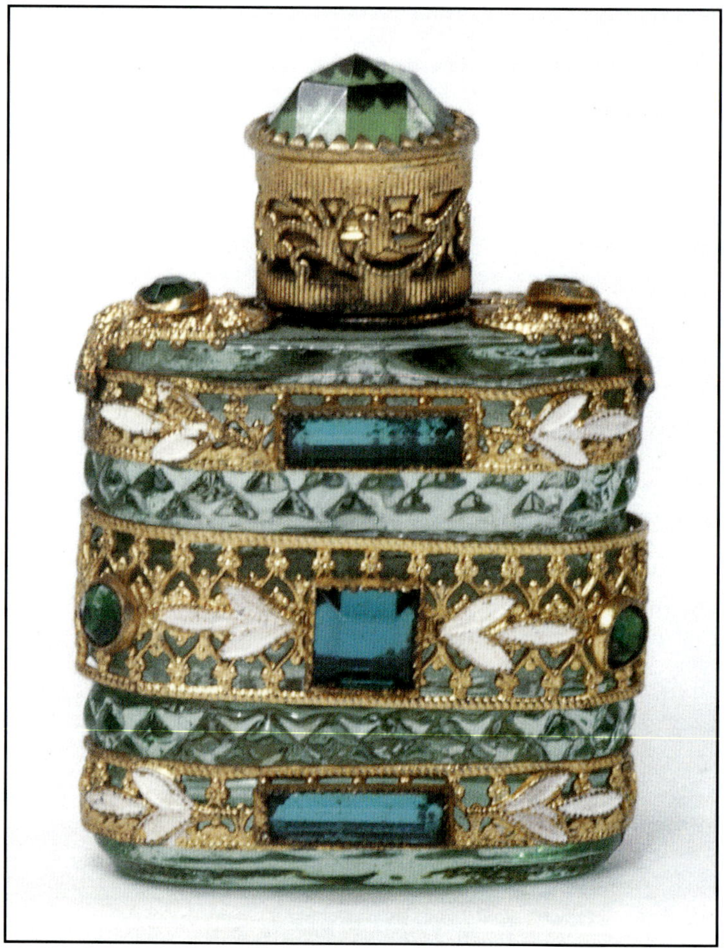

This filigree banded bottle is formed on a green, pressed base and decorated with faceted green stones and white enamel work. The cap has a metal tag and the base has a small, round paper label reading "MADE IN CZECHOSLO-VAKIA." 1.875". $175-225.

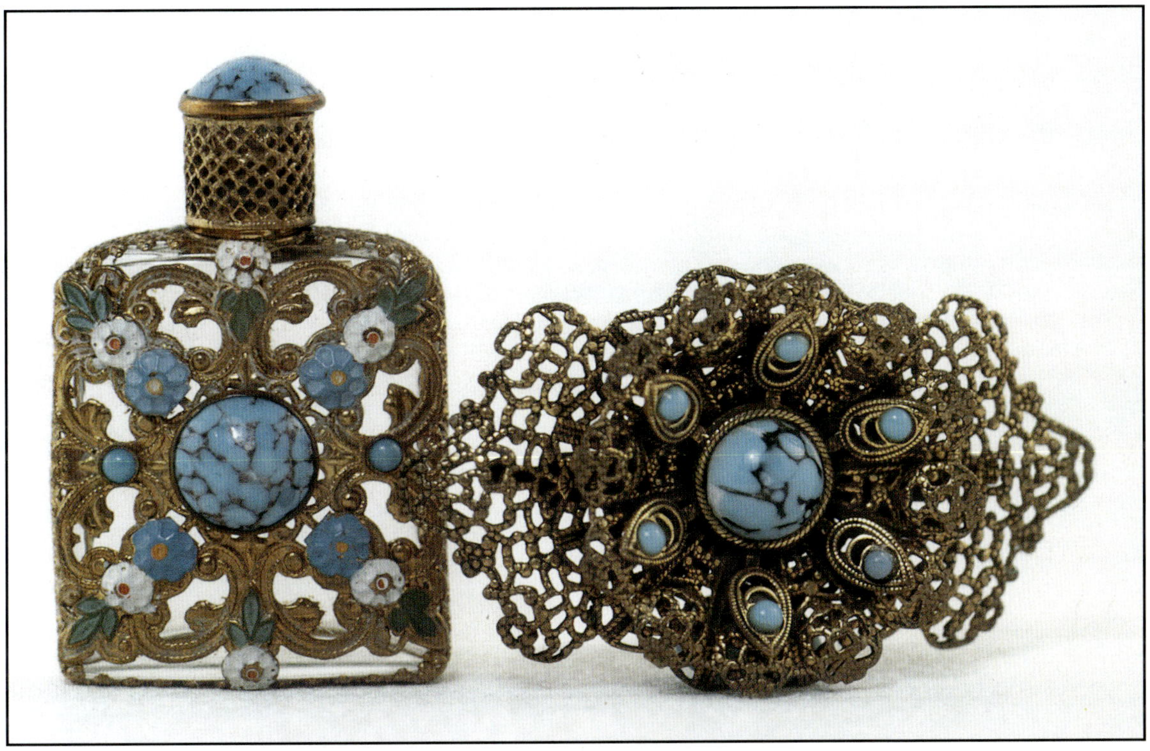

This unmarked bottle is adorned with turquoise center and capstones. The enamelwork is elaborate and colorful. Because of the cap style and the differences in the enamel work, the author believes this bottle to be Austrian. 2.25". $150-200. The unmarked pin has a similar turquoise center stone. $35-55.

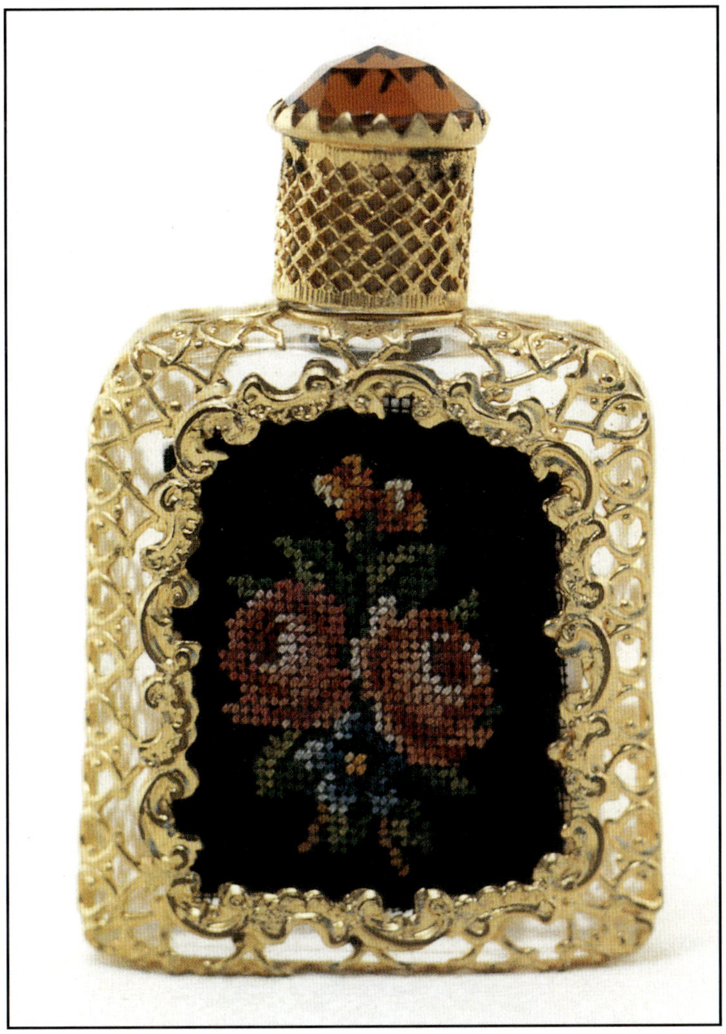

Another unmarked bottle with a mesh cap, petit point needlework flowers, and amber faceted capstone. Probably Austrian. 2.25". $150-200.

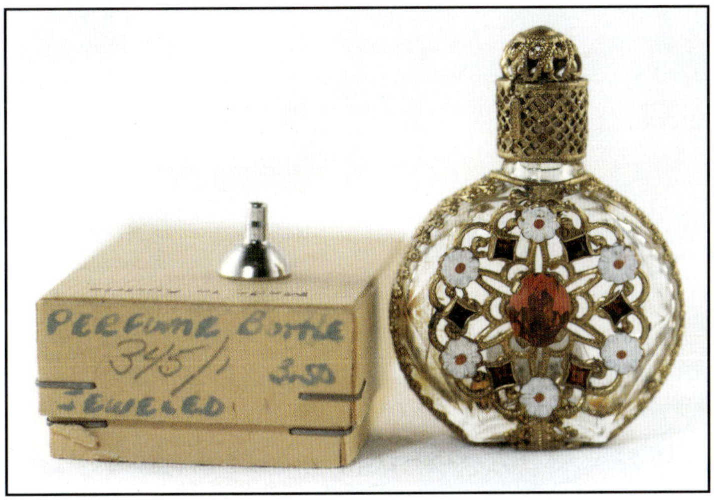

This purse bottle and its box are marked Austria. The back of the bottle is slightly concave and is molded with a flower outline. A tiny silver funnel accompanies the bottle in the box. Note the original sale price printed on the box of $3.50. 2.25". $150-200.

Hinged Purse Bottles

Related to the caged purse bottles, hinged bottles are usually made of two completely separate components: the filigree case that is hinged on one side and has a clasp closure on the other, and the bottle itself. A hinged bottle like the first one pictured here is shown in a 1938 Irice ad in Jones-North's book (1999, p. 114). Shown in the same ad is a portion of what appears to be a hinged basket. Irving W. Rice imports have the embossed name Irice in the metal base. Some of the inner bottles have caps that are marked with a metal tag.

Pictured in an ad from 1938 (Jones-North, 1999, p. 114), this hinged bottle has the Irice mark in the metal of the base. The inner bottle has a plain cap and lifts free of the base. The case is 2" in height. $200-300.

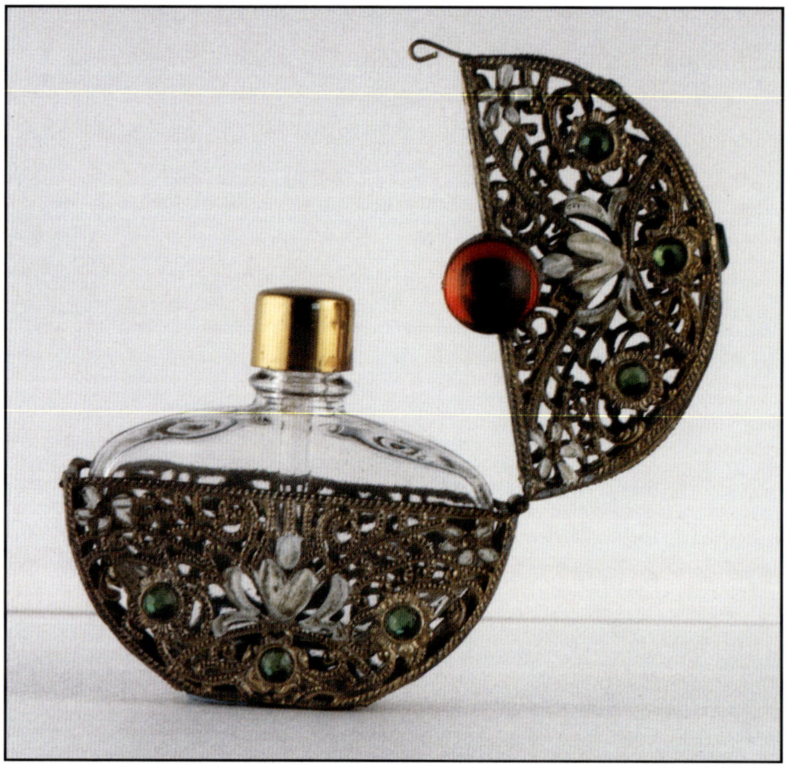

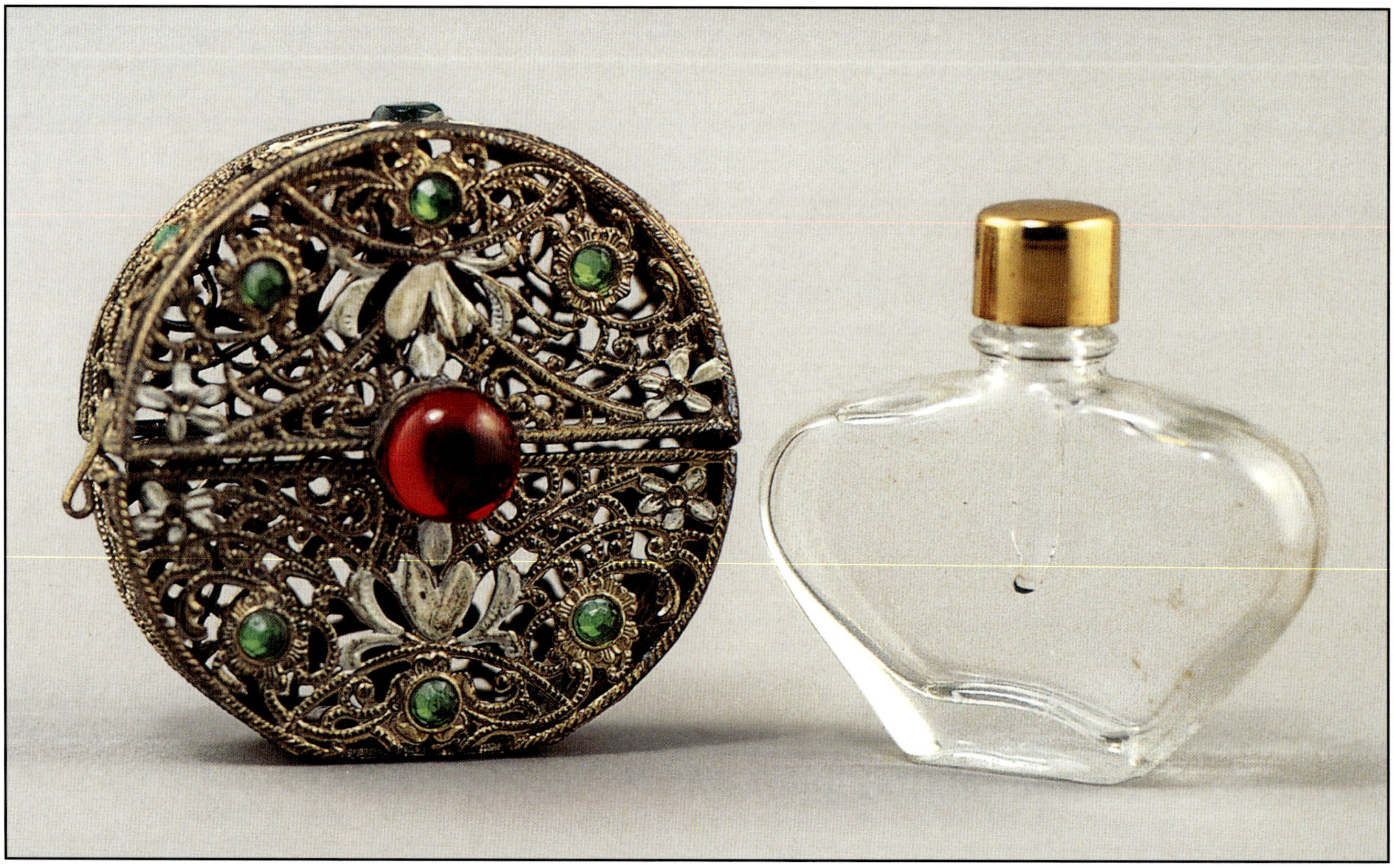

Three views of another hinged bottle decorated with a pink carved rose and pink stones. The inner bottle has a pink "moonstone" capstone. The bottle neck is metal covered: the cap is marked. 2". $300-350.

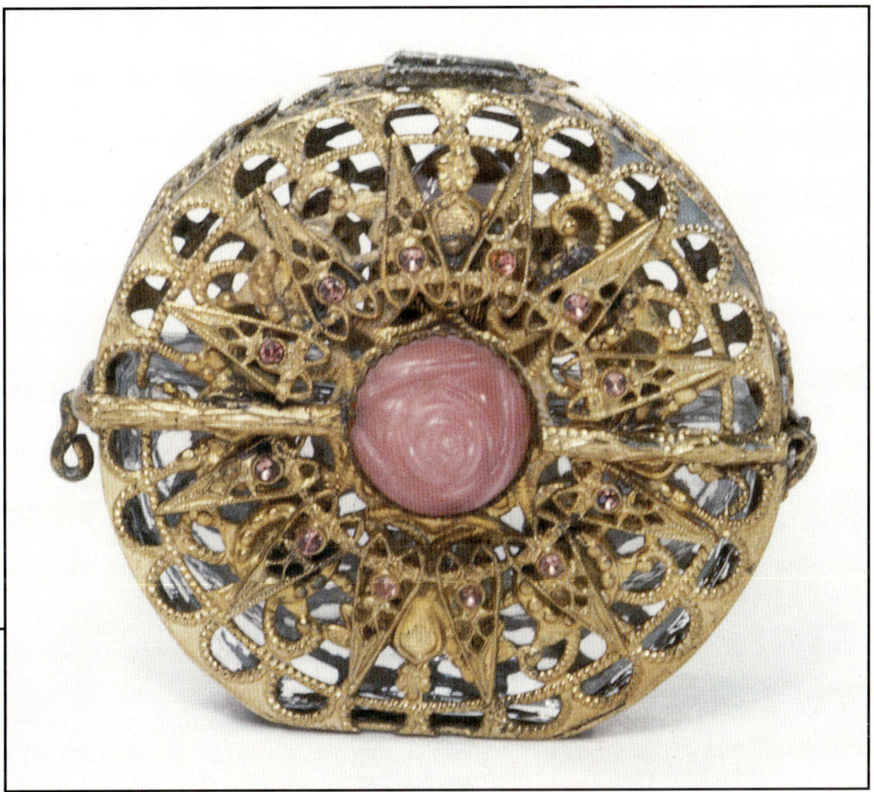

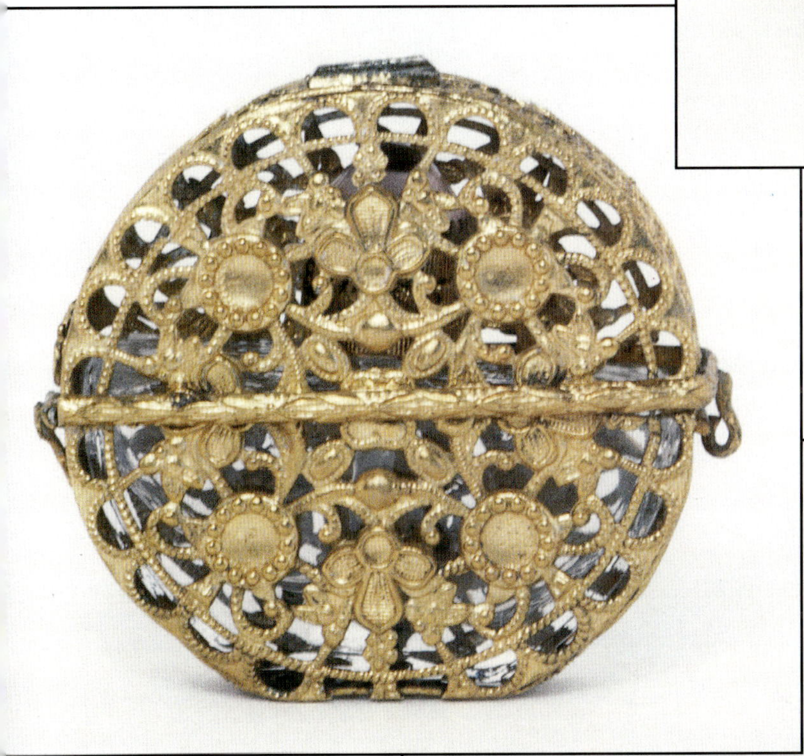

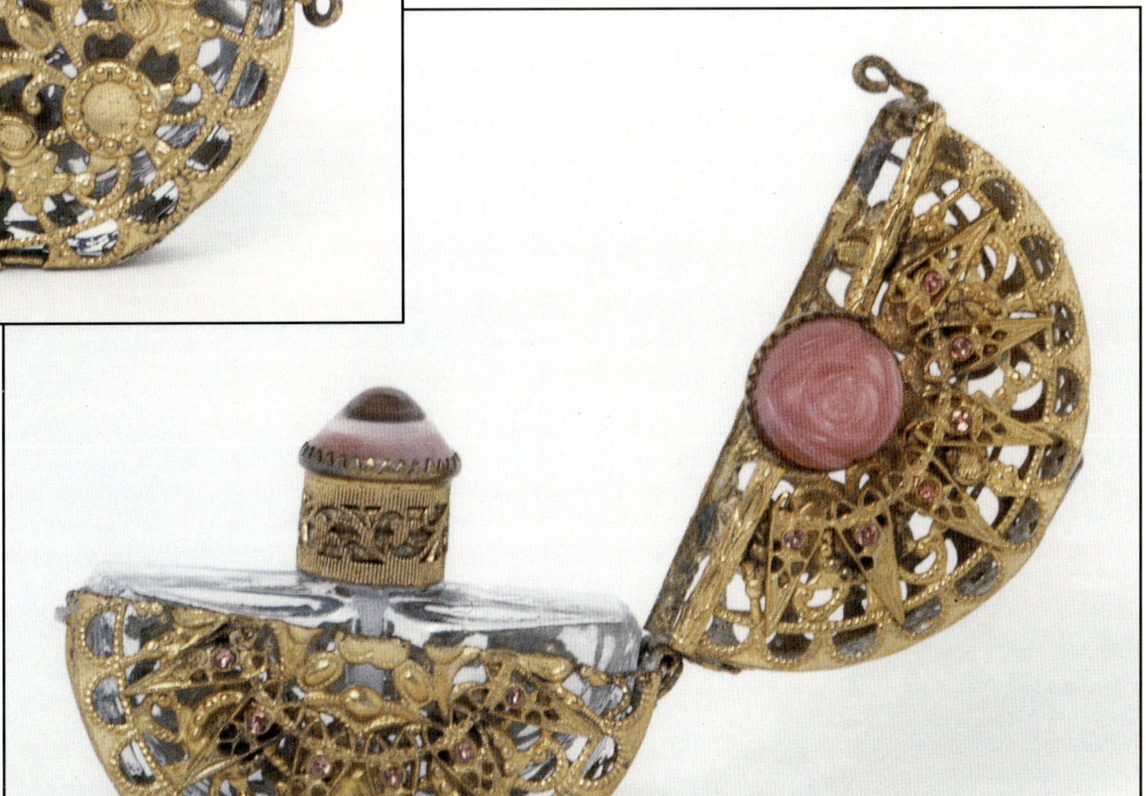

Footed hinged bottle holder. Decorated with green, turquoise, and cobalt blue stones, this 2" case is marked "Irice" in the base. This same caging was sold with other colored "gem" combinations. $150-200.

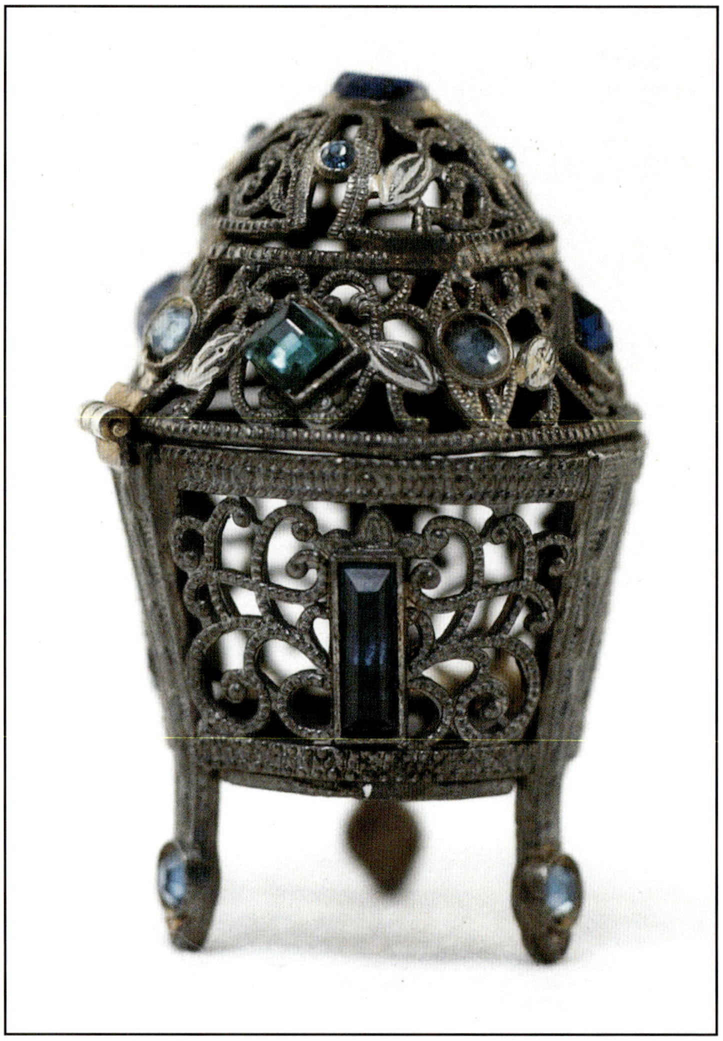

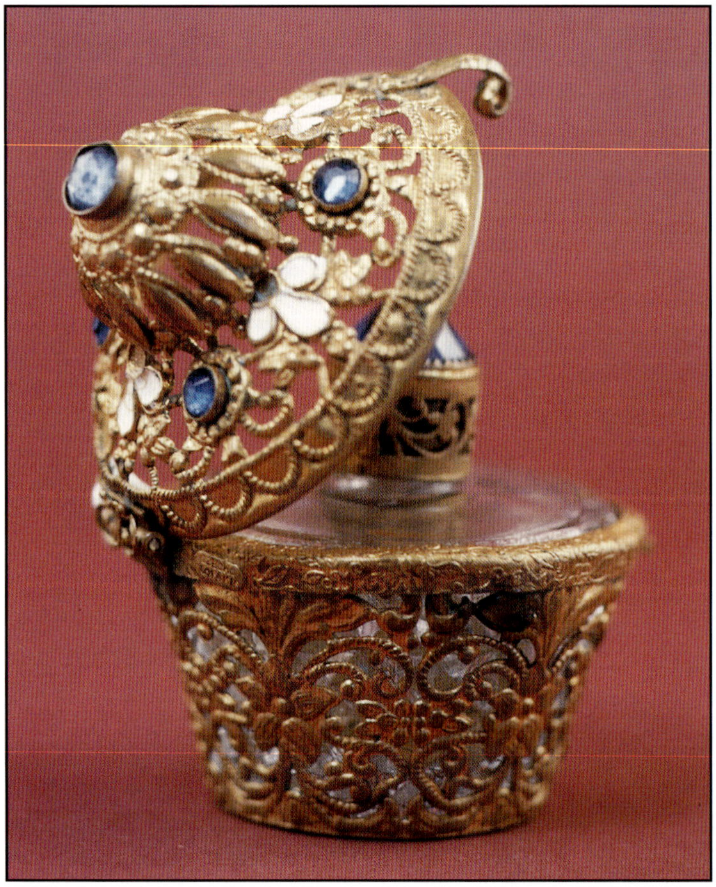

Hinged basket. The basket and the inner cap are both marked " Czechoslovakia." The basket crimps over the bottle, fixing it in place. 2". $275-325.

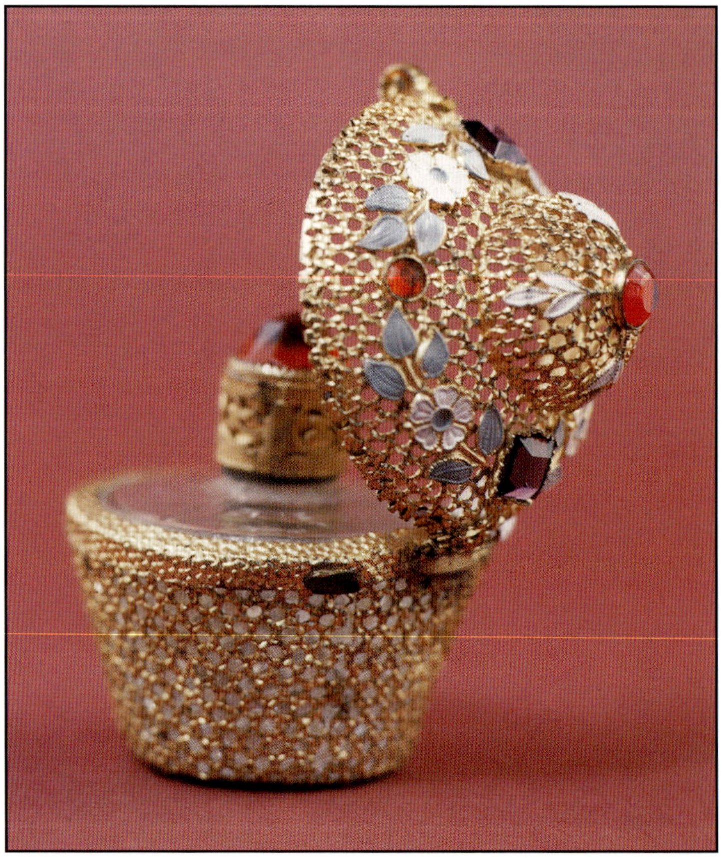

Trapped in a metal mesh basket embellished with enamel work plus amethyst and ruby gems, bottle and basket are both marked (also pictured in the 1938 ad, Jones-North, 1999, p. 114.). 2". Very rare. $300-400.

Related to the hinged bottles are solid metal holders with covers connected to the holder by a delicate-looking chain. The holders originally contained a glass vial with a glass stopper with a long glass dauber. The holders are marked in the neck, "MADE IN CECH.SLOV." The small round holder shown with its tiny glass vial is marked, "MADE IN FRANCE."

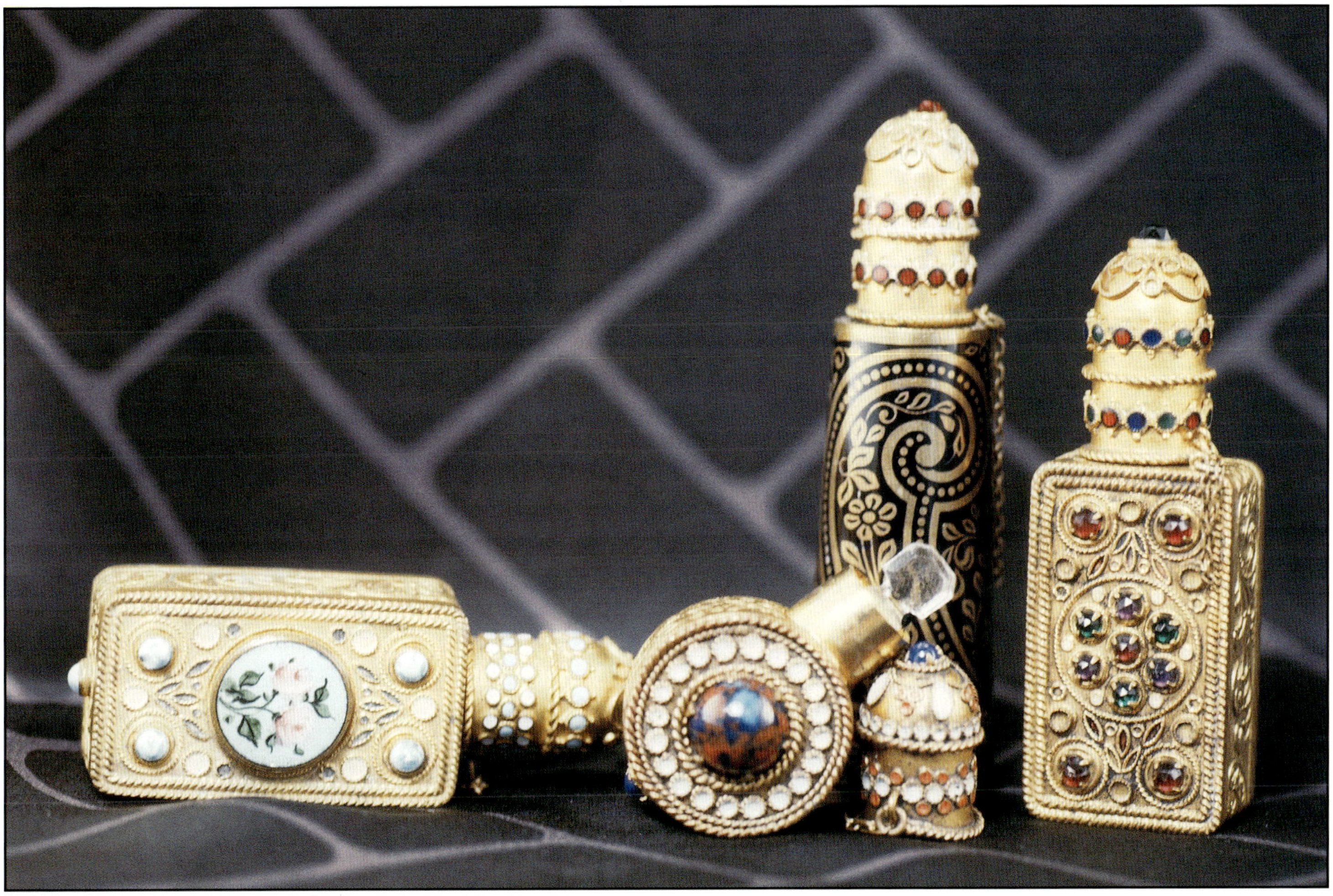

Perfume vial holders. These bottles, with their covers held by a delicate chain, covered and protected a small glass vial with glass stopper. Left: Rose enameled medallion featured opaque and mottled turquoise stone. The dots on the cover are enameled. 2.625". Back center: Black swirled enameling on brass. Red enameling on the cover, red glass gem on the top. Filigree applied to the cover. Right: Multi-colored glass stones are set into the front and back of this case. The cover has multi colored enameled work and a red glass capstone. Both this and the center bottle have open work on the bottom. 2.375". All three are marked in the neck "MADE IN CECH.SLOV." $125-175 each. Front center: This smaller bottle cover is clearly related to the other three cases, but is marked "France." 1.75". $200-250.

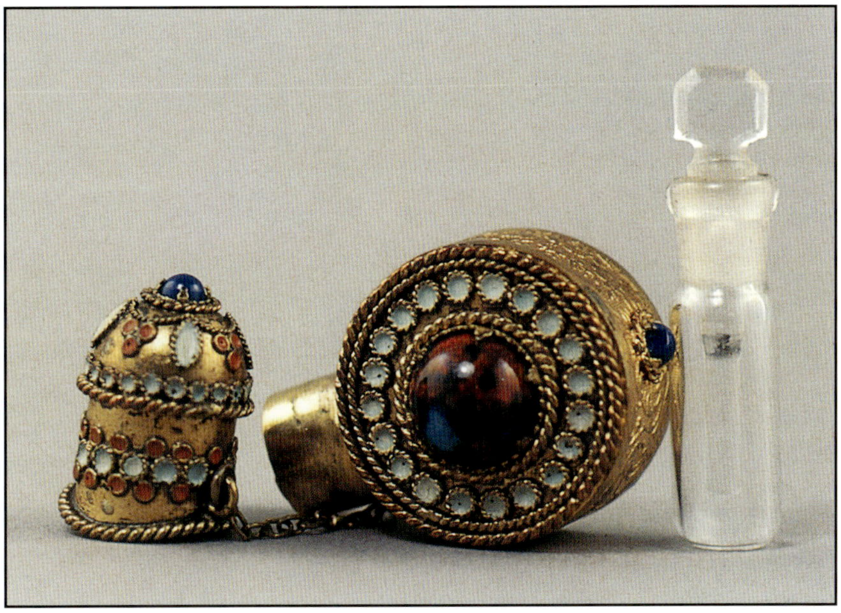

Another view of the smaller bottle cover marked "France," shown with its vial and stopper.

Shown here because it shares some characteristics with the vial holders is a unique round, single-footed metal bottle. The enamel work is similar and the cobalt glass sets feature painstakingly applied detailing. The five pearls are prong set. The cap unscrews for applying perfume, and the neck base unscrews for filling the bottle. It is unmarked, and though it resembles the Czech holders, its origin is unknown.

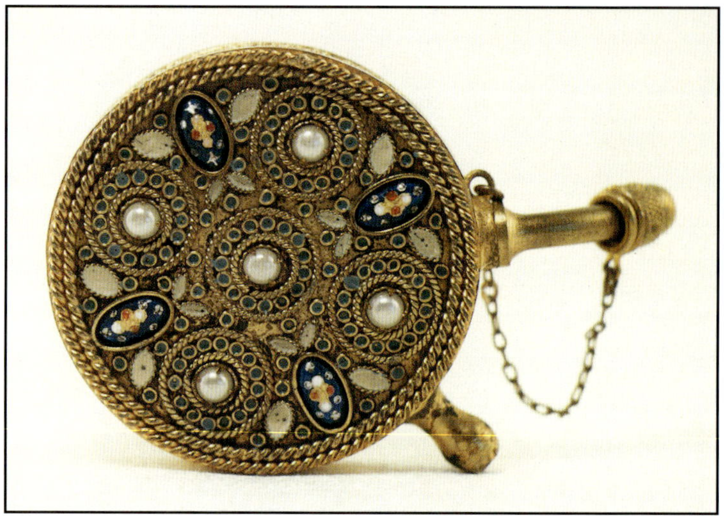

Unmarked, this unusual bottle remains a mystery. It shares some characteristics with the previous covers. The pearls are prong-set, the blue beads, which are lamp worked with applied glass dots, are bezel set. The enamel work is similar to the Czech and French holders. The neck unscrews for filling.

Jaco Bottles

Thanks to Donna Everitt, a perfume bottle collector from Indiana, this book contains a copy of a brochure from Jablonex Czechoslovak Export Company Ltd., or "Jaco." This product catalog, dated between 1953 and 1961 (when the company used that name), shows pictures of forty-eight purse or dresser bottles. Three types of caps are pictured here, which we now know were still being used after the nationalization of the industry. These are the "cut-away" cap that is the most commonly found on purse bottles, a "leaf and berry garland" cap, and a plain (non-jeweled) "coin and bangle" cap. Though most of the caps shown apparently do not have metal tags, a few tags can be seen in the brochure pictures. These are round, rather than the usual rectangular tags found on older bottles. The bottles were sold with a paper "hang tag" identifying the company and the country of origin, although few of these "hang tags" remain. The Jaco purse bottles do have metal, threaded necks affixed to the glass, and the screw caps have glass daubers.

The catalog bottles that have the lowest sequence of item numbers, that is, 6 F 23001 through 6 F 23012, are shown as small purse and dresser bottles with cut glass bases. In contrast to most of the other bottles pictured, they are dainty and in the old style. Many have finer filigree and feature a "carved" glass flower medallion. Dresser minis have colored or clear faceted stoppers with daubers; purse bottles have a capstone with a pierced floral design of the same mottled colored glass as the focal stone on the bottle. One of the photographed Jaco bottles from this early sequence has an acid mark in a circle in the polished base.

Several of the bottles pictured in the brochure are made to be worn as jewelry and hang from a bar pin, reminiscent of a popular earlier Victorian style—though the Victorian pin bottles are much smaller and lighter. Even the smallest of the Jaco bottles would have been too heavy to wear from a practical standpoint. Perhaps for that reason, few of these bottles seem to have survived.

The metal encasements for these bottles are generally not enameled. (The exceptions are the card suit and the mushroom bottles.) The designs are bold, large metal flowers with glass leaves or a small cabochon center stone. While a few faceted gems are present, they do not dominate the design and are sometimes completely absent. Themes other than card suits and mushrooms include flowers, sports, birds, insects, and a flying dragon. Though most metal cages are formed over unrefined pressed glass blanks, some have a polished bottom surface or a polished "window" in the design.

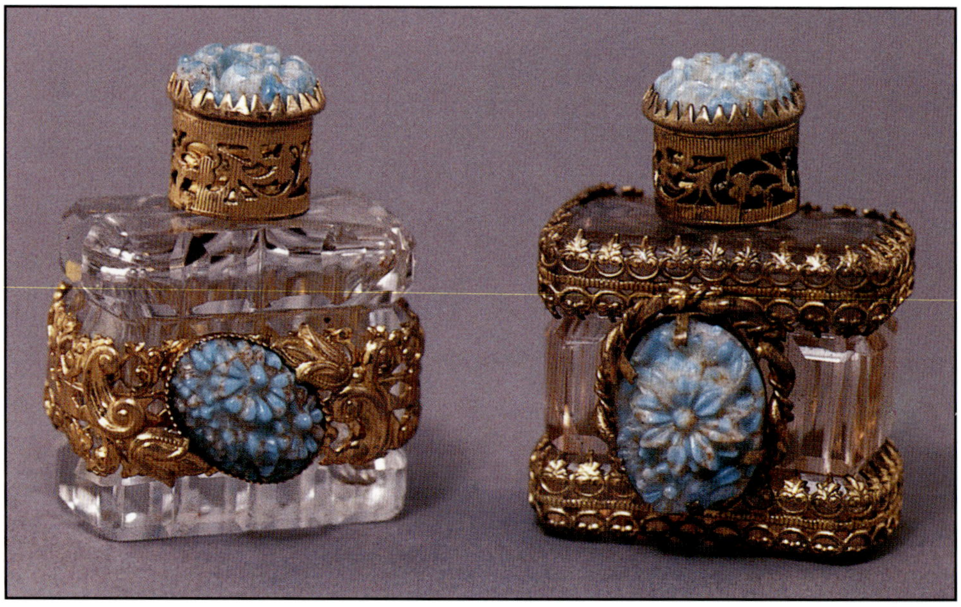

Two Jaco bottles, matching serial numbers 01 and 02 in the catalog. Left: Clear, "ice cube" bottle has a center band with a mottled turquoise glass medallion. 1.625". Right: Pink ice cube cut glass base. A similar medallion is mounted between base and top filigree bands. The base has an acid mark. The capstones on both bottles are pierced, mottled turquoise glass. 1.75". $175-225 each.

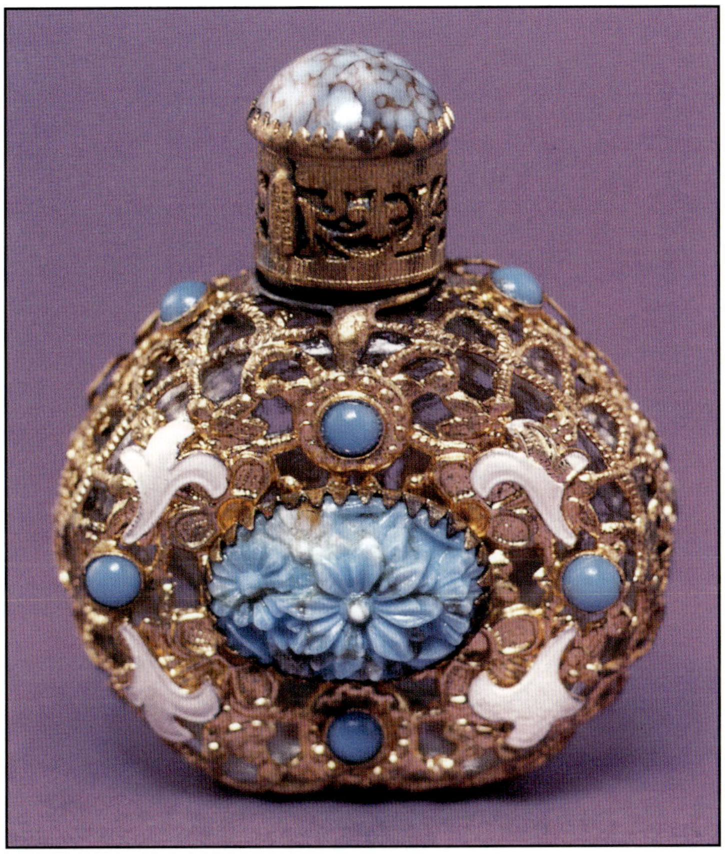

Purse bottle with a medallion of mottled turquoise that is strikingly similar to the one on the previous Jaco bottle. This bottle is marked in the cap. 1.875". $150-200.

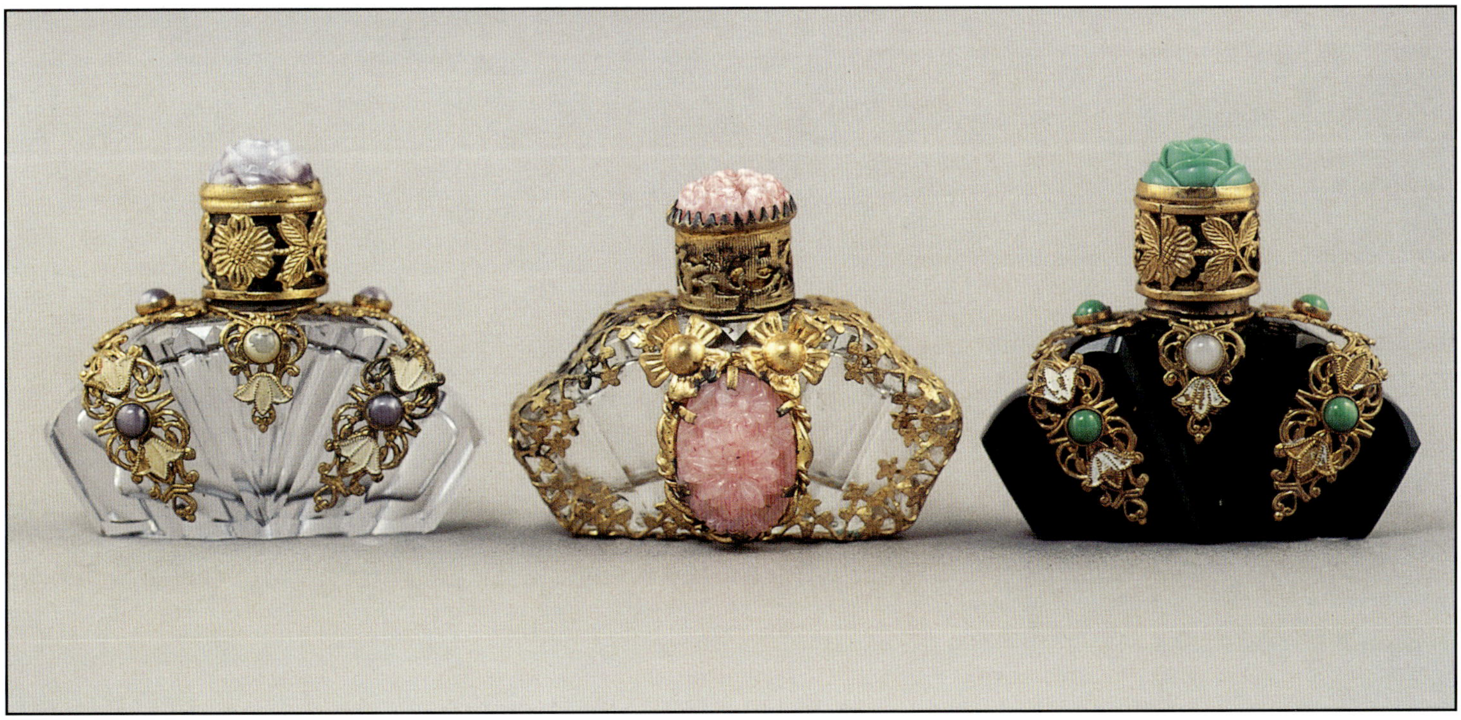

Compared with two early cut glass purse bottles, it is obvious that the Jaco bottle (in the center) came from the same mold. 1.625". $175-225.

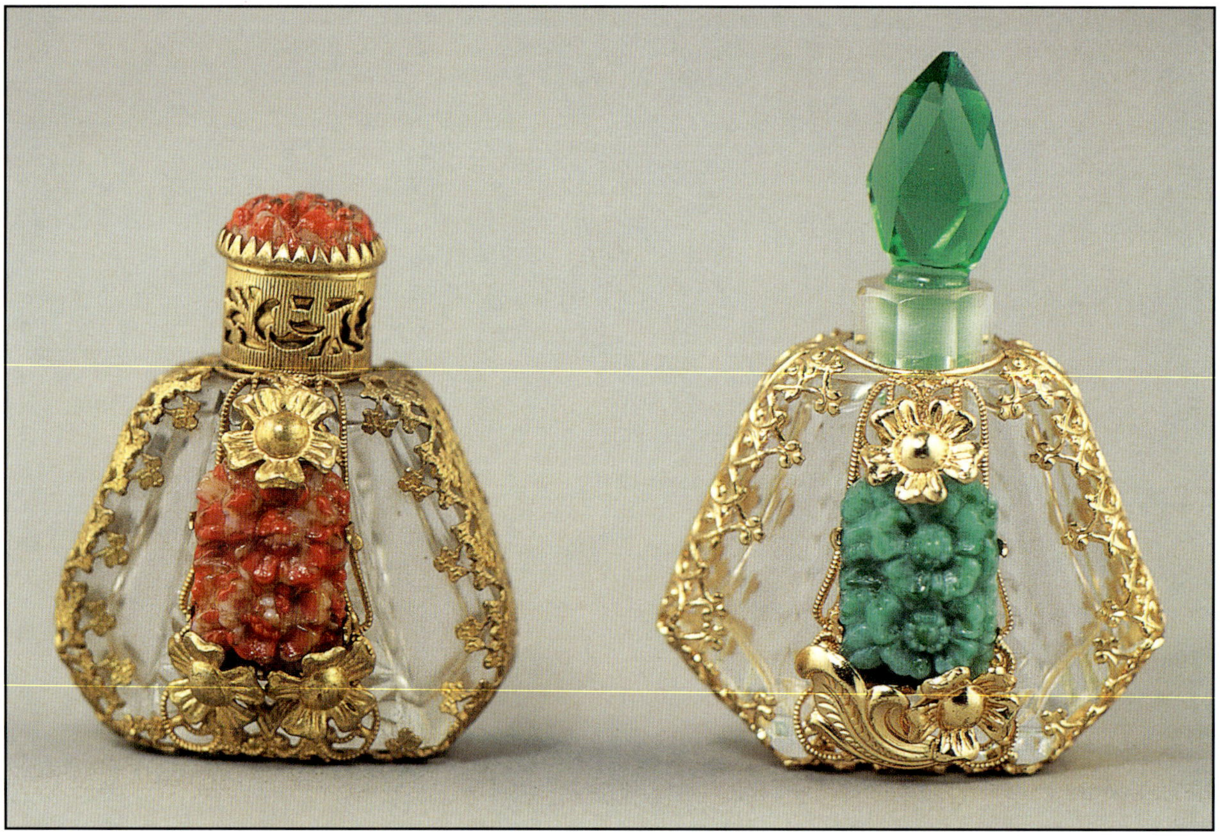

Two clear, cut, Jaco bottles with different top treatments. Left: Red, 1.875". $175-225. Right: Green, 2.375". $175-225.

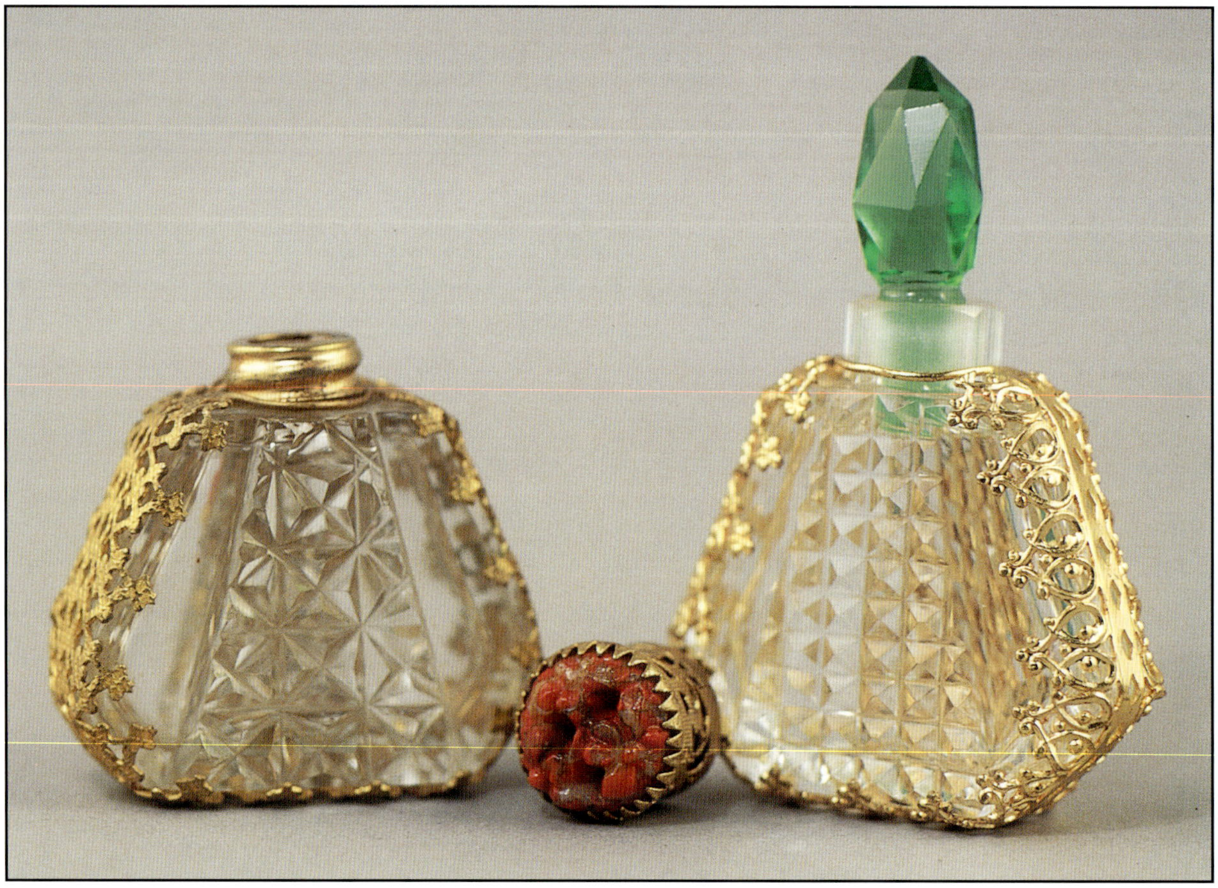

Back view. Note that the center cuts are different.

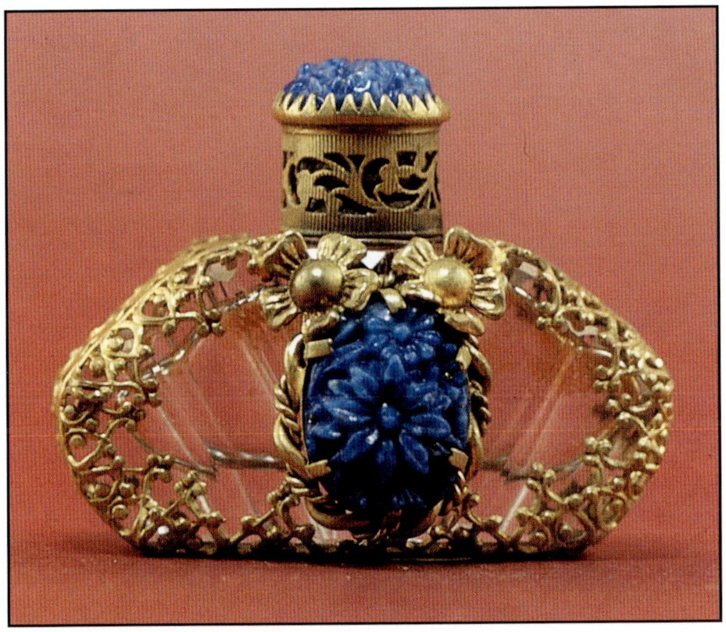

A familiar style, but with lapis. 1.625". *Courtesy of Earline Kopriva.* $175-225.

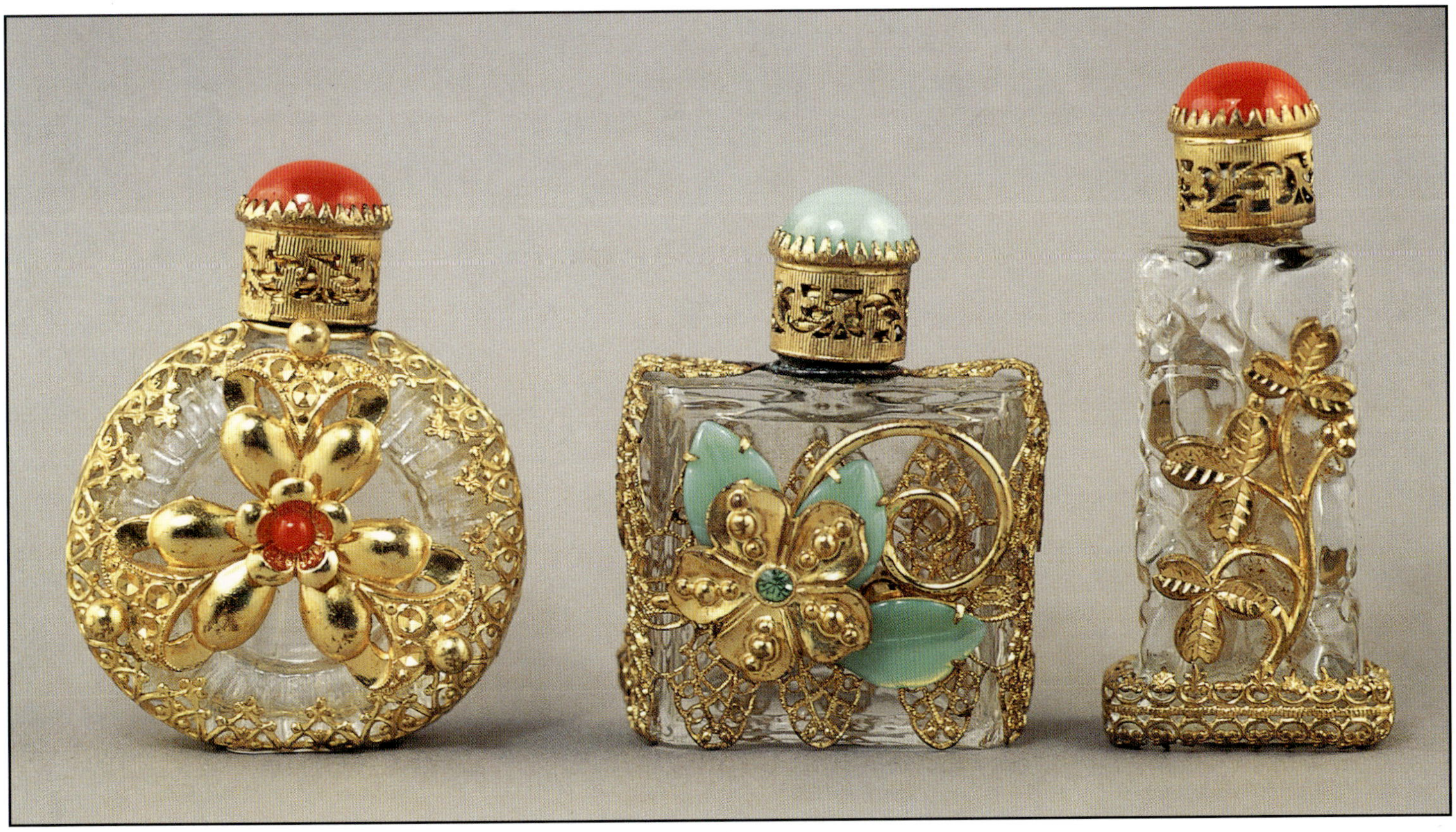

Three caged Jaco purse bottles. Left: Shown on the catalog cover in blue, this bottle has a polished, round window in the back. 2.125". Center: 2" filigree over a rough blank, gold flower has prong-set green glass leaves, matching green capstone. Right: Three-leaf clovers rise from a filigree base over a rough blank. The bottom, however is polished. All of the above have metal necks, daubers. $100-150 each.

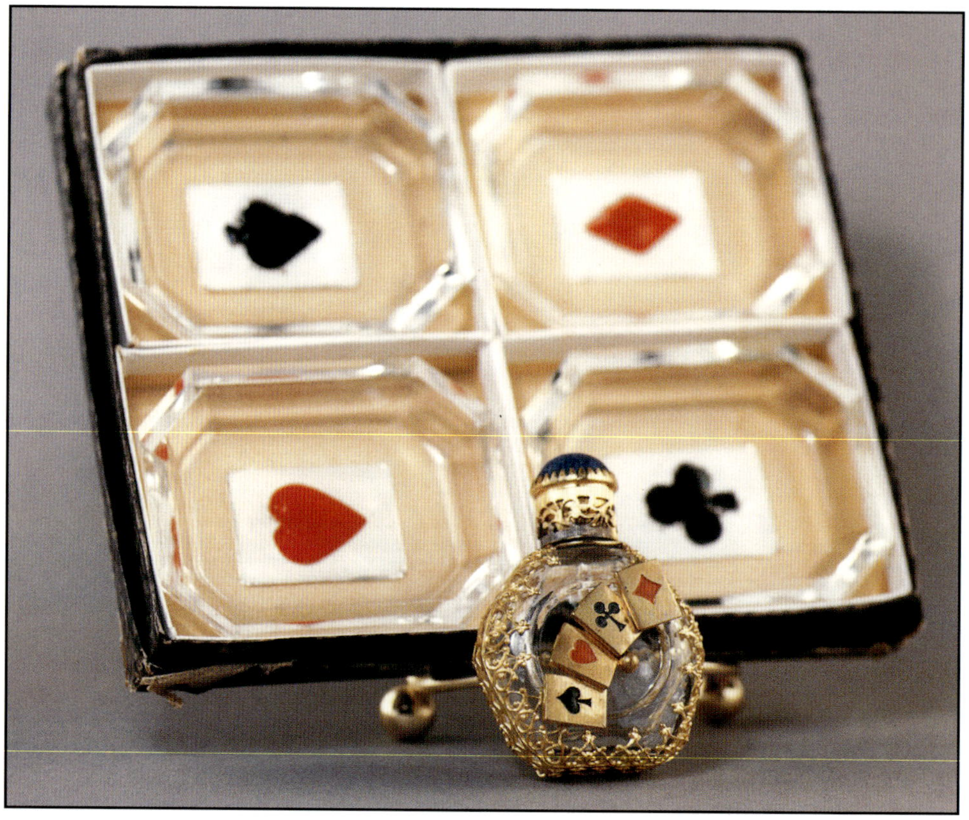

Cards and card suits are a recurring theme. This Jaco card suit bottle is prized by collectors. 2". \$350-400. Shown with a boxed bridge favor or ashtray set. \$50-100.

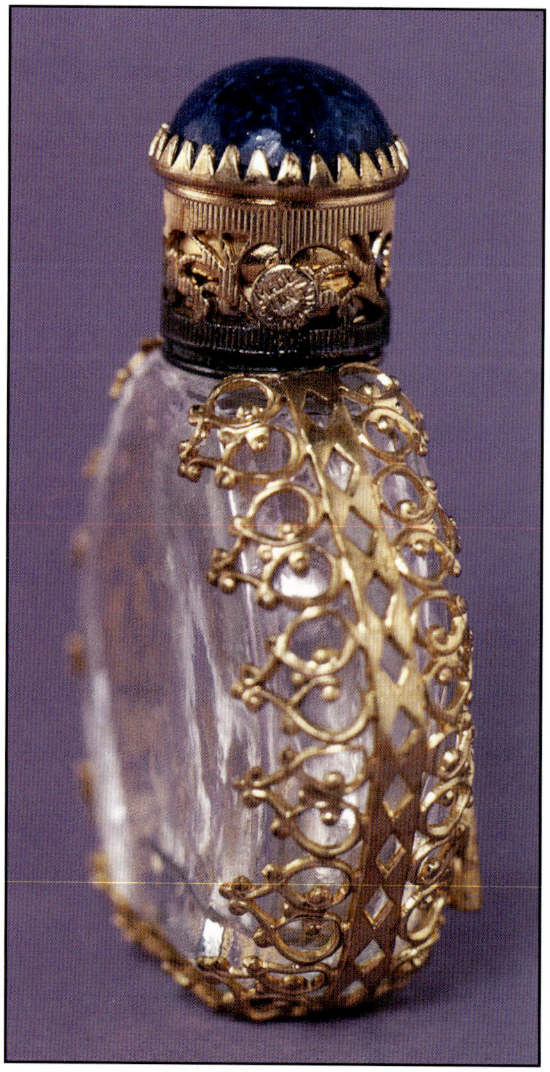

Close up of card suit cap with round metal tag reading "MADE IN CZECHOSLOVAKIA."

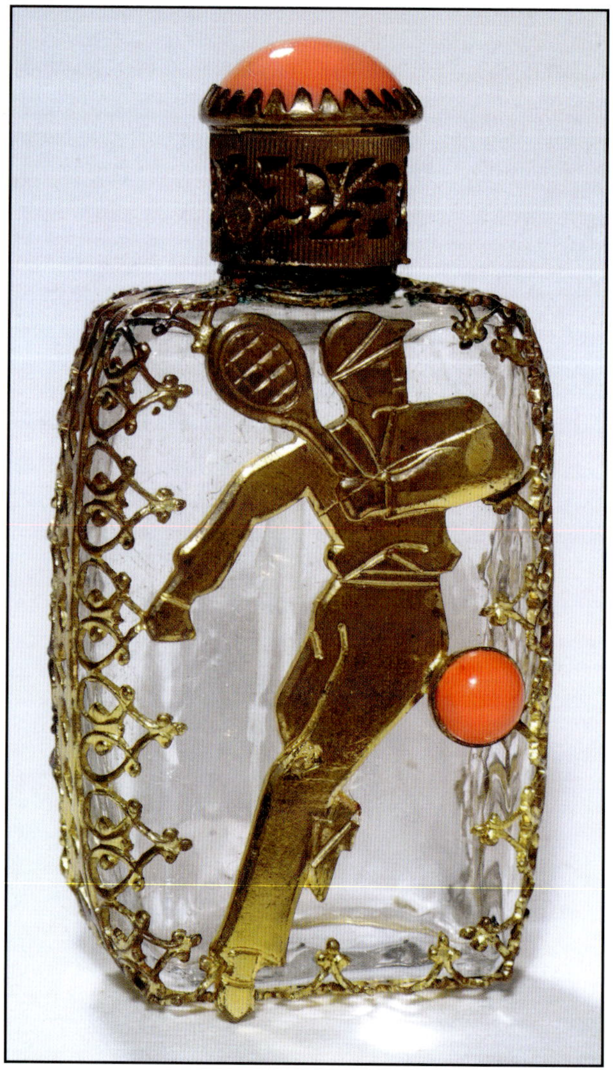

Rare clear glass purse bottle with band of metal filigree and metal tennis player on front with coral glass tennis ball. Filigree screw cap topped with smooth coral jewel. 2.375". *Courtesy of Don Orban. Photo by David Kirk of Kirk Photography.* \$350-400.

Jablonex Catalog

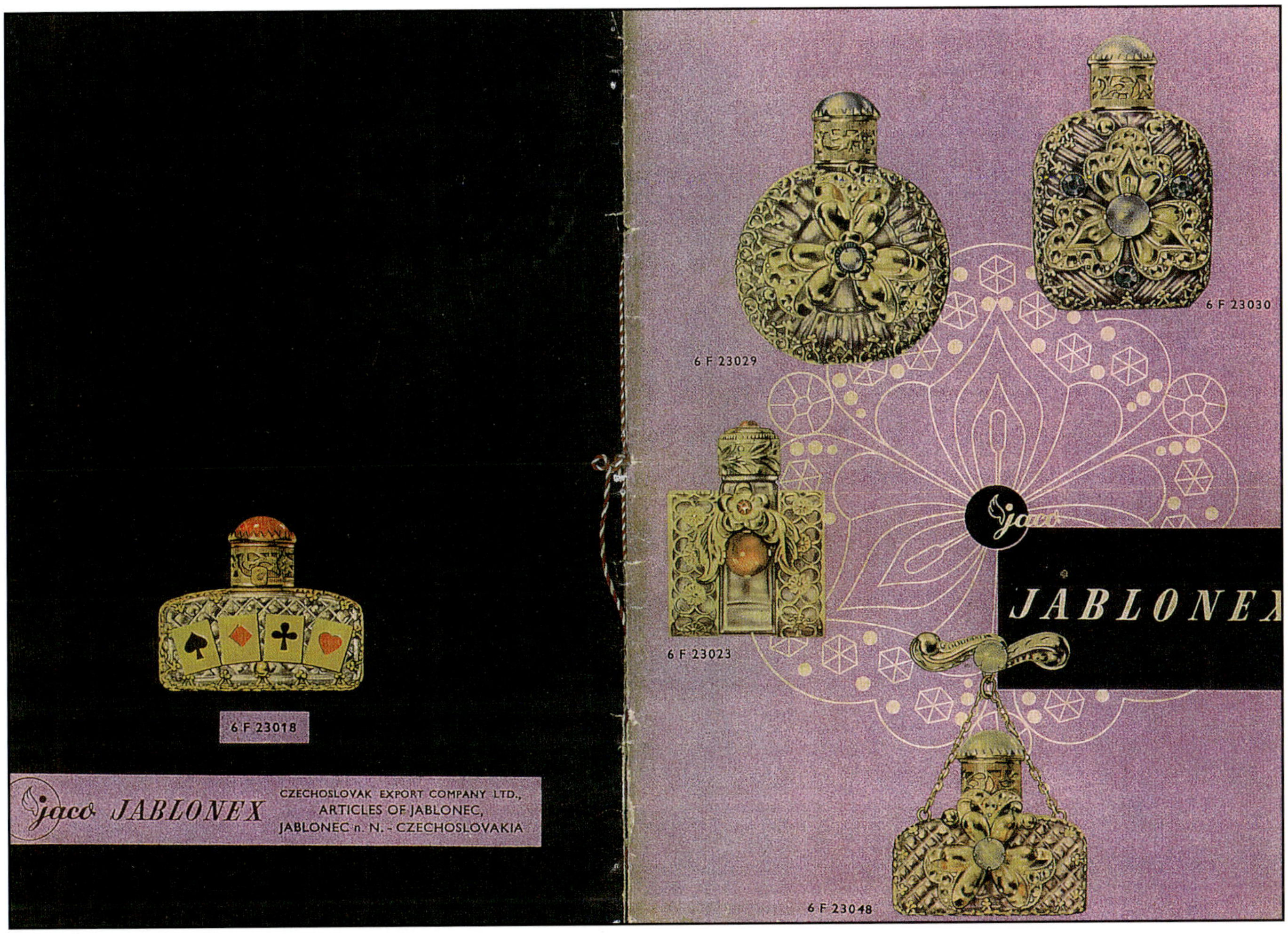

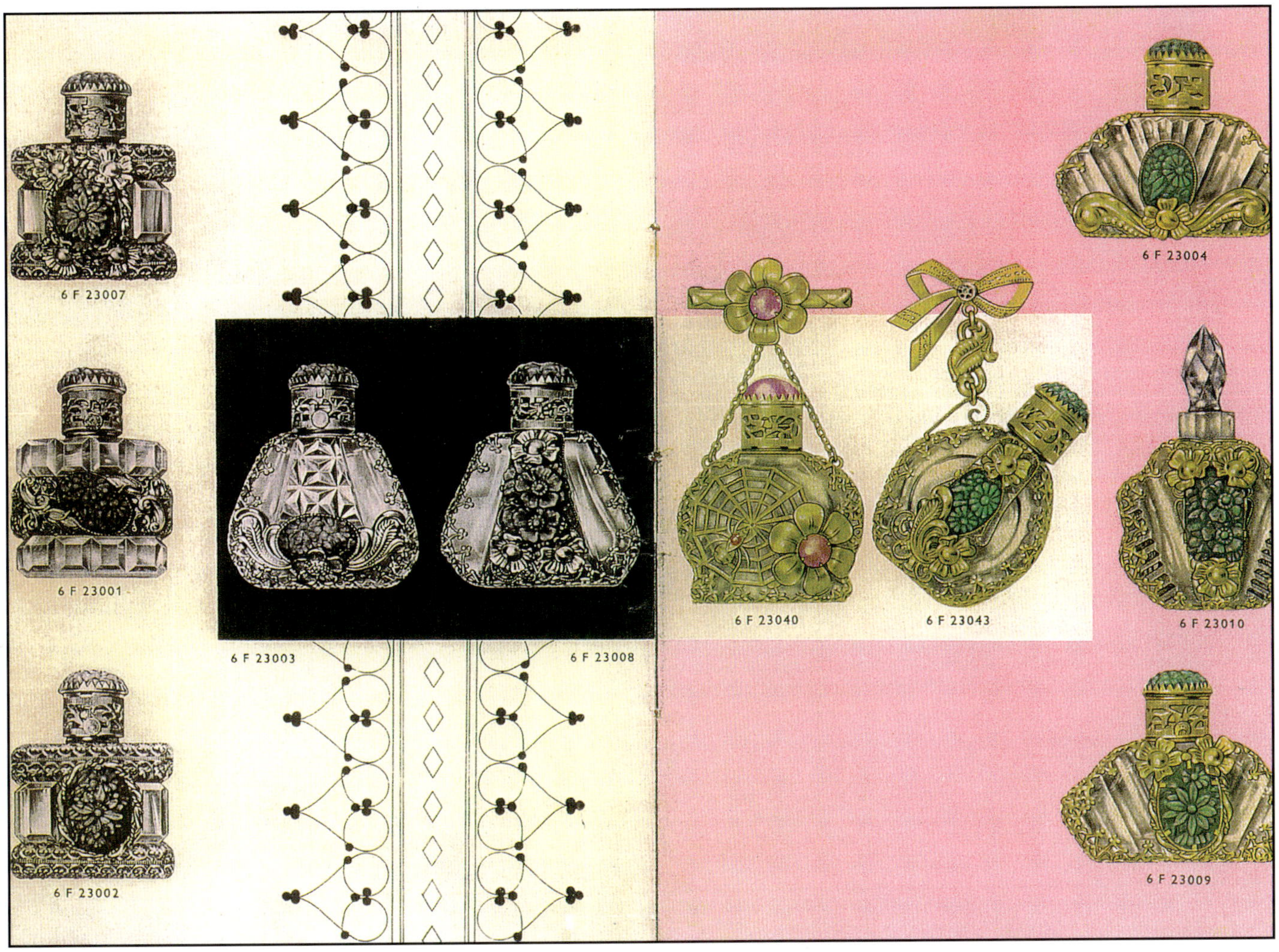

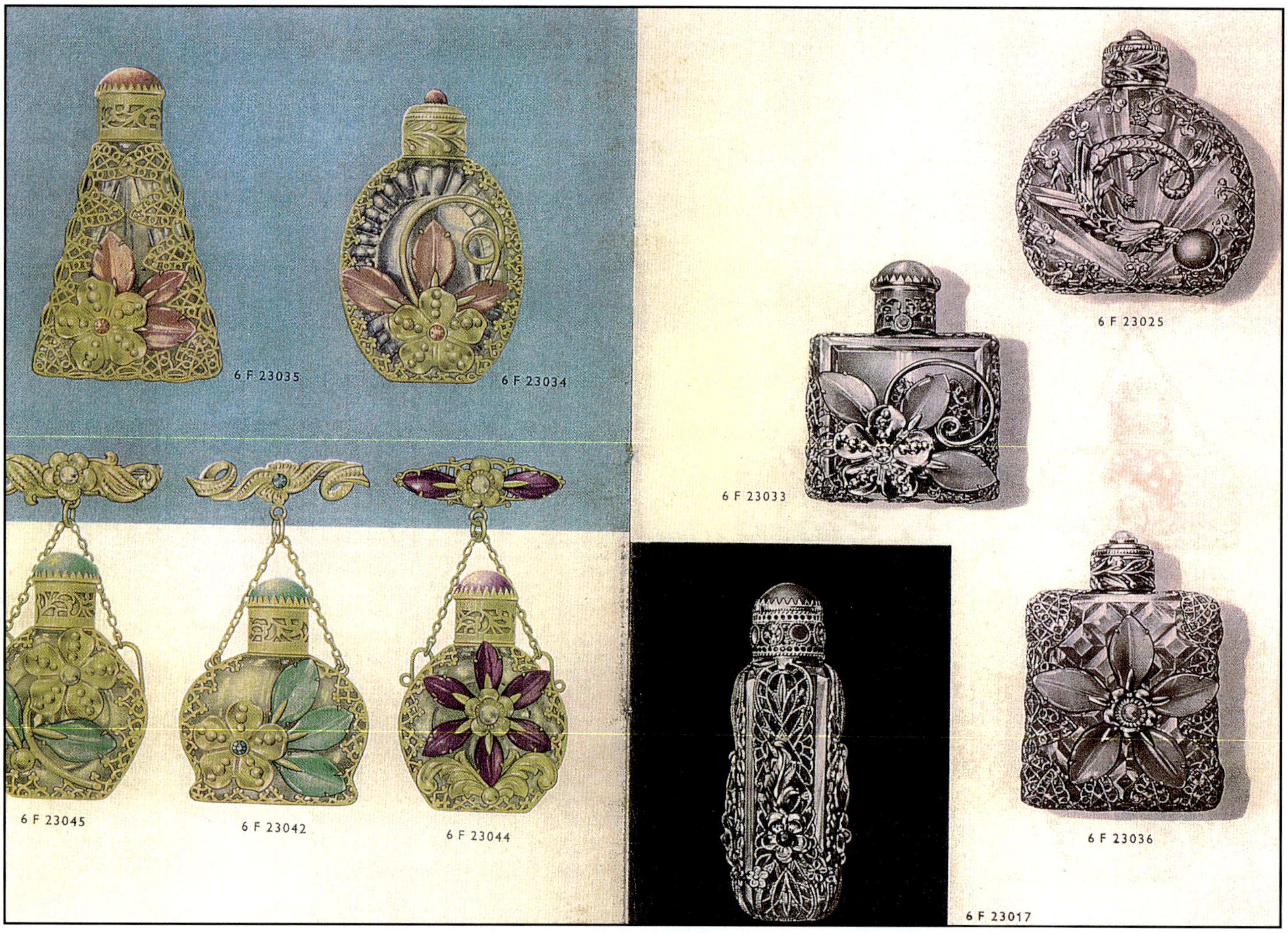
6 F 23035
6 F 23034
6 F 23025
6 F 23033
6 F 23045
6 F 23042
6 F 23044
6 F 23036
6 F 23017

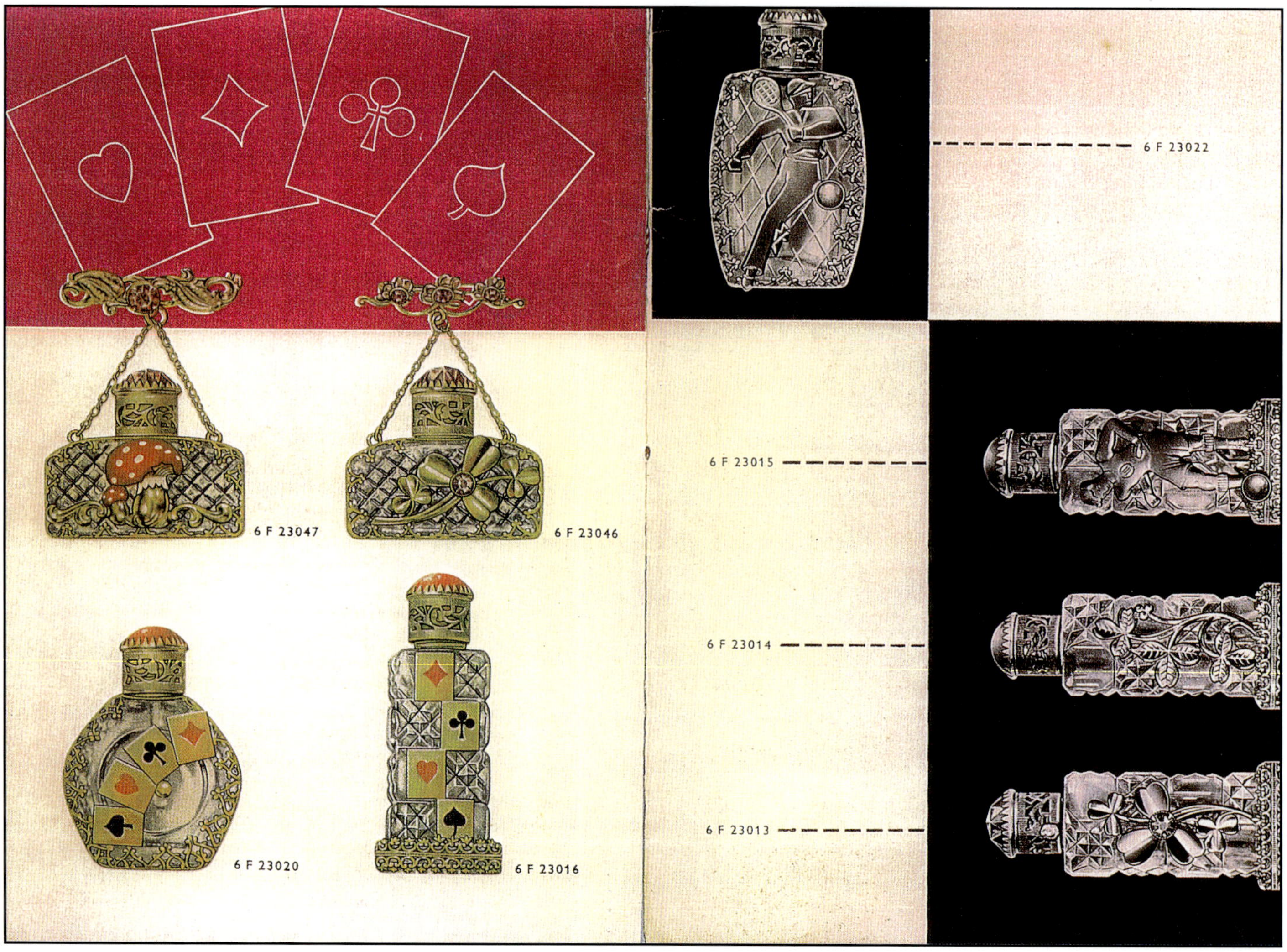
6 F 23022
6 F 23047
6 F 23046
6 F 23015
6 F 23014
6 F 23013
6 F 23020
6 F 23016

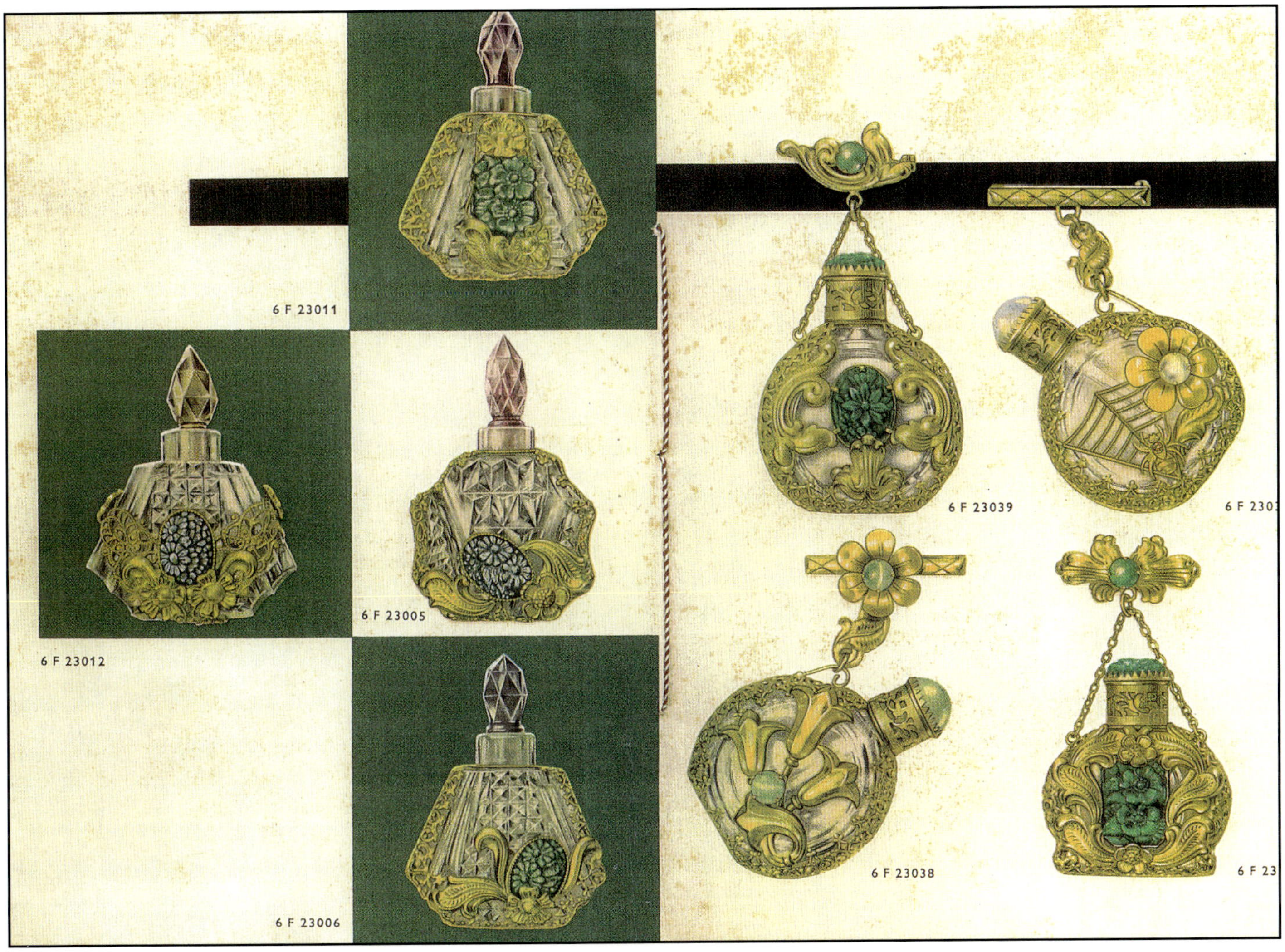
6 F 23011
6 F 23012
6 F 23005
6 F 23006
6 F 23039
6 F 23038

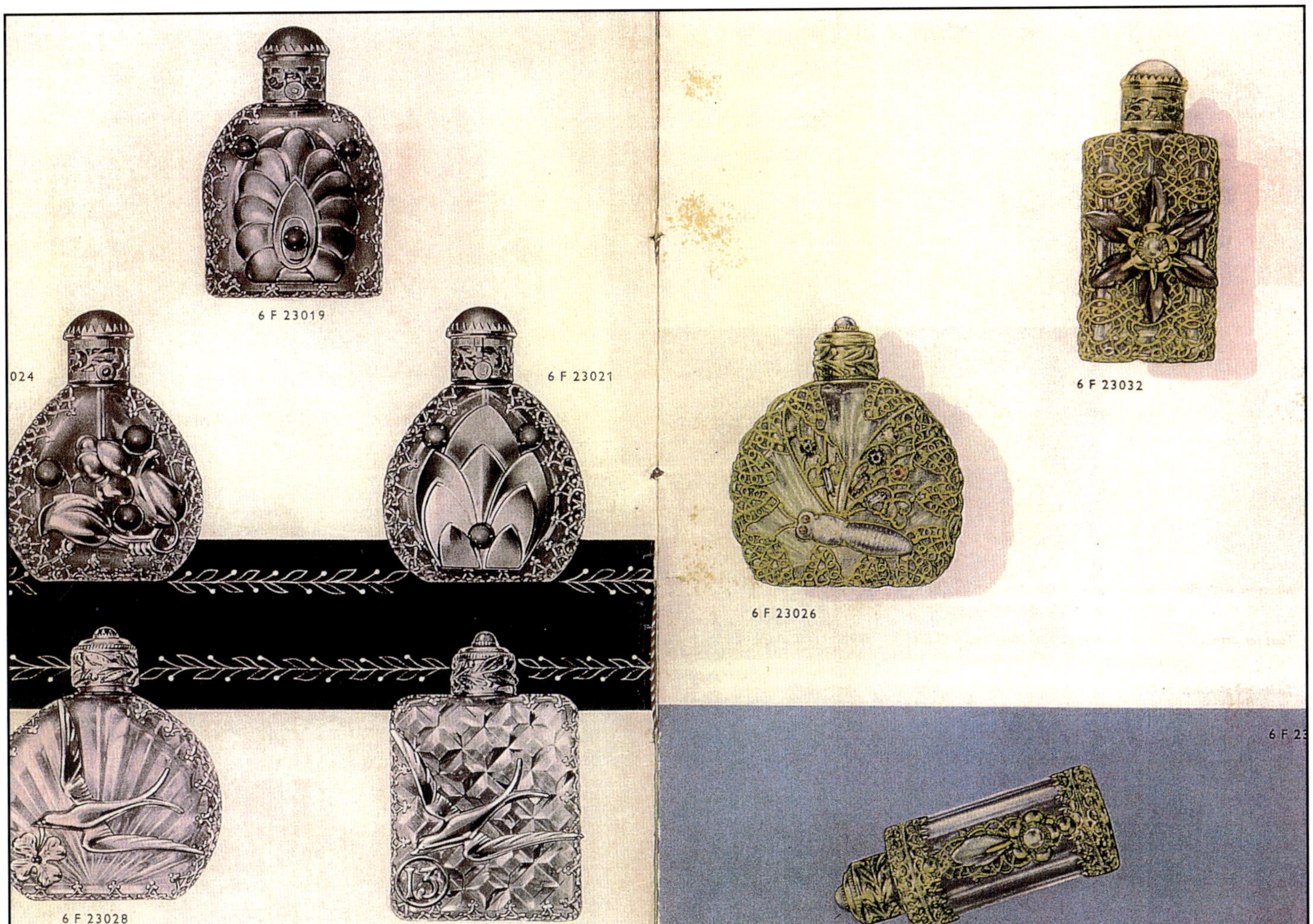
6 F 23019
6 F 23021
6 F 23032
6 F 23026
6 F 23028
6 F 23027

Micro Mini Purse Bottles

Micro bottles can be found on the market, however it is difficult to determine their origin or the era of manufacture. The pictures in this section group some of these bottles as they are commonly attributed. A few were marked permanently or still have tags or labels, which helps narrow the range of possibilities. Many of the bottles pictured have a finger ring or a bar pin clasp and could be worn. Some are for carrying in a purse.

The bottles pictured in the first picture are all unmarked. They are shown with a six-inch ruler to give perspective. Most have been speculated to be Czechoslovakian or Austrian because of the lacy filigree and jewel work. In the top row, the middle bottle is stamped in an identical pattern to the middle bottle two rows below it. The top bottle is finer, encasing black glass. It has tiny red brilliants in the enameled flower centers. The lower bottle encases a clear bottle base. The red dot flower centers are enameled.

The left bottle in the second row from the top has a hinge holding the filigree over a small round mirror. The middle bottle has a blue central medallion with a courtly couple in gold. The left bottle in the third row from the top is shaped like an acorn, with the gold colored acorn cap decorated with a spattering of tiny green gems. Its counterpart on the right in the same row was purchased from a dealer in Prague.

On the bottom row, left, the filigree is as delicate as a spider web and the cabochon stones are an unusual intense orange, not a color typical in Czech stones. On the far right in the bottom row, the bottle has heavier, more modern looking filigree and is more reminiscent of the 1950s Jaco styles.

Most of these bottles could be purchased for from $50 to $100.

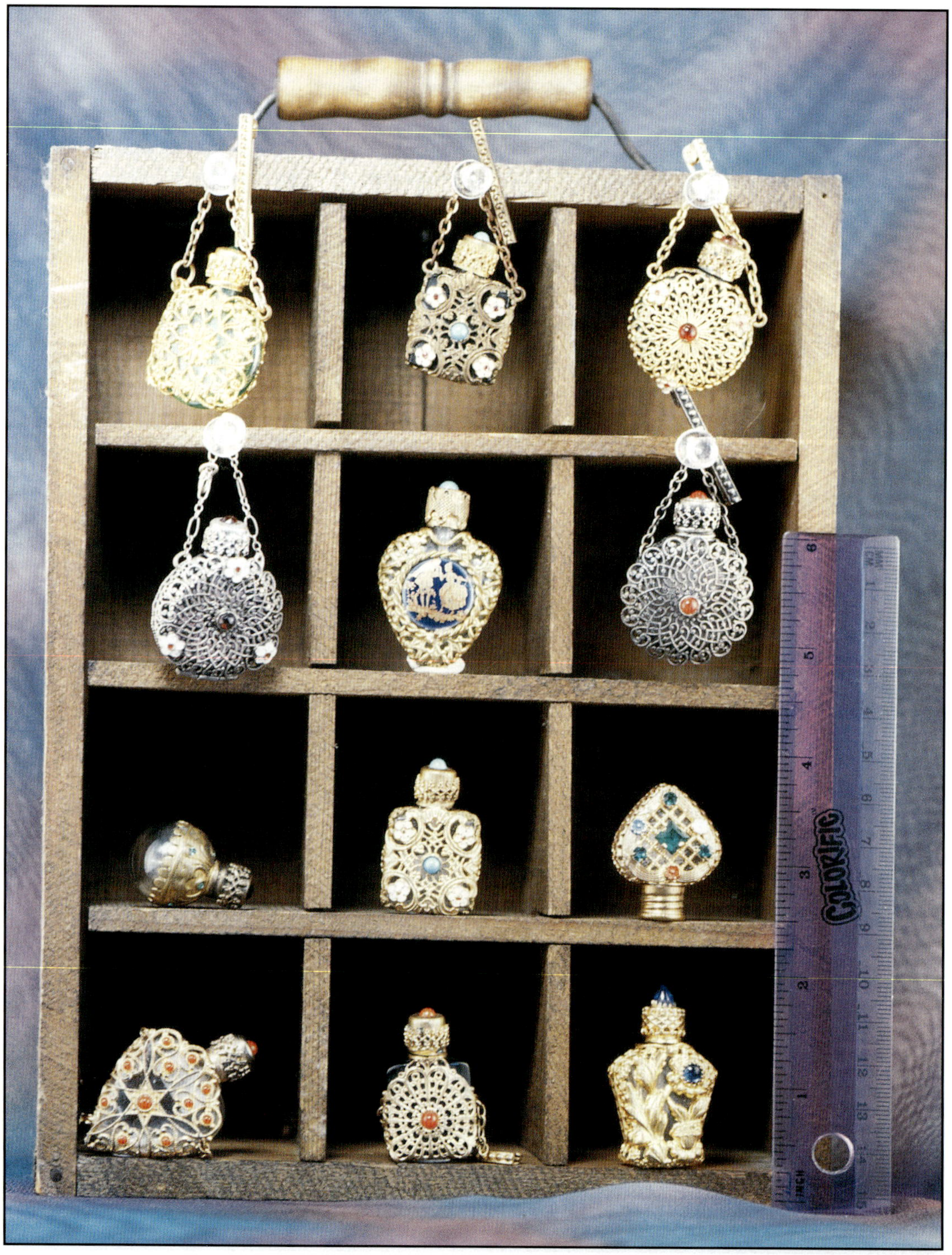

Pictured next is a menagerie of bottles with petit point stitchery patterns. The hang tags shown on two declare them to be made in Austria. The hand mirror is unmarked, but very fine and purchased from a dealer in Prague.

Most of these bottles have a clear plastic protective cover over the fronts. Those with black backgrounds do not have the cover, nor does the largest bottle with white background. The mirror is covered. Bottles in this grouping range in value from $25 to $125.

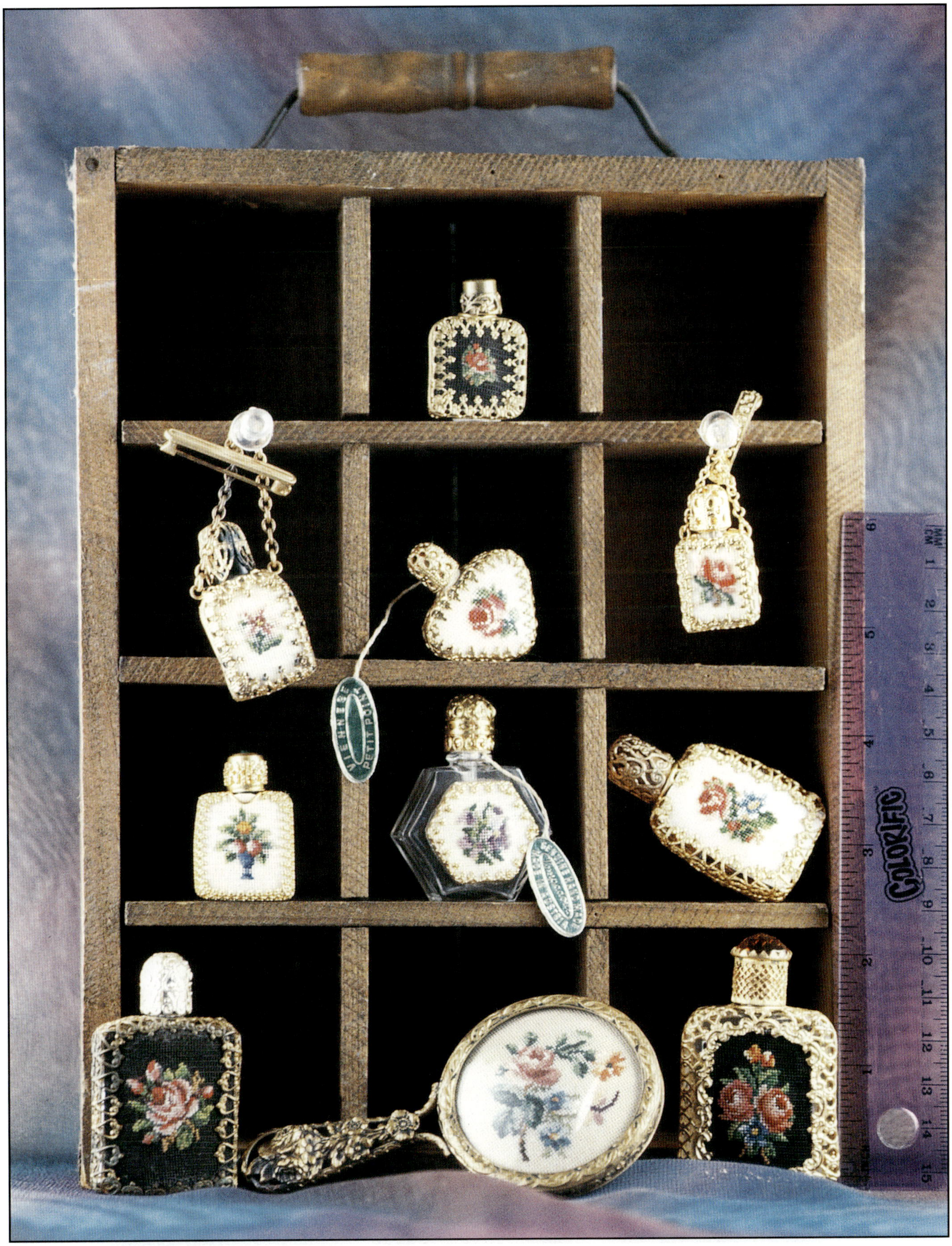

In the next group, the two larger black bottles are from the same mold. The one with the dog has a label on the back reading "Geneve." In the second row from the top, the bottle on the left is marked "Limoges France." The center bottle has no markings, but has a similar medallion on the back. The bottle on the right is loose in its silver-appearing caging. It is unmarked. All the other bottles are marked "France" in raised letters in the glass base. The value range is $50 to $125 each.

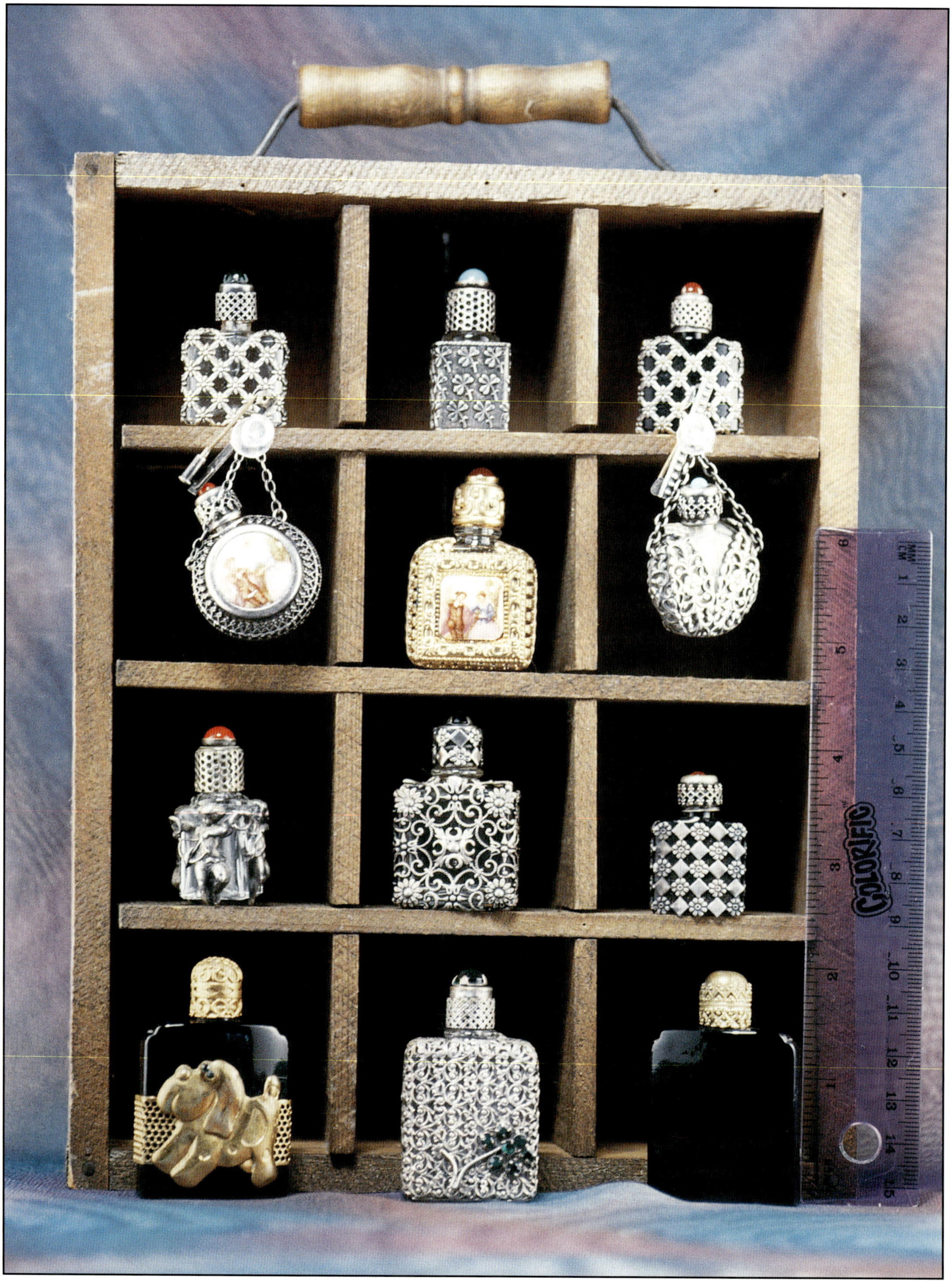

This final grouping highlights small bottles from Germany. In the top row, the bronze-helmeted bottle on the left is unmarked, but its complementary companion on the right has a silver tag on the back of the filigree that reads, "Western Germany." The vial in the center is marked "Germany" in the cap.

The second row from the top holds marked vials on the left and right. The orange heart-shaped bottle with pink rose decals, hand painted embellishments, and mercury dauber is unmarked.

The bottom row contains three identically shaped bottles with different refining finishes. The bottle on the right, with the bird in a branch, is marked "Germany." The other two are unmarked. Values range from $35 to $125.

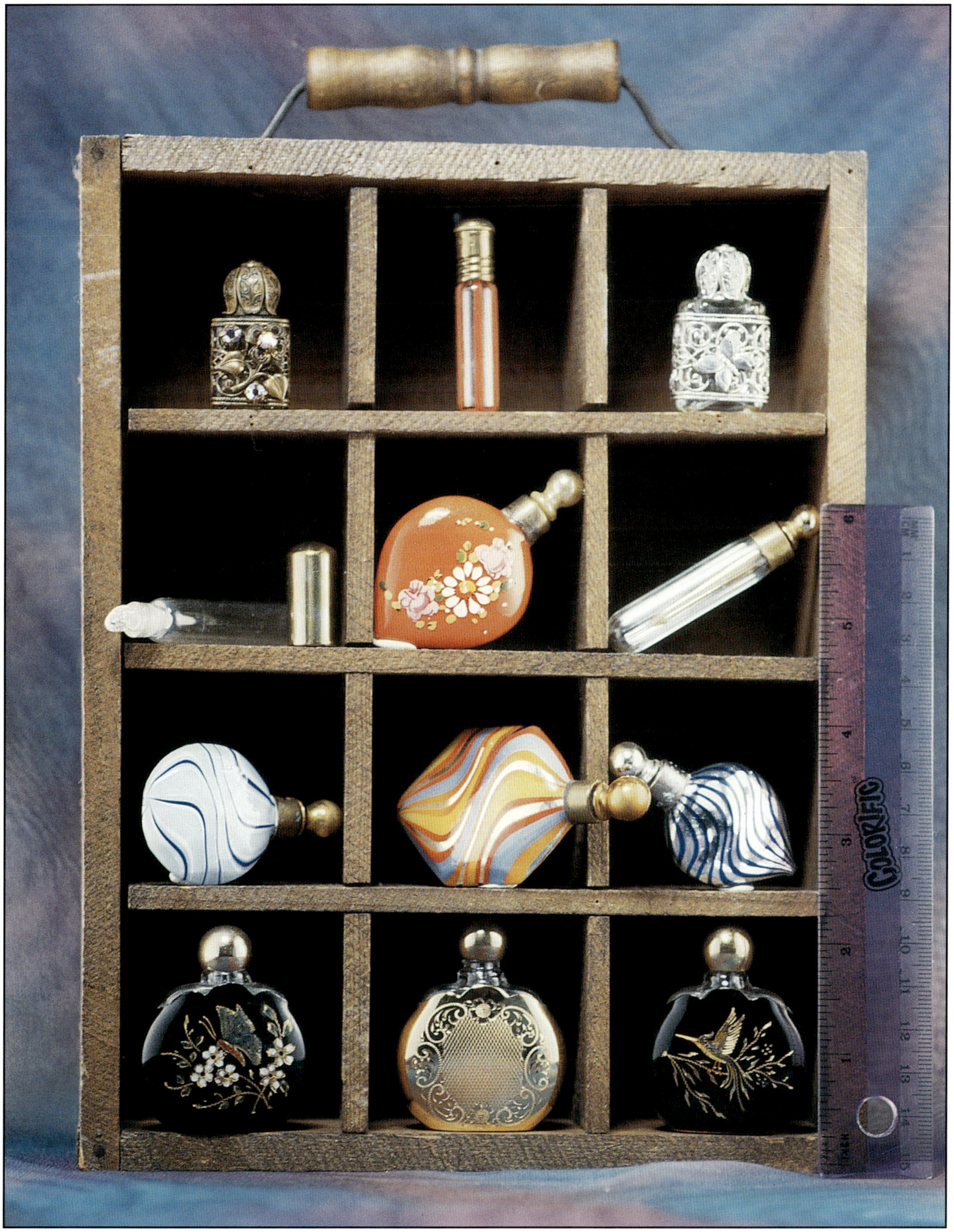

Teal bottle with a hinged top and stopper hangs from a finger ring. Marked with a paper sticker. 1.75". $200-300.

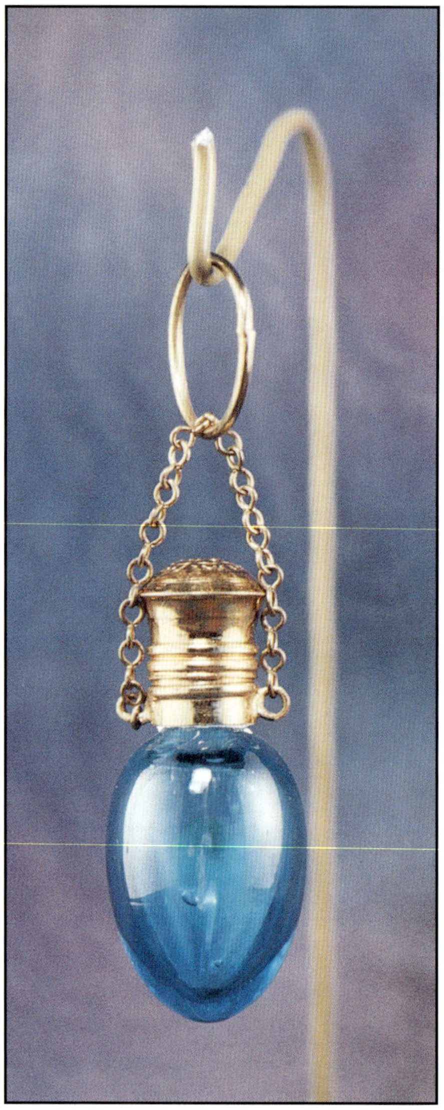

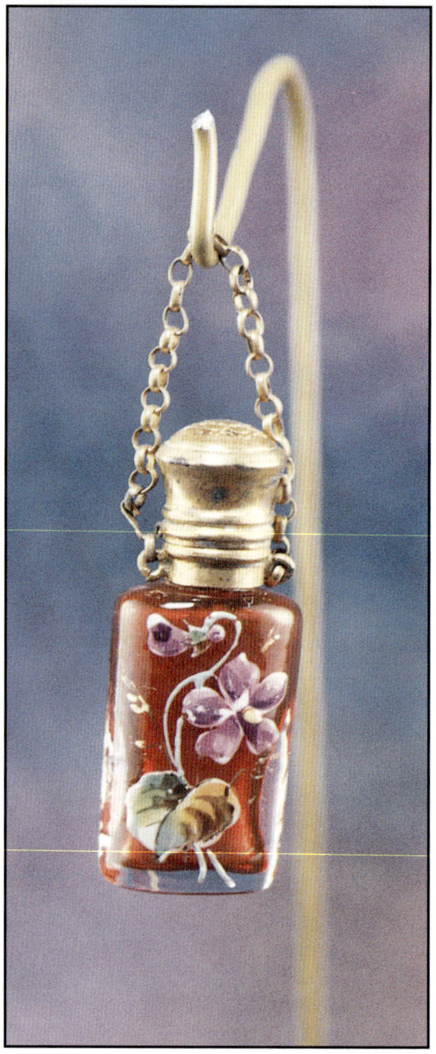

Clear cased over red, enameled violet spray, hinged top with chain, inner stopper. 1.875". $300-500.

Iridized green bottle with enameled violets, hinged top, and finger ring. 2". $300-500.

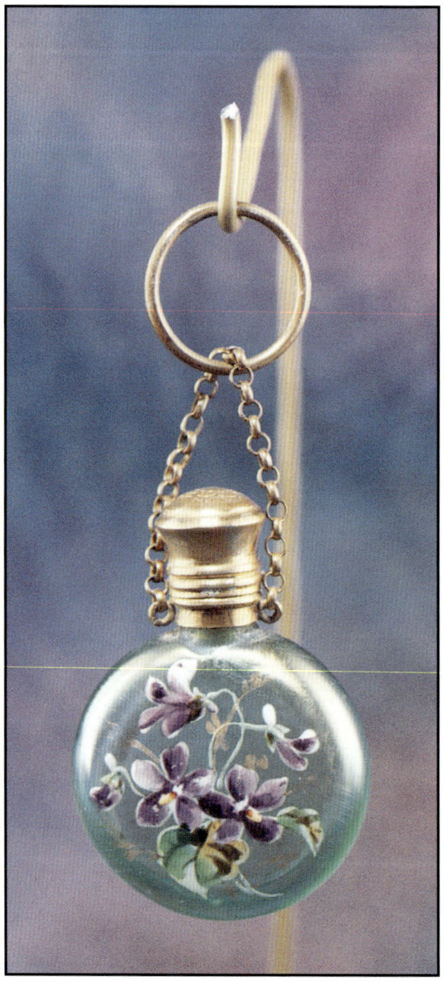

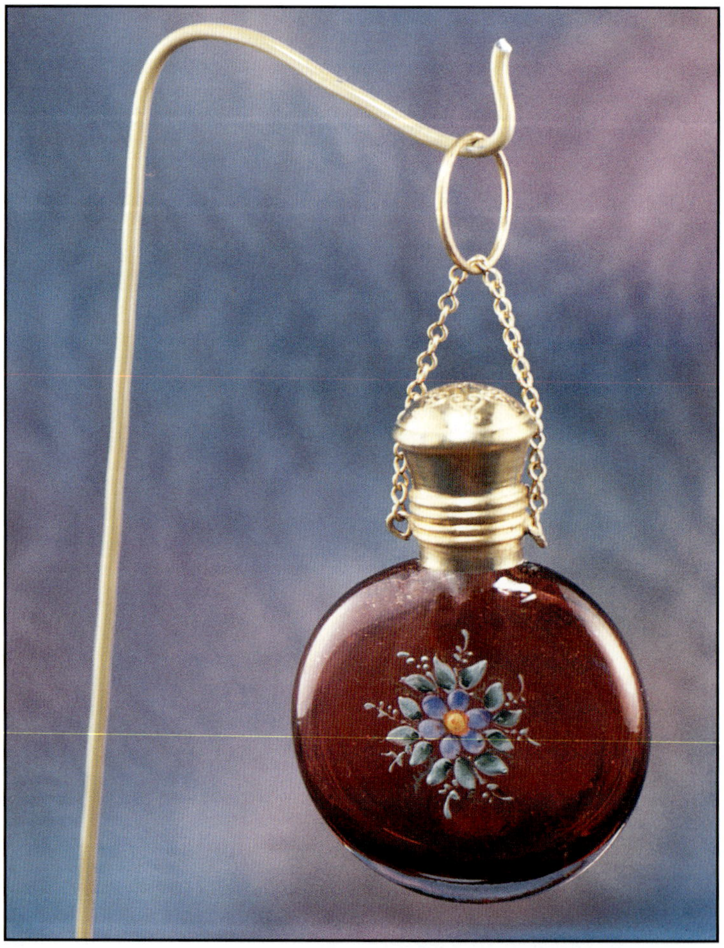

Clear cased over red, enameled flower with leaves, hinged top, inner stopper, chain and finger ring. Marked "Made in Czechoslovakia" and "Hall House New York" on paper stickers. 2.875". $200-300.

Cap Styles

This section offers a summary of the most common caps found on Czechoslovakian purse and dresser minis of the 1920s and '30s. Since perfume bottles have continued to be produced—some from original molds and often with similar embellishments—knowledge of the caps and the times they were used is key for determining whether a bottle originated in the period between the world wars, in the period after the industry was nationalized (1948-1969), or during the modern era. And, though many of the older caps were marked with a tiny metal tag reading "Czecho" or "Czecho-Slovakia," a few cap styles appear consistently with no marking at all. It is obviously beneficial for collectors to know which those typically are.

Some cap styles were found only on Irice pressed glass purse bottles and some styles are only on caged purse bottles. Some, however, are found on many varieties of bottle bases. It would be nice to have more "original information" available to help know by whom and how different caps were made and distributed for the bottles. What we do have is the sample of bottles that have survived. Of course, who knows what switching of caps has occurred over time from various owners? We examine and draw our best conclusions based on our sample.

Czech caps are usually ornate and complement or set off the design of the bottle. The showy outer cap fits over and is fixed to a simple threaded under cap, and though most are gold colored metal, a few are silver. Caps are often tarnished or discolored at the base, especially those that were actually used to seal perfume in a "working bottle" (as opposed to one that served only as decoration). The question is always asked if the discoloration can be removed. The best answer that I have found is that though cleaners can improve the appearance of the metal, it will not remove the damage of corrosion. That being said, these bottles are seventy to eighty years old and ought not to look like teenagers. Cleaners should be used with care so that they do not damage the metal or the stones.

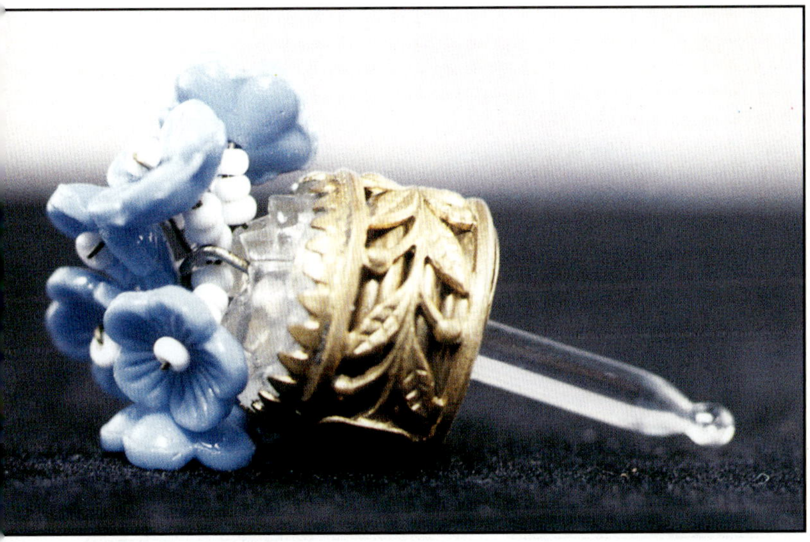

Side view of a purse bottle cap.

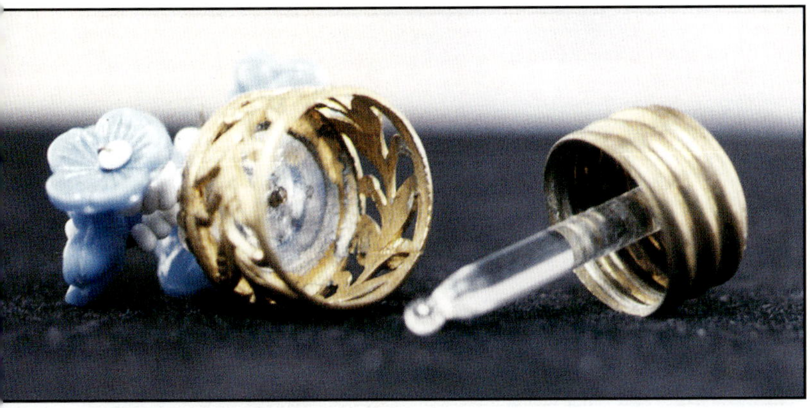

View showing outer and inner cap.

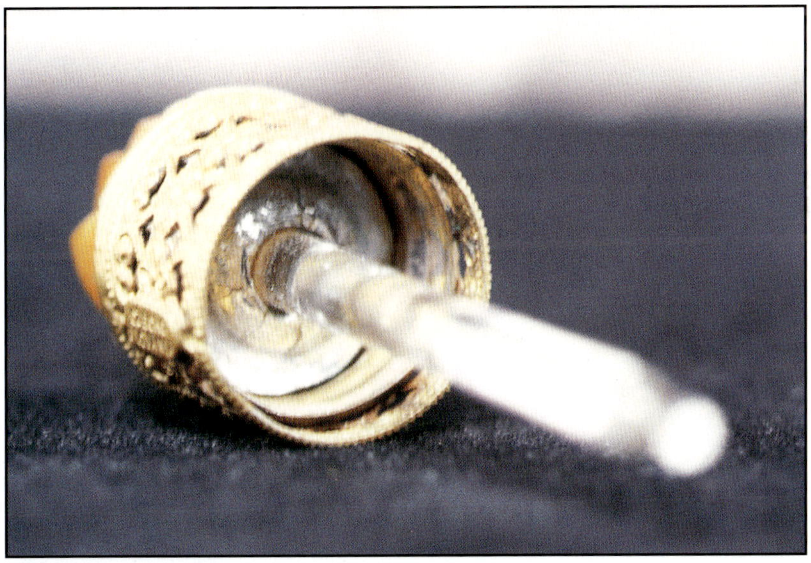

View showing cap interior.

Iríce and Dangle Style Caps

The "bold flower" cap design is found on some of the most desirable Irice pressed glass bases. Doll dangle bottles feature this cap with an opaque glass faceted capstone and a double chain affixed to a metal loop at the center top. Fruit dangles with transparent, colored faceted capstones have matching colored glass fruit, also hanging by double chains from a metal loop found on the center top of the capstone. Shoe dangle bottle caps use the same cap design, but are topped with a convex metal cap "crown" studded with multi-colored jewels that match tiny, multi-colored jewels set in the toes of colored opaque glass Dutch shoes. The bold flower design also forms a "collar" around the neck for the animal head bottles. These caps are all marked with a metal tag and the bottle bases are all embossed with the Irice identifier. The bold flower top can also be found on a higher quality cut glass base, embellished with enamel work and jewels. It is shown with two bottles of similar quality but with coin and bangle caps.

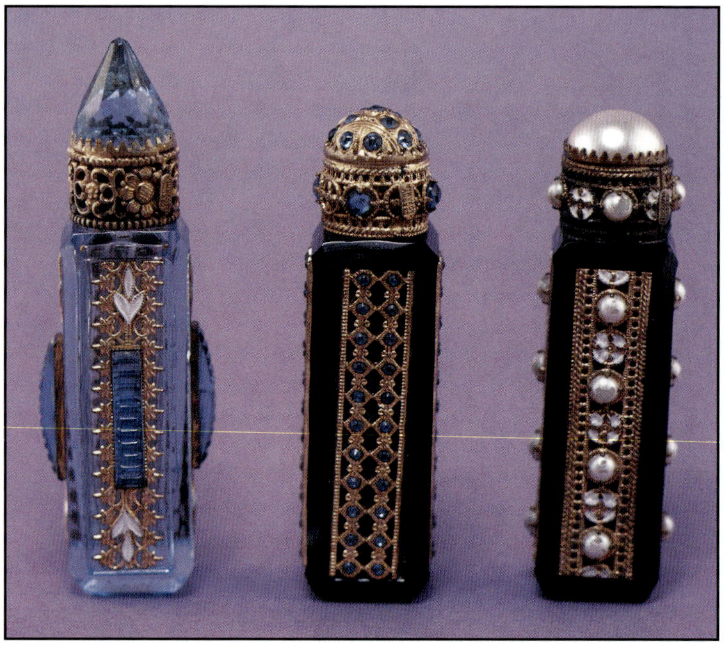

Bold flower (left) and coin and bangle caps (center and right) with fancy detailing on cut glass bottles.

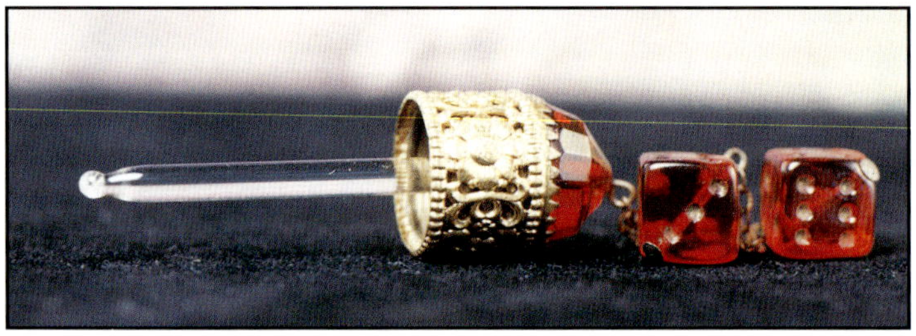

Bold flower cap with red dice dangle.

The "coin and bangle" top has a metal stamped design consisting of alternating circles of the same size, one resembling a coin stamped with a five-petal flower and the next circle worked with an open cross. These form the base for a variety of capstone "sets." On some "coin and bangle" caps, glass gems are prong set onto the "coin" part of the design. Metal tags appear on the jeweled caps, but do not appear on the plainer (non-jeweled) caps.

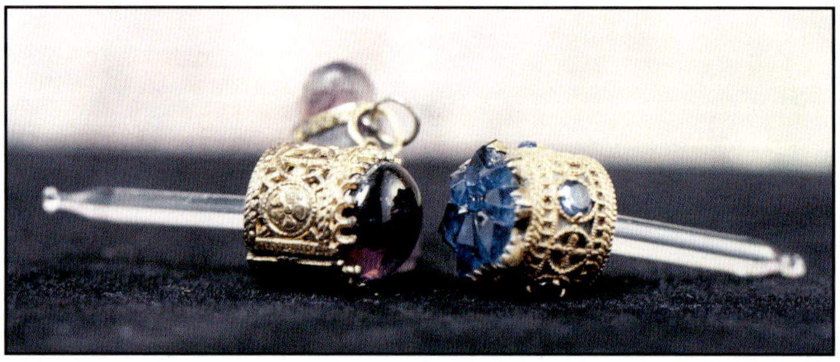

Coin and bangle caps: left is unmarked and without gems, right has set stones and a metal tag.

Painted pinch bottles (three sided) and a few other styles of Irice bottles that are caged in metalwork have similar fancy crown caps with faceted, jeweled capstones. The caged bottles are stamped "Irice" in the bottom metal piece. The pinch bottles, though distinctive, are unmarked. A striking similarity, besides sharing the same cap style and the bright, vivid faceted capstones, is that these bottles are among the smallest, most ranging from between 1-5/8" to 1-7/8" in height and from 1" to 1-1/8" at the widest point.

Irice imported bottle sets, again, have pressed glass bases and trays or stands that grouped the bottles together. Some of these sets came with plain, brass colored metal caps with jewels set in the tops. These sets and the painted pinch bottles probably were presented as low end items and may have been marked with paper tags that have since been removed.

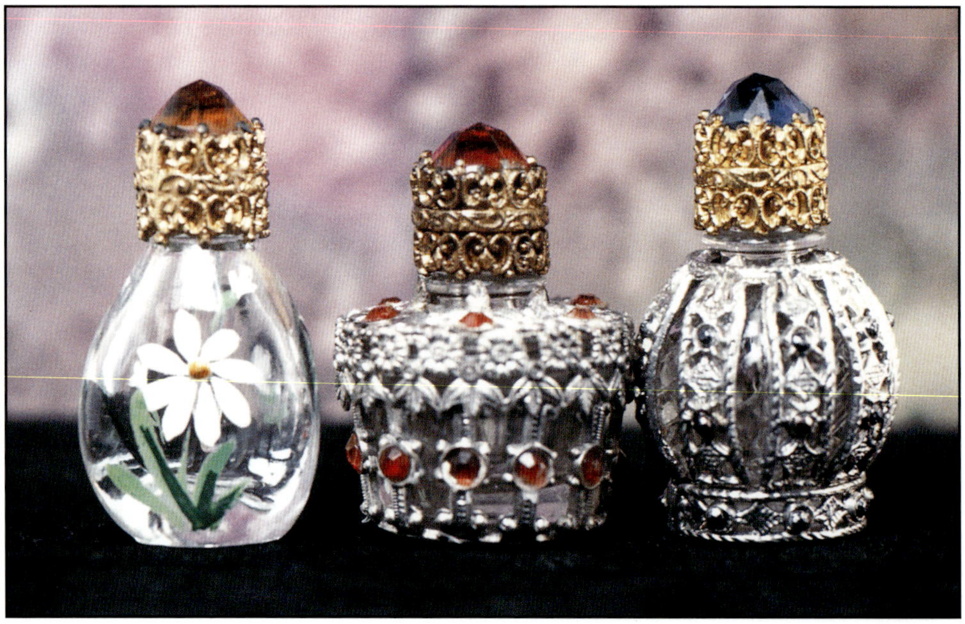

Crown caps with faceted capstones. The pinch bottle on the left is unmarked. Center and right bottles are embossed Irice in the base.

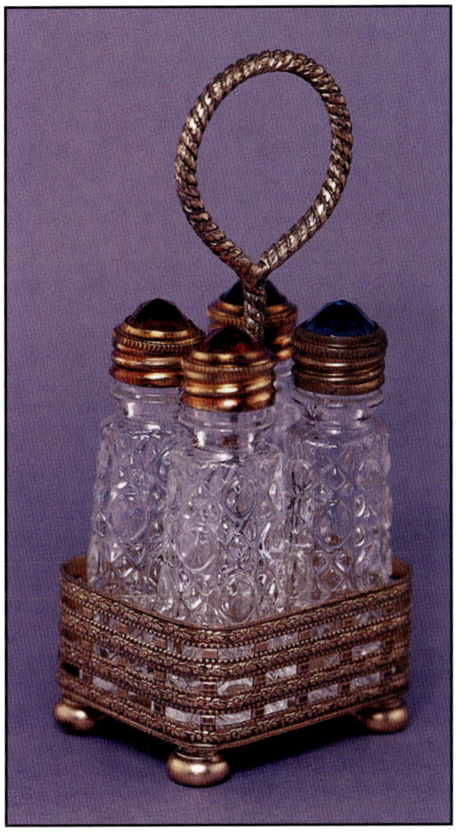

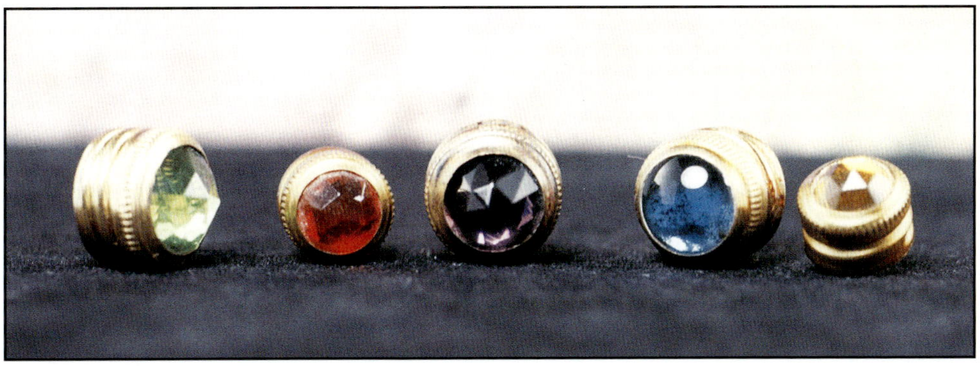

A variety of plain caps.

A basket full of Irice bottles with plain caps and red, yellow, green, and blue faceted capstones.

The twin bottles pictured on the jeweled mirror tray are made of pressed glass with "made in Czechoslovakia" and "Irice" embossed in the base of each bottle. The cap on these bottles, also marked with a metal tag, is smaller than those on purse bottles or on Irice dangle bottles. It is a "grape leaf wreath" cap with a foil backed, clear faceted glass gem in the top. Other assorted caps do have metal tags, as shown below, but are not found in significant numbers.

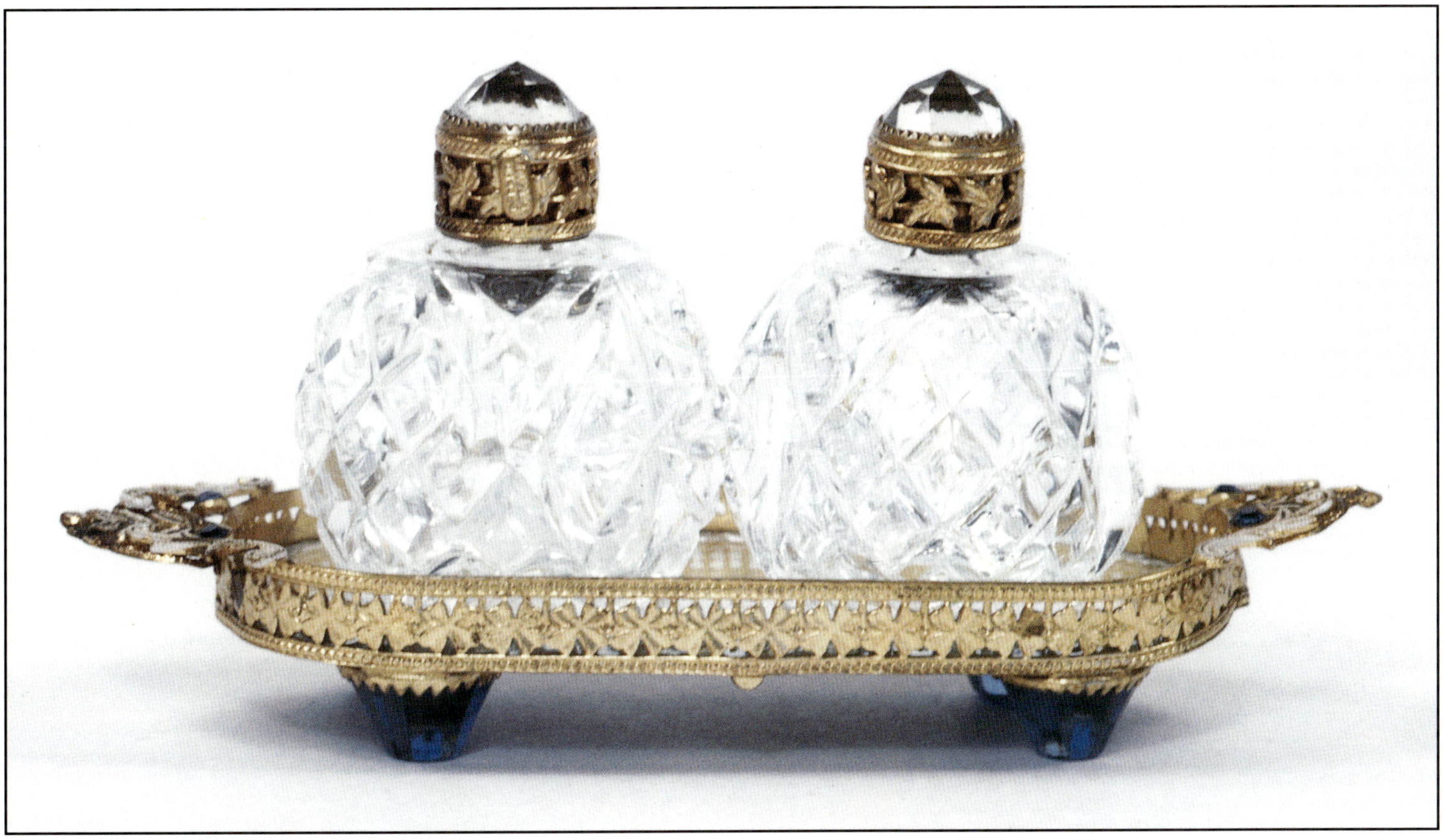

A twin set on a mirrored tray. The bottles are pressed glass and the caps are marked.

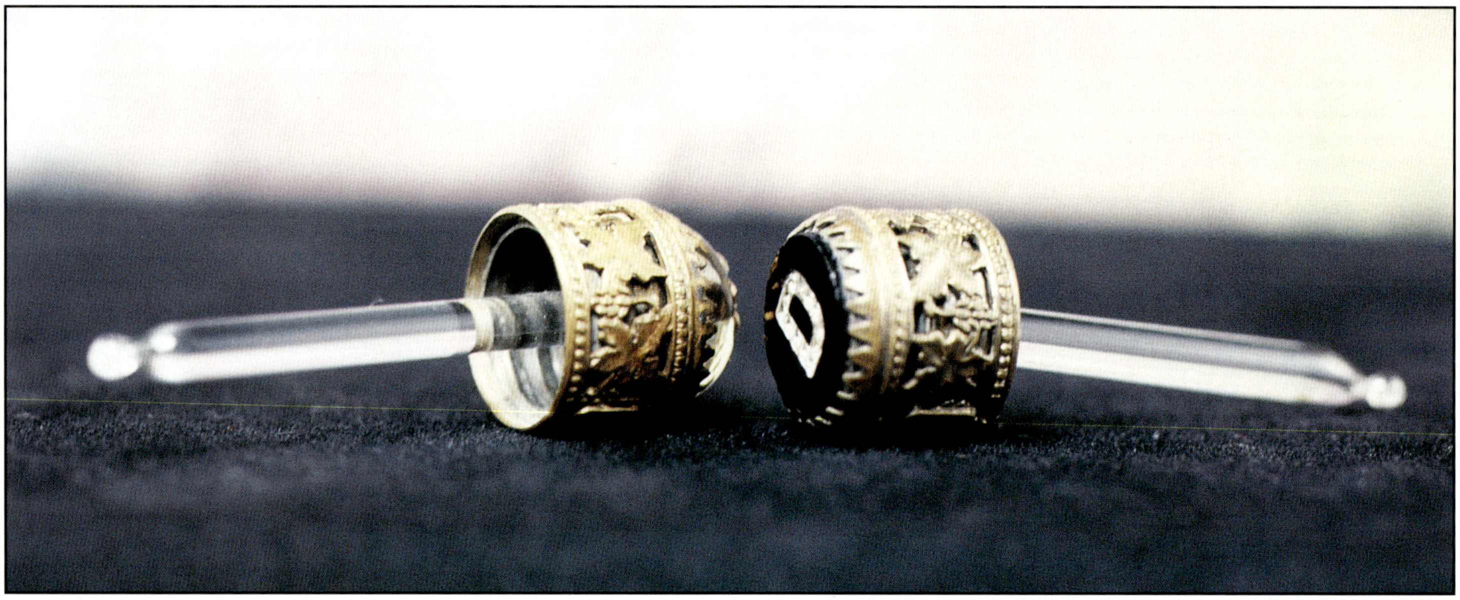

Two grape leaf wreath caps, marked.

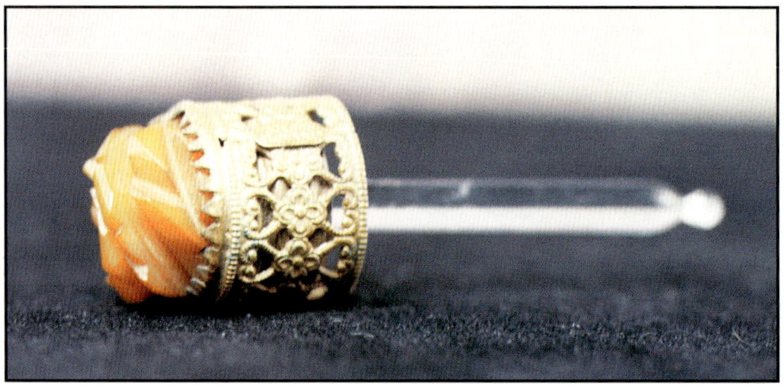

A floral wreath cap with a carved coral rose capstone, marked.

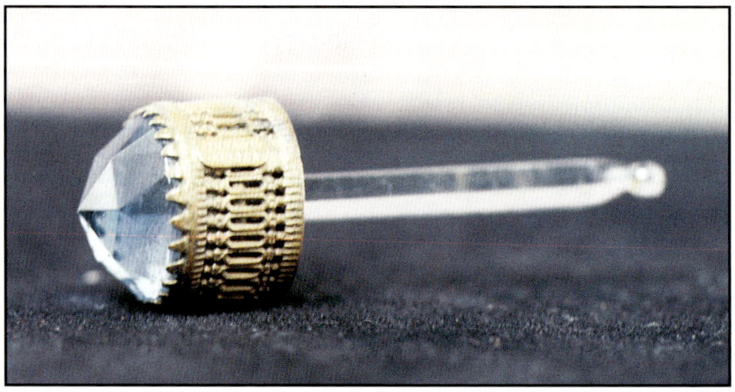

A mesh cap, marked.

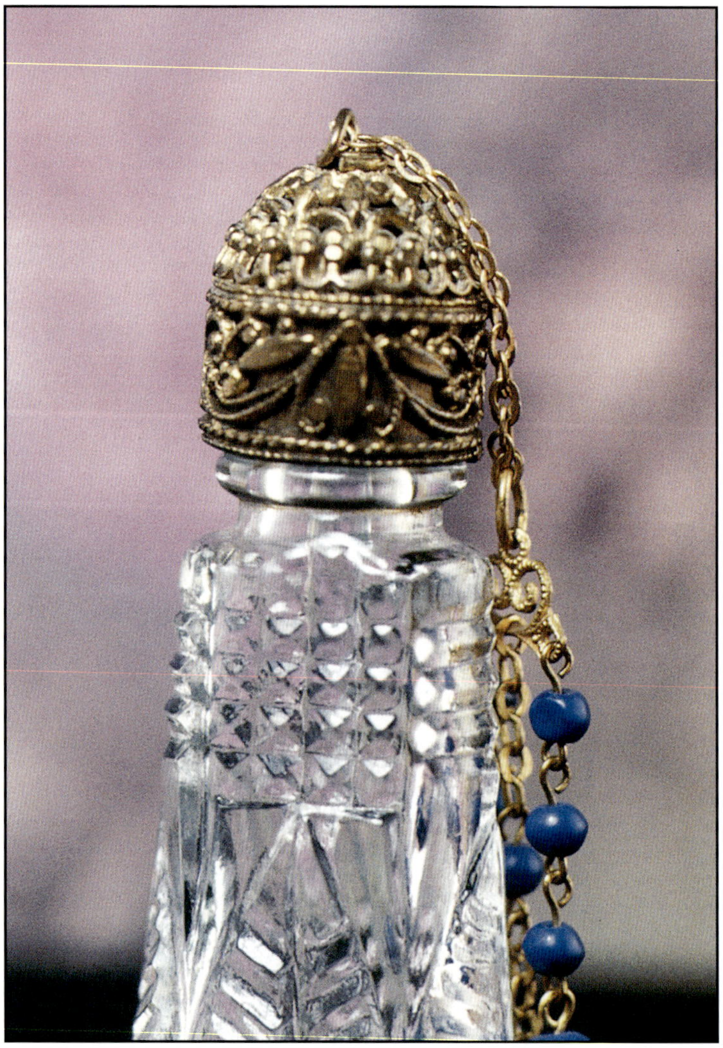

Elaborate cap with a dragonfly design, unmarked.

Another cap found without identifier tags is the "railroad track" cap. It appears with a variety of dangles and ornaments on the pressed Irice bases, including geometric shapes, birds, and other animal dangles. In each case, the capstone is in harmony with the dangle. There is speculation among collectors that the unmarked caps and dangles were produced more recently than caps with the metal tags. The more obvious seams and lack of gem embellishments would appear to support that theory.

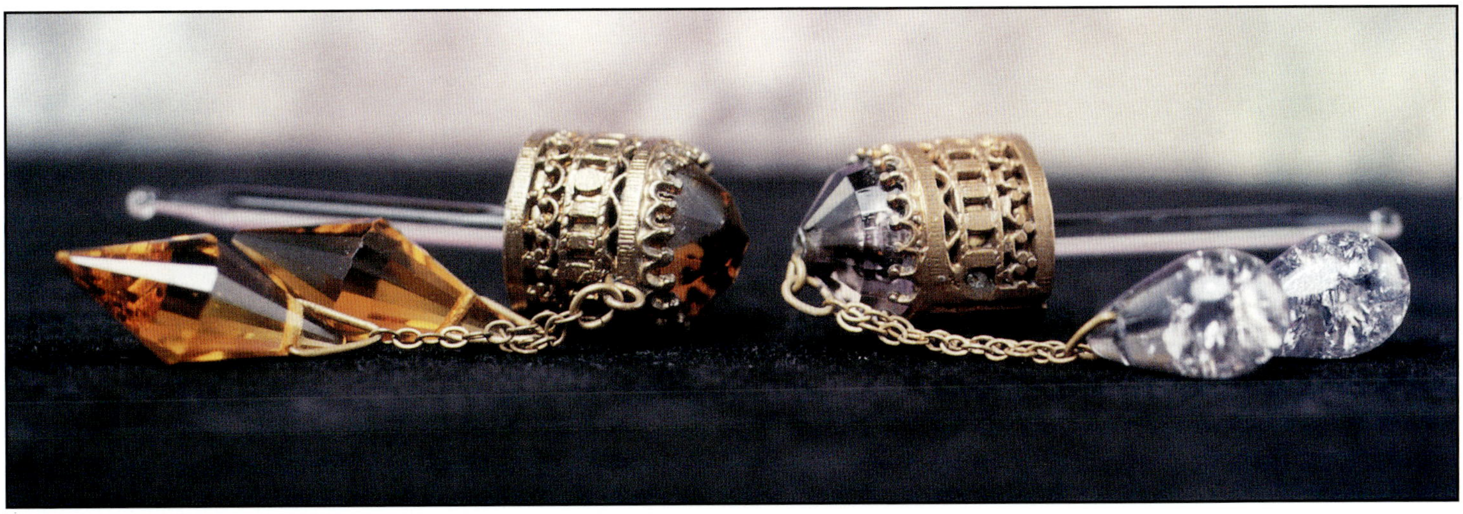

Two railroad track caps. These have a variety of dangles and are the most common of the unmarked caps.

Purse Bottle Caps

The most common of the caged purse bottle caps is the "cut-away" design. The toothed flange at the top holds the capstone, which is most often akin to the focus stone on the bottle front. The second most common cap has a "zipper" band around the center of the cap and a row of tiny "three leafed clovers" above and below the center band. Both of these caps are usually marked with a tiny metal tag.

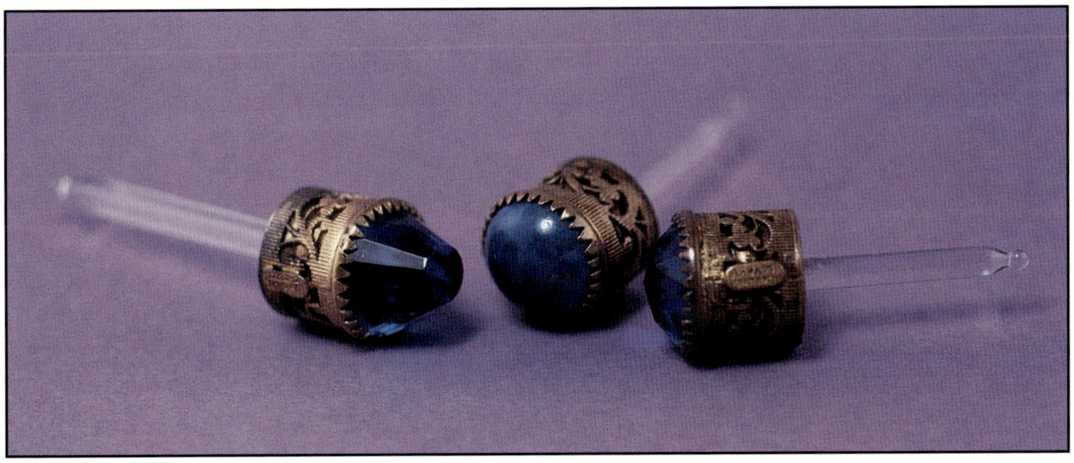

Three examples of cut-away caps. These are the most common caged purse caps and are marked.

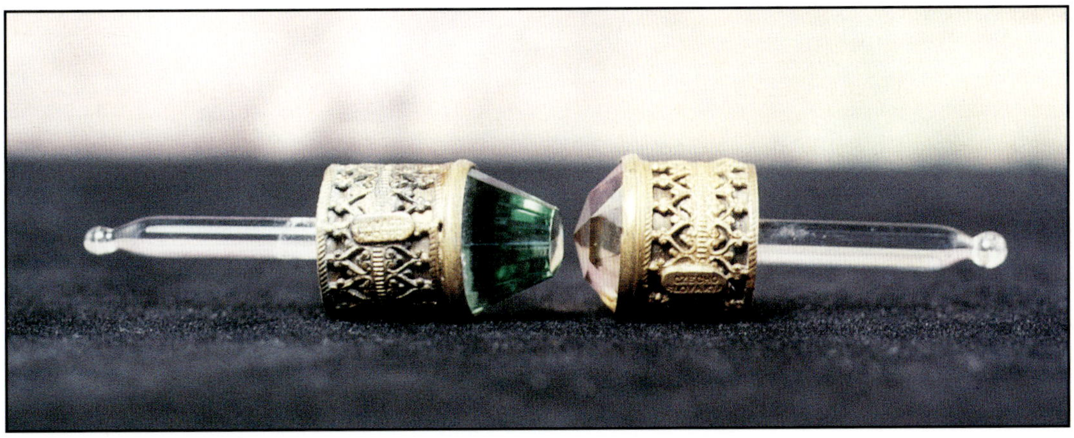

Zipper caps have fine detailing and are common on caged purse bottles. Marked.

A third and less common purse bottle top has a simple metal mesh over-cap. Of the three pictured here, none is marked on the cap. The top with the green stone accompanies a bottle with a metal tag on the caging at the back of the bottle. The two other caps go with bottles that are completely unmarked, but because of the styling, could be Austrian

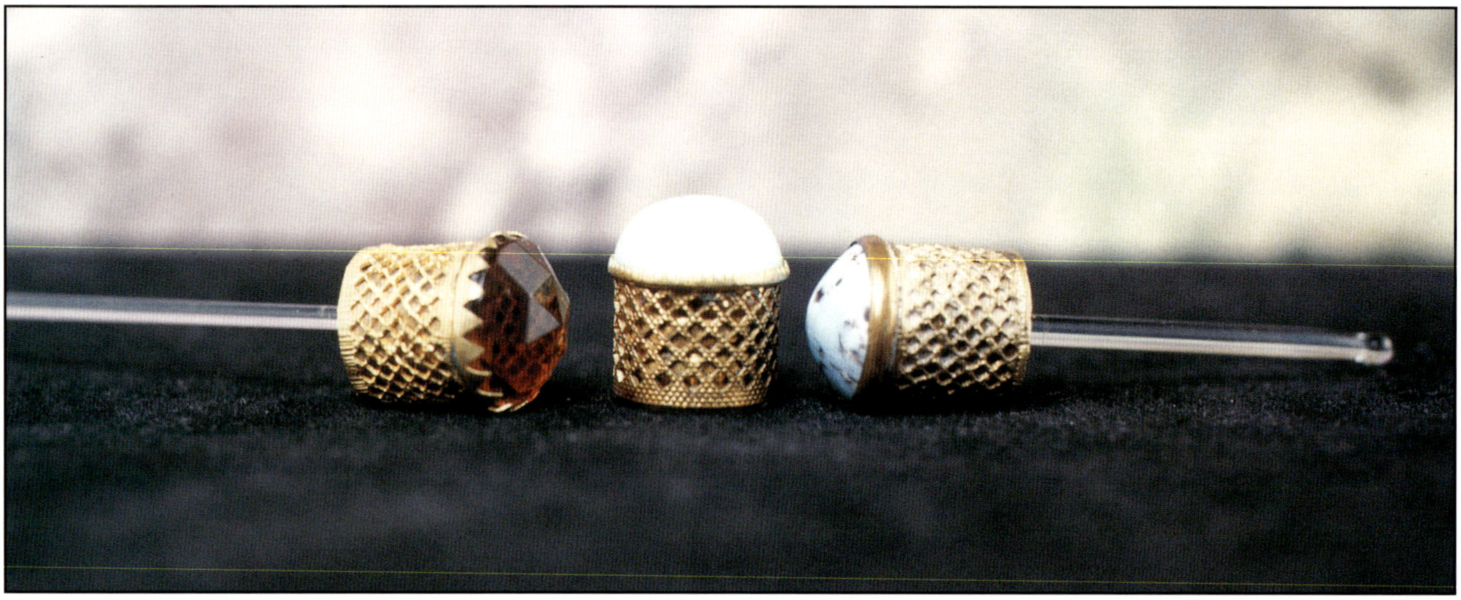

Mesh caps from caged purse bottles. The middle one came from a marked bottle, left and right are likely Austrian.

The next photo shows a variety of caps from Ingrid purse bottles. Bakelite caps (shown in both black and red) were pictured in the early advertising copy and would designate that the bottle came from the mid to late 1930s. The blue rose cap came on an acid marked bottle, and the opaque green cap has a metal tag. For those reasons, I conclude that these were from early bottles as well. I believe the plain caps to be from the 1930s because one came from a lapis bottle, which was not made again until recently. The gold circle cap (third from the left) accompanied the bottle shown with the paper label, and was probably a 1940s or '50s bottle.

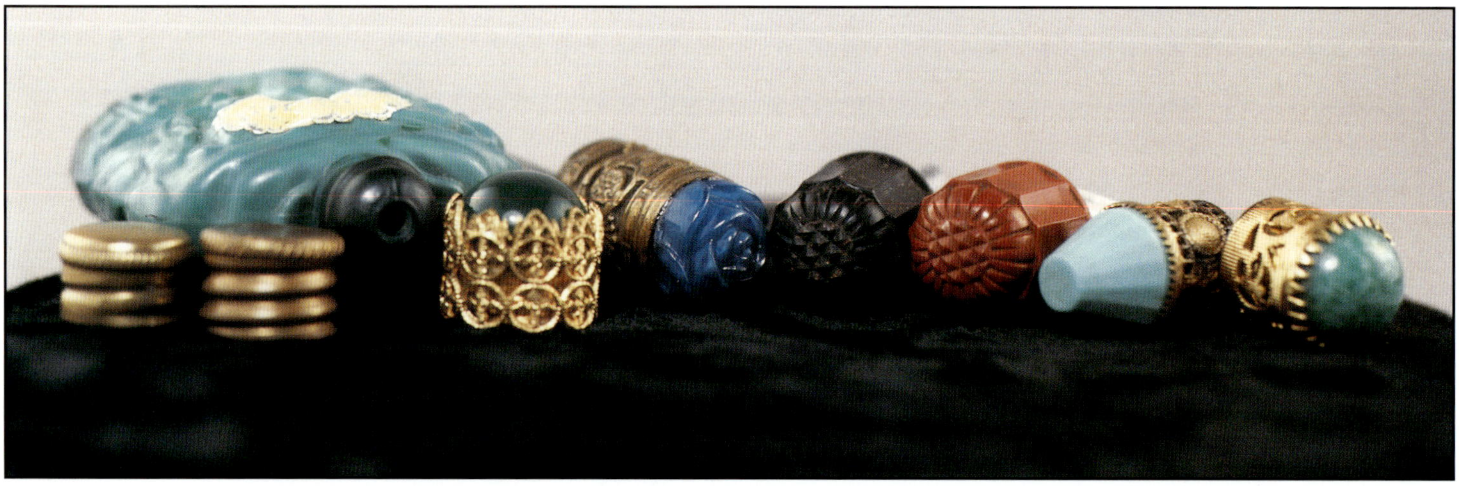

Ingrid purse bottle caps. The red and black Bakelite are mid to late '30s. The gold cap, third from the left, is probably the newest—from the 1940s or '50s—and goes on the green bottle with the Ingrid sticker.

Caged purse bottles that were produced in the 1960s resemble earlier prototypes in that the filigree, enamel, and gem work are very similar. The difference is in the caps. The cap metal is not open filigree, although the stamped design is similar. Most capstones are smaller and were glued in place. Additionally, the cap fits onto glass threads at the bottle's neck, rather than metal threads found on the earlier bottles.

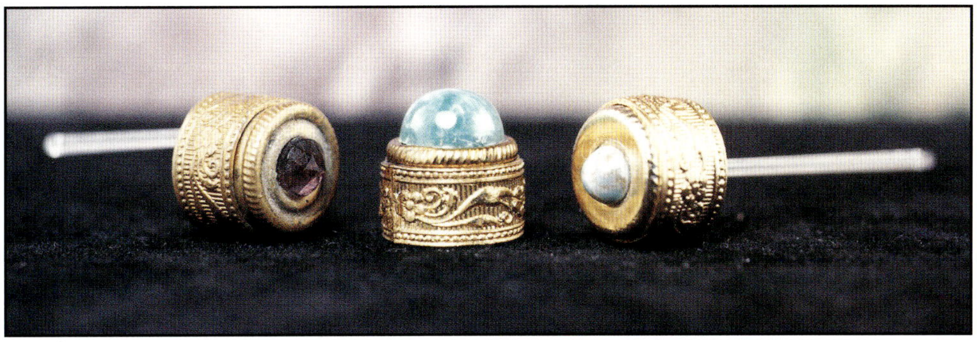

Caps from 1960s caged purse bottles. Note that the cover has the cut-away pattern, but is solid. Capstones are often smaller and glued on.

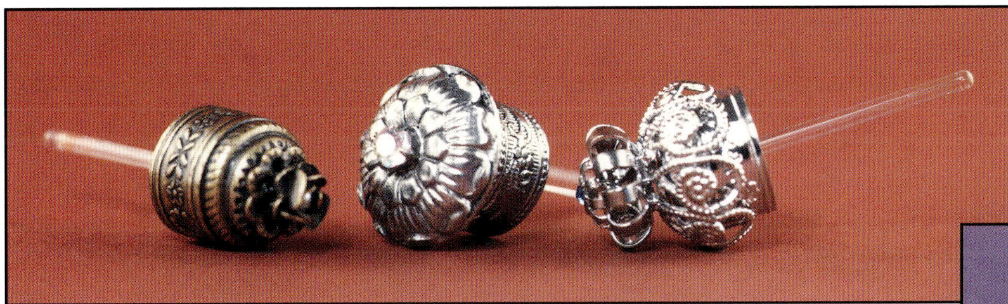

Caps from bottles made in the 1990s to the present. Note that these appear more often in silver color and can be elaborate.

Contemporary bottles come with a variety of cap styles. Those from the 1990s resemble the 1960s caps and are found in both gold and silver. It appears that the caps have become more ornate, yet still different from the early purse bottles. Just since the spring of 2005, some purse bottle caps from the Czech Republic have begun mimicking the cut-away style. The one I purchased lacks both a capstone and a dauber.

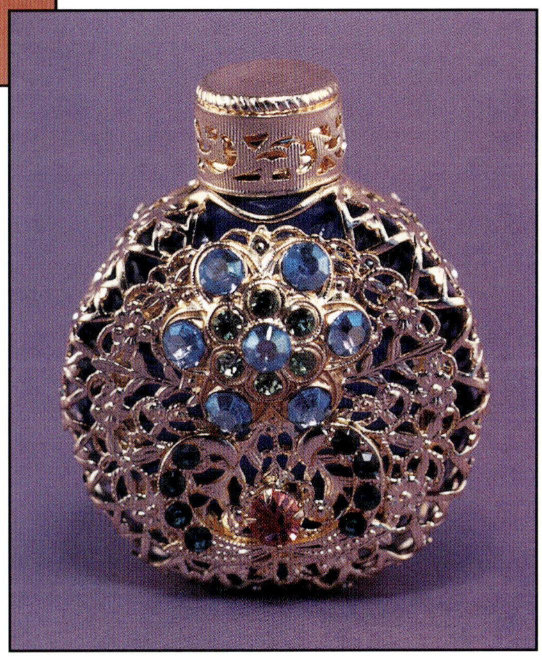

This new production bottle's cap has the old cut-away style, but lacks both a capstone and a dauber. It was said to be "new old stock." 2". Less than $25.

Micro minis with filigree and jewels, though unmarked, have been generally attributed to Czechoslovakia. They have a different look from those that are embossed "France" in the base. In my study of other small perfume bottles, I have found indicators that parts sometimes came from different sources and were assembled and given an "origin" name at that point. The next photo offers substance for the assumption that the filigree and jeweled micro minis were, indeed Czech. Of the five bottles pictured, only the one on the far right is marked and it is French. The four remaining are thought to be Czech. Two caps on those are identical to the cap on the French bottle; the other two caps, however, are miniature versions of the Czech cut-away caps found on caged and jeweled purse bottles. I would argue that the cut-away caps were an earlier production, and that at some later point, both the French and the Czech craftsmen came to acquire their caps from the same source.

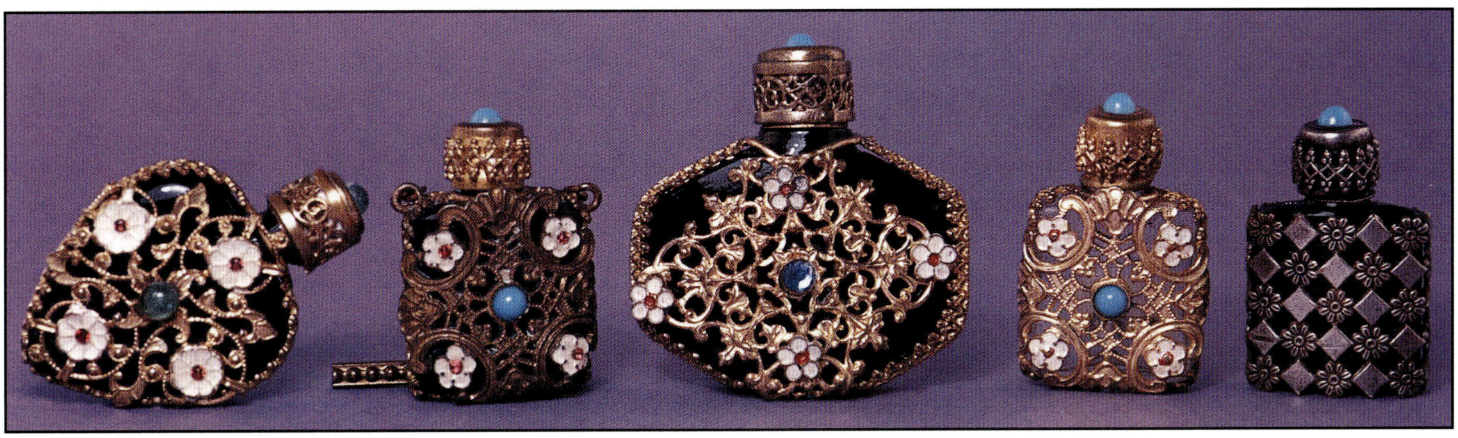

Micro mini bottles showing cut-away and "French style" caps. Heart, 1.75". $125-150; bar pin, 1.375". $125-150; center: 1.75". $50; clear Czech, 1.375". $100-125; French, 1.25". $50-100.

Part II

Dresser Bottle Minis

Dresser bottles, as opposed to purse bottles, were fitted with glass stoppers rather than screw caps. Most of the stoppers, with somewhat elongated plugs, originally had a glass rod—a dauber—affixed to the base. The stopper, when turned into the mouth of the bottle, "locked" into place and "sealed" the bottle. Dresser bottles were made to be placed on a surface rather than to be carried on the person. The glass stoppers used on Czech bottles were finer, more attractive, and more permanent than corks, which were often used in early perfume bottles.

The stoppers on dresser bottles were made separately from the bottles, but ground to create a tight fit for the individual base. They were an important complement to, or extension of, the bottle's design. Some of the same popular designs were made to "top" several bottle styles. Some stoppers were so elegantly created that they took on a life of their own and are now sought after as the primary focus of collectors.

Dresser bottles varied in size from the very small and delicate dram and mini bottles, to medium sized, large, and very large. The problem with setting a specific measurement to define each category is that categorizing is not so simple. If one defines by height, how does one classify a tiny bottle with a tall stopper or a short, clunky bottle? It seems that one would have to consider factors other than height, such as content volume and general delicacy of design. Thus, the divisions in this chapter should be considered a bit flexible.

Dresser bottles came in a variety of colors, both transparent and opaque. They were cut, cased, enameled, decorated with filigree and gems, and were in general, works of art to adorn the dressing table.

Cut Glass Minis

Long overlooked as collectors sought out their larger, more elaborate "cousins," these delicate and eye-catching small crystal dresser bottles made in Czechoslovakia entered the country in "thousands of thousands of dozens" (Jones-North, 1999, p. 104) and are now coming into their own with collectors. They are generally less expensive to purchase, yet many have all the color, detailing, and hand finish work of their larger counterparts. And, they take less room to display.

These clear and colored minis were originally touted as inexpensive gifts or card party favors. Importers encouraged shop owners to profit doubly—from the sales of the empty bottles and from the perfume sold to fill them. The tiny bottles of fine cut glass, a dram or two of provocative scent...what could make a more appealing, luxurious, essentially feminine, yet relatively inexpensive gift? Or, a nicer way to pamper oneself!

How expensive were they? The dram bottles often retailed for half a dollar. Other minis ranged from that to a dollar; a rare, more elaborate mini might go for as much as two dollars. Bought by merchants for $3.75 a dozen, depending on the size of the lot, the profit on a fifty-cent bottle was about eighteen to twenty cents.

The smallest and simplest of the cut glass stoppered bottles were "perfumettes." They came in simple shapes of a half or full circle with flat front and backs, rectangular or ball-shaped, but always with radiating or faceted cuts. Typical stoppers were faceted balls or elongated prisms in usually clear, but sometimes in colors. The perfumette bases were predominantly crystal clear, blue, pink, green, amethyst, and opaque black. This particular style of bottle apparently was not made in yellow. Yellow does appear in other styles of minis. Red was virtually never found in mini bottles, but was occasionally used for stoppers or for twin trays if the stoppers were also red.

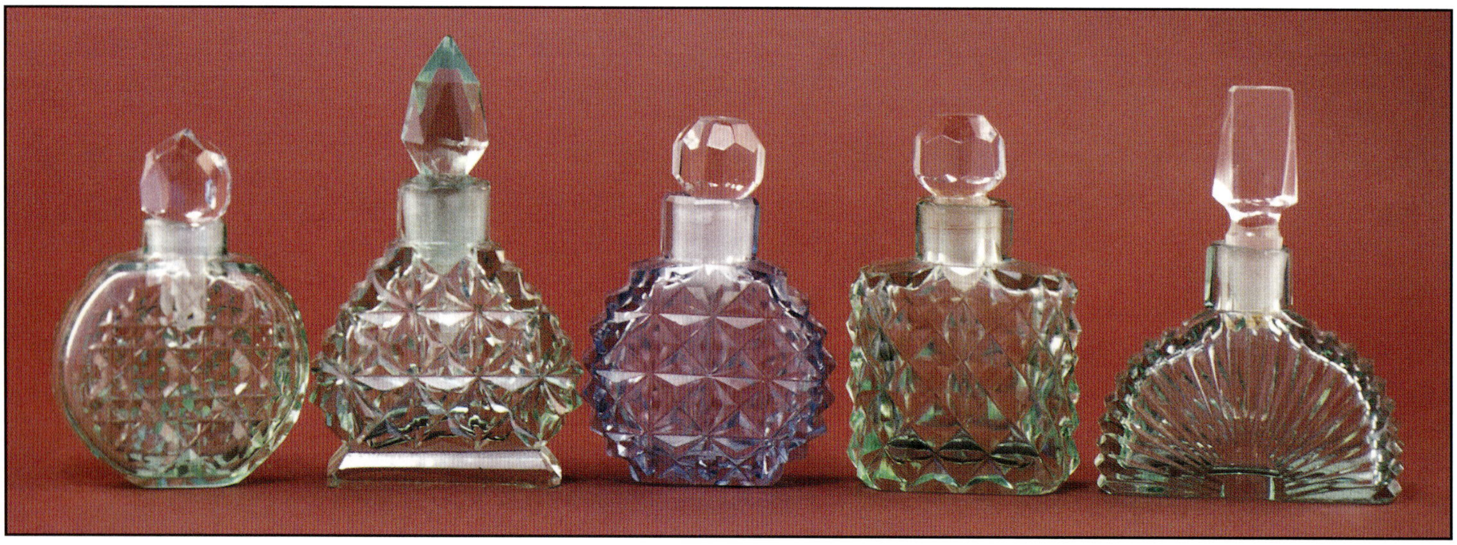

Perfumettes, ranging in height from just under 2" to 2.375". The far right bottle has a mismatched top. From left: XOXO patterned green. $100-125. Footed prism topped green. $150-175. Amethyst, round. $125-150. Squared green. $100-125. Half-moon green. $50-100.

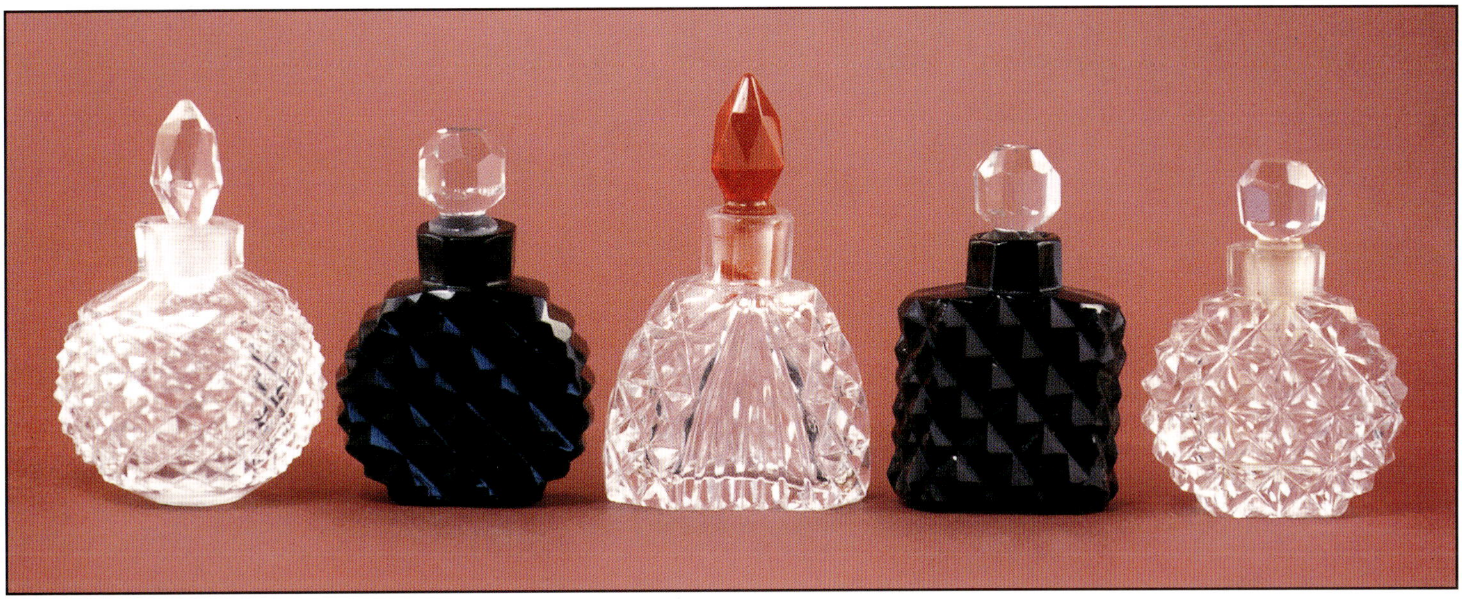

More perfumettes. From left: Hobnail ball base, prism top. 2". $150-175. Round, opaque black. 1.875". $125-150. Cut, clear base; red, prism top. 2.375". $150-175. Opaque black cut square. 2". $125-150. Round, clear, cut. 2". $100-125.

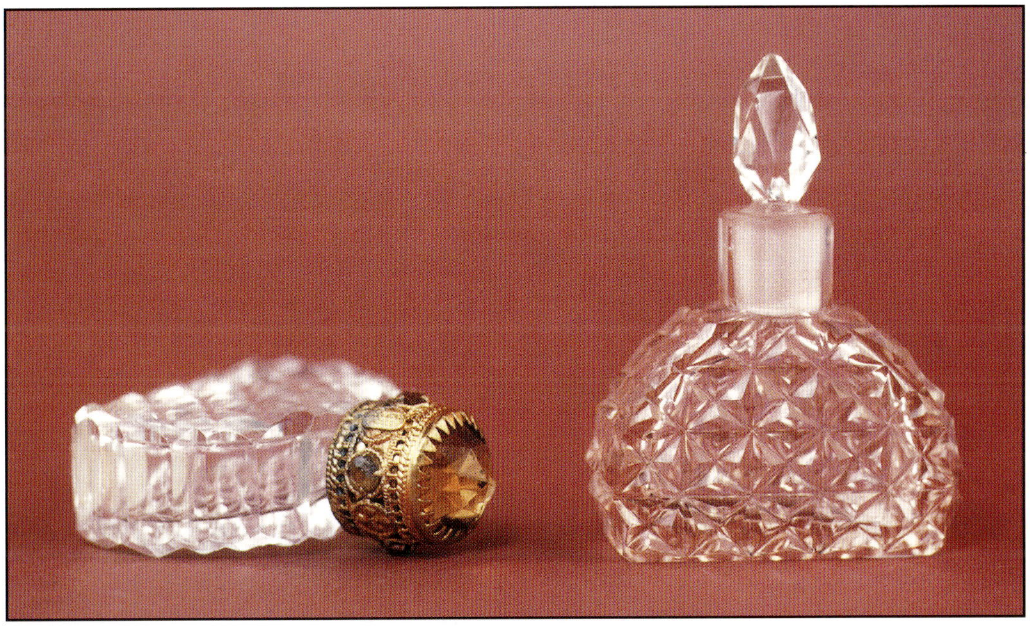

Two bottles with the same base design. The purse bottle has a coin and bangle cap with amber stones. $125-150. Dresser bottle has a pink base, clear prism top. 2". $150-200.

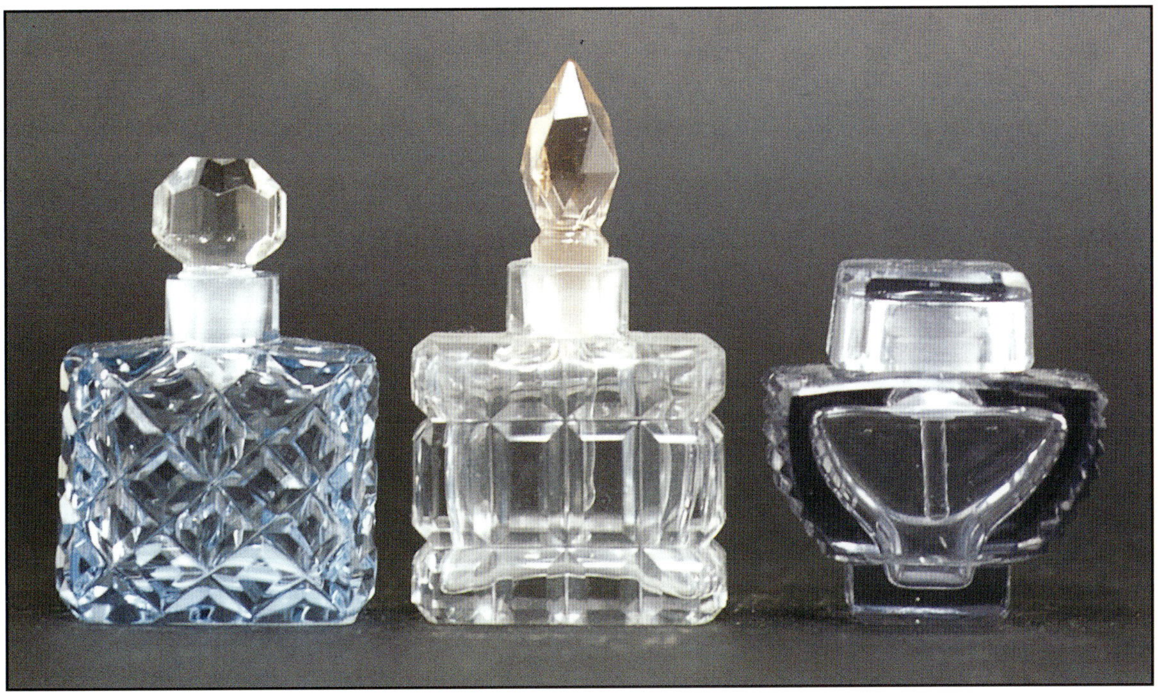

Left: Blue, squared perfumette. 2". $150-175. Center: Clear, cut, "ice cube" with prism top. 2.125". $150-175. Right: Amethyst, cap-over style stopper. 1.5". *Courtesy of Earline Kopriva*. $175-225.

The term "Lilliputian" was used in some advertising and appeared to describe tiny versions of some of the popular commercial perfumes. One can find Czech minis that resemble perfumes by Guerlain, Ciro, Lentheric, and Lucien LeLong. (Jones-North, 1999, p. 14, picture, p. 104) Lilliputian bottles are a similar size and capacity of perfumettes, but are more delicate and refined in appearance.

Most minis fall in a general classification of dresser bottles by virtue of larger, taller, and more elaborate stoppers. The variety of styles and interchangeable pieces on these bottles soon becomes apparent to the collector. The same top design can sometimes be found on a variety of bases, and identical bases can sport several different styles of tops. The bottle and top can be found in the same color, but often only one part is colored and the other part is clear. One could assume with a high degree of accuracy that, except for black, if the colored base has an entirely different colored top, they were not originally sold as a pair.

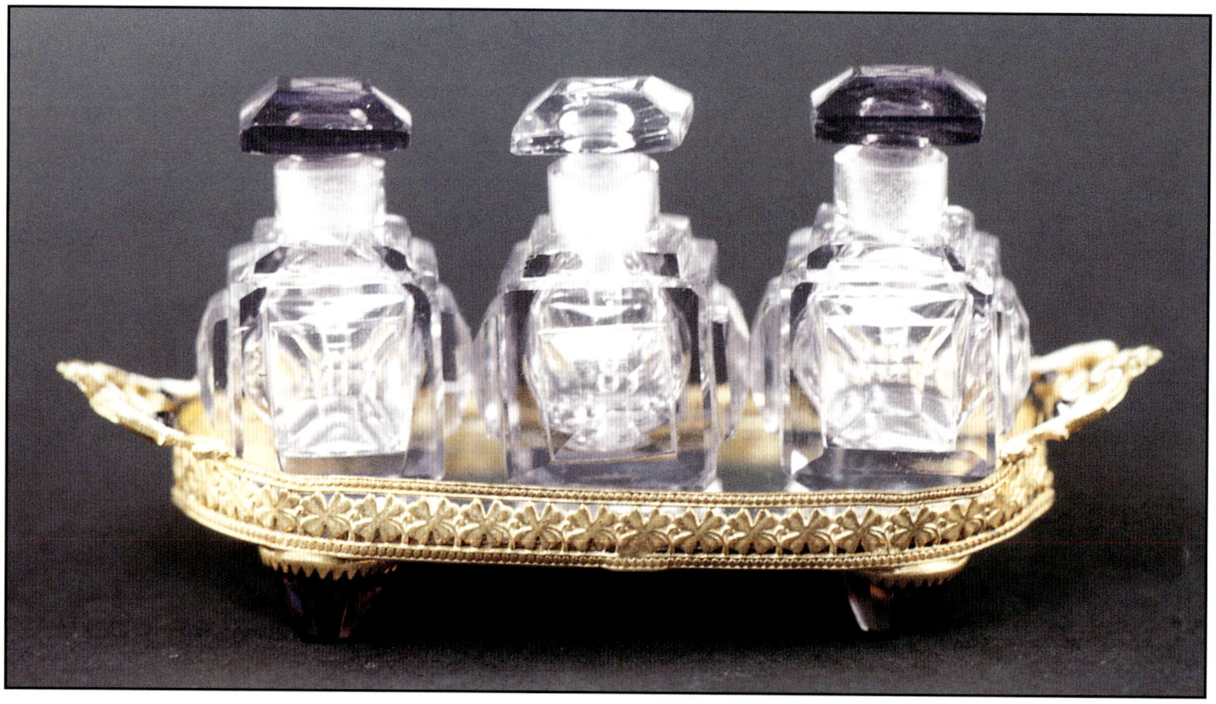

Three cubes in a row. 1.375". $125-150 each. Filigree, jeweled mirrored tray, $100-125.

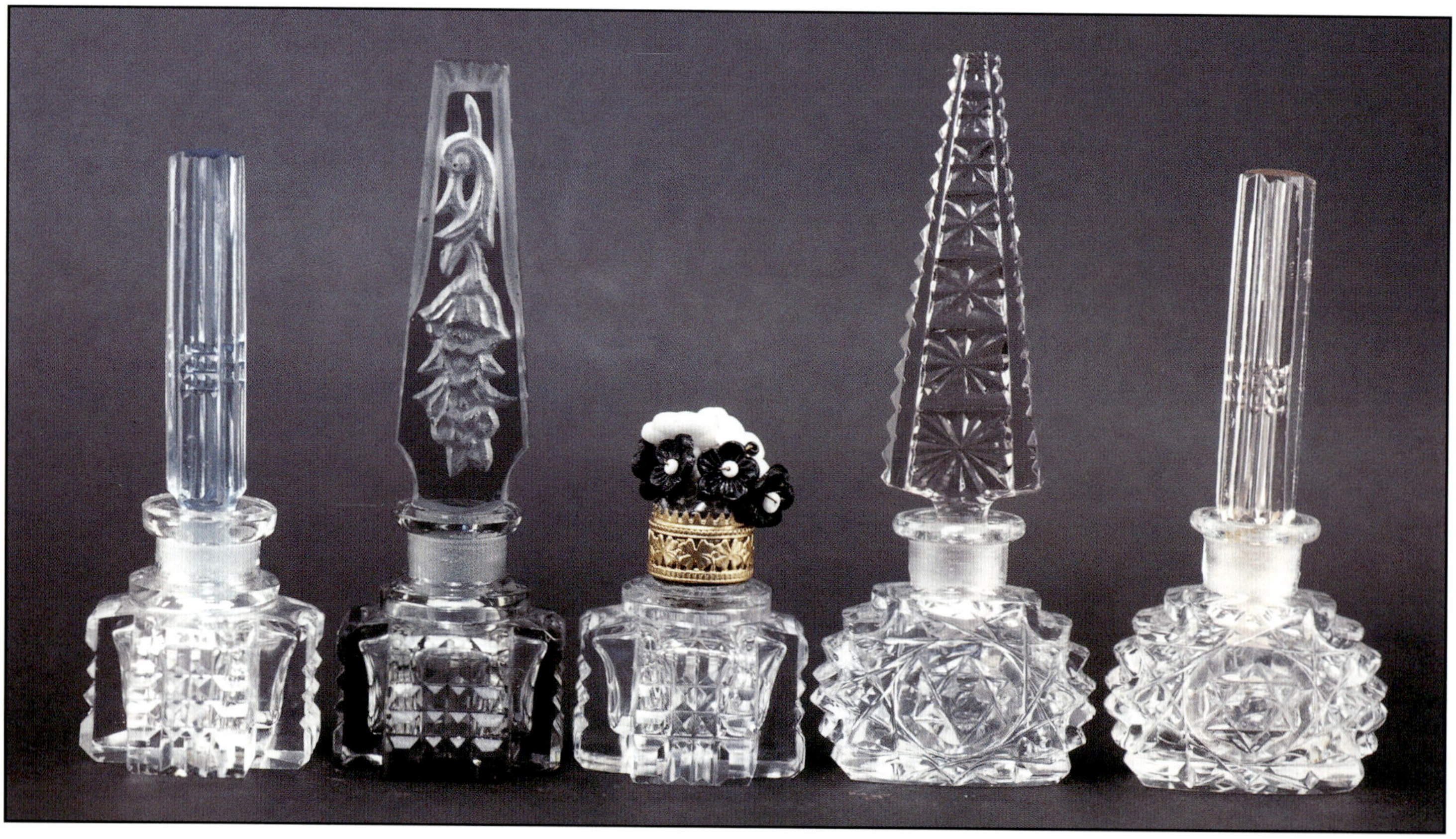

From left: Cross-shaped base in clear; cut, tall blue top. 3.25". $150-200. Same base shape in smoke, floral intaglio top. 3.5". $175-250. Same base shape in clear with a bead flower cap in black and white. 2". $150-200. Round, clear, star-cut base; tall, geometric cut tall stopper in amethyst. 4". $150-200. Same base, tall, pink cut top same as the first bottle in the set. 3.25". $150-200.

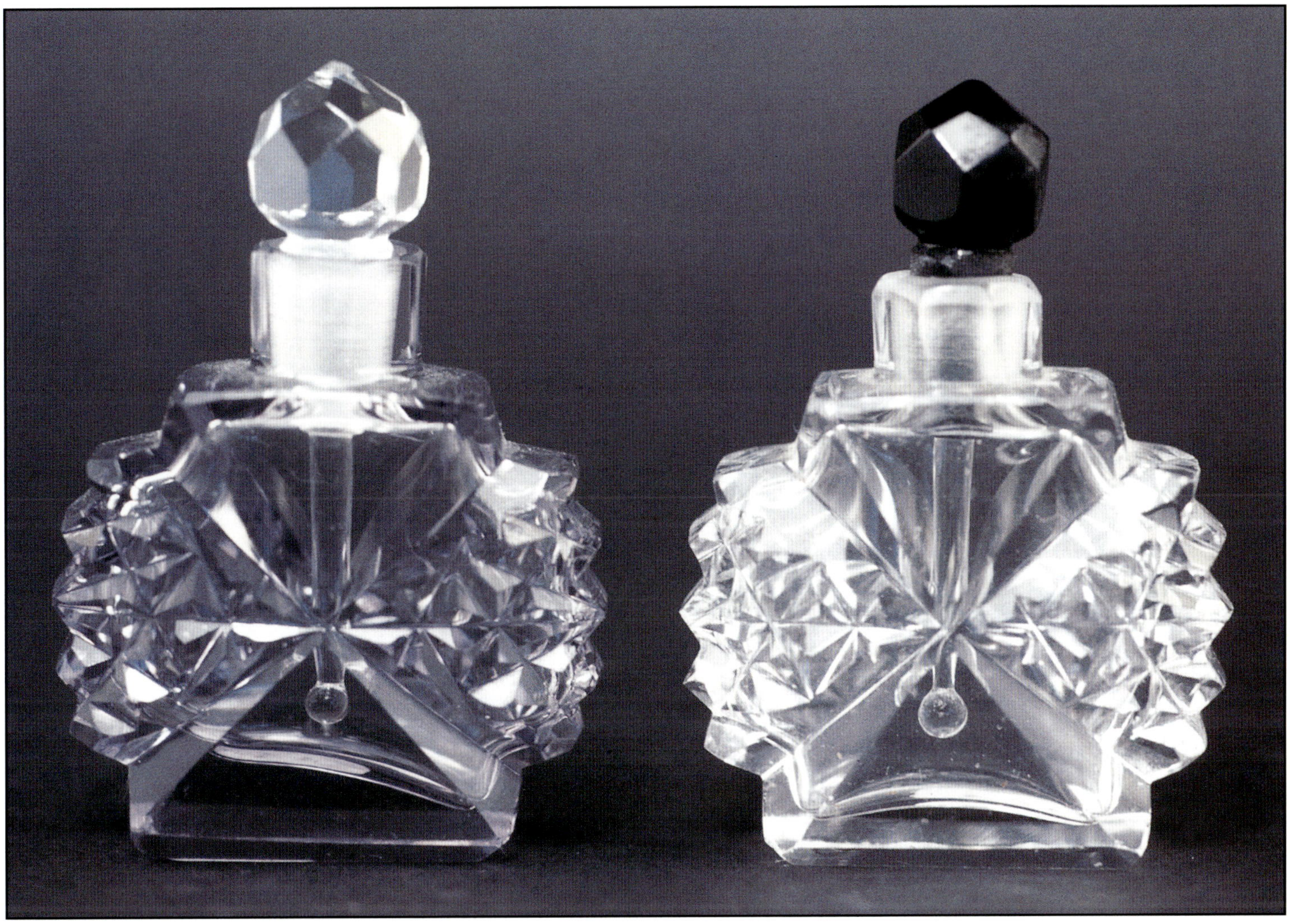

The same bottle in different colors. Left: Amethyst mini, clear top. 2.25". $150-200.
Right: Same base in clear with an opaque black top. 2.25". $150-200.

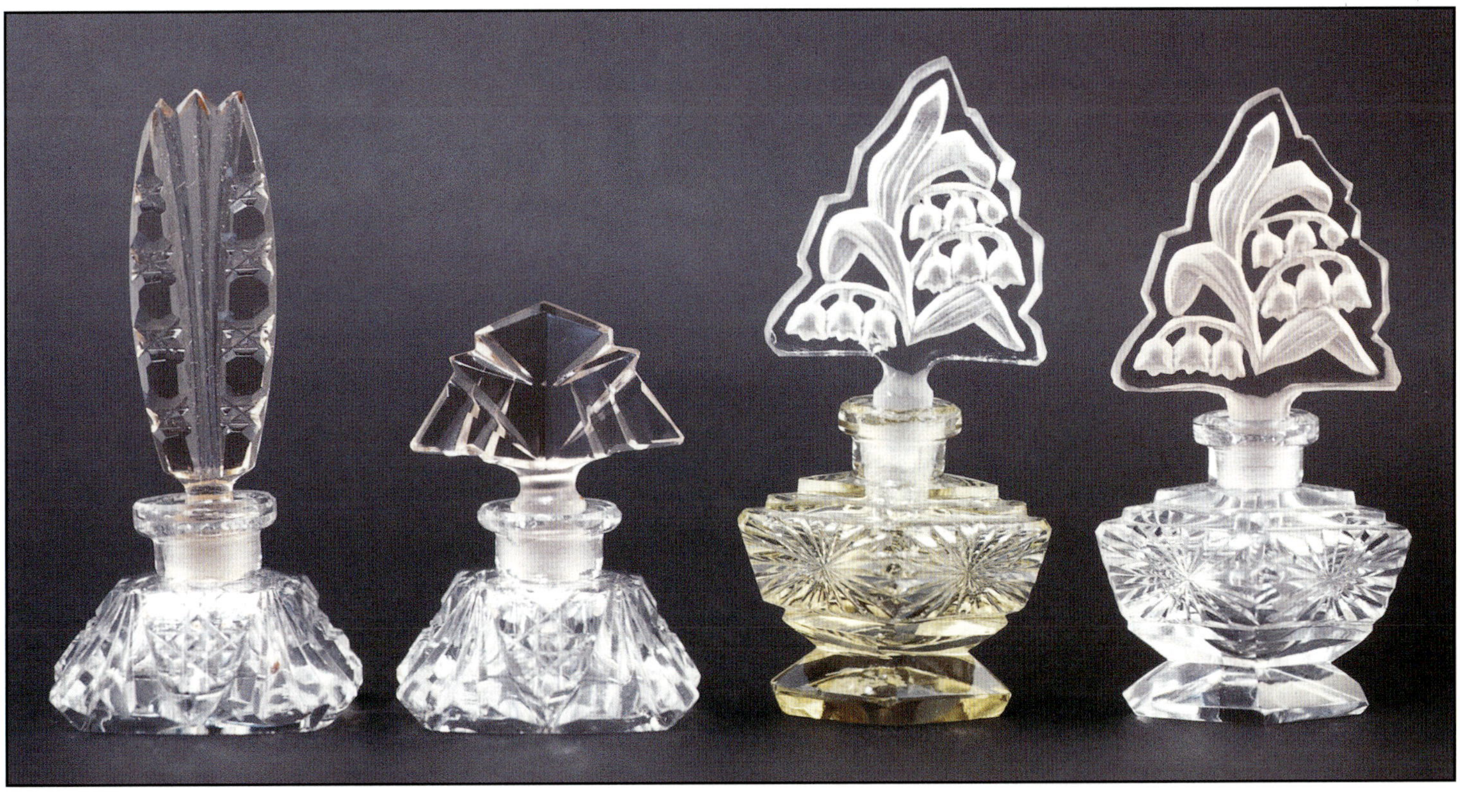

From left: Clear, cut base; tall, pink, geometric cut top. 3.25". Same base; pink "winged" top. 2.25". Yellow footed, cut base; triangular, clear lily-of-the-valley intaglio top. 3.5". Same base in clear; same top in pink. 3.375". $150-200 each.

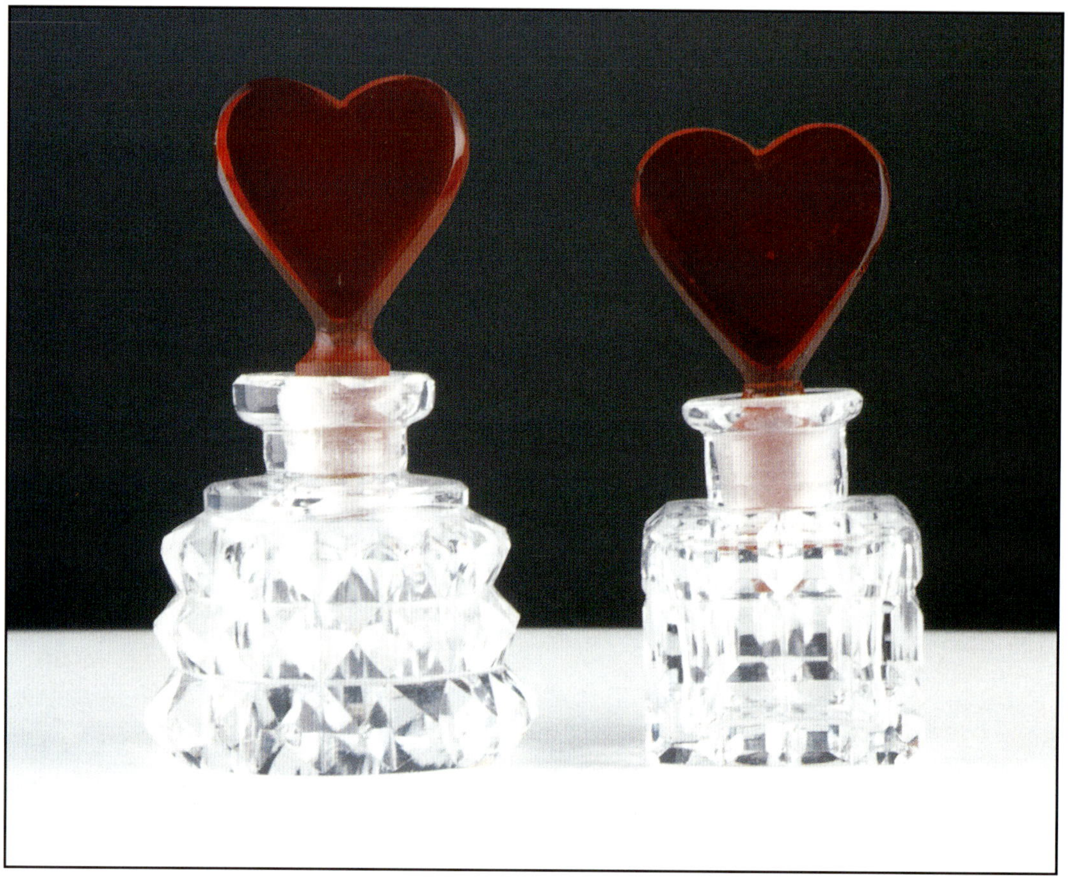

Left: Clear base, red heart top, Morlee sticker. 2.625". $150-200. Right: Small, square base with red heart stopper. This was probably one of a set of four as seen in an ad in Jones-North, (1999, p. 104). (Aristo bottle sold by Marshall Fields) 2.25". $150-200.

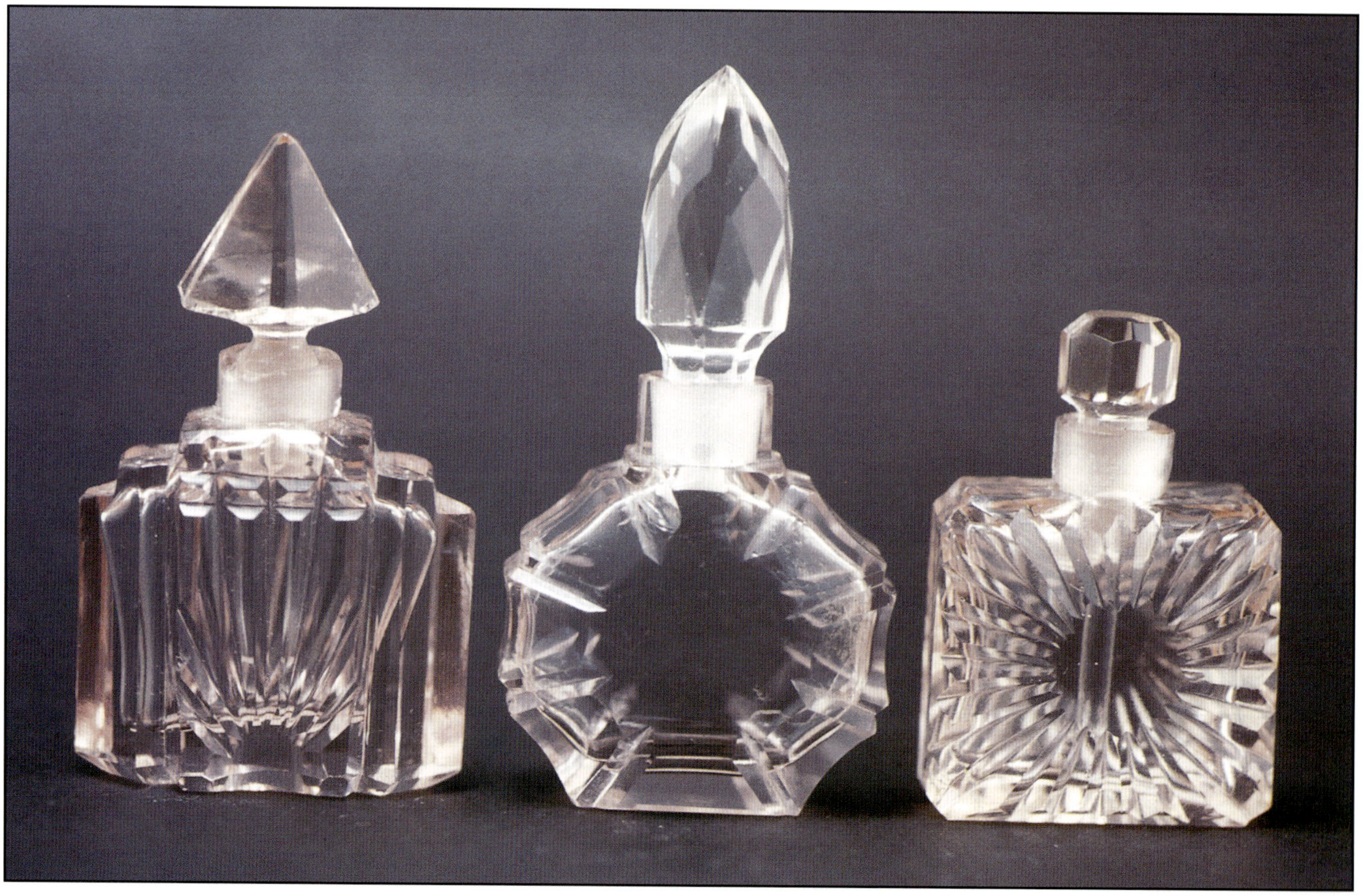

"Lilliputian" or dram bottles, pictured in the ad from Jones-North (1999, p. 104). Left: Pink, cut base; pointed, winged pink top. 2.5". Center: Pink, cut, base; clear, cut, elongated prism top. 2.5". Right: Pink, round "window" radiating cuts; pink, squared prism top. $150-200 each.

Bohemian glass had a long-standing tradition of fine quality. Many references in the earlier advertising copy shown in Jones-North (1999, pp. 89-120) trades on that reputation. Copy from the mid to later '30s begins to use the name "Czecho Slovakian" as that emerging name became more familiar.

Most of the mini dresser bottles are hand cut and polished in geometric designs.

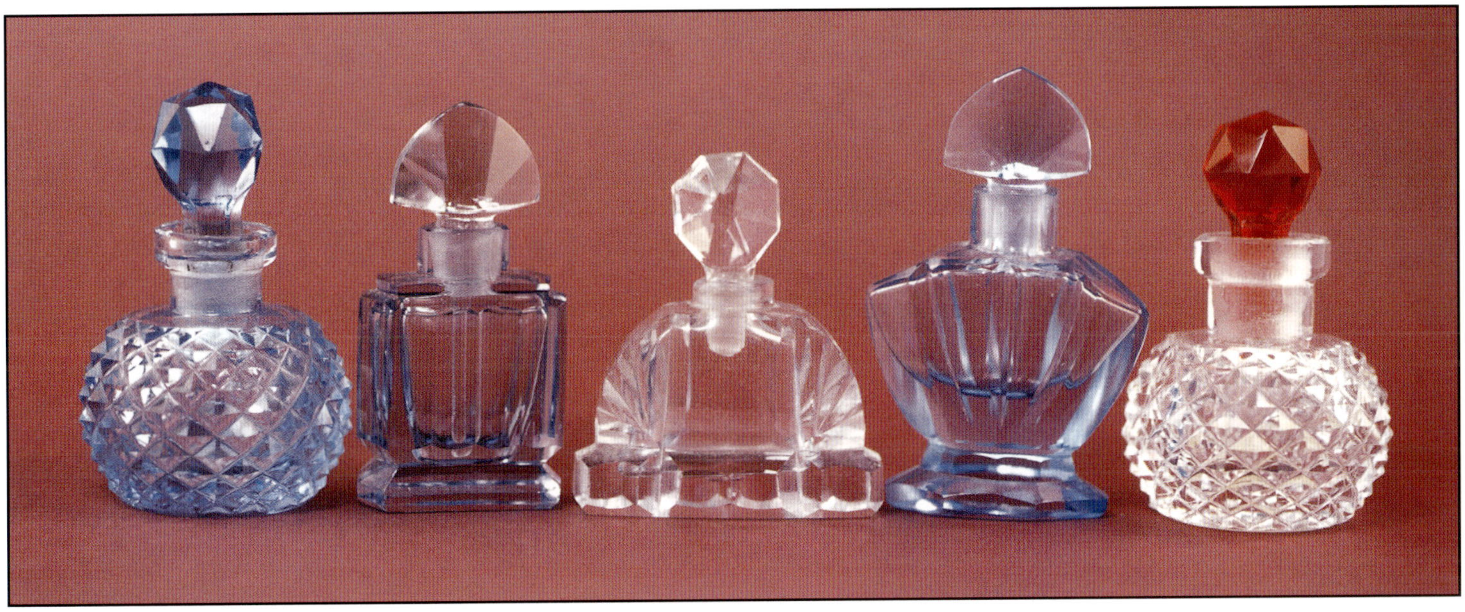

More from the Aristo, Marshall Fields Ad. From left: Blue, hobnail cut; prism top. 2.375". $150-200. Amethyst, fan top. 2.375". $200-250. Clear, sitting figure. 2". $150-200. Sloped Shalimar-shaped; blue fan top. 3". $200-250. Clear, hobnail cut; red prism top. 2.375". $150-200.

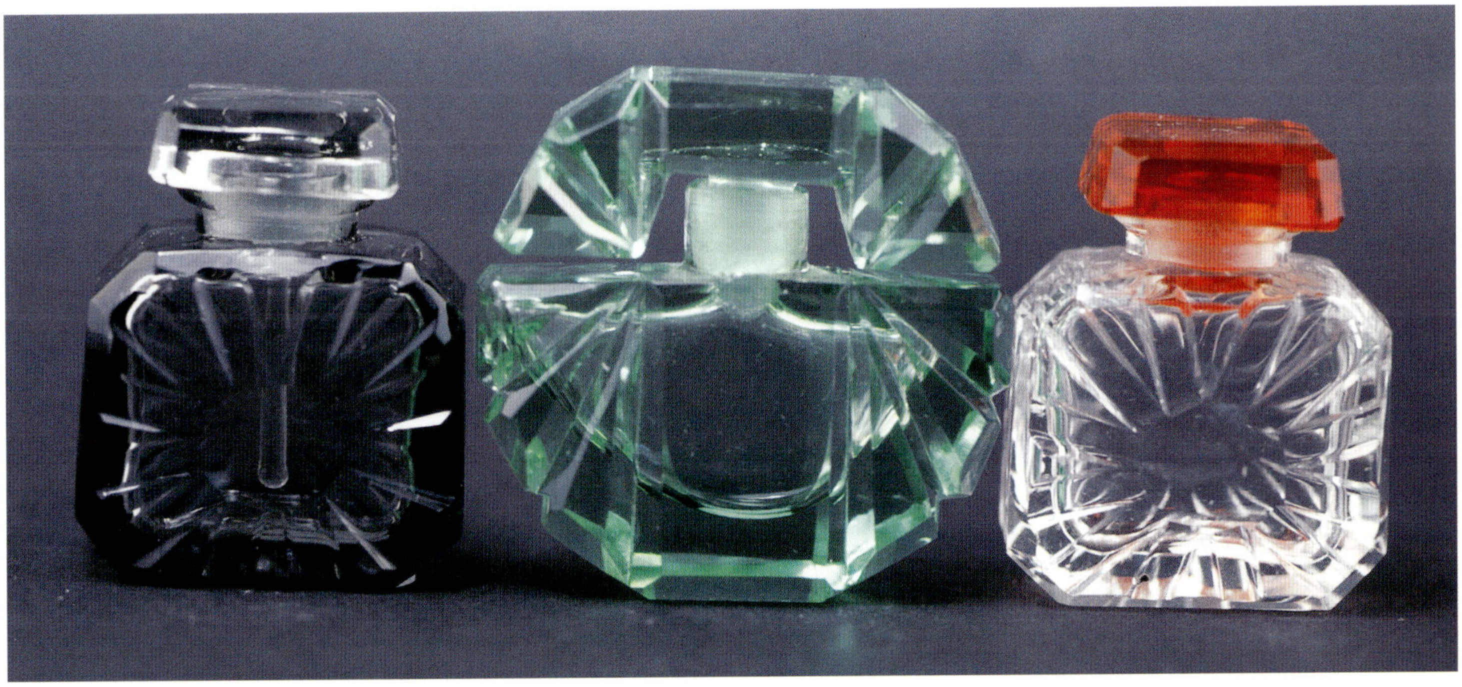

Three cap-over styles: Smoke colored bottle and top. 1.625". $150-200. Green cut with green cut over top. 1.625". $200-250. Red topped. 1.625". $150-200.

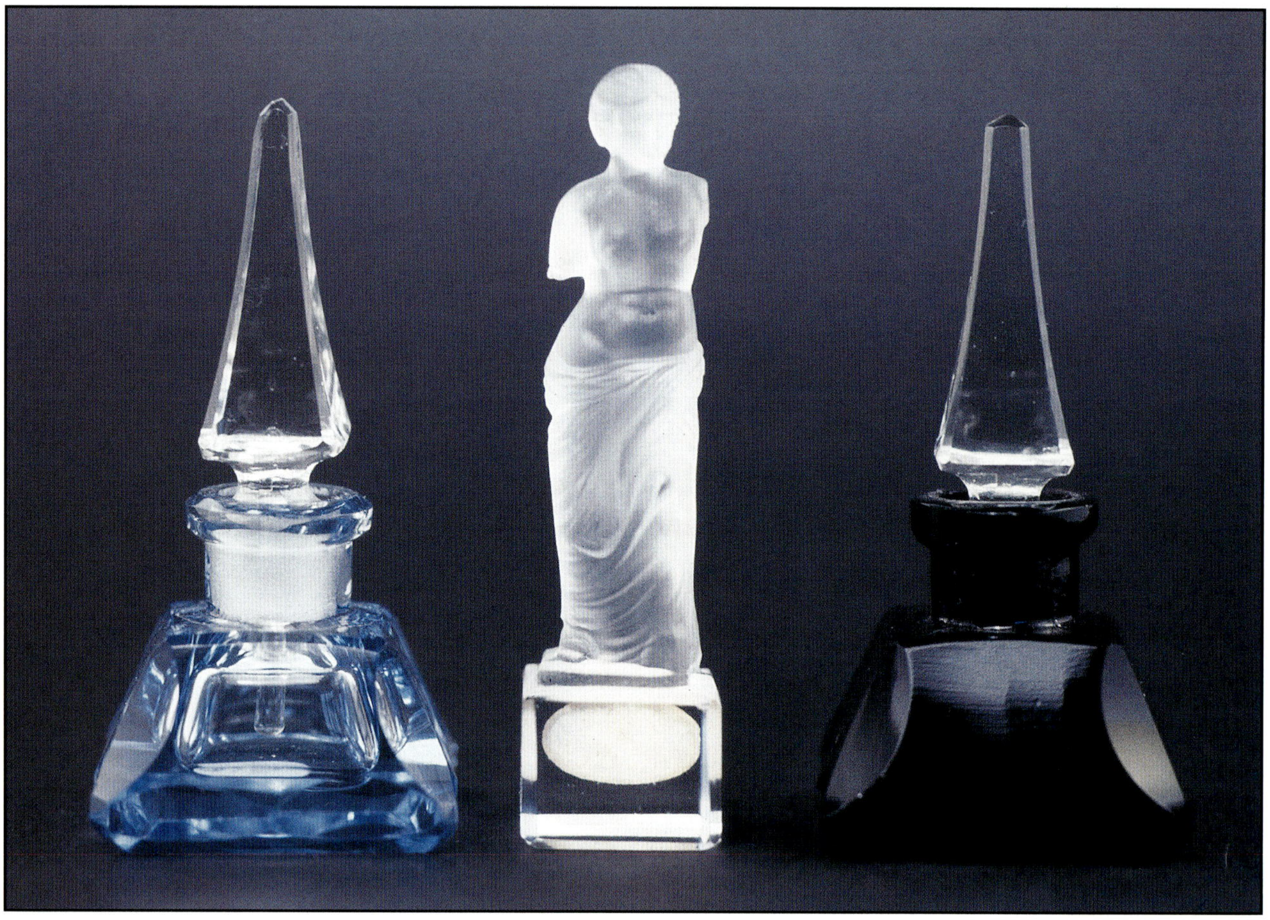

Two Irice minis; originally sold for $.59 (Jones-North, 1999, p. 96). 2.75". $150-200 each. The Venus figurine in the center is 2.875" tall and is marked Czechoslovakia with a paper label. This figure was also found as a stopper on some larger dresser bottles. $100-125.

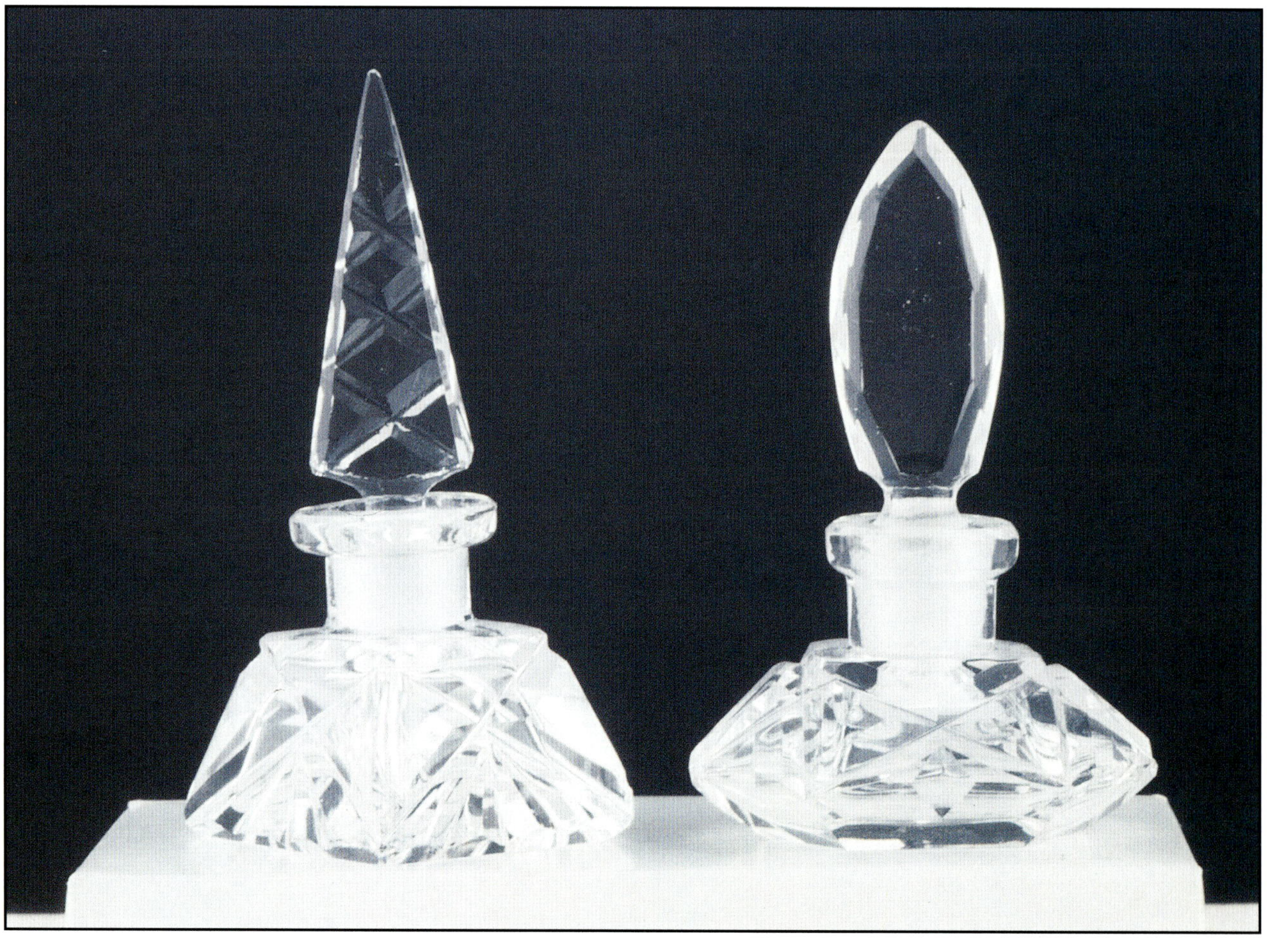

Additional Irice minis. Left: Cut clear base and top. 3". Right: Clear, shaped like lips; clear feather top. 2.75". $100-150 each.

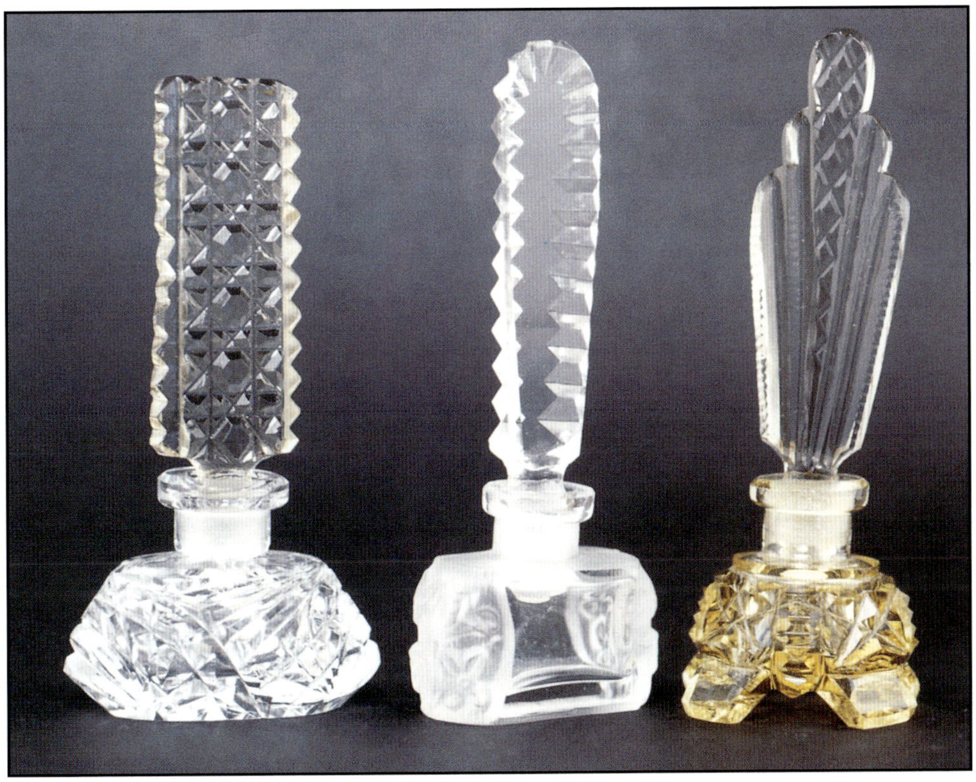

Left: Cut clear geometric base; yellow geometric top. 3.625". $150-200. Center: Clear, frosted base; tall, feather cut top. 3.875". $150-200. Right: Yellow geometric base; yellow geometric top. 3.875". $175-225.

Clear, cut base. Amethyst spire top with amethyst colored dauber. Tip of the stopper possibly broken off. 3". $100-125.

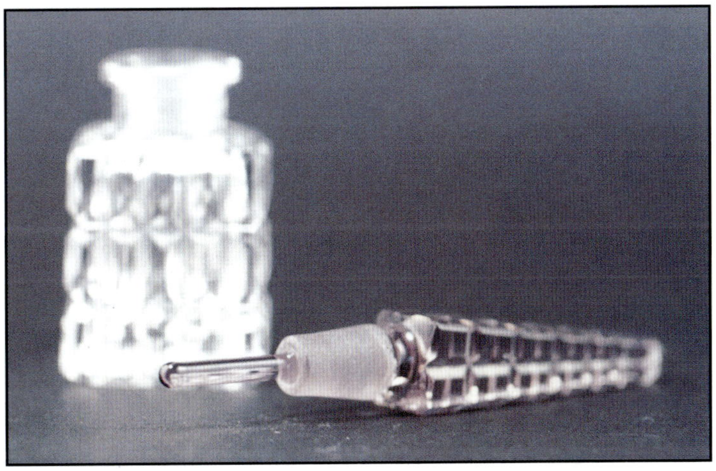

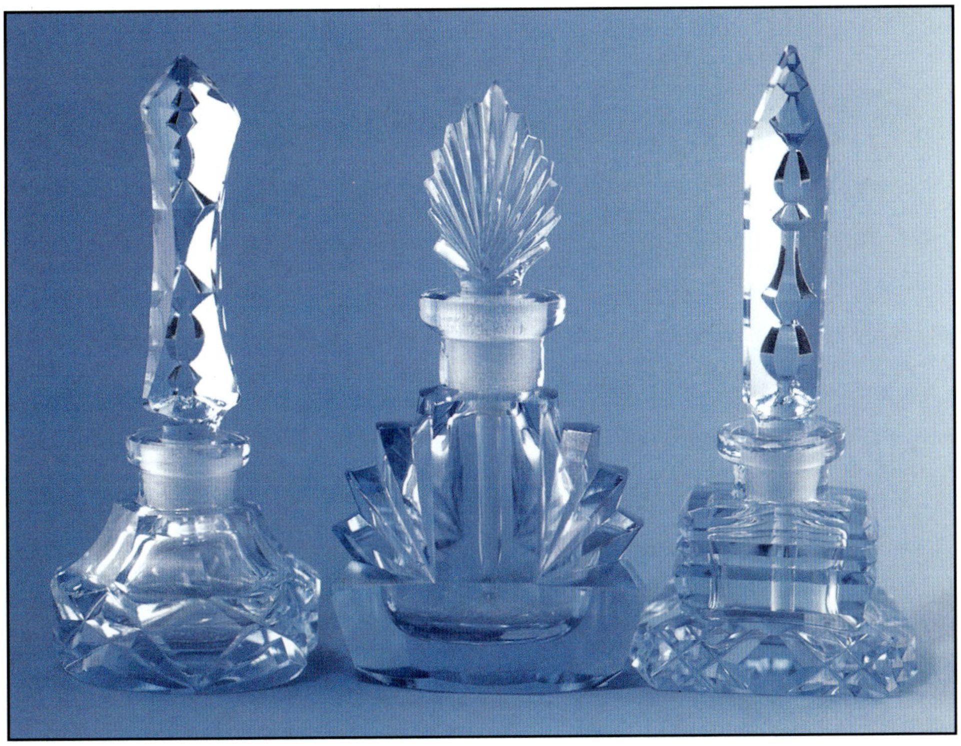

Three blue cut glass minis and tops. The outer two have triangular stoppers with the back "corner" edge shaped to form the pattern viewed from the front flat surface. Left: 3.25", $175-200. Center: 3", $150-200. Right: 3.5", $175-200.

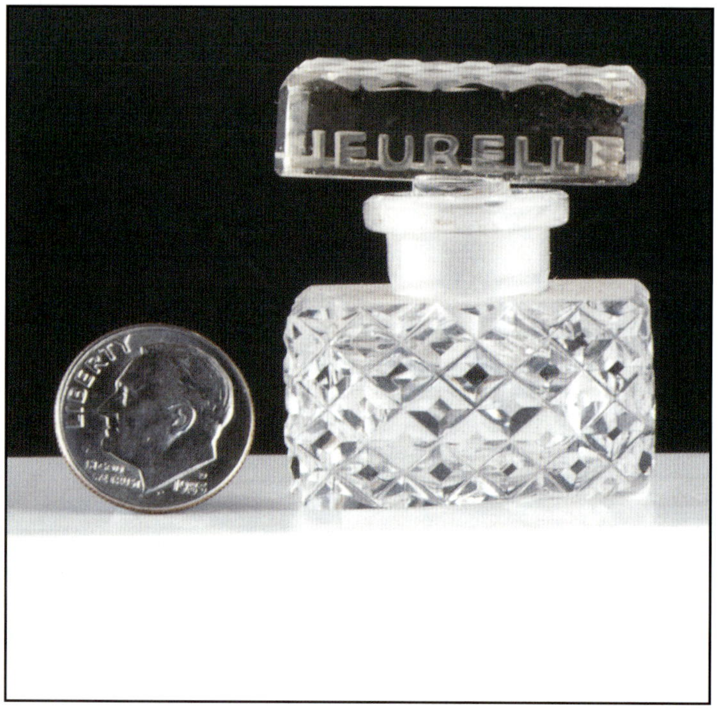

Cut glass base; pale yellow top reads "Jeurelle" for a commercial perfume. 1.675". $100-150.

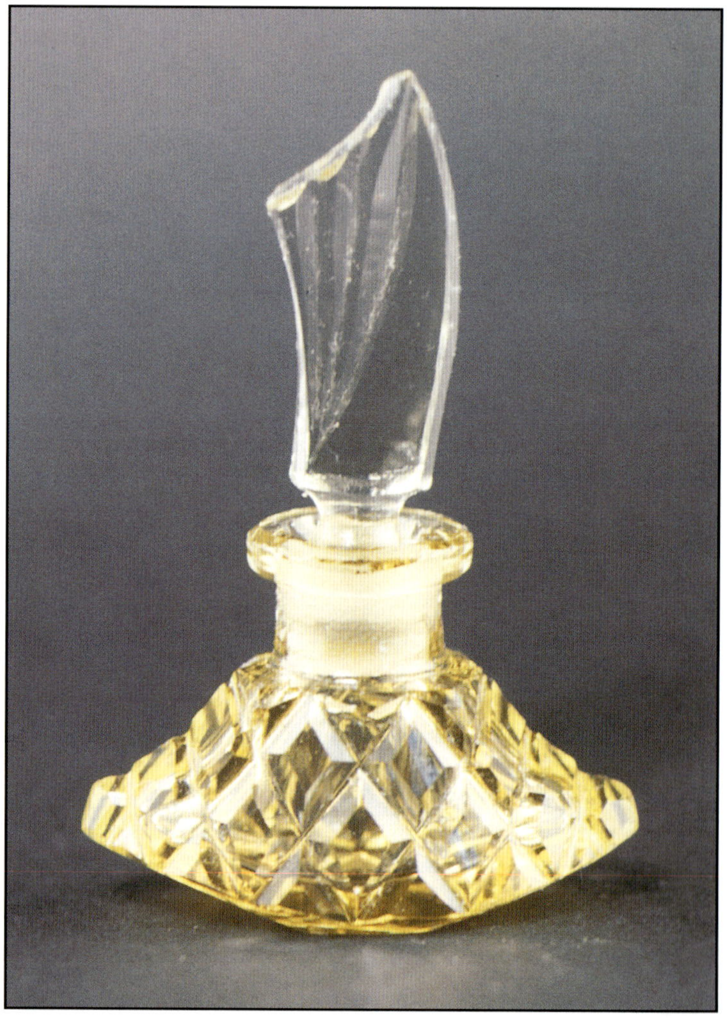

Amber cut bottle and asymmetrical top. 4". $200-250.

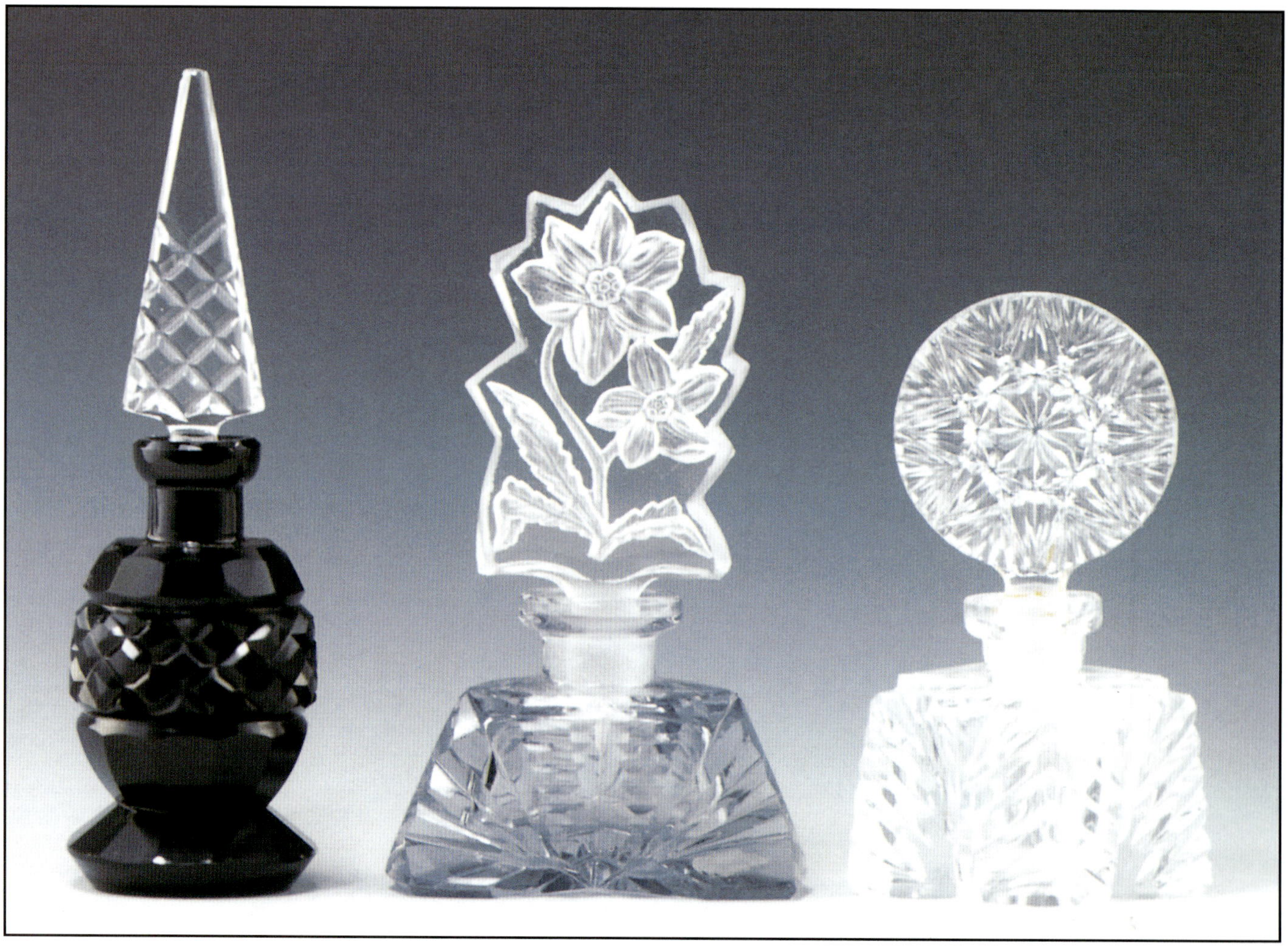

Three minis. Left: Opaque black base with a clear, geometric cut stopper. 4". Center: Amethyst cut base with a floral intaglio stopper. 3.75". Right: Clear mini with a highly cut base and round starburst stopper. 3". *All courtesy of Earline Kopriva.* $125-200 each.

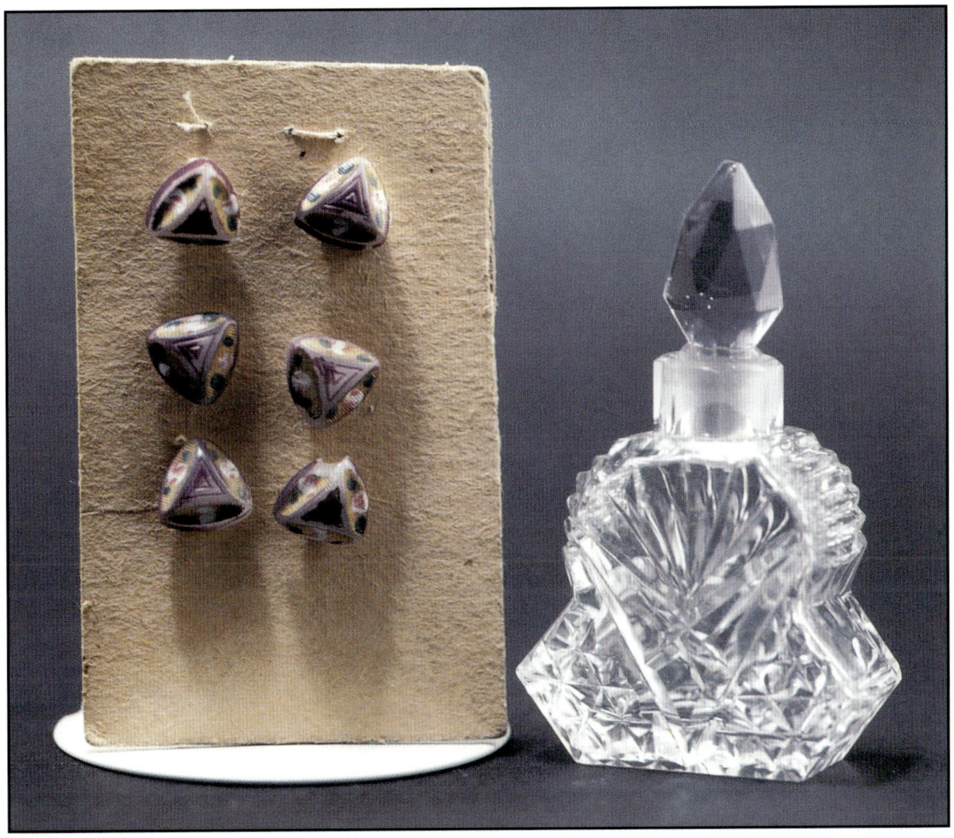

Cut glass, violin-shaped bottle with amethyst prism stopper. 2.25". $150-175. Shown with a card of antique glass buttons. $10-15.

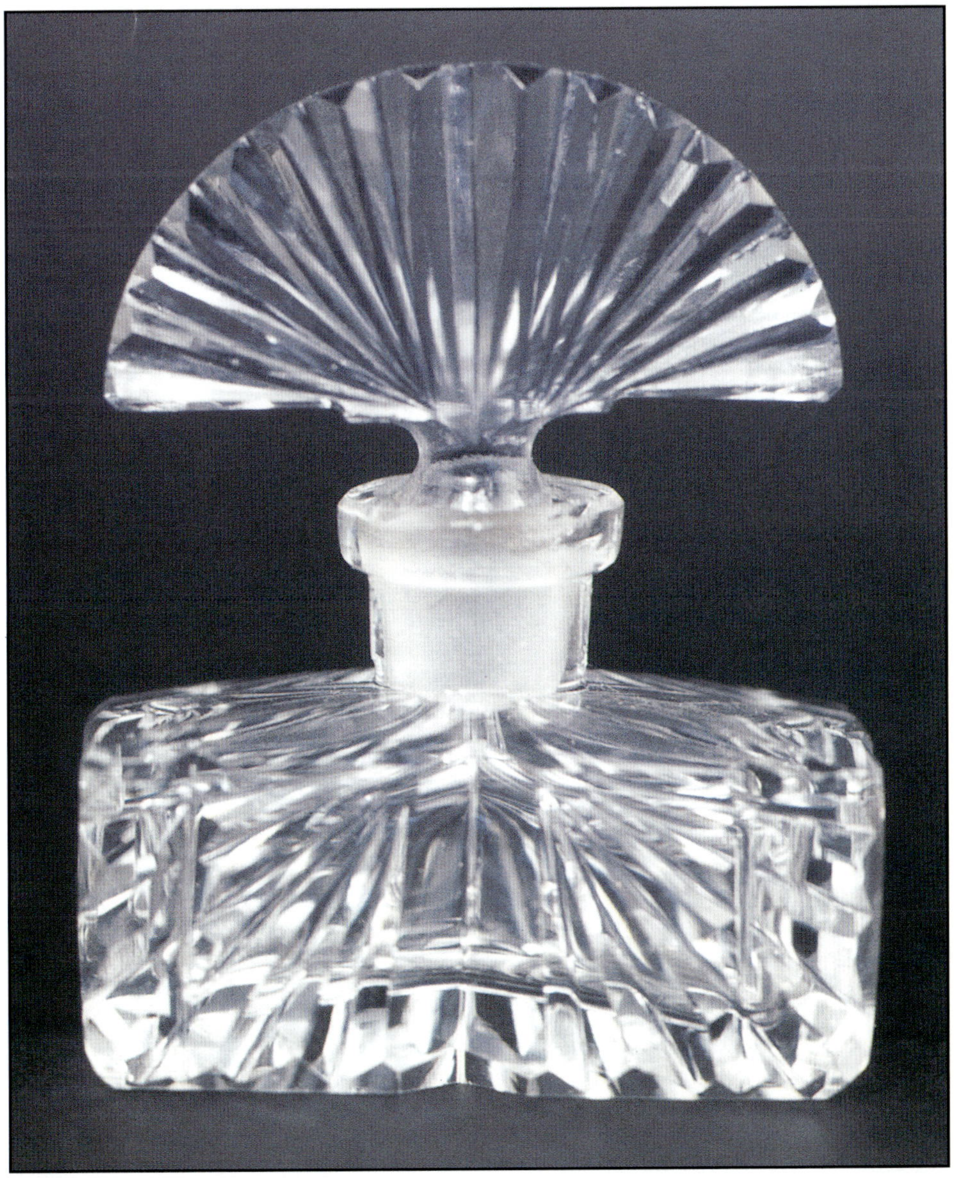

Clear cut glass base with amethyst cut fan stopper. 2.5". $200-250.

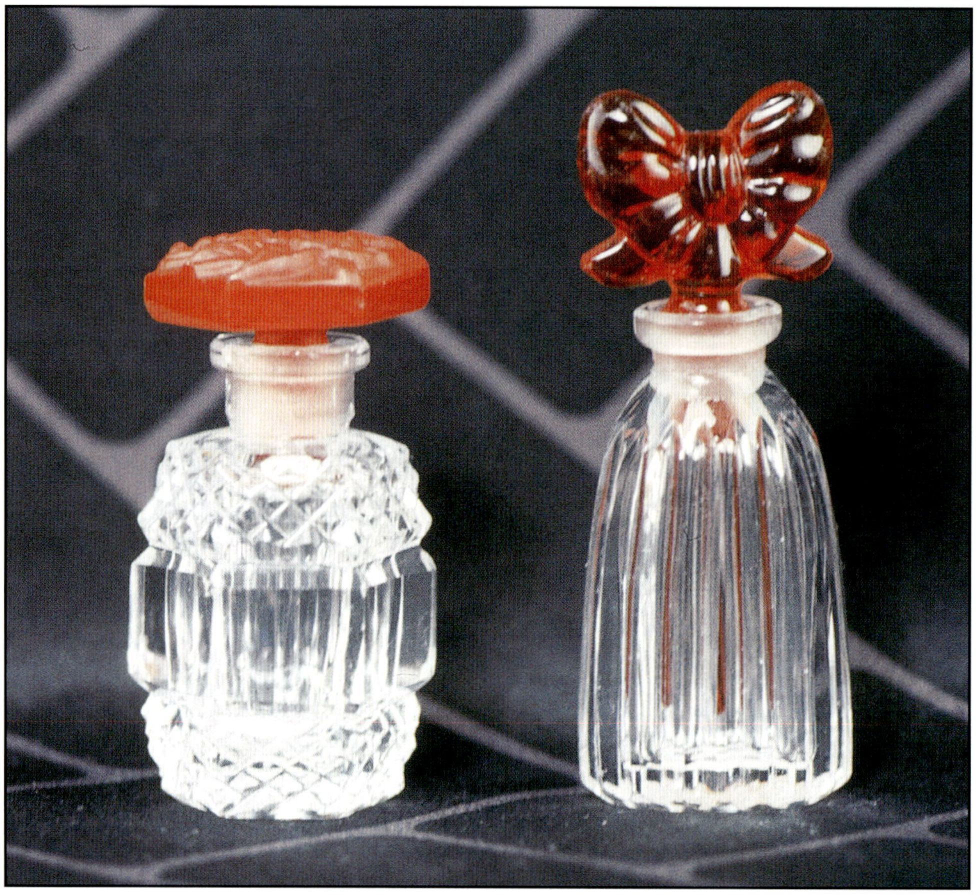

Left: Clear, geometric cut base; unusual opaque red floral top. 1.875". $200-250. Right: Molded clear base, unusual molded transparent red bow top with red dauber. 2.5". $250-300.

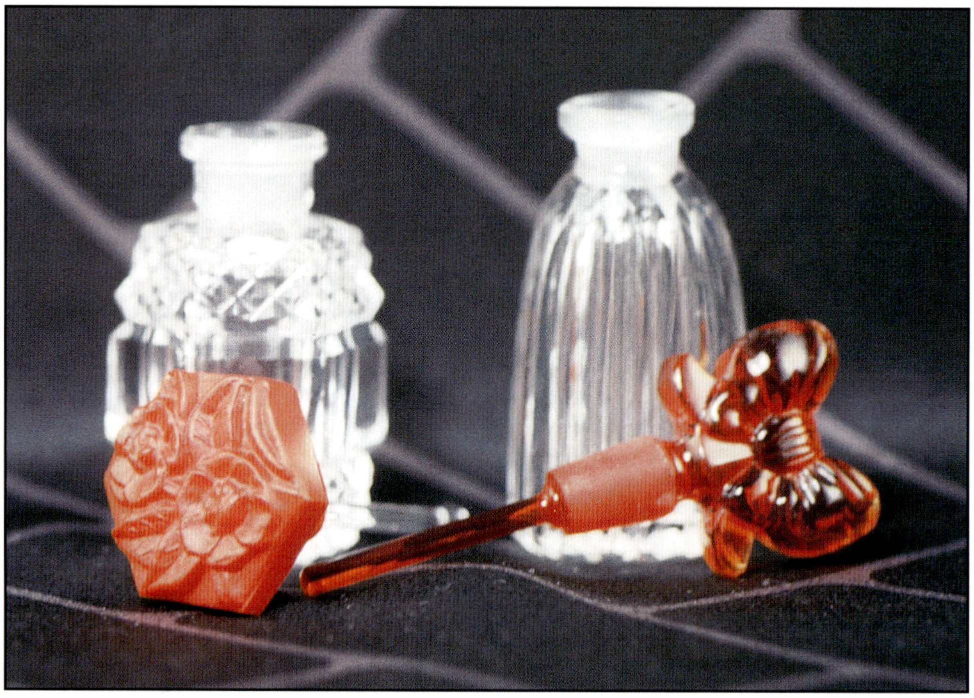

Same bottles, showing top detail.

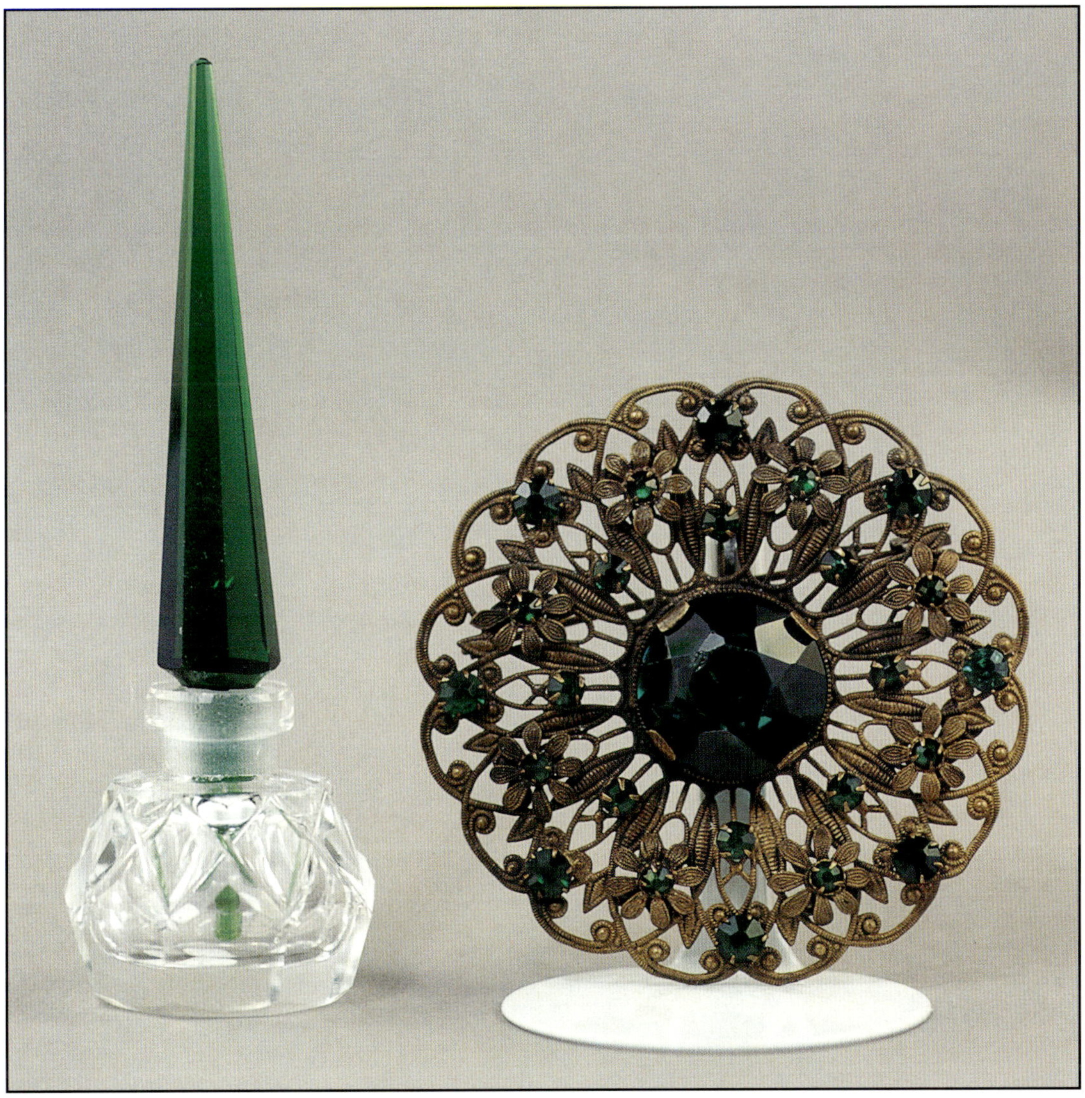

Clear, cut crystal base; unusual emerald green spire stopper with green dauber. 4". $250-300. Shown with a marked filigree and "emerald" brooch. $50-75.

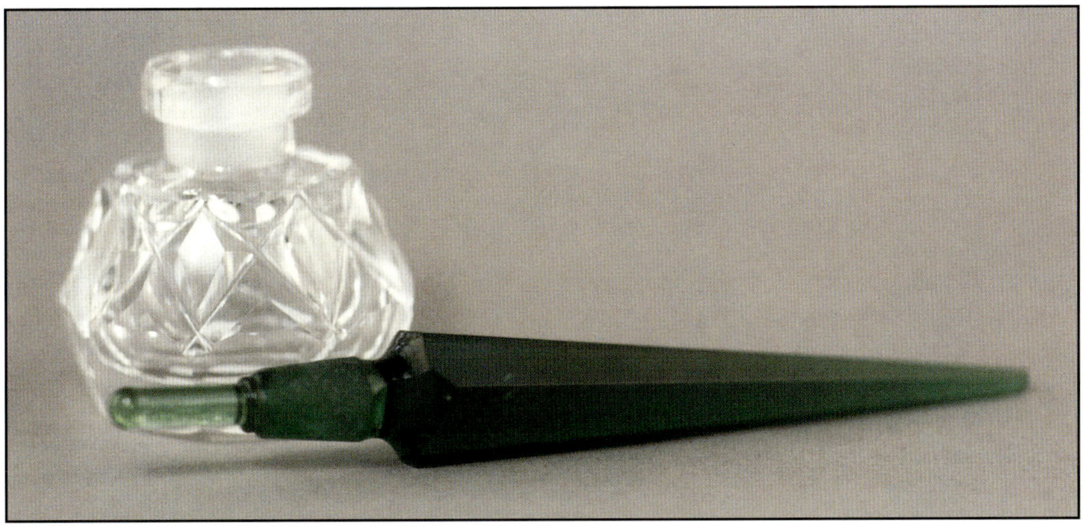

Same bottle, showing stopper detail.

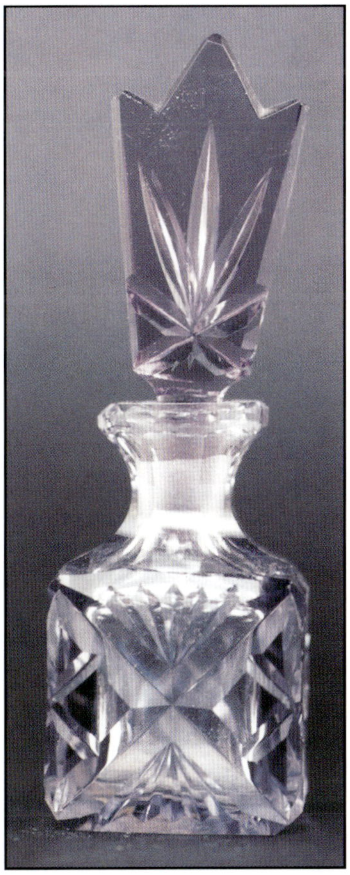

Amethyst cut glass bottle and stopper. 4". $150-200.

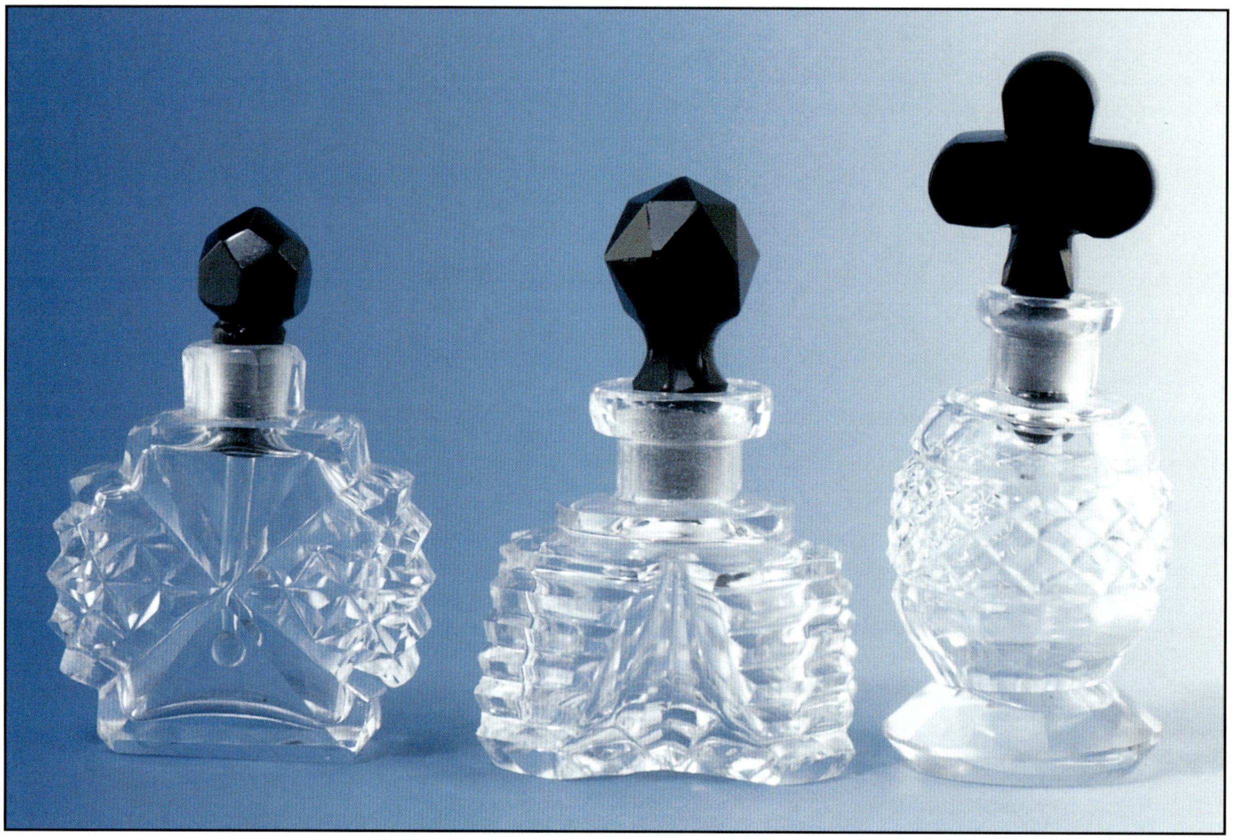

Three clear, cut glass bases with opaque black stoppers: Left: 2.25". $150-200. Center: Heavier base, larger prism top. 2.5". $150-200. Right: Club card suit top. 3". $175-225.

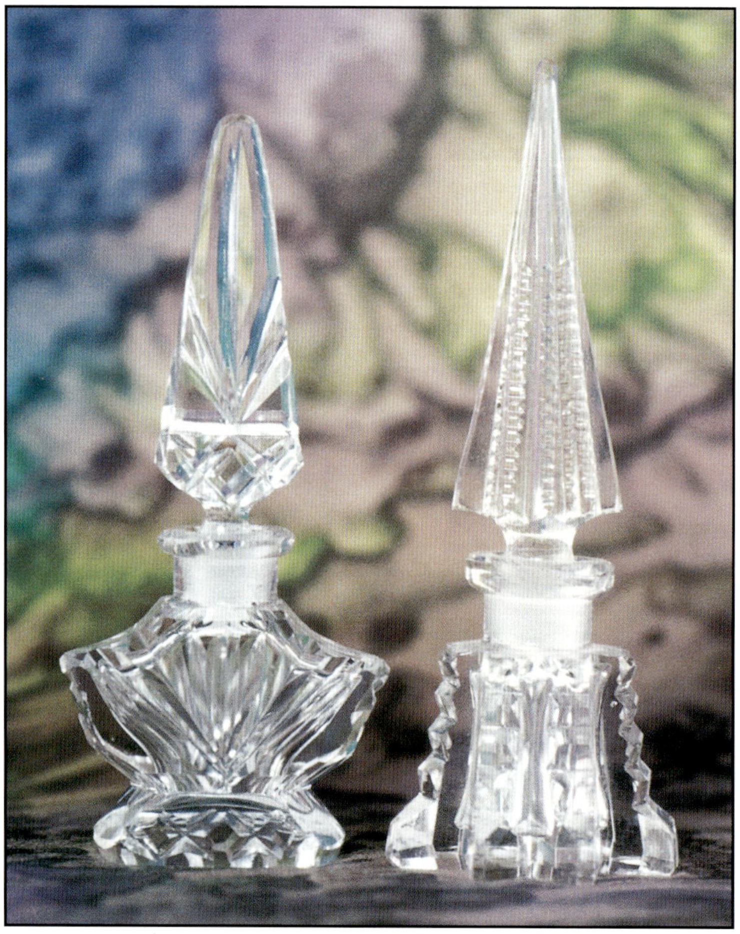

Two clear geometric cut bases and tops: Left: Simple cuts. 3.625". $150-200. Right: Ornate cuts. 4". $150-200.

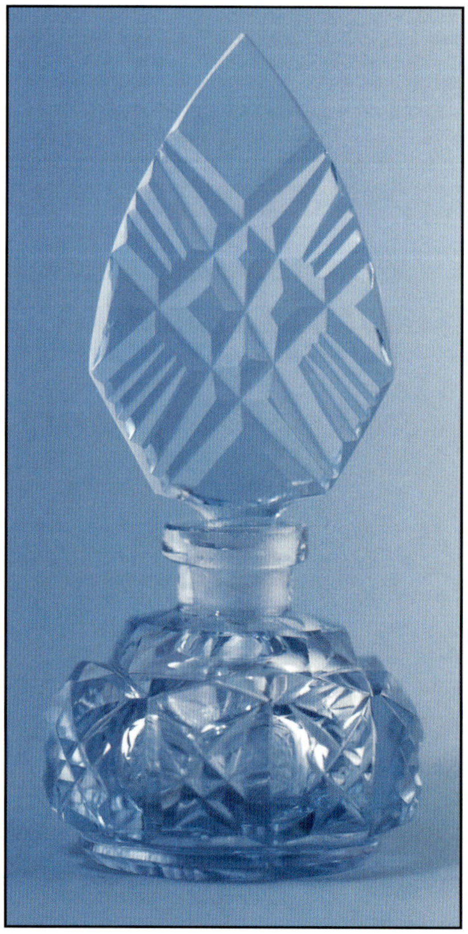

Blue cut glass mini, matching top. 3.75". $200-275.

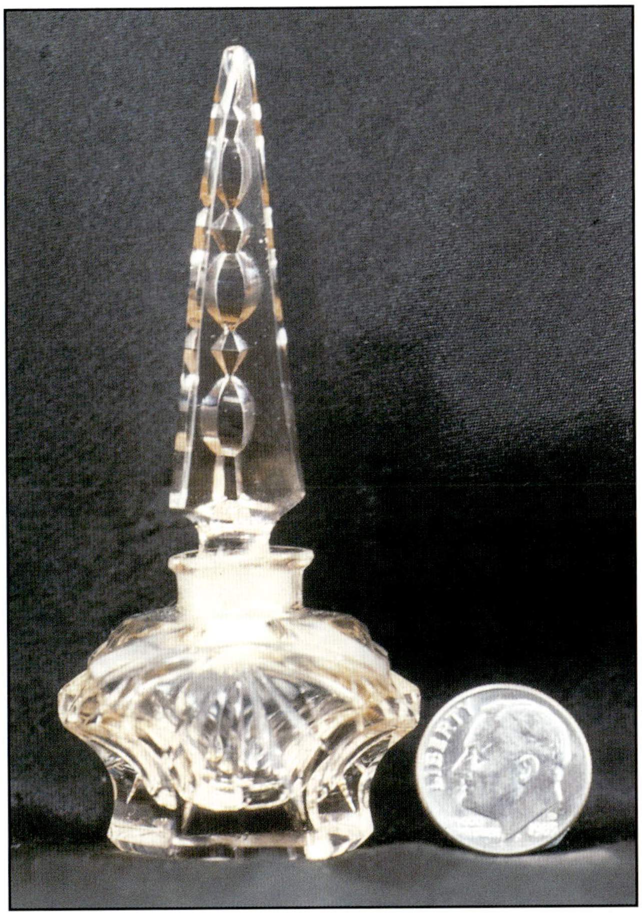

Pink cut glass mini, triangular top, cut from the back corner. 3.75". $175-225.

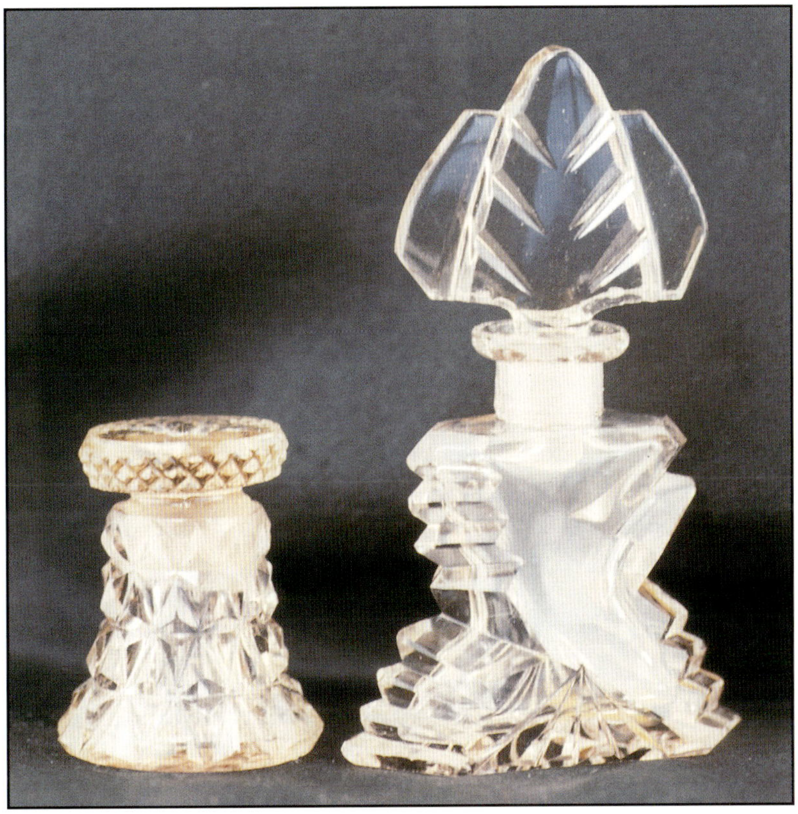

Two pink cut glass minis, matching tops: Left: Short bottle with an unusual, wide neck. 1.625". $100-150. Right: Asymmetrical cut bottle. 3.5". $125-175.

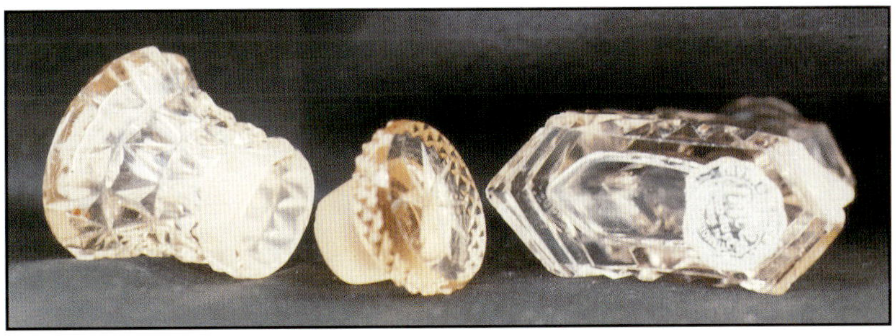

Showing previous bottles' cap detail and black and silver "Irice" sticker on the bottom of the larger bottle.

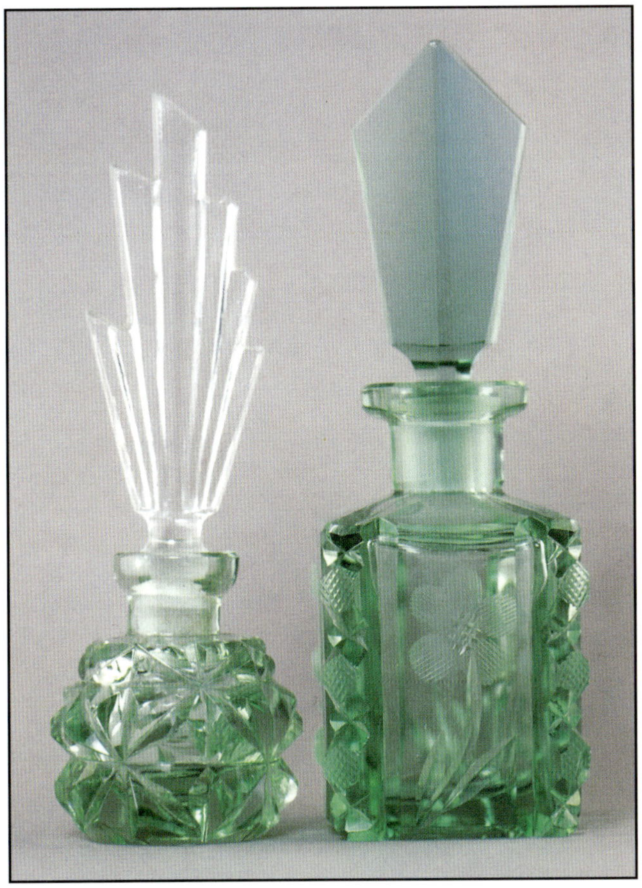

Two green cut glass bottles: Left: Clear cut glass top. 4.5". Right: Etched detail in base; green, simple faceted stopper. 4.625". $125-175.

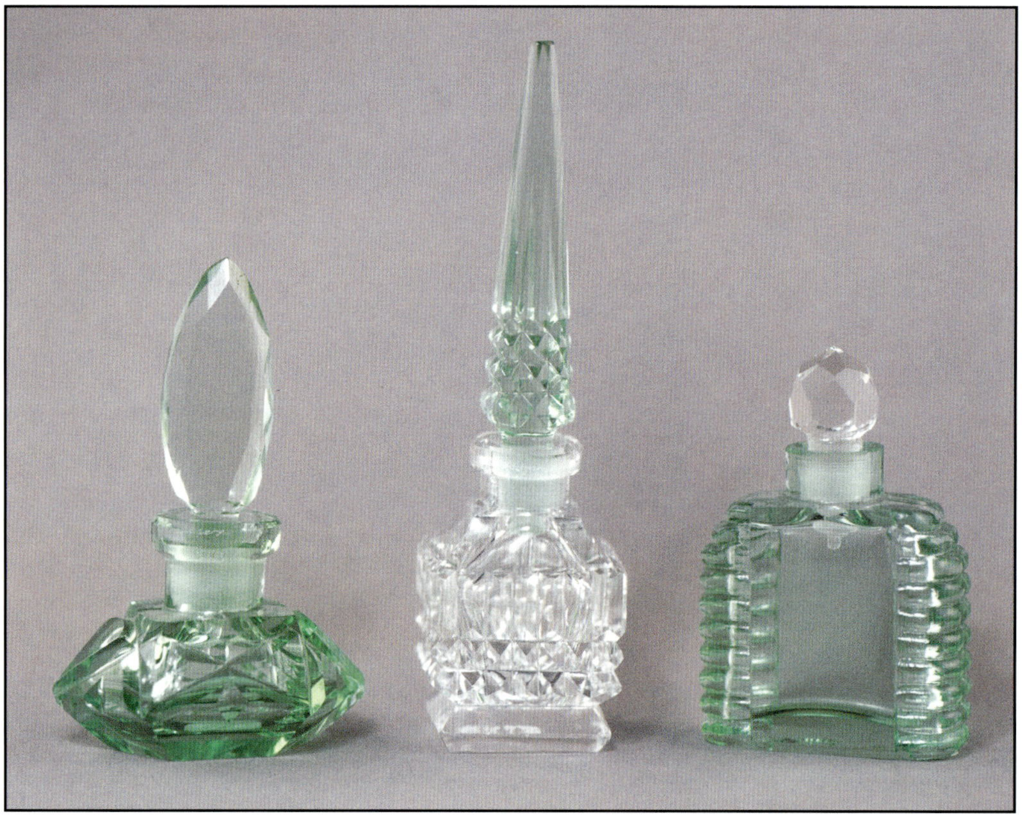

Three green minis. Left: Irice lip shape with a feathered stopper. 2.75". $100-125. Center: Clear, cut, footed base with tall green spire stopper. May be a "surviving" twin. 4". $125-175. Right: Green cut and molded base; clear, prism stopper. 2.25". $75-100.

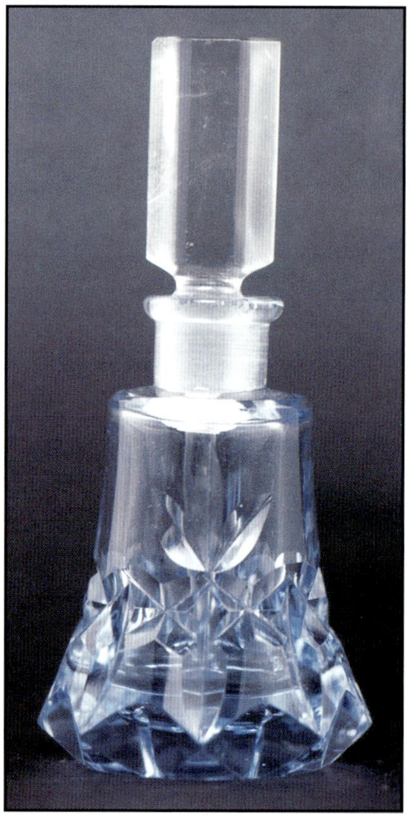

Blue cut base, clear cut stopper. 4". $125-175.

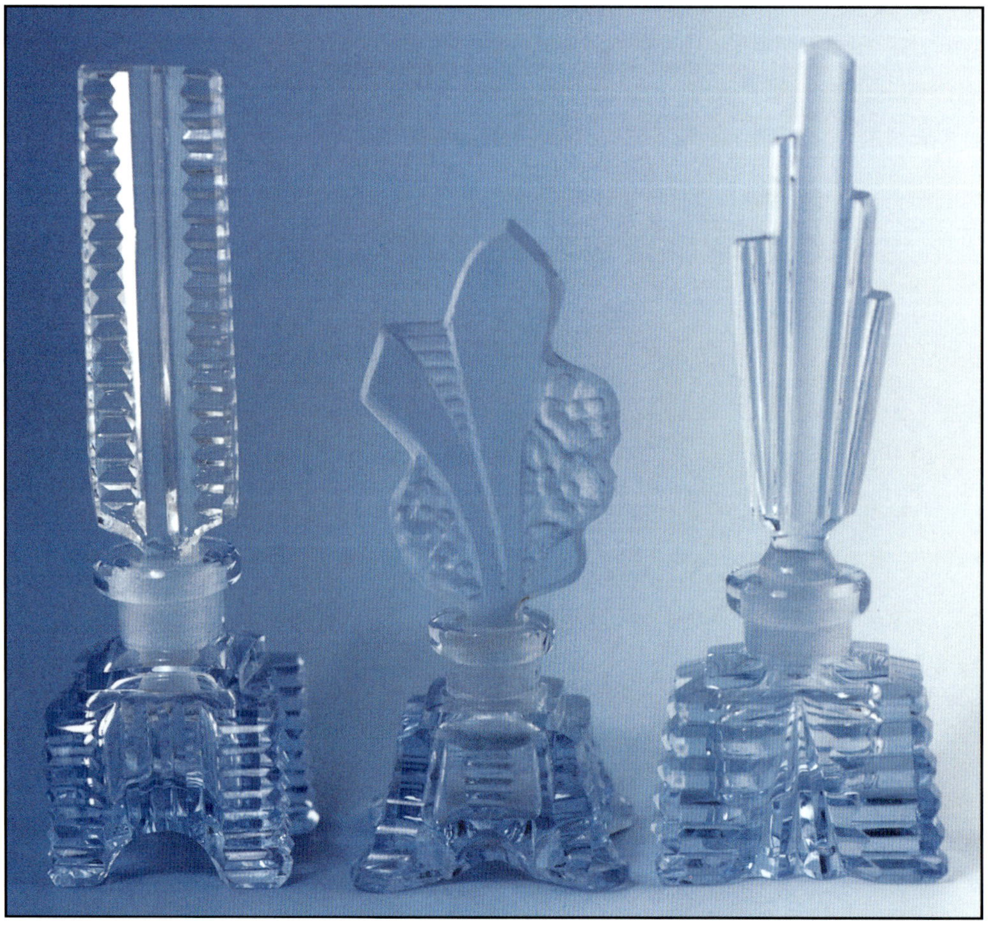

Three blue minis. Left: Blue cut base; clear, cut stopper. 4.5". $150-200. Center: Blue cut base; frosted intaglio and cut stopper. 3.375". $200-250. Right: Stair-step cut blue base; blue cut stopper. 4". $150-200.

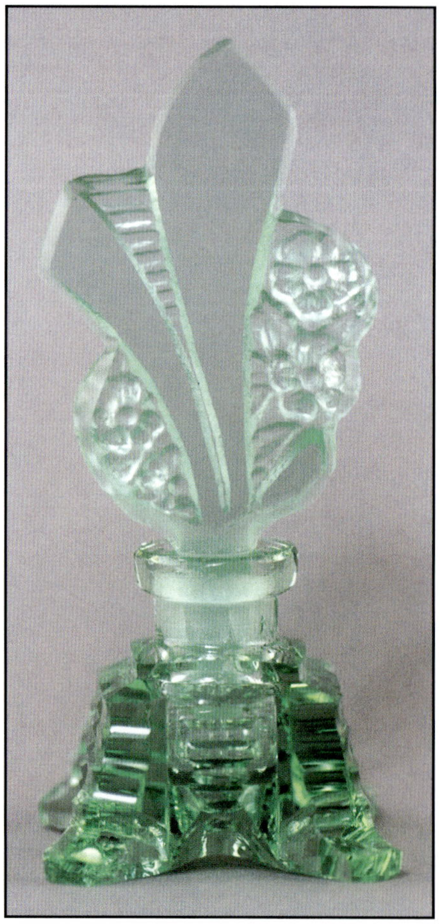

Green cut glass mini, identical to center bottle in the previous photo. 3.375". $200-250.

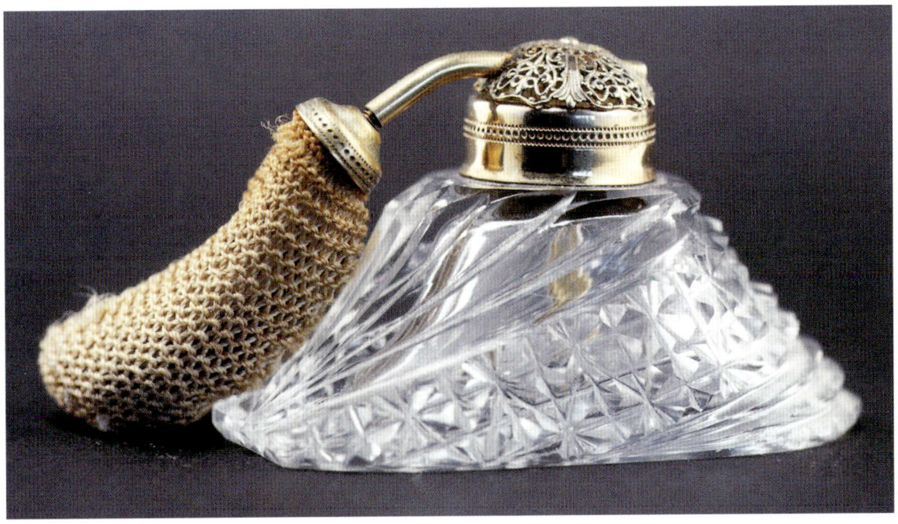

Cut glass base, mini atomizer. Some chips and other damage. 2". $50-100.

Blue trapped air mini, with a clear trapped air top. This bottle can also be found in a larger size. 2.5". $200-250.

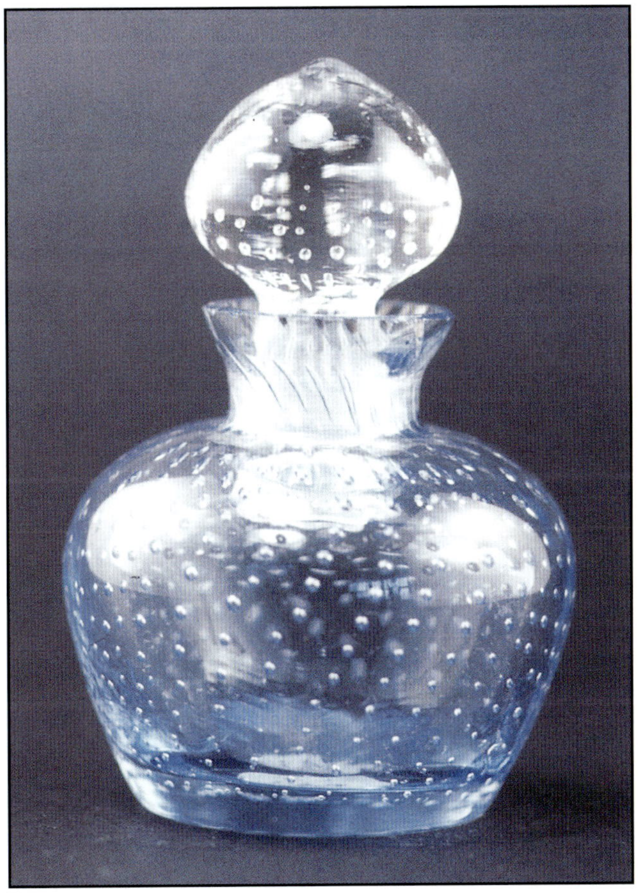

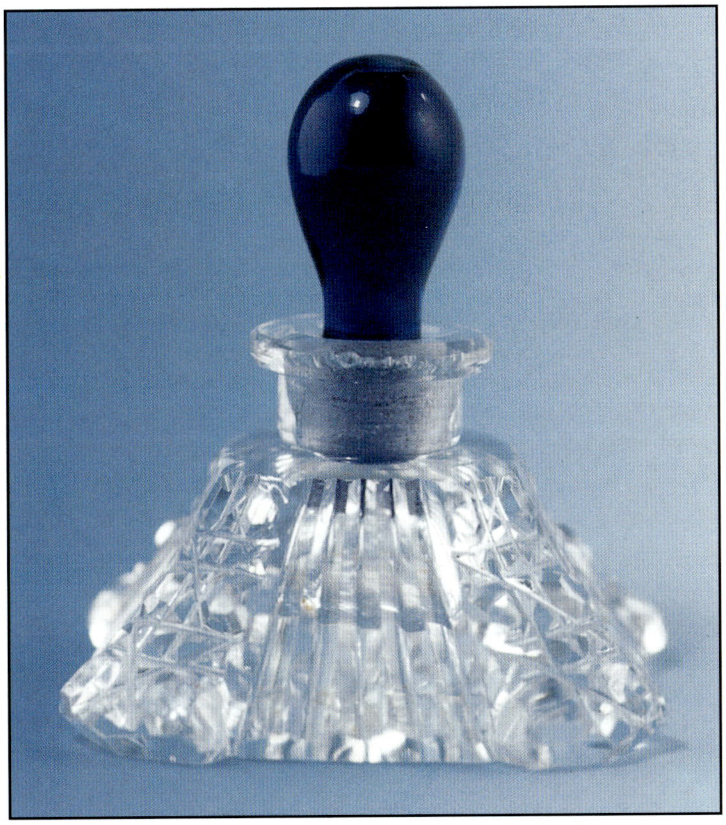

Cut glass base, unusual cobalt blue teardrop top. Shown as found; the top is a snug fit, once had a dauber. 2.25". $100-150.

Left: Clear, cut bottle with a light yellow geometrical edge-cut stopper. 3.5". $150-200. Center: Blue, simple geometric cut bottle and top. Paper label, "Made in Czechoslovakia." 2.375". $100-150. Right: Light yellow bottle base with a clear crescent stopper. 2.25". $150-200.

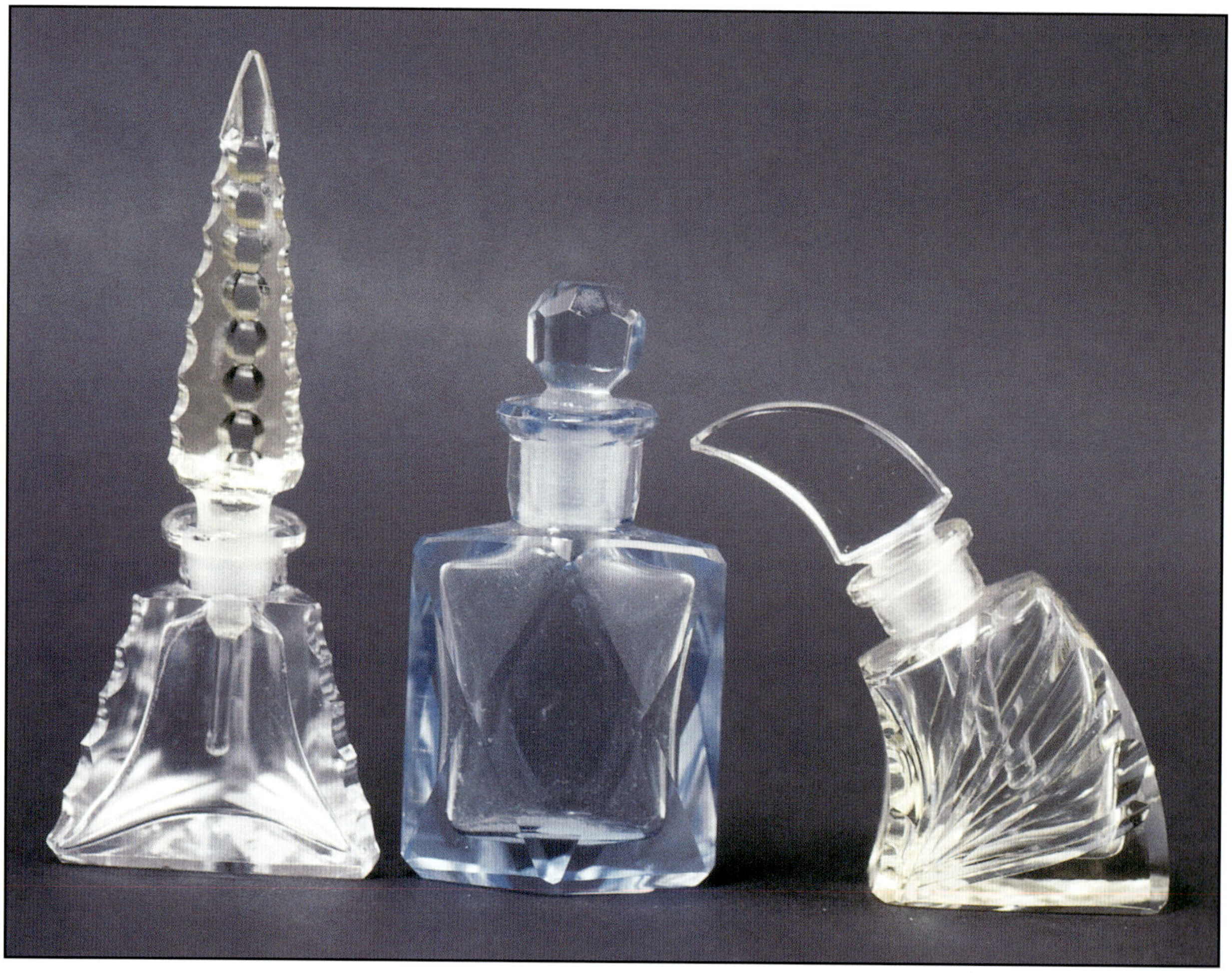

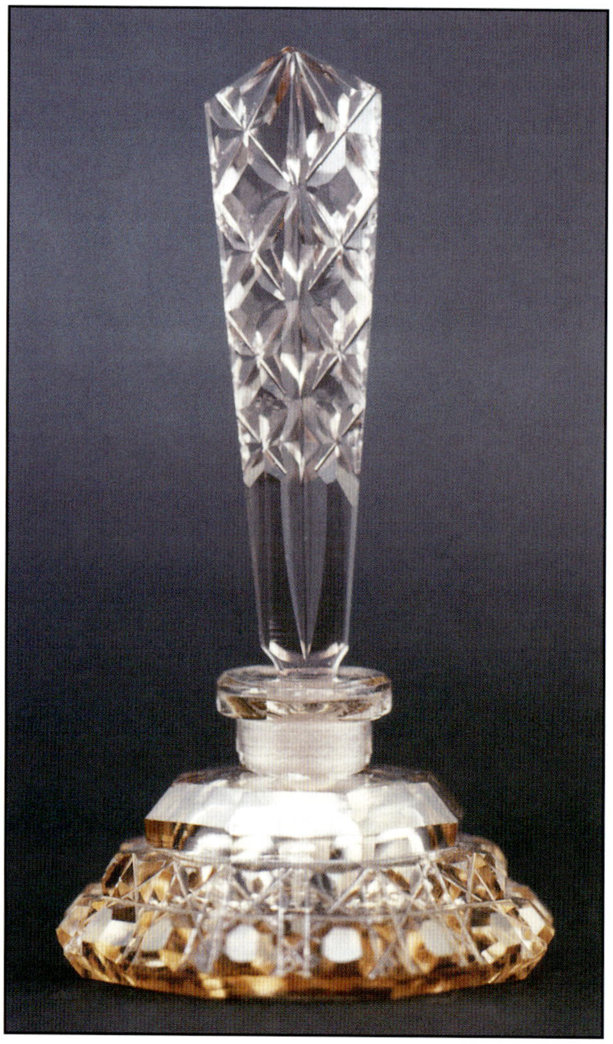

Tall, spire topped pink cut mini. 3.75". $125-175.

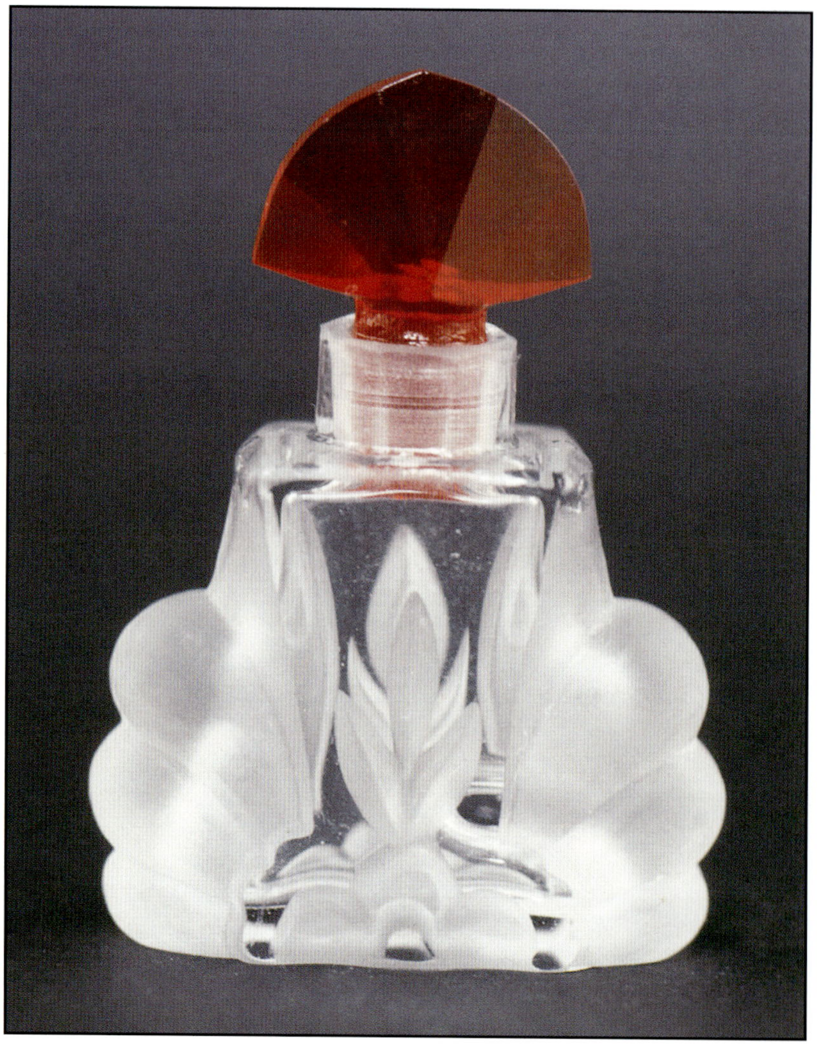

Clear and frosted bottle with red fan top. 1.375". $125-175.

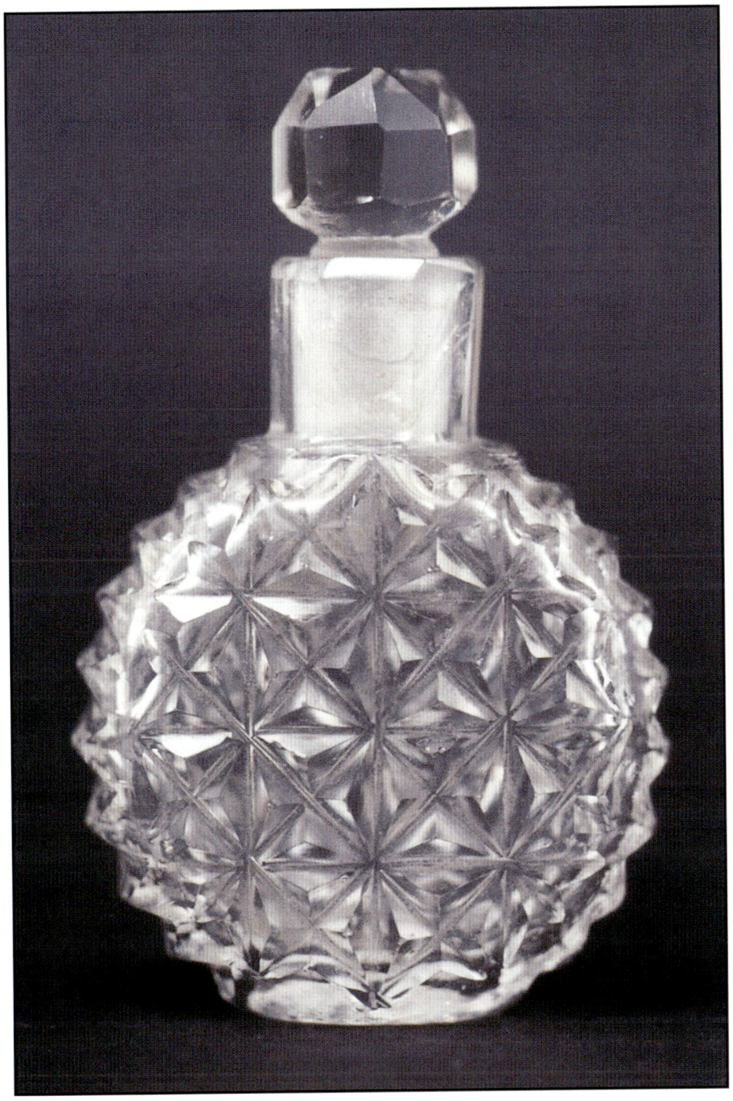

Clear diamond cut, prism top. 3.625". $100-125.

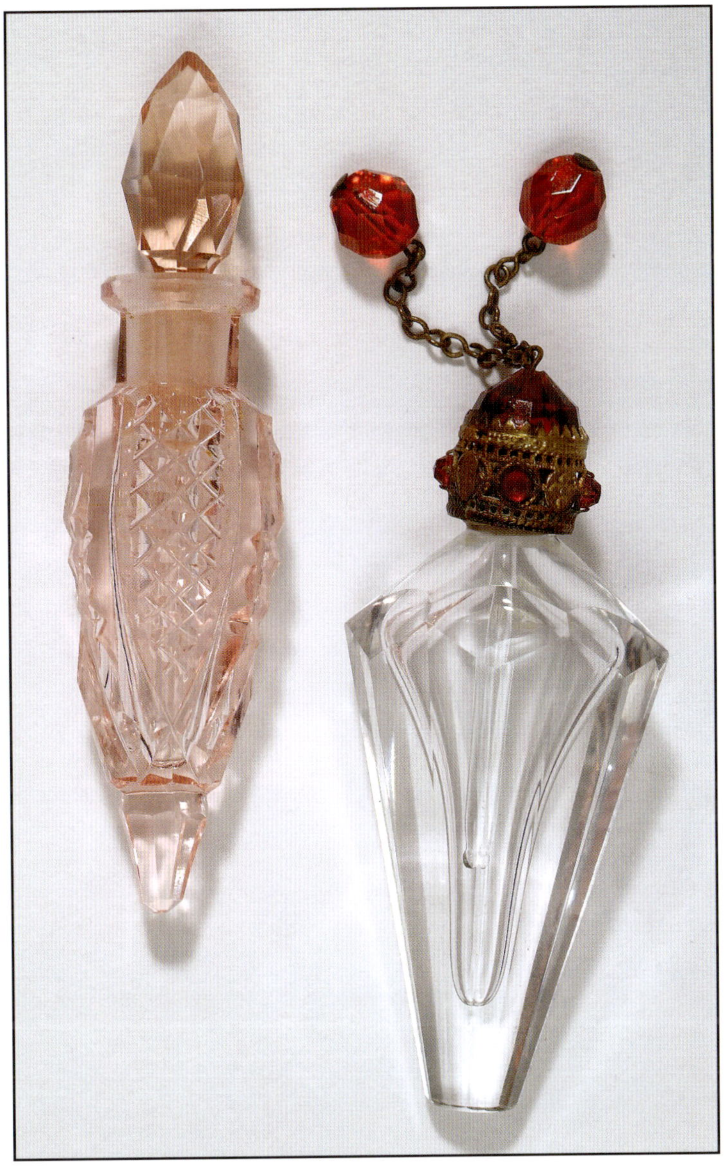

Fully cut pink crystal laydown bottle with prism cut ground stopper. 3.875". $150-175. Clear, cut crystal laydown bottle; filigree screw cap with red jewels and red glass dangles. 3.25". $200-250. *Courtesy of Don Orban Photo by David Kirk of Kirk Photography.*

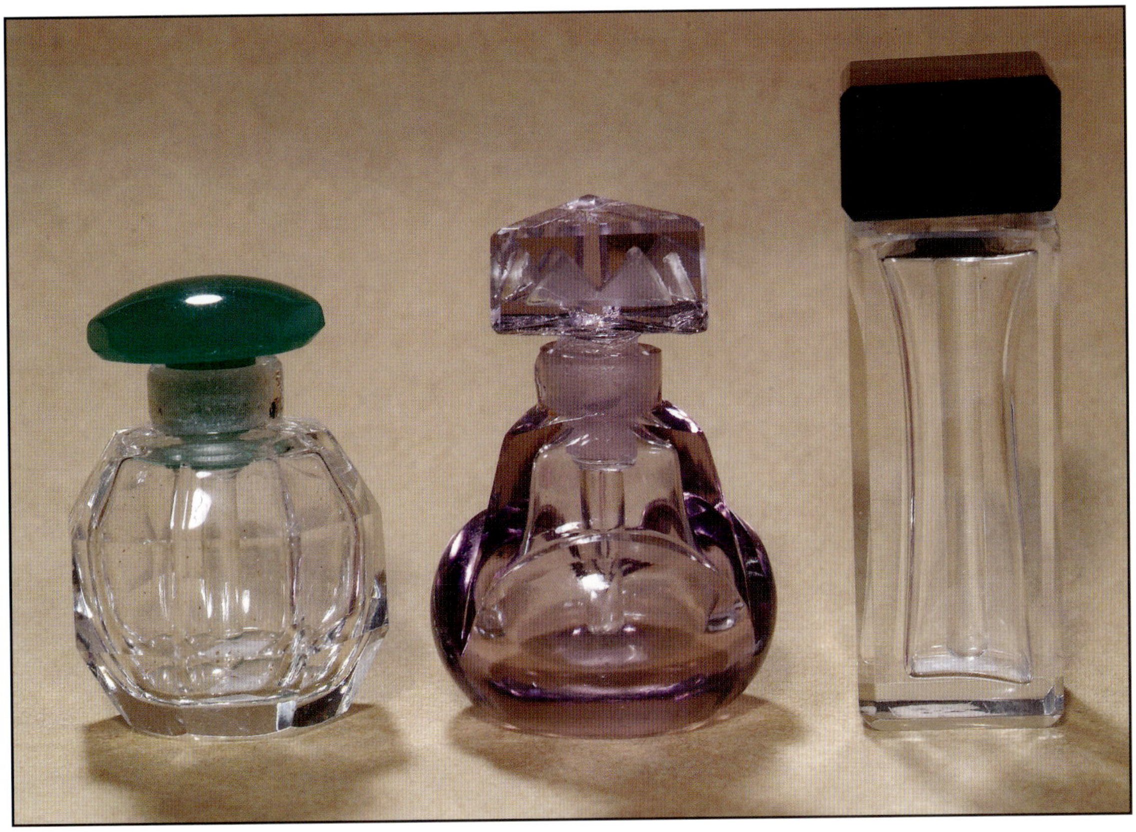

Three mini bottles. Left: Clear cut/faceted ball-shaped bottle with unusual semi-opaque blue-green glass octagonal stopper with glass dauber. 1.375". Center: Purple cut glass bottle with triangular stopper decorated with frosted intaglio triangles. Glass dauber. 1.5". Clear, polished rectangular bottle with beveled edges. Matching black glass stopper sets over neck and has long dauber. 2". *Courtesy of Don Orban. Photo by David Kirk of Kirk Photography.* $150-175 each.

Intaglio and Figural

Intaglio designs were popular, too. They featured designs molded below the surface of the bottle or stopper and acid treated to frost the molded portions. Handwork to remove mold lines and enhance the design was followed by polishing the flat surfaces.

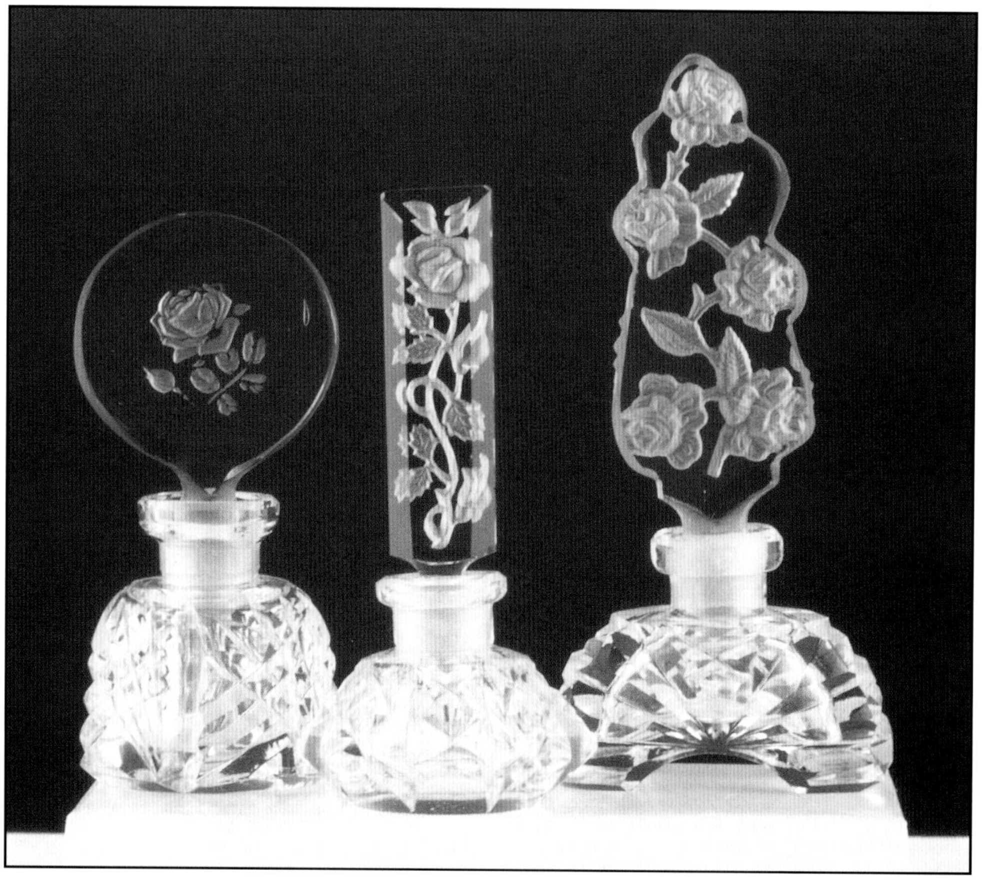

Roses, roses, roses! Three cut glass bases with amethyst, floral intaglio tops. Left: Single rose. 3". Center: Sister's friendship roses, beveled edge. 3". Right: A cloud of roses. 3.75". $175-275 each.

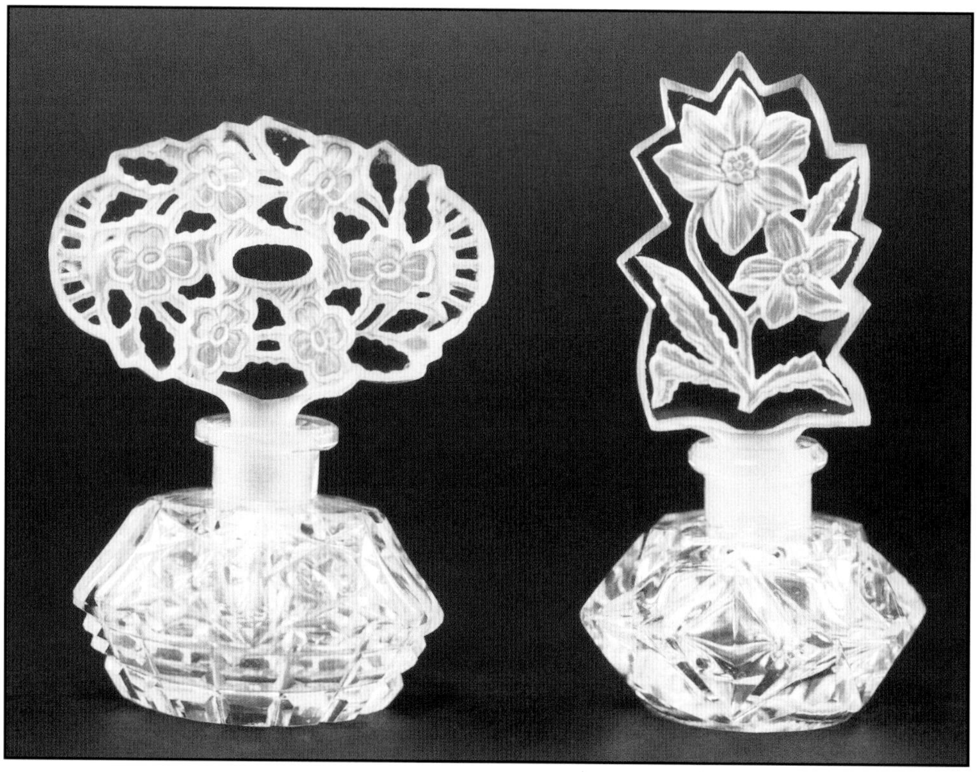

Left: Clear, cut base, pierced floral stopper. 3". Right: Opened flower and foliage. 3.5". $150-250 each.

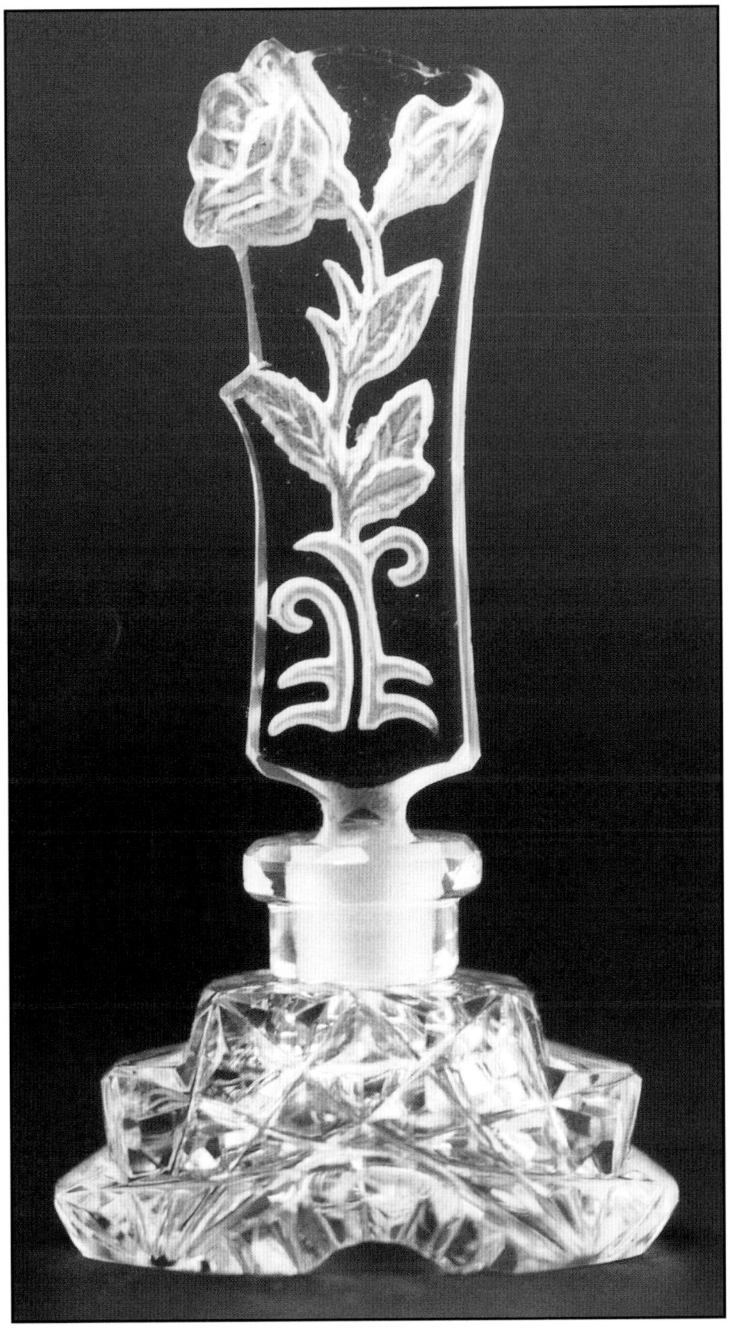

Clear, cut bridge-like base with a tall, thorned rose. 4.875". $150-250.

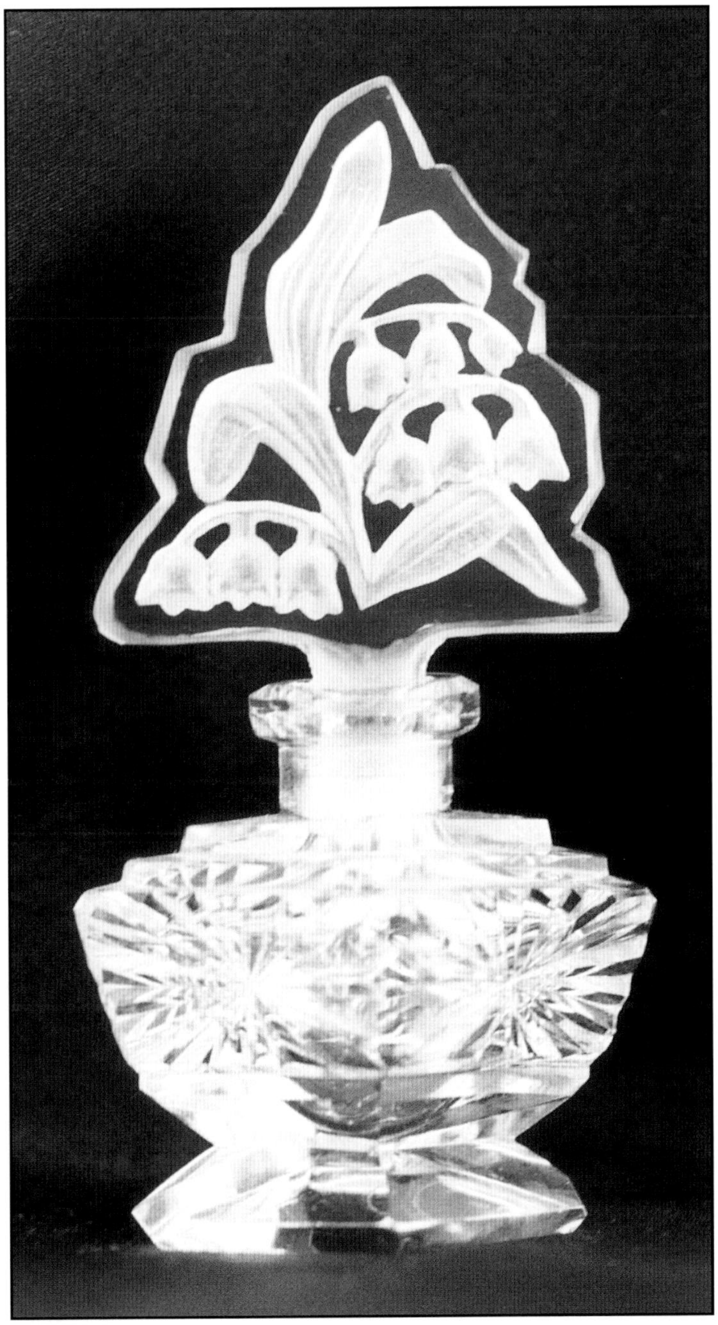

Shown at the beginning of this section with its yellow twin (see page 93), this style is shown in Jones-North (1999), p. 103 in a McCoy, Jones and Westlake advertisement. The flowers are lily-of-the-valley. 3.375". $150-200.

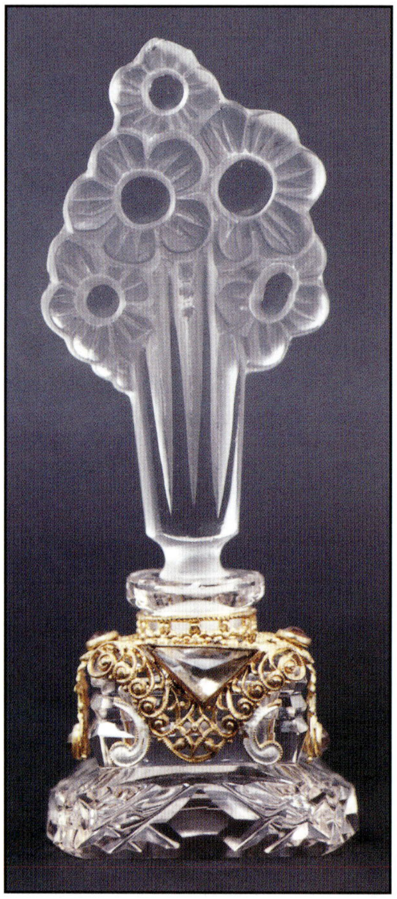

A clear bouquet of daisies forms the stopper on this pink, filigreed, jeweled base. 4". $250-300.

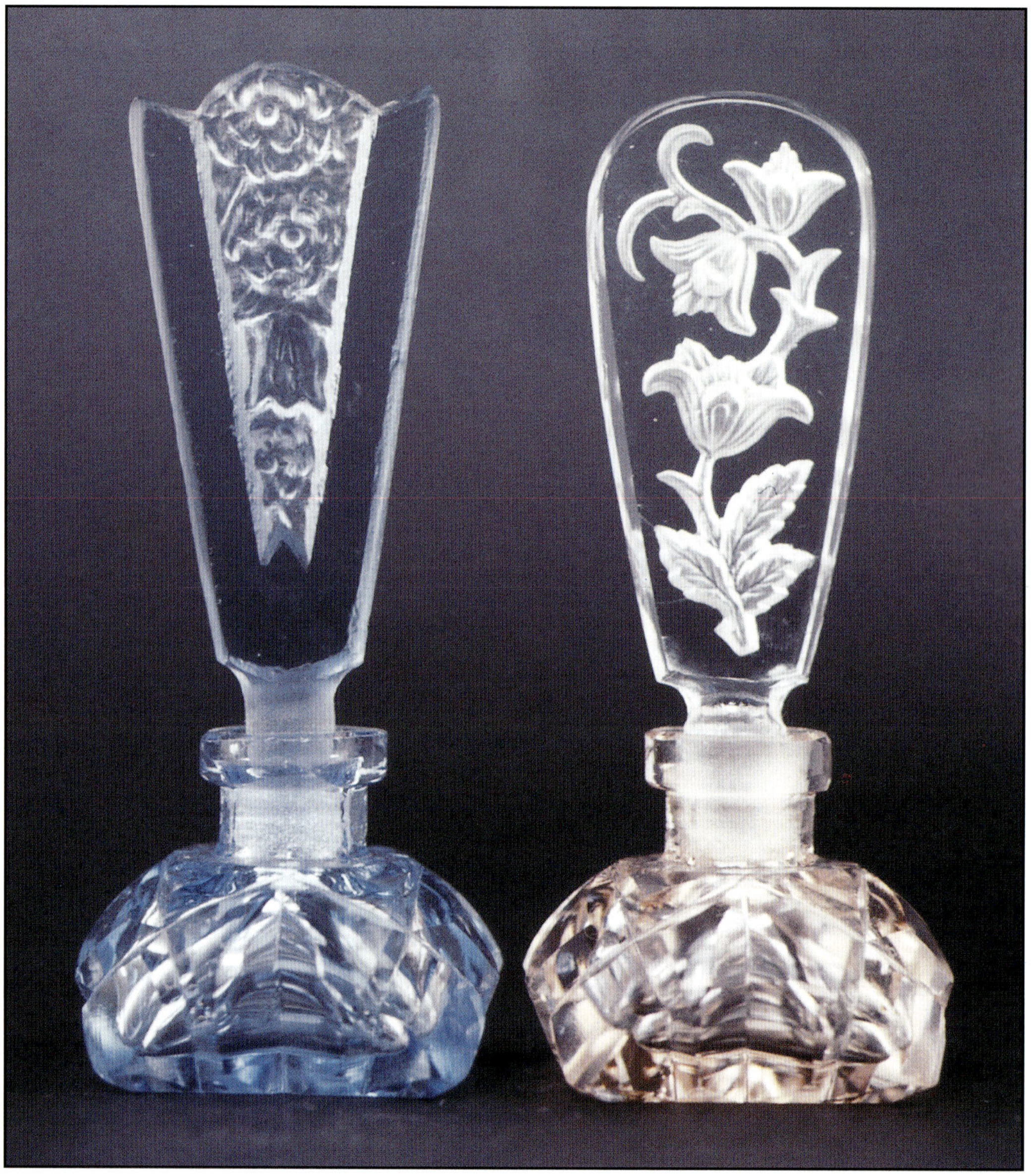

Left: Blue cut glass base with blue floral stopper. 3.625". Right: Same base in pink with a clear blooming vine stopper. 3.5". $200-250 each.

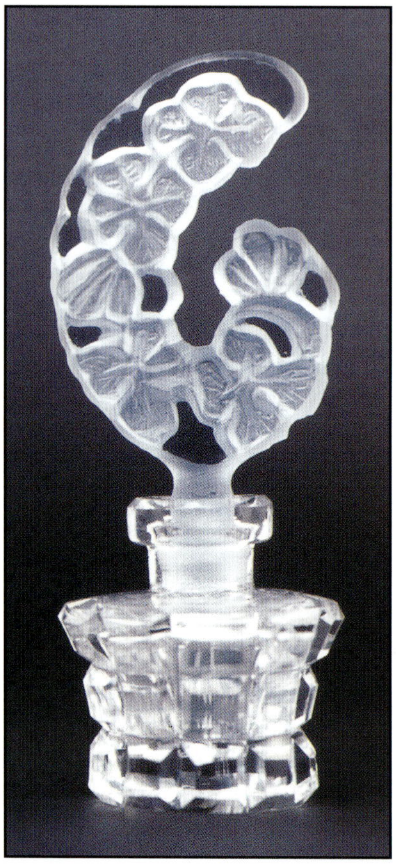

Clear, cut base with a "C" shaped stopper; a drift of flowers in an unusual soft blue. 3.875". $200-250.

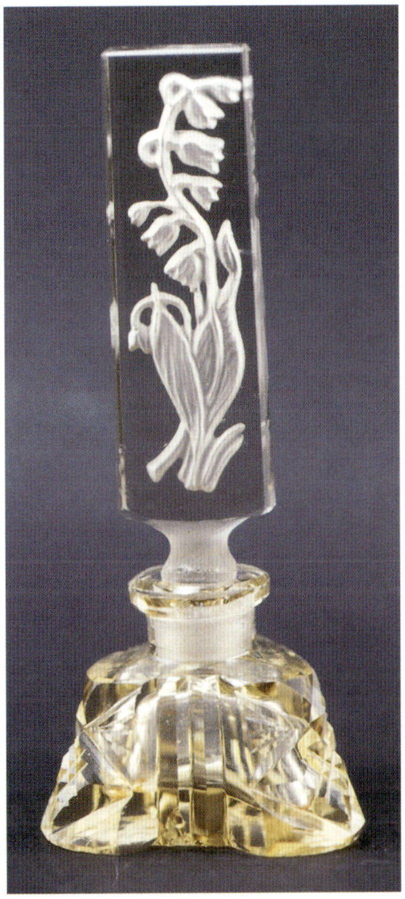

Yellow, three-sided base with a yellow, floral intaglio stopper. 3.75" $200-250.

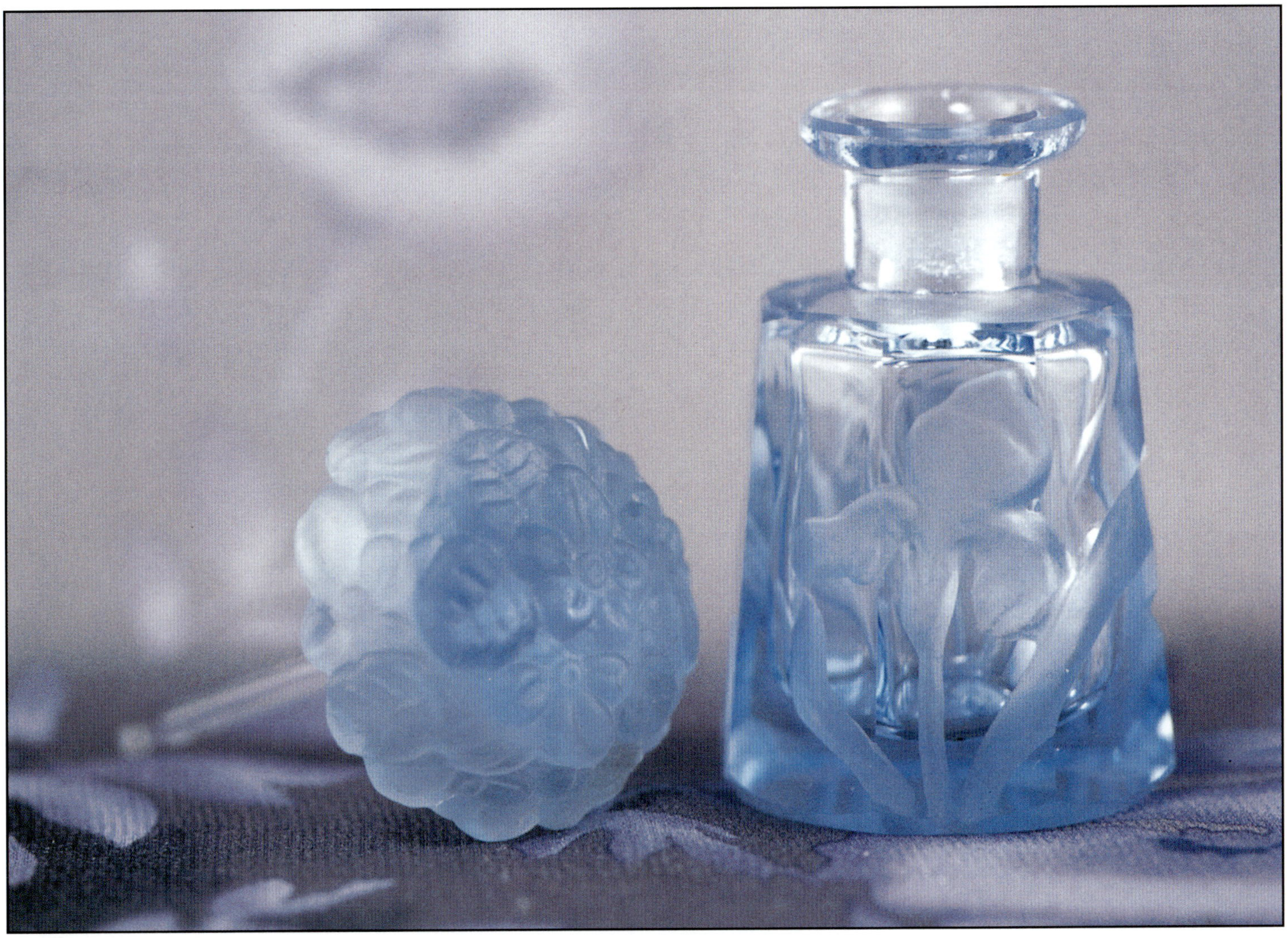

Intaglio iris are molded and frosted in the base of this bottle. The stopper is a molded cap of flowers. 2.875". $300-400.

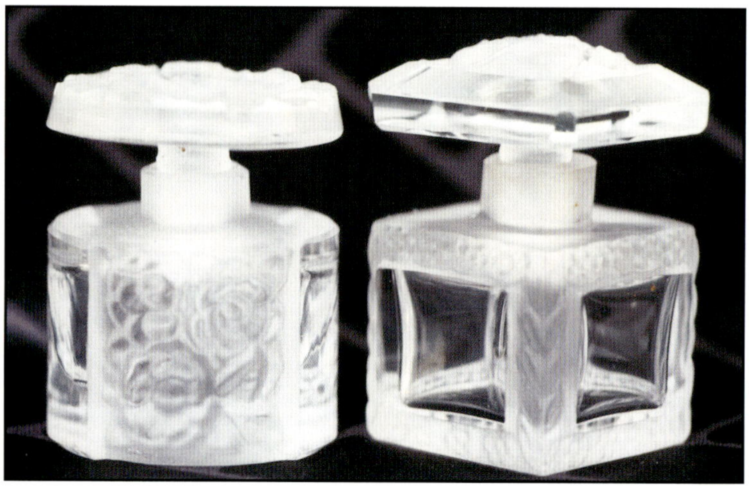

In a similar style, reminiscent of Lalique, these two bottles of clear, cut, frosted and polished glass form windows in the sides. The frosted caps show floral detail. Left: 2". Right: 2.125". $300-400 each.

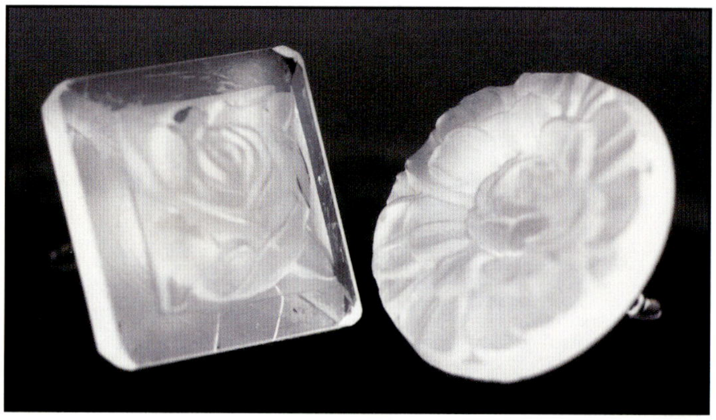

A view of the stoppers from the two previous bottles.

Figural bottles, like the Madame Pompadour bottle and the dog, are rare. Only a few stopper designs included human figures for the mini bottles. These few are hard to find.

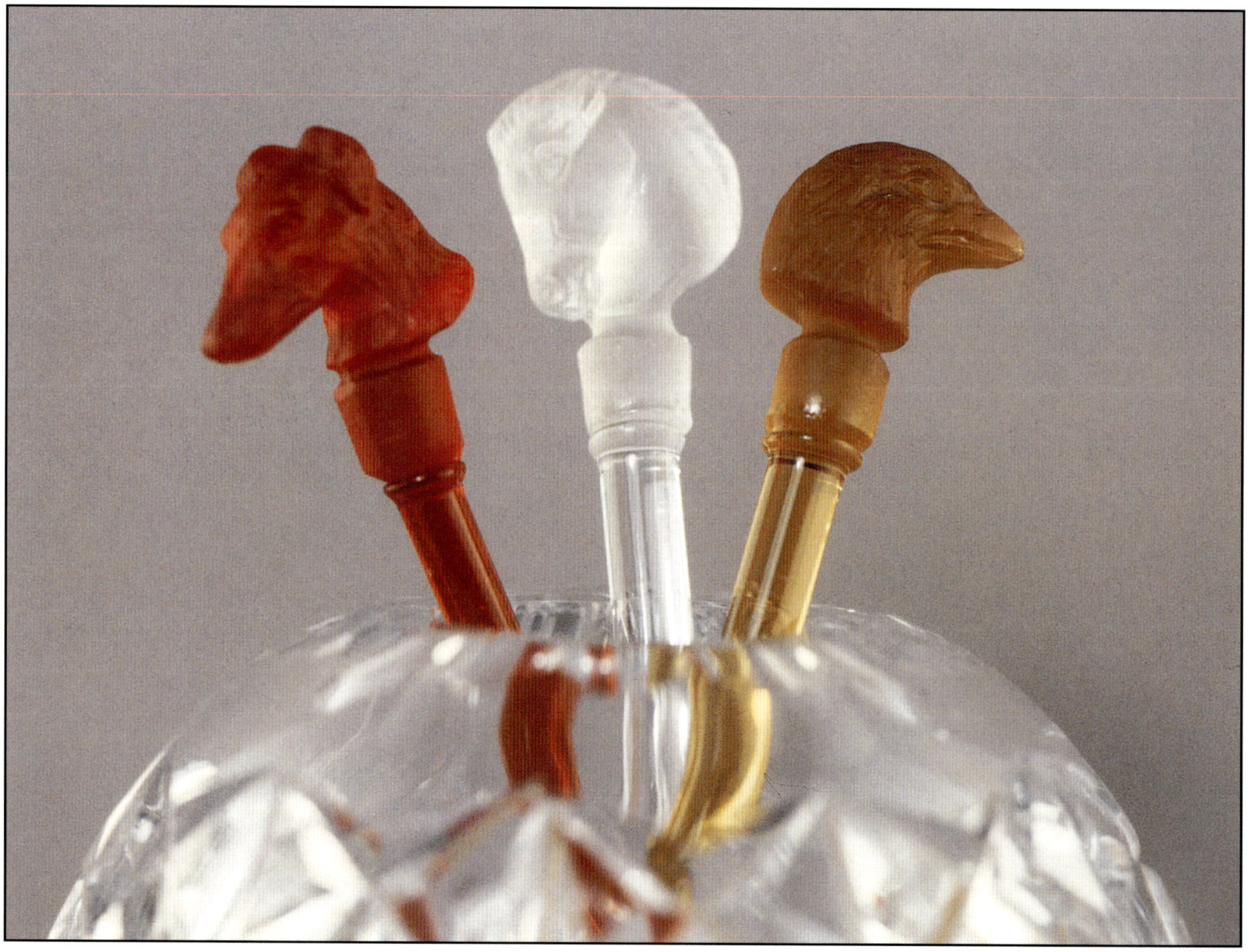

Swizzle sticks with animal heads similar to those found on some figural minis. $50-100 each.

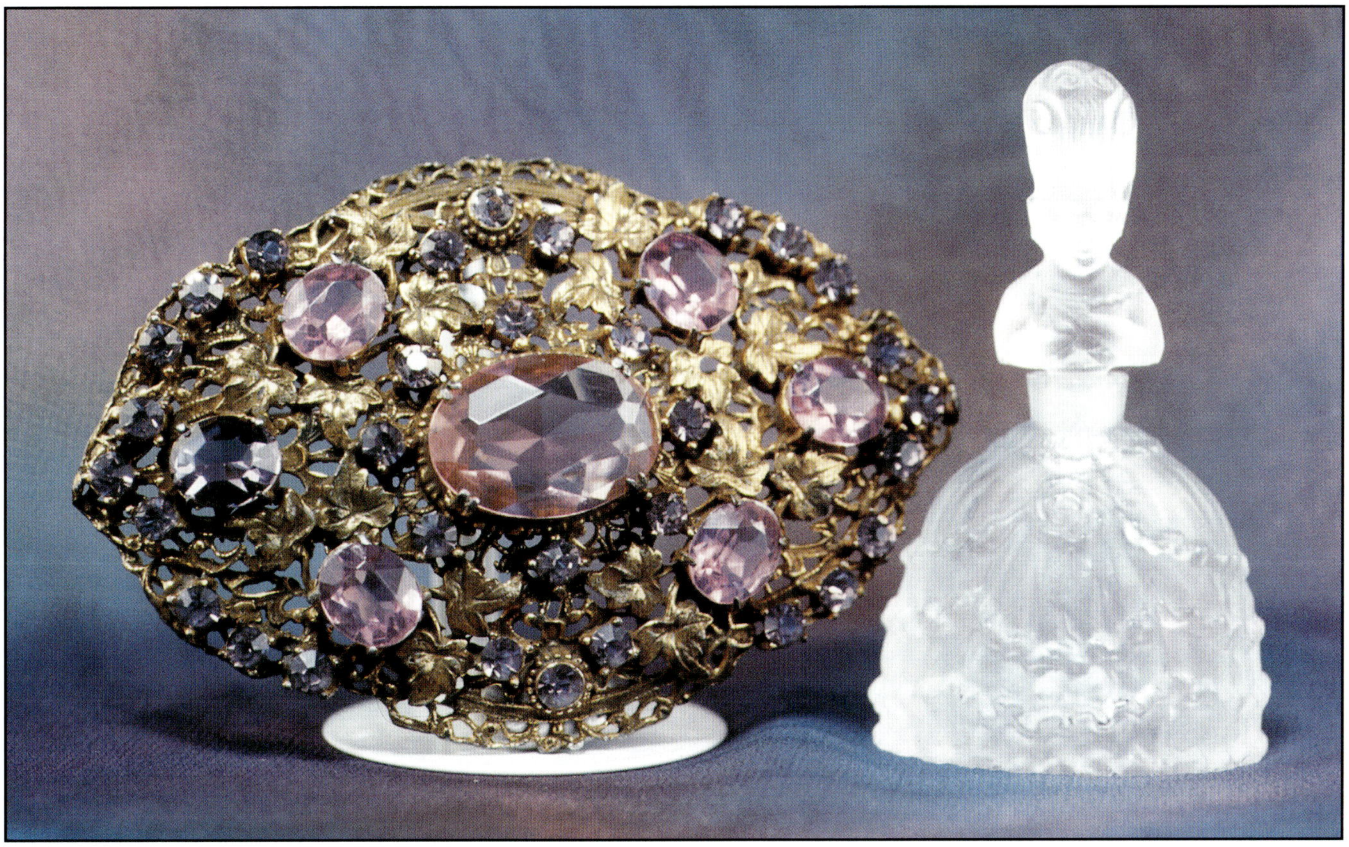

Rare miniature of Mme. Pompadour, molded and frosted. 3". $700-900. Shown with a large filigree and amethyst brooch. $75-100.

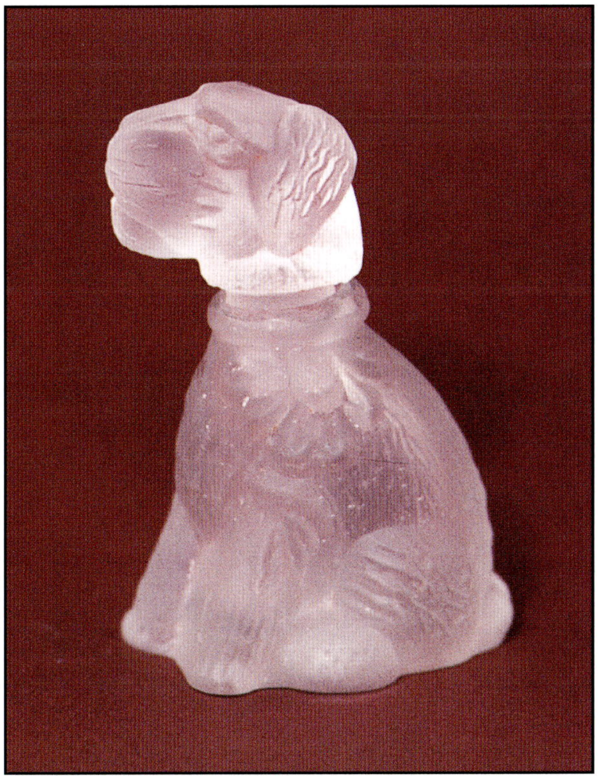

Molded, frosted dog. 1.75". $250-300.

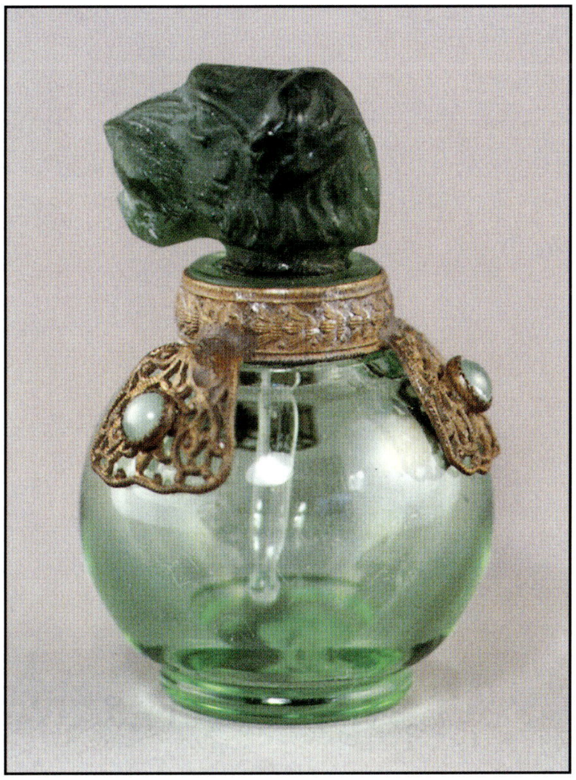

The same dog head mold in frosted green serves as a stopper for a clear, green, filigree jeweled base. 2.125". $350-450.

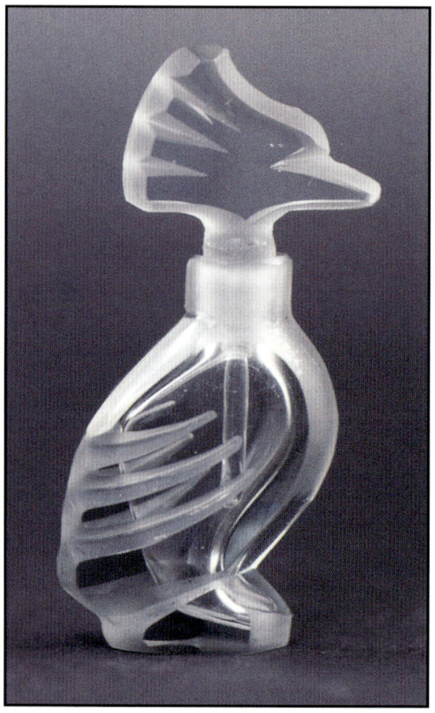

This woodpecker bird is fashioned out of smoke colored cut glass. 2.25". $200-300.

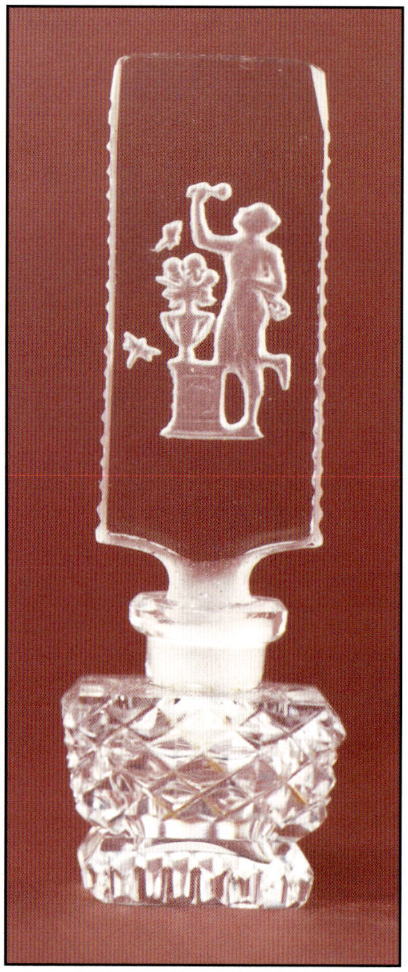

Clear, cut base and top. The classical stopper with a figure holding a flower. The knee rests on a pedestal, on which also stands an urn full of flowers. Two dragonflies hover. This is a fairly common figural stopper, appearing in this squared top shape as well as shaped or rounded. 3.875". $250-350.

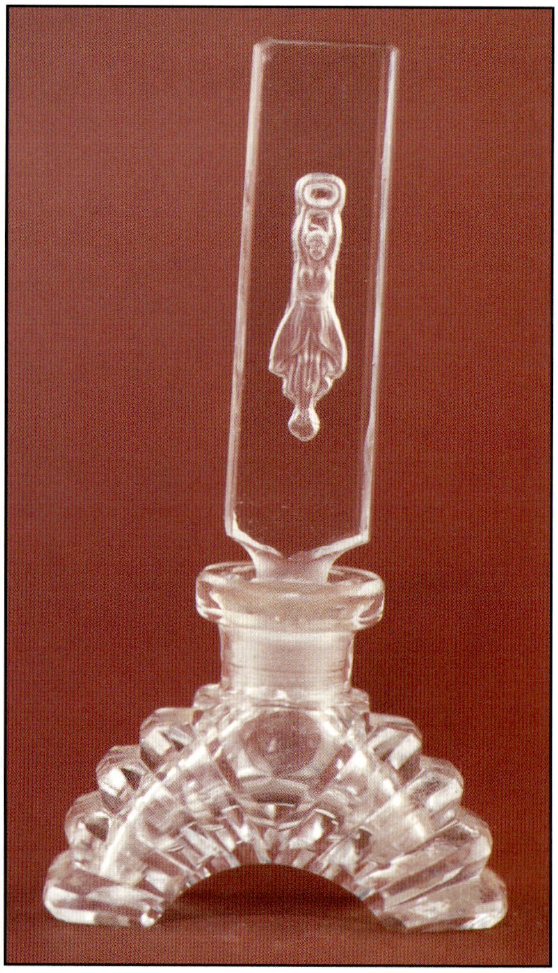

A clear, bridge base. The stopper features a woman holding a tambourine over her head. 3.5". $275-375.

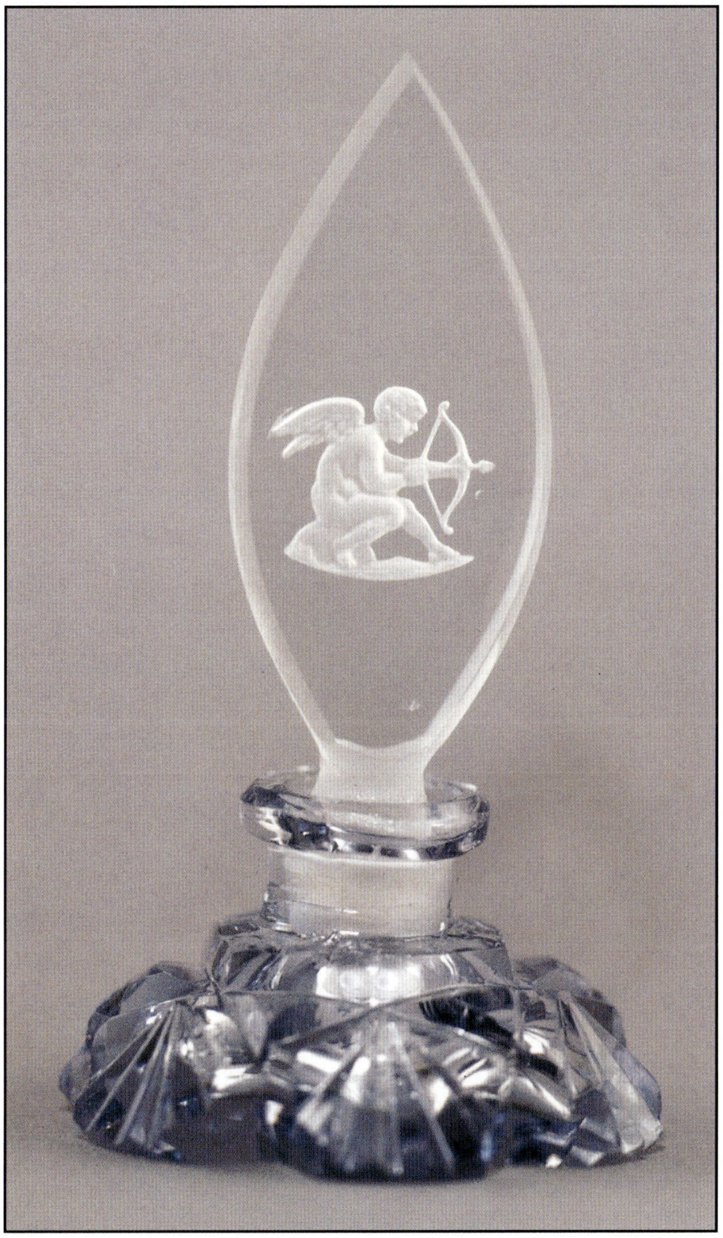

The base is amethyst cut glass. On the stopper, winged Cupid sits on a rock with his bow and arrow armed and ready. The stopper is clear, cut glass. 3". $375-450.

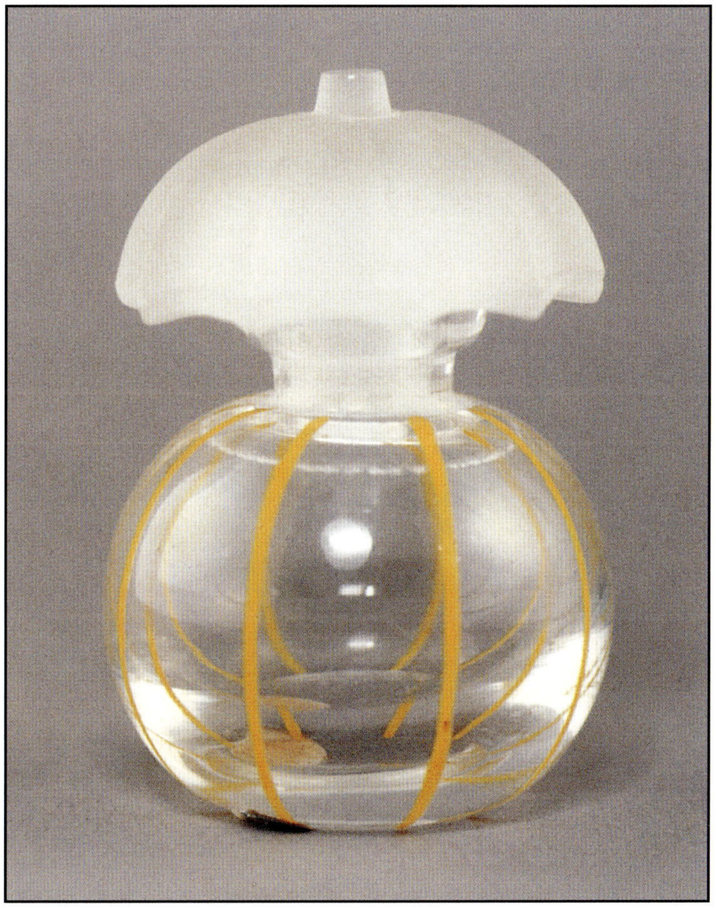

Applied yellow lines decorate this crystal ball. A frosted umbrella forms the stopper. This bottle is acid marked, but also has a Morlee paper label. 2.25". $150-200.

Filigree and Jeweled

Stoppered minis with filigree and jewels are considered desirable by collectors. If part of the design is also figural, the value is even higher. Bottles were generally acid marked in the base, but most are also marked with a metal tag in the filigree. Often the tag is the same oblong "button" found in the cap of purse bottles, but it can also be an almost invisible tiny line set onto a line in the filigree edge. Often it spells out the entire word "Czechoslovakia."

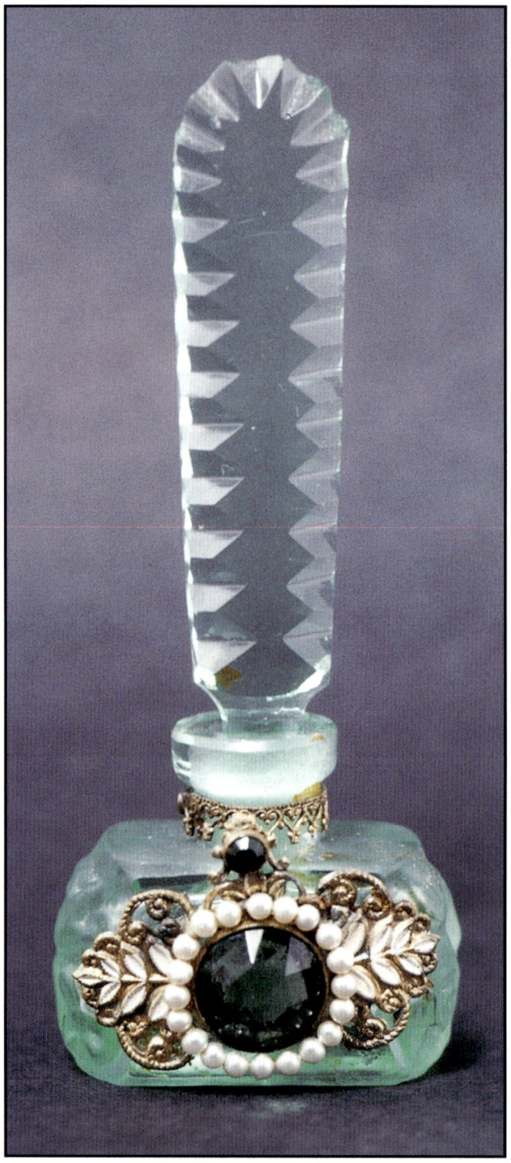

Green clear and frosted cut glass base, topped by a tall cut green feather stopper. This bottle has a dark emerald center stone wreathed with pearls in a filigree and enameled setting. 3.875". *Courtesy of Earline Kopriva*. $300-400.

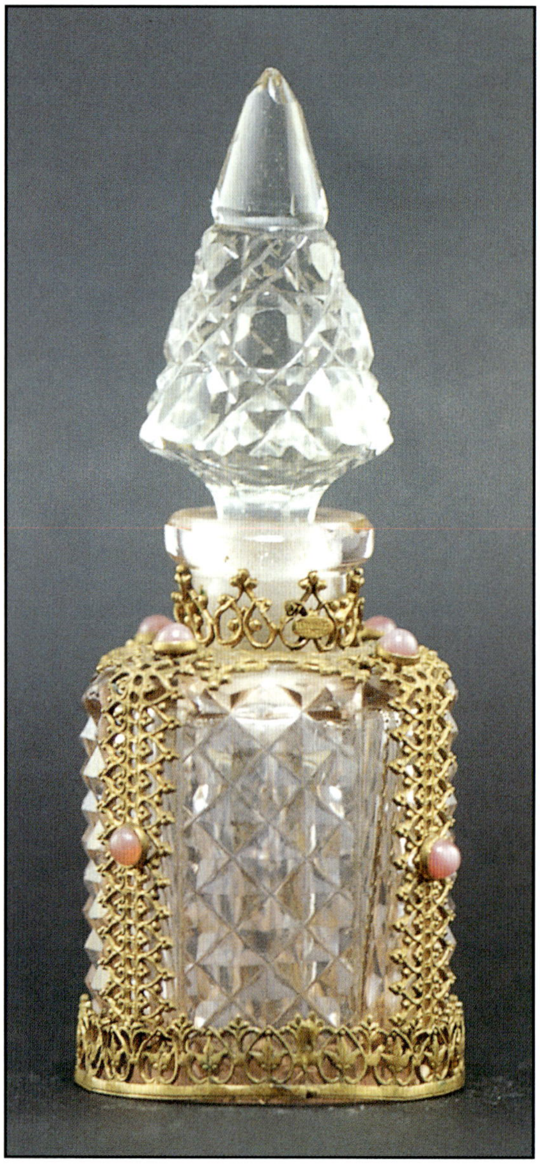

Edged in filigree and pink cabochon stones, the base bottle is pink cut glass. The stopper is clear, cut glass. 4". *Courtesy of Earline Kopriva*. $300-400.

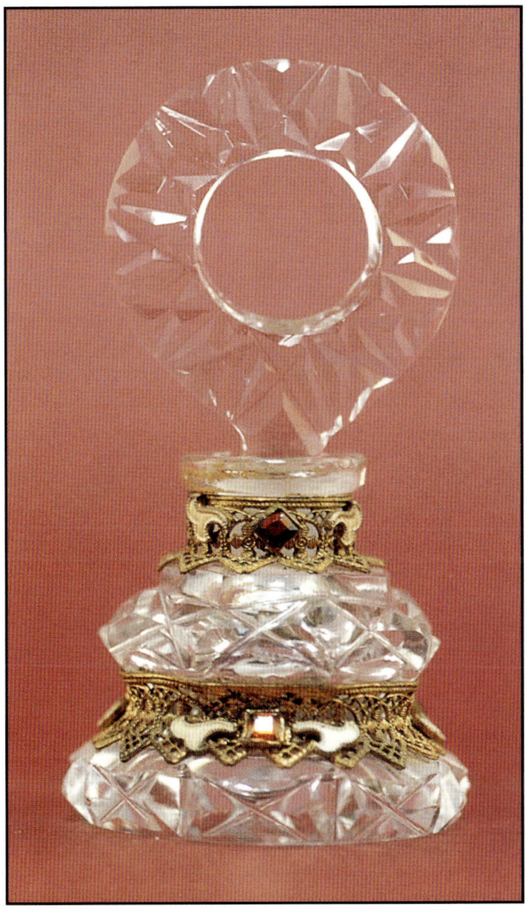

This clear, cut bottle with an open circle stopper is set off with bands of filigree, enameling, and pink, faceted stones. 3". *Courtesy of Earline Kopriva*. $300-400.

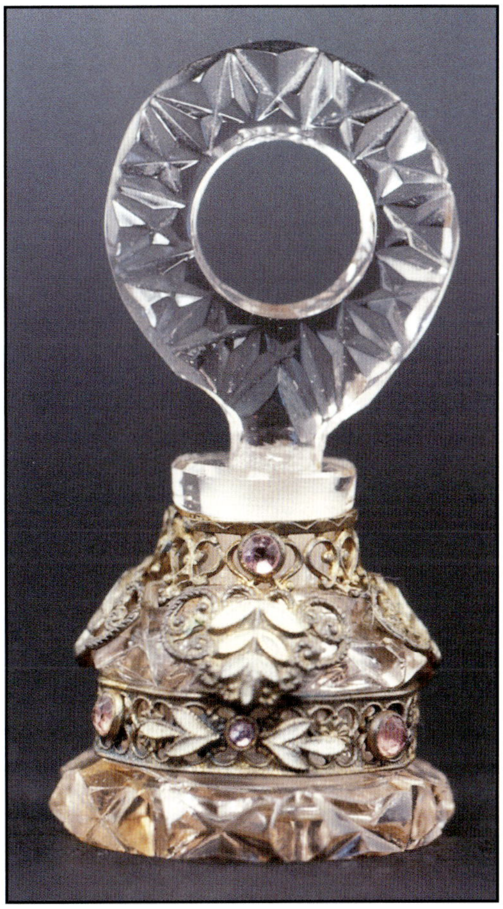

The same bottle with a pink cut glass base and added filigree and jewel work. 3". $300-400.

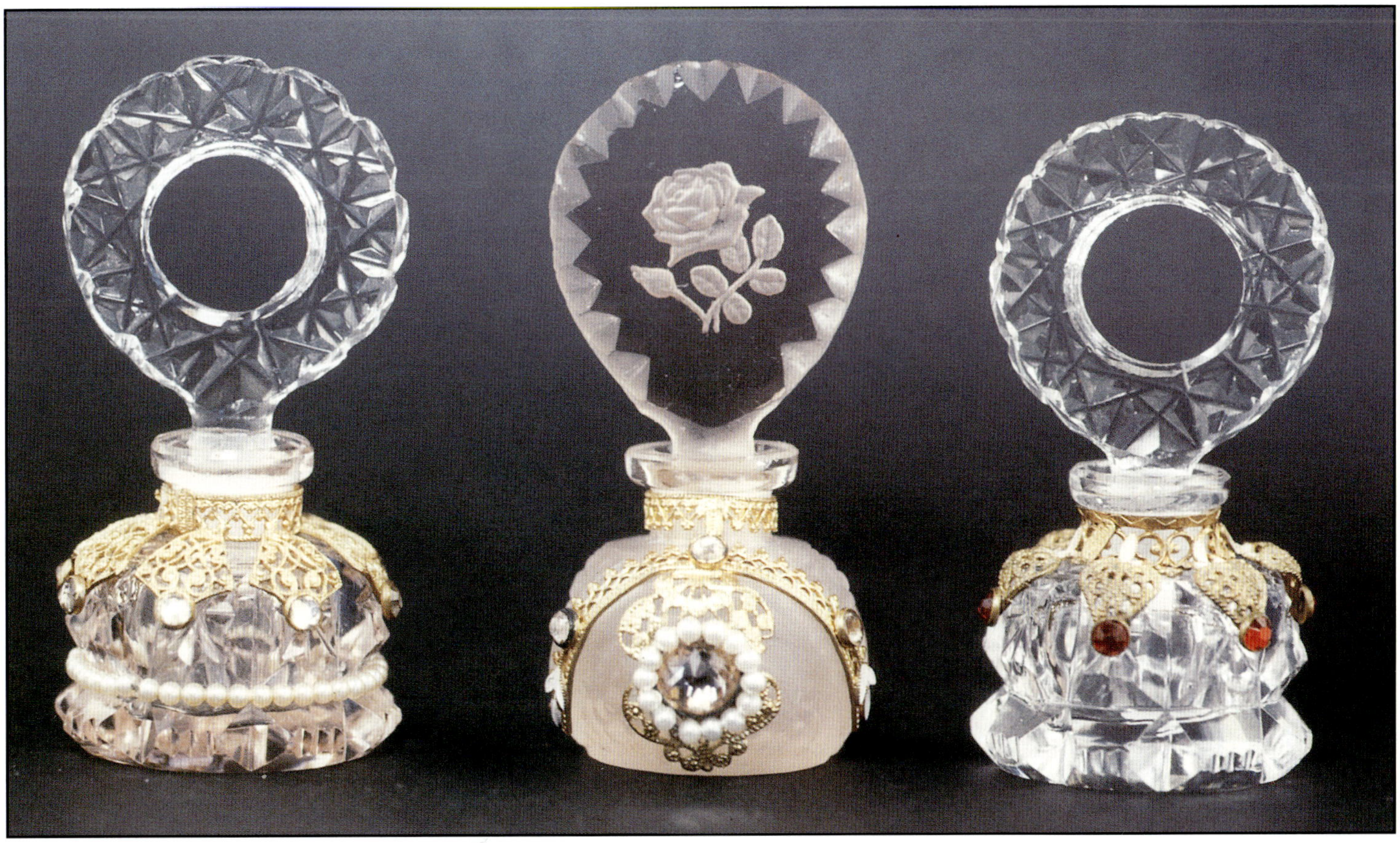

Though the outer bottles resemble the preceding two, they are different in design and are slightly bigger around. Left: Pink cut glass base, with jeweled filigree, pink faceted stones, and a belt of pearls. 3". Center: The frosted pink base has a subtle braided design complementing the filigree. The pink center gem is wreathed with pearls. The filigree is attached to the bottle only by the neckband. 3". Right: The same bottle as on the left, but in clear, cut glass with filigree and red gems. 3". $300-400 each.

Left: Opaque black butterfly bottle with opaque green gems and a pearl set in the filigree. Clear, cut fan stopper. 2.75". $450-550. Right: Opaque black cut bottle with a center band and opaque green carved medallion. The stopper is green cut glass with an intaglio floral design. 4.25". $300-400. Shown with cut opaque black and green crystal beads. $50.

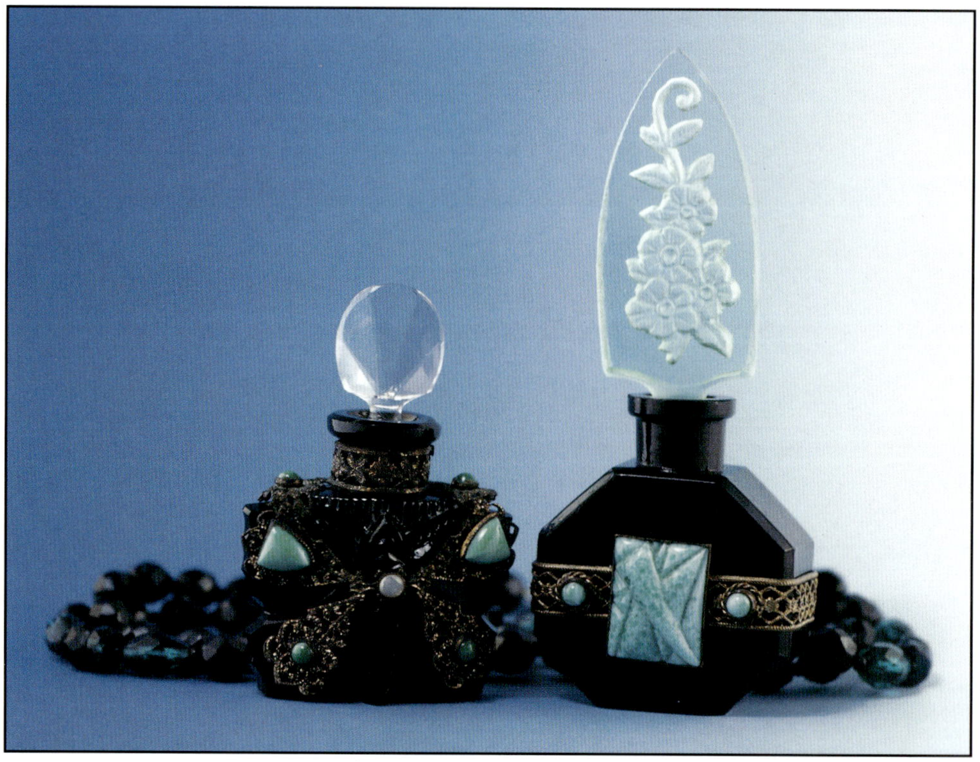

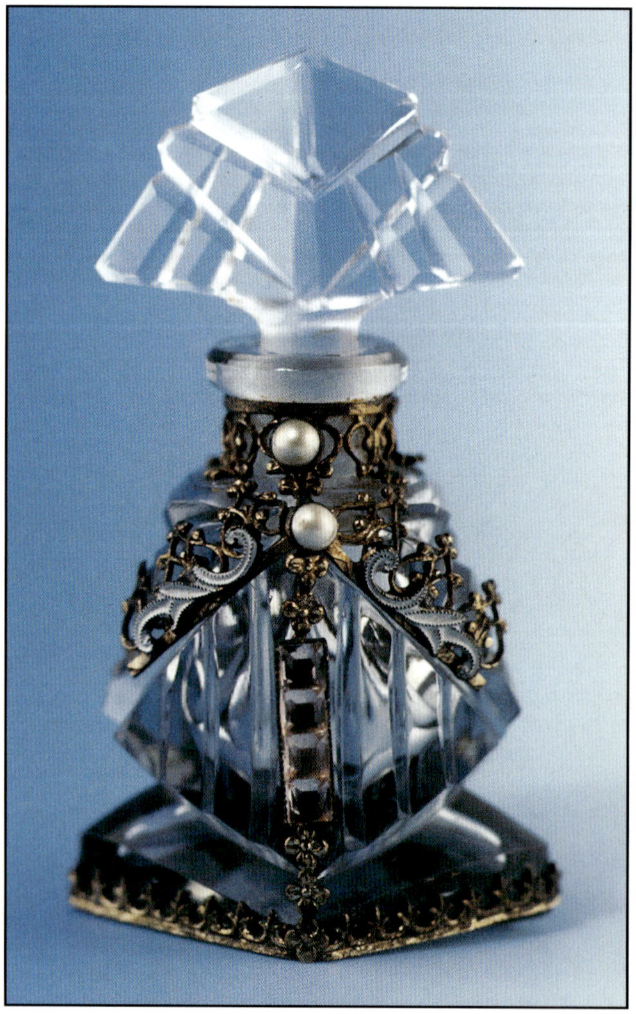

This smoke, cut glass bottle is enhanced with filigree, enameling, pearls, and a row of pink gems down the front. The center front filigree attaches to both the neckband and the filigree band around the base. The stopper is clear cut glass. 3". $350-400.

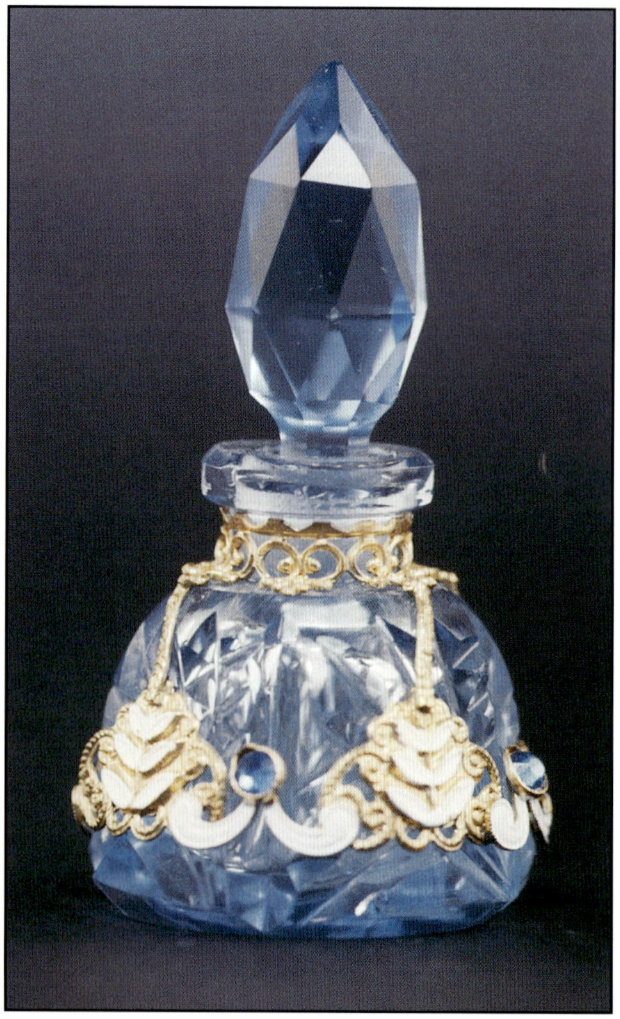

Blue cut glass bottle and base. Enameled filigree with blue, faceted sets. The stopper is a blue faceted prism. 2.75". $250-350.

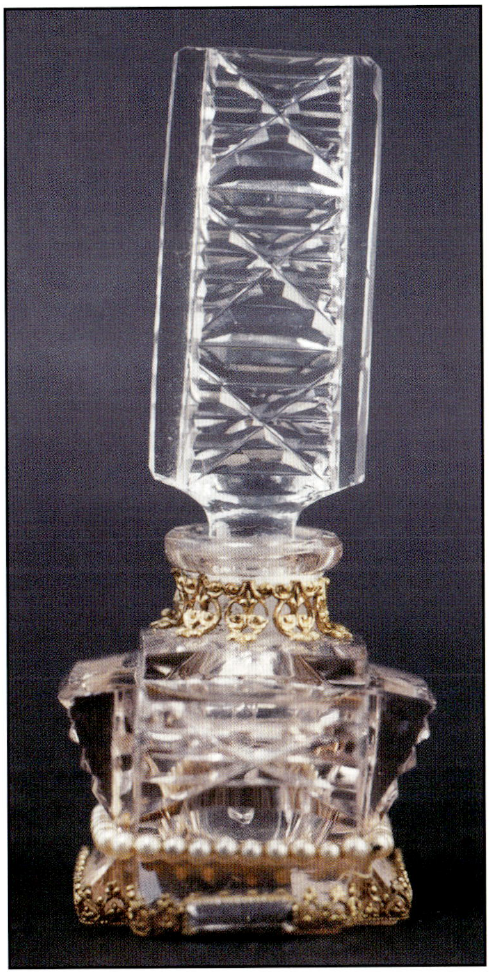

Pink cut glass base. This bottle has three bands of decoration, the bottom with a single oblong pink jewel, a belting of pearls, and a dainty filigree collar. The stopper is clear glass with deep geometric cuts. 3.25". $350-400.

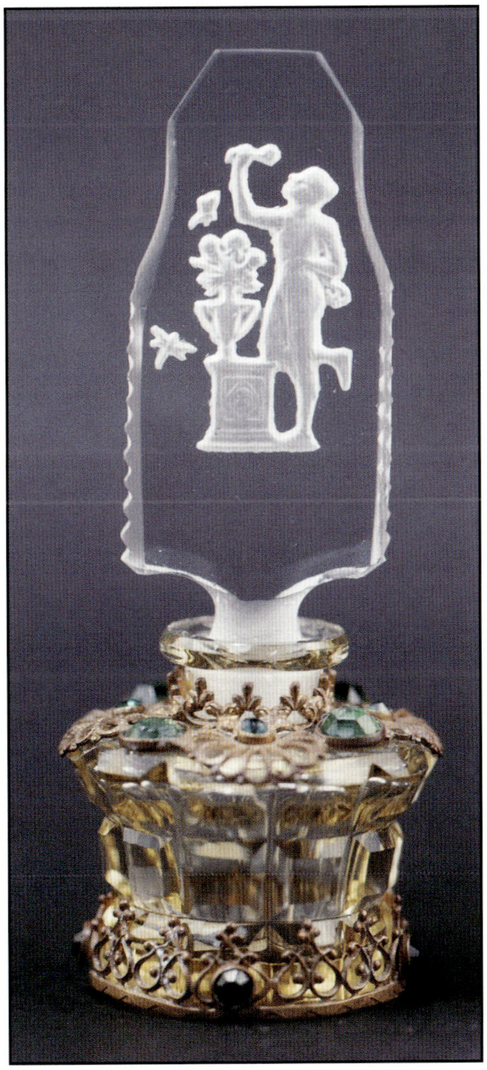

The filigree with its green gems spills over the shoulders of this yellow cut glass bottle and surrounds the base. The figural stopper is from a squared mold, but has been shaped by cutting. 3.75". $400-500.

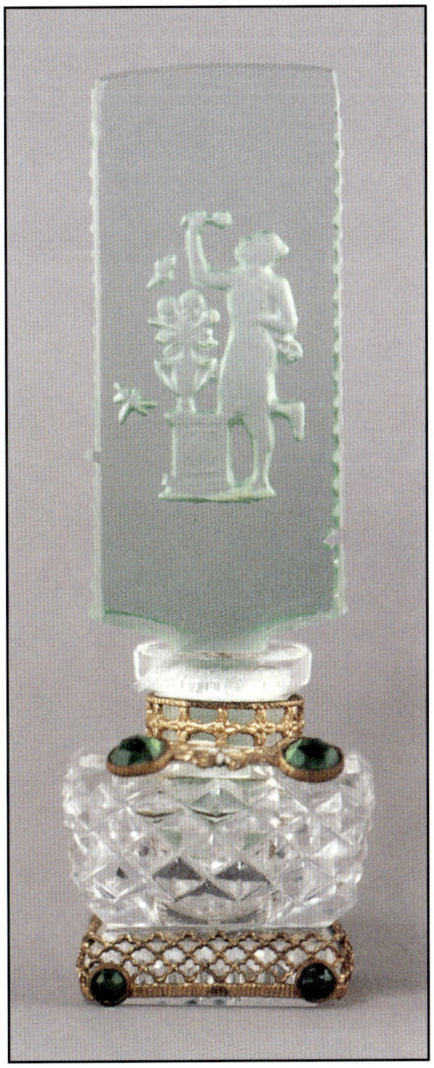

The clear, cut base has simple filigree at the neck and around the bottom. The green cut intaglio stopper is in its original squared form. 3.75". $400-500.

The decorations on the shoulder filigree of this bottle are formed of glass beads—a small green flower bead with a pearl attached to the center. An enameled leaf is attached to each side of the filigree. The band at the base has a green faceted gem at each corner. Green cut glass feather stopper. 4". $350-400.

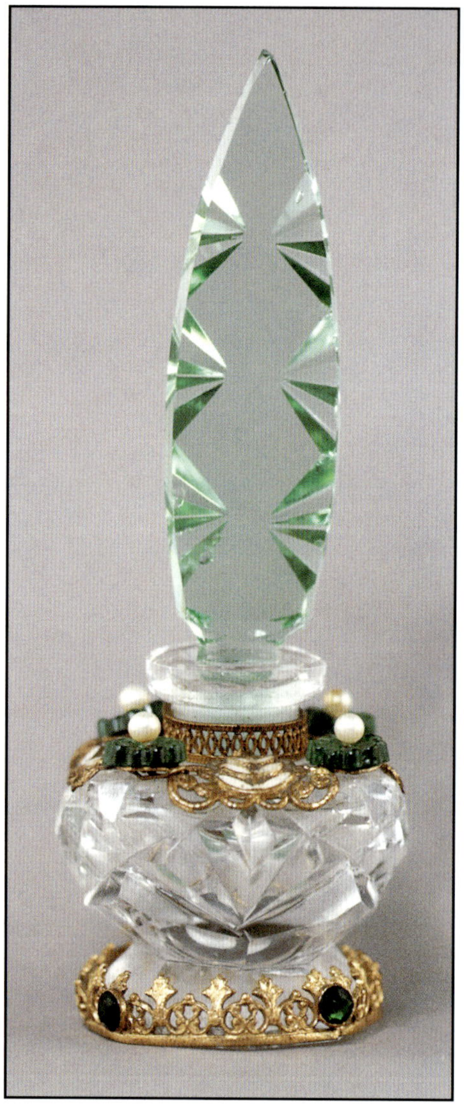

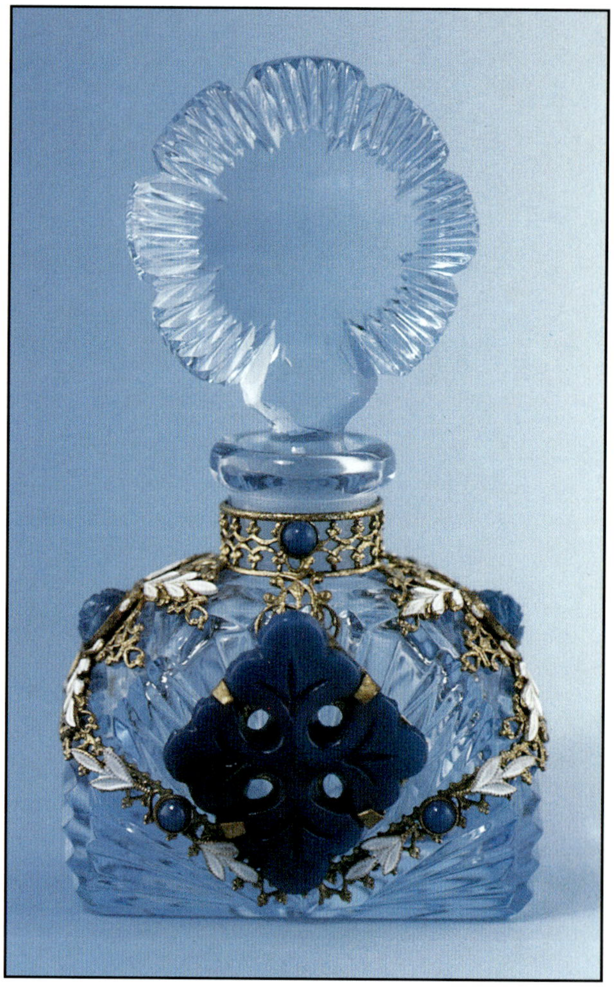

Blue cut glass base with filigree and enamel work, blue cabochons, and a large prong-set pierced lapis glass medallion. The stopper is a clear blue floral circle with edge cuts. 3.5". $350-400.

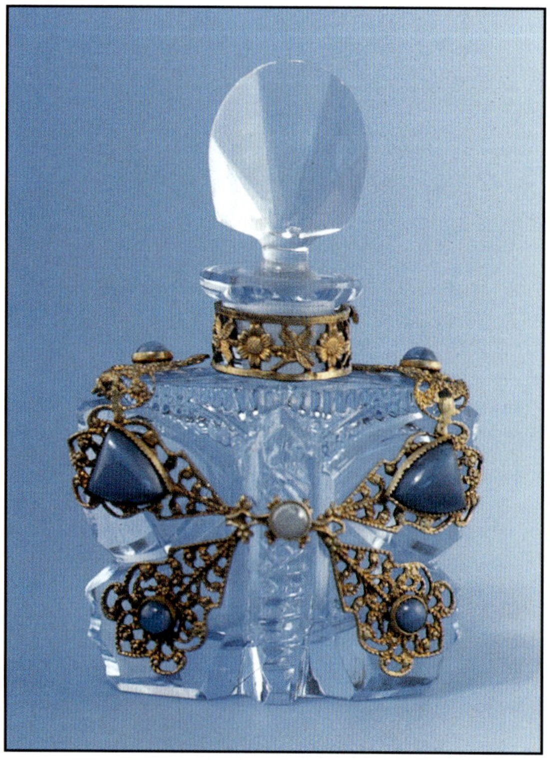

Blue cut glass butterfly bottle with lapis stones and cabochons on the filigree. Clear, cut glass fan stopper. These butterfly bottles were made in several colors and in at least two sizes. 2.5". $350-400.

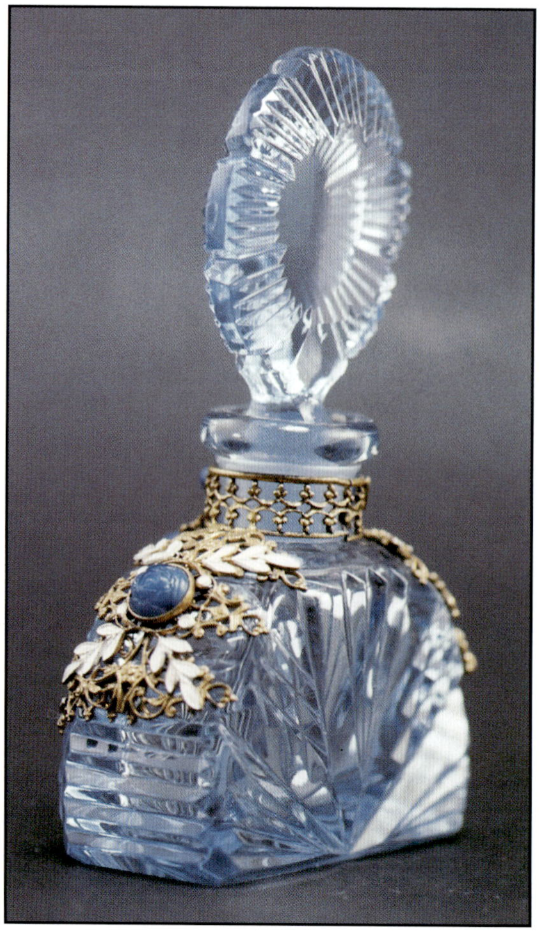

Same bottle showing side detailing with enameling and carved lapis roses.

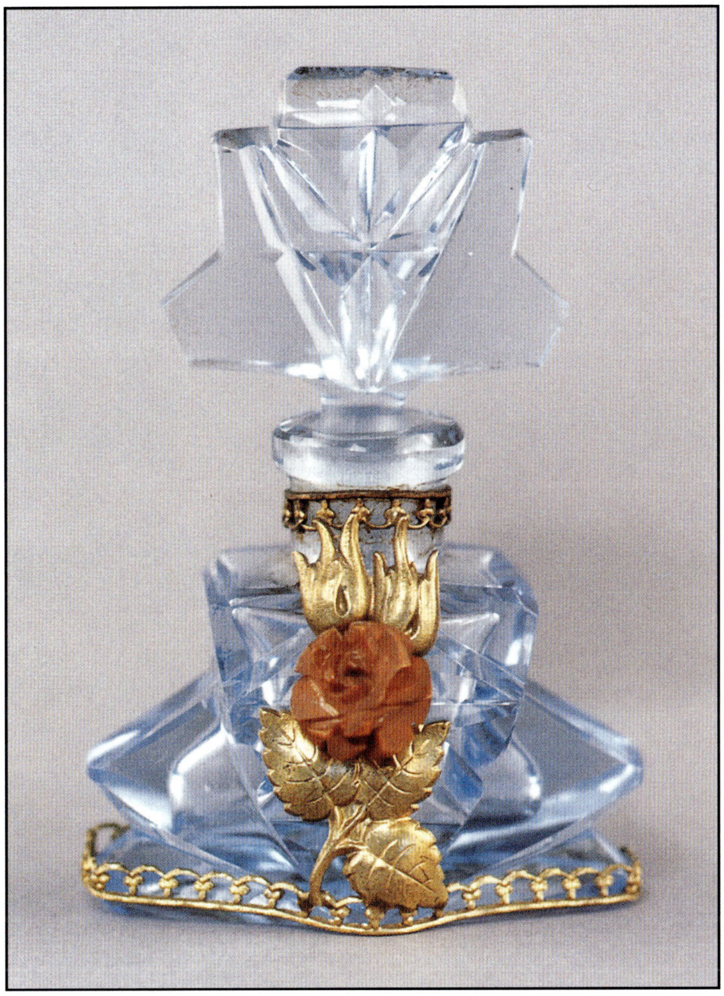

Joining at the center is a filigree piece of rose leaves below and closed buds above, with a full-blooming carved coral rose as a centerpiece. The stopper is blue cut glass. 2.75". $200-300.

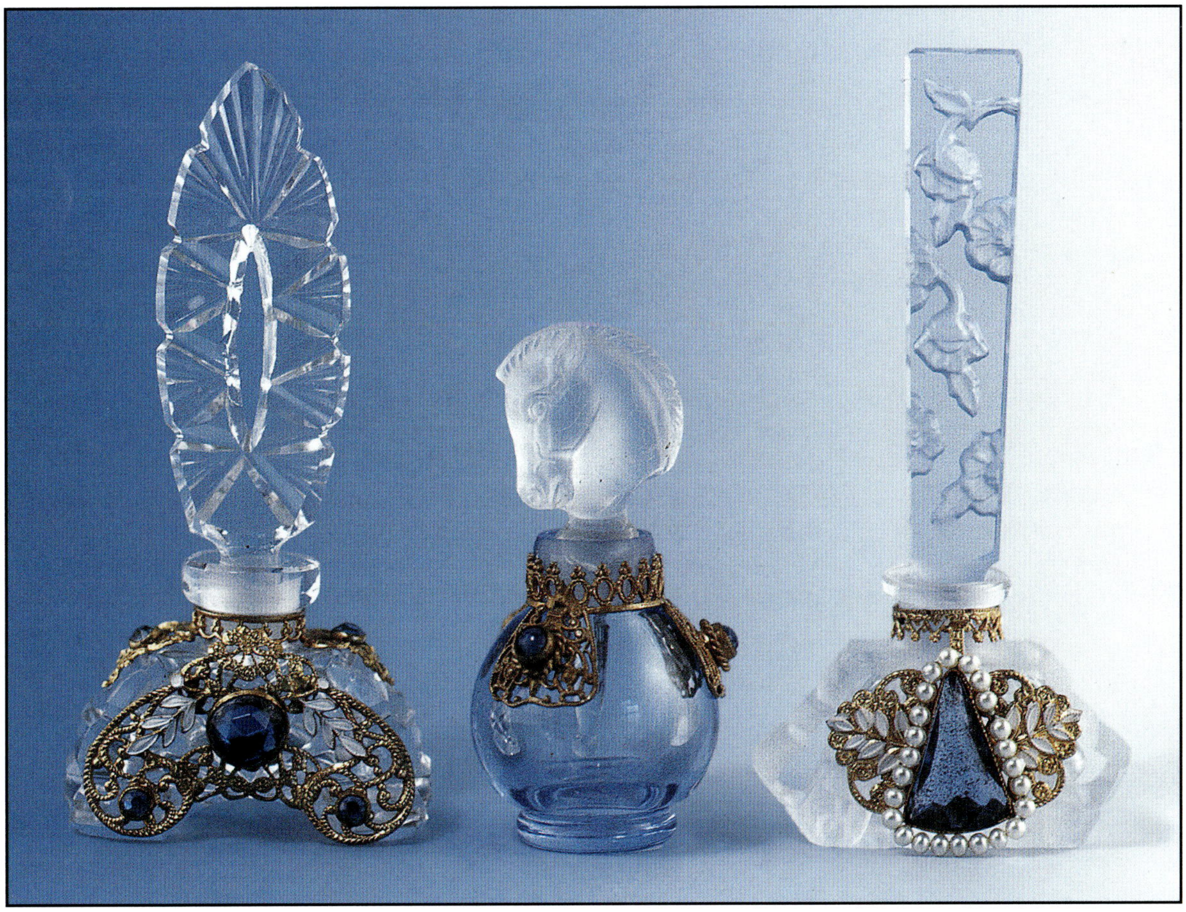

Left: Clear, cut bridge base with filigree and blue faceted gems. Clear, cut, pierced stopper 3.5". Center: Frosted horse head stopper over a round, polished blue base with three sections of filigree and lapis cabochons. Right: Clear, frosted base with enameled filigree and a triangular blue faceted stone in a frame of pearls. The stopper is blue with a run of intaglio flowers. 3.5". $300-$400 each.

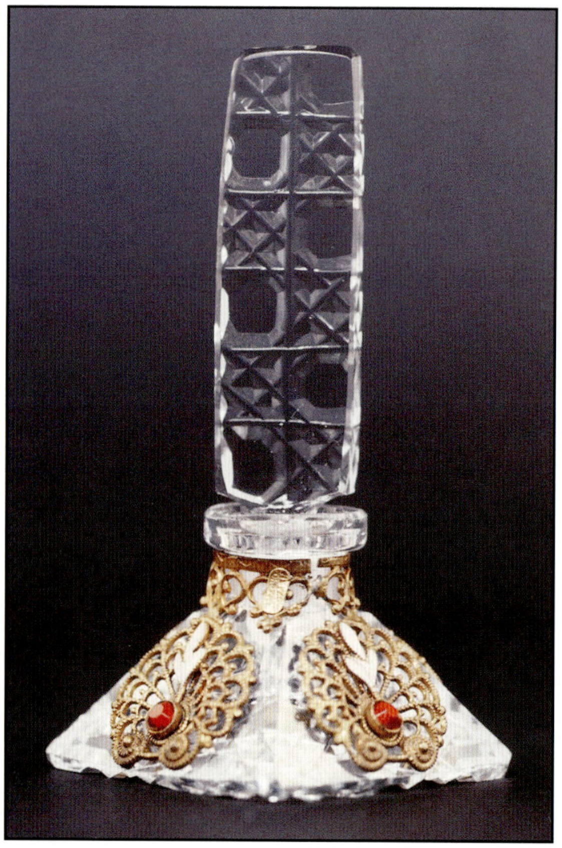

The clear glass underside of this bottle carries out the XOXO theme of the clear stopper. Panels of enamel work and filigree cover each smooth, polished side of the pyramid shape. The stones are red and facet cut. 3.25". $200-300.

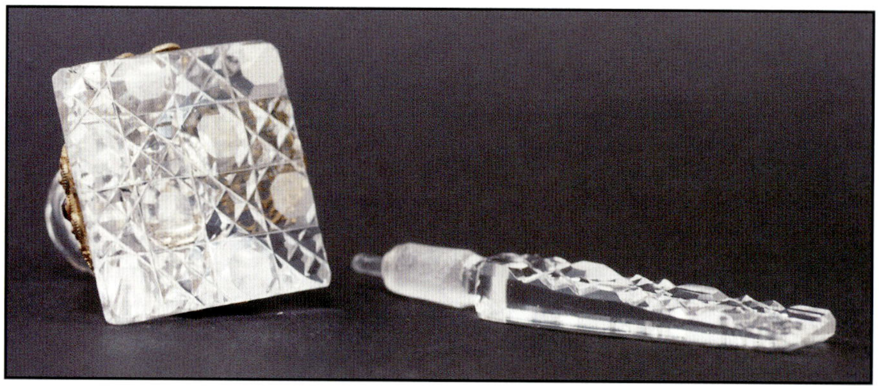

Another view of the same bottle, showing the cuts of the bottom and the stopper surface.

Right:
Filigree and red stones sit on the top of this bottle, with its tall, cut, coffin-shaped intaglio swirl stopper rising above. 4". $300-350.

Far right:
The amethyst cut glass "cloud" stopper holds a lily-of-the-valley spray settling into a cut glass bottle with delicate bands of enameled filigree and amethyst faceted stones. 3.75". $300-400.

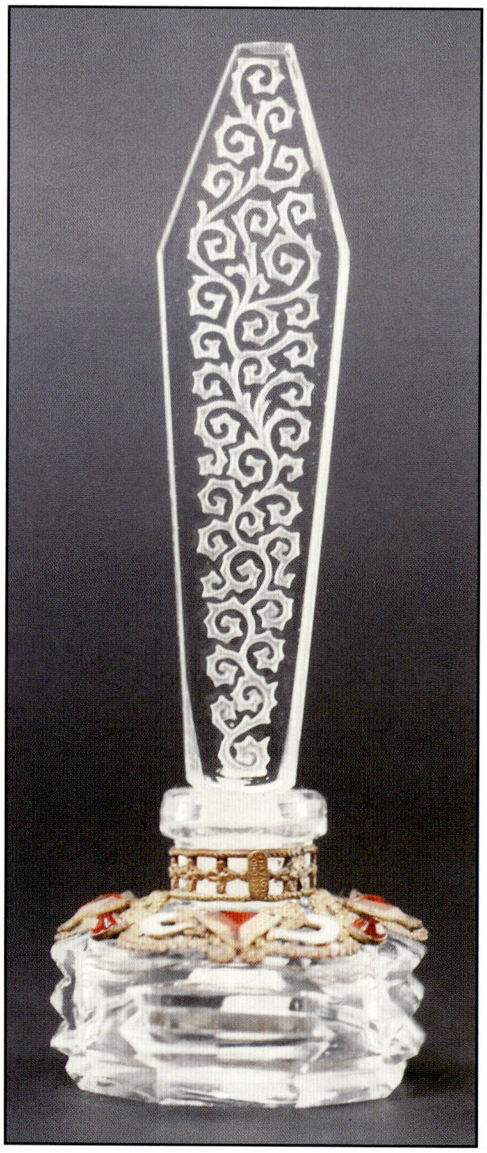

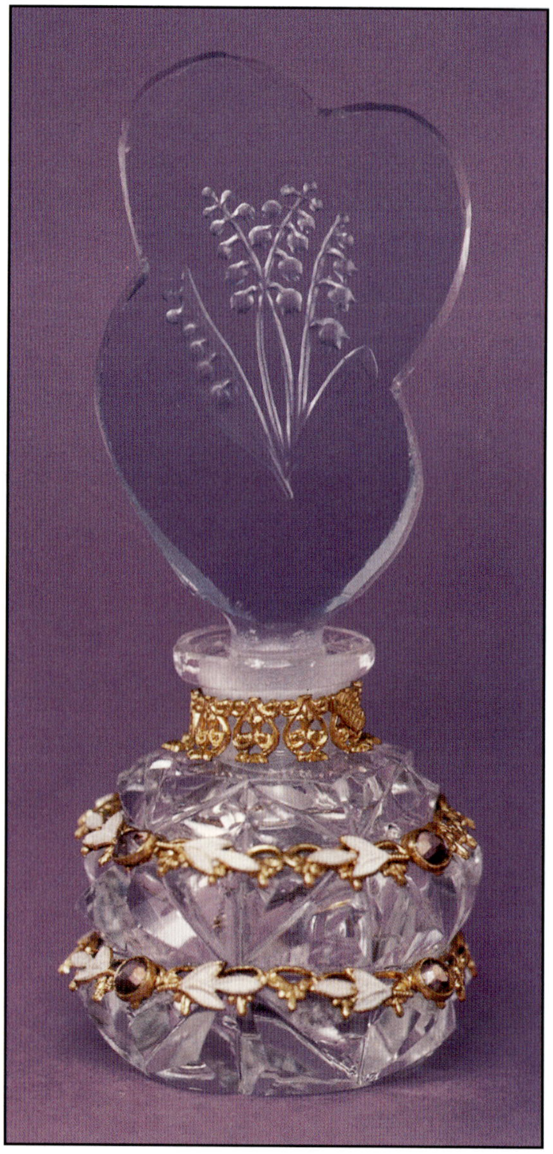

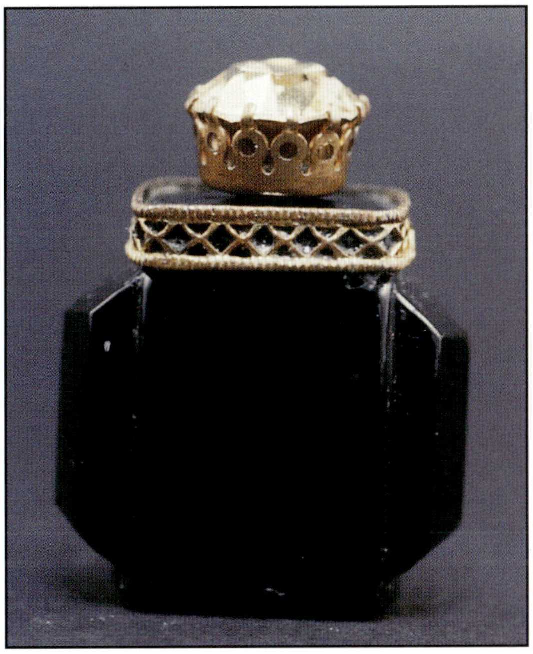

The ultimate micro-mini, this opaque black base holds a yellow faceted gem that comprises the entire stopper. The dauber is plastic. No marks. 1.375". $75-125.

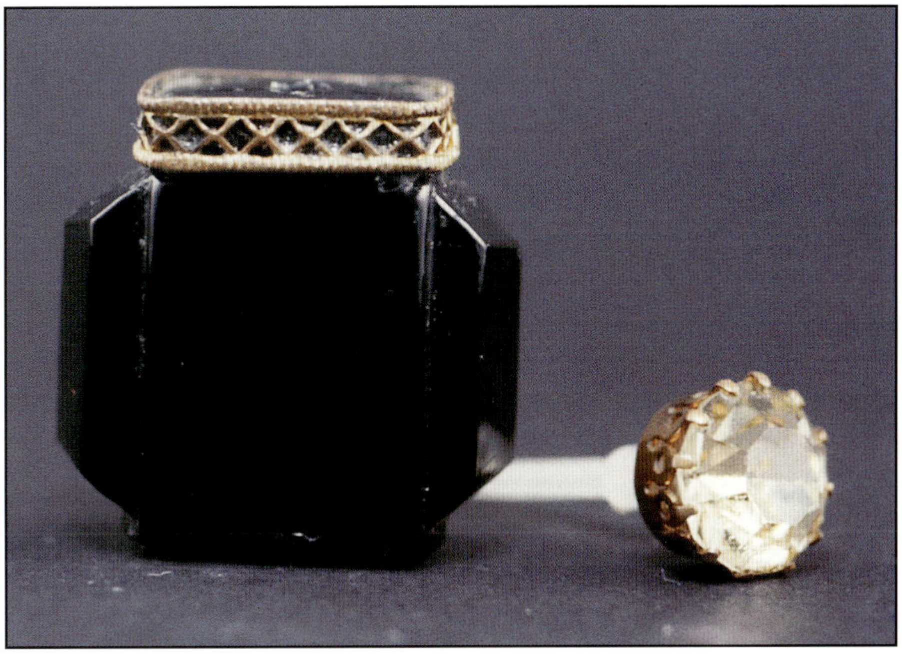

View of stopper.

Multiple Sets

Since such a variety of colors and styles were available to the consumer, these tiny perfumes could be bought individually or the consumer could "assemble" sets of their own by selecting two or more bottles with some common characteristics—color, size, or pattern. The advantage would be to easily identify the different scents that filled them. Importers also had packaged sets or groupings of bottles that were sold together, often on a glass tray or ormolu stand. Theses are known as twin, triplets, or quad sets. The advertising also referred to them as "families" or "clusters."

Multiple sets offer a special challenge for the collector and can be found in a wide range of prices, sizes, colors, and cluster styles. The Irice Company presented baskets and cages for groupings of pressed glass purse bottles. Some were even sold on tiny jeweled, mirrored trays.

The finer sets, of course, are made of cut glass and rest on cut glass trays that are usually the same color as the tops. Complete multiple sets are hard to find because pieces have been broken or separated over time. Completing sets can be done, however, and the separate bottles are fine "stand alone" pieces in the meantime.

In general, cut glass is preferred over pressed; color, over clear; and complete sets with more components are preferred over twins. Rare or unusual sets readily claim the collector's interest.

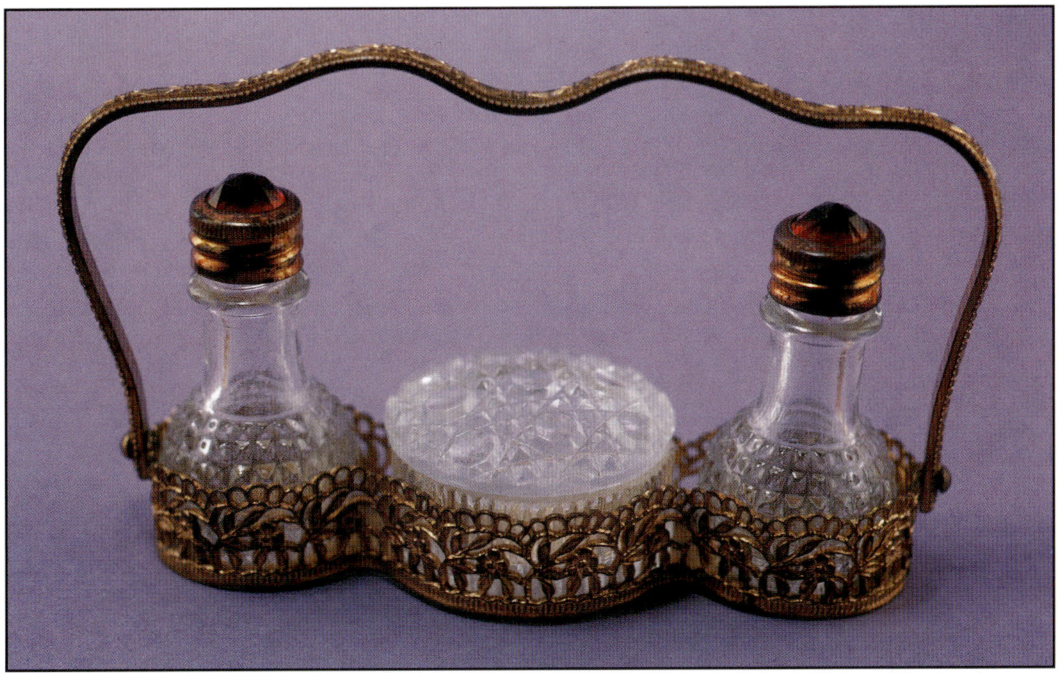

Irice basket and unusual set includes two Stubby bottles with red jeweled caps and a tiny glass box in the middle. The box could be used for a ring or for face powder or rouge. The box top is cut and polished; the bottles are pressed. 2.75". $250-350.

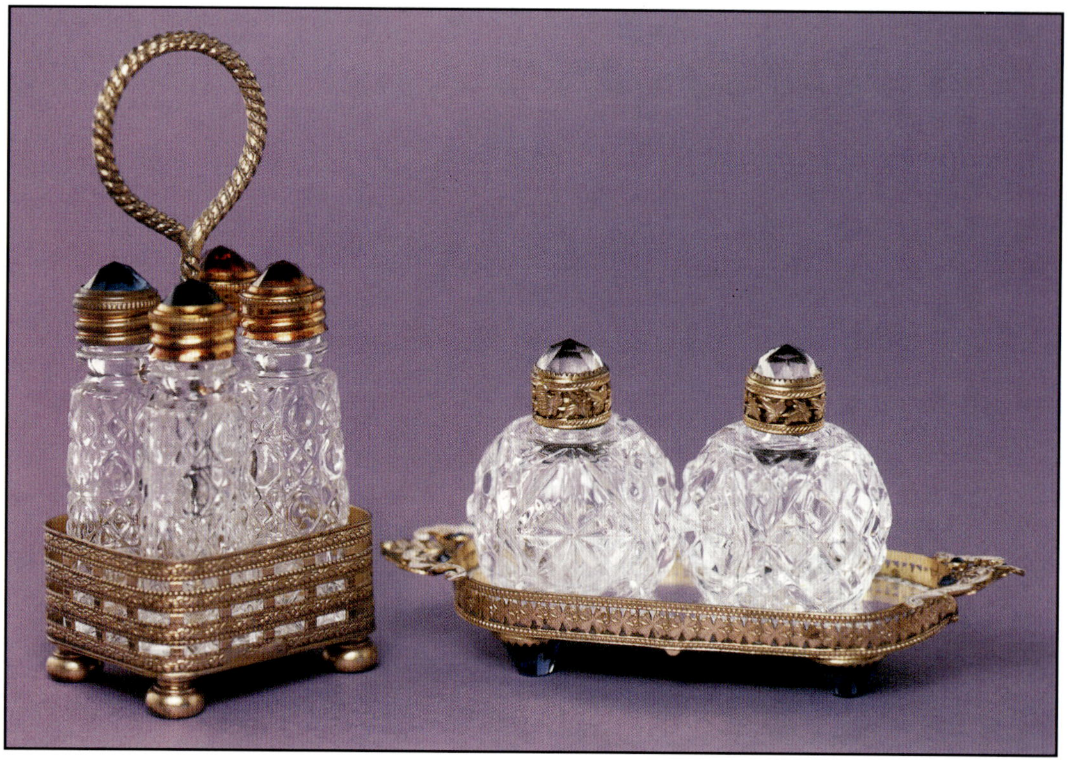

Left: A quad set of tall Irice purse bottles with a rainbow of colored tops rests in this basket with a metal handle. 4.25". $150-200. Right: Clear, pressed glass Irice purse bottles with gem-topped screw caps were sold on a jeweled, filigree, mirrored tray with faceted gem feet. 2.25". $125-175.

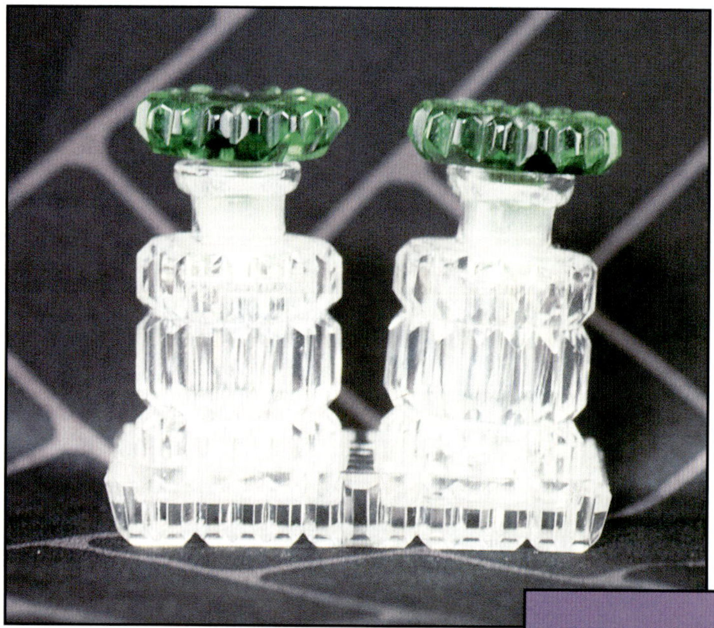

Green topped twin set, collected piecemeal. This set should have a matching green tray to be correct. 2.25". $150-250.

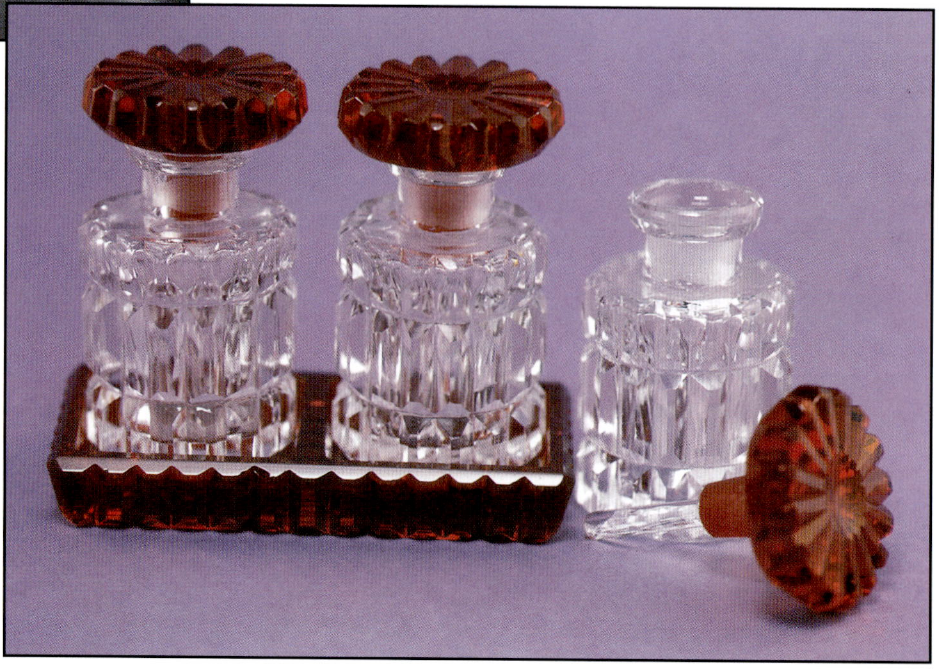

Clear twins with red, flat tops and a red tray. Red is a less common color and harder to find. The extra bottle shows an intact dauber. This style set was pictured in Irice advertising from 1937. (Jones-North, 1999, p. 106) 2.25". $350-450.

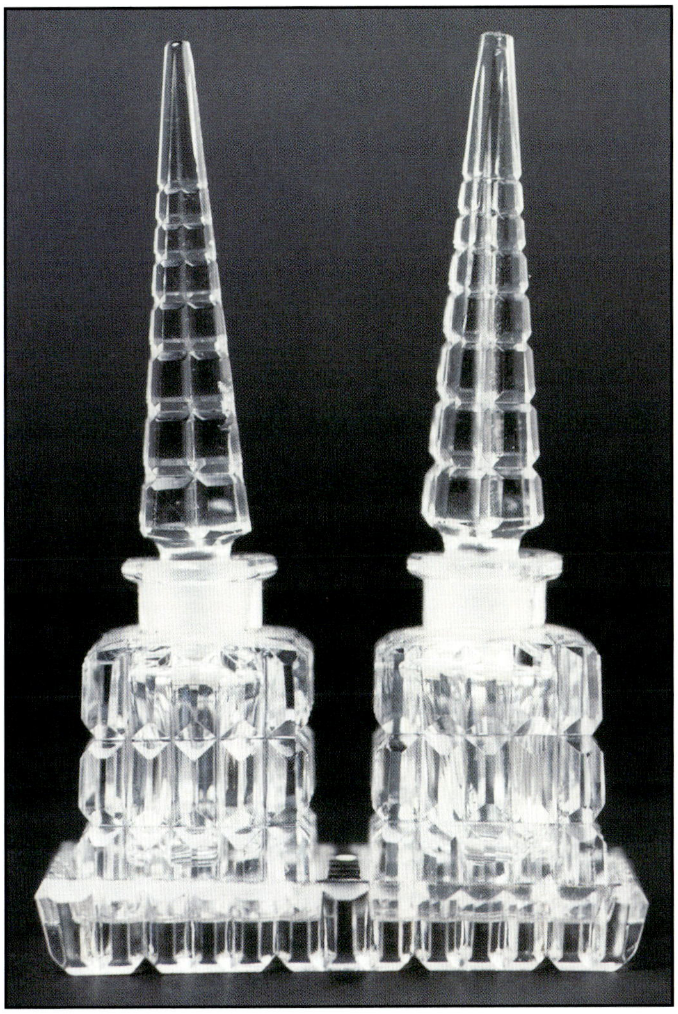

Clear cut glass twin set with barrel bases and four-sided cut glass spire tops. 4". $200-300.

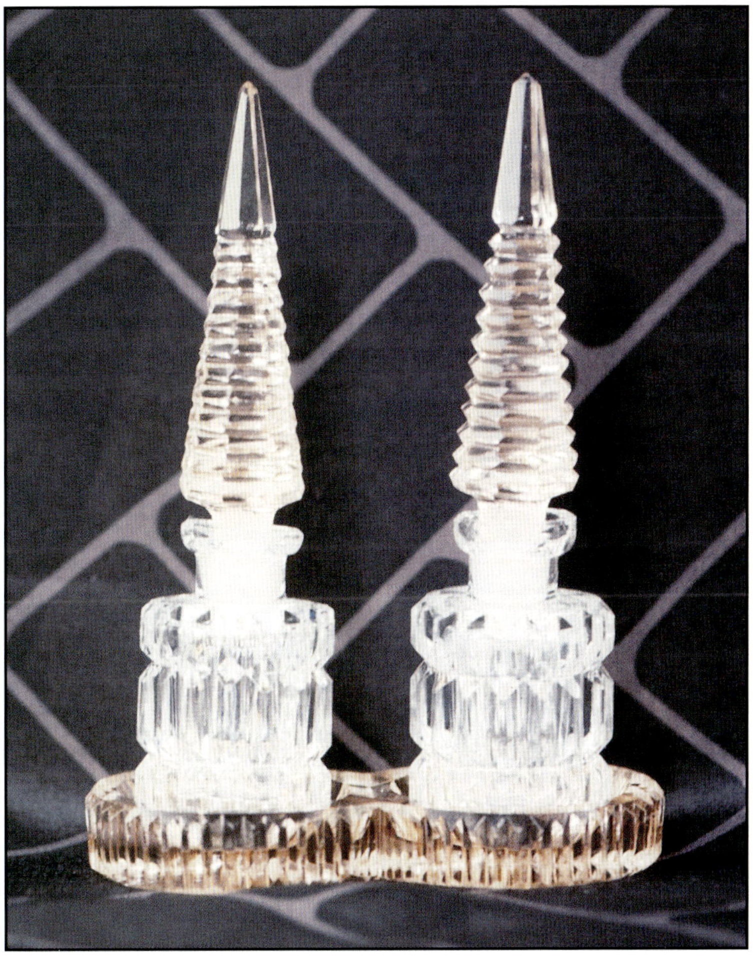

Pink twins in a figure eight tray. Tops are cut, but form a rounded pattern in the spires. 4.25". $250-350.

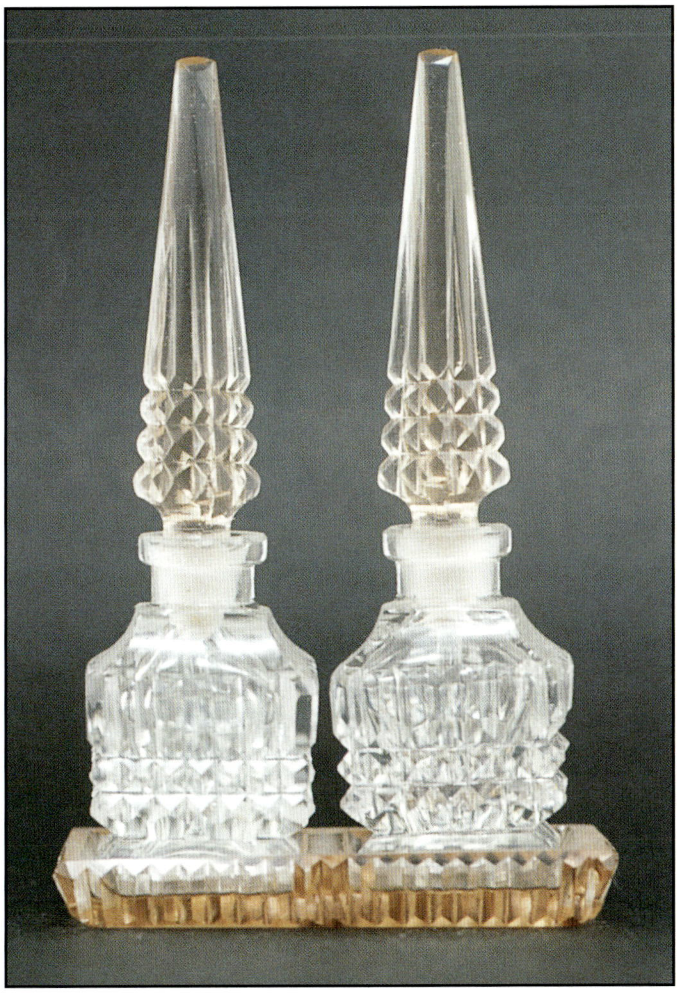

Clear, footed bottles in a pink squared tray. The pink spire tops are cut differently again from the preceding sets. 4.25". *Courtesy of Earline Kopriva*. $250-350.

Aristo triplet set with opaque black tops and tray. The underside of the tray has a cut starburst in the center and is acid marked. 2.5". $550-750.

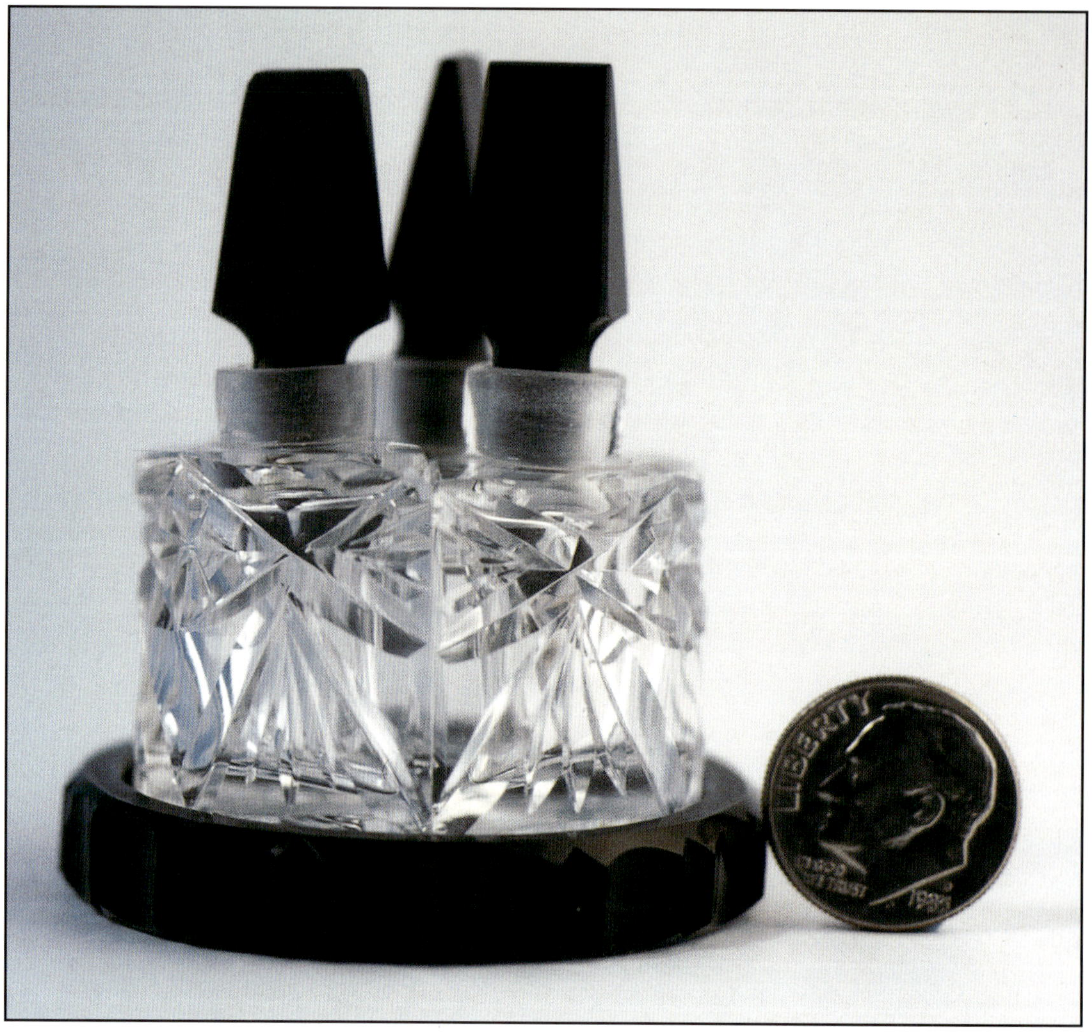

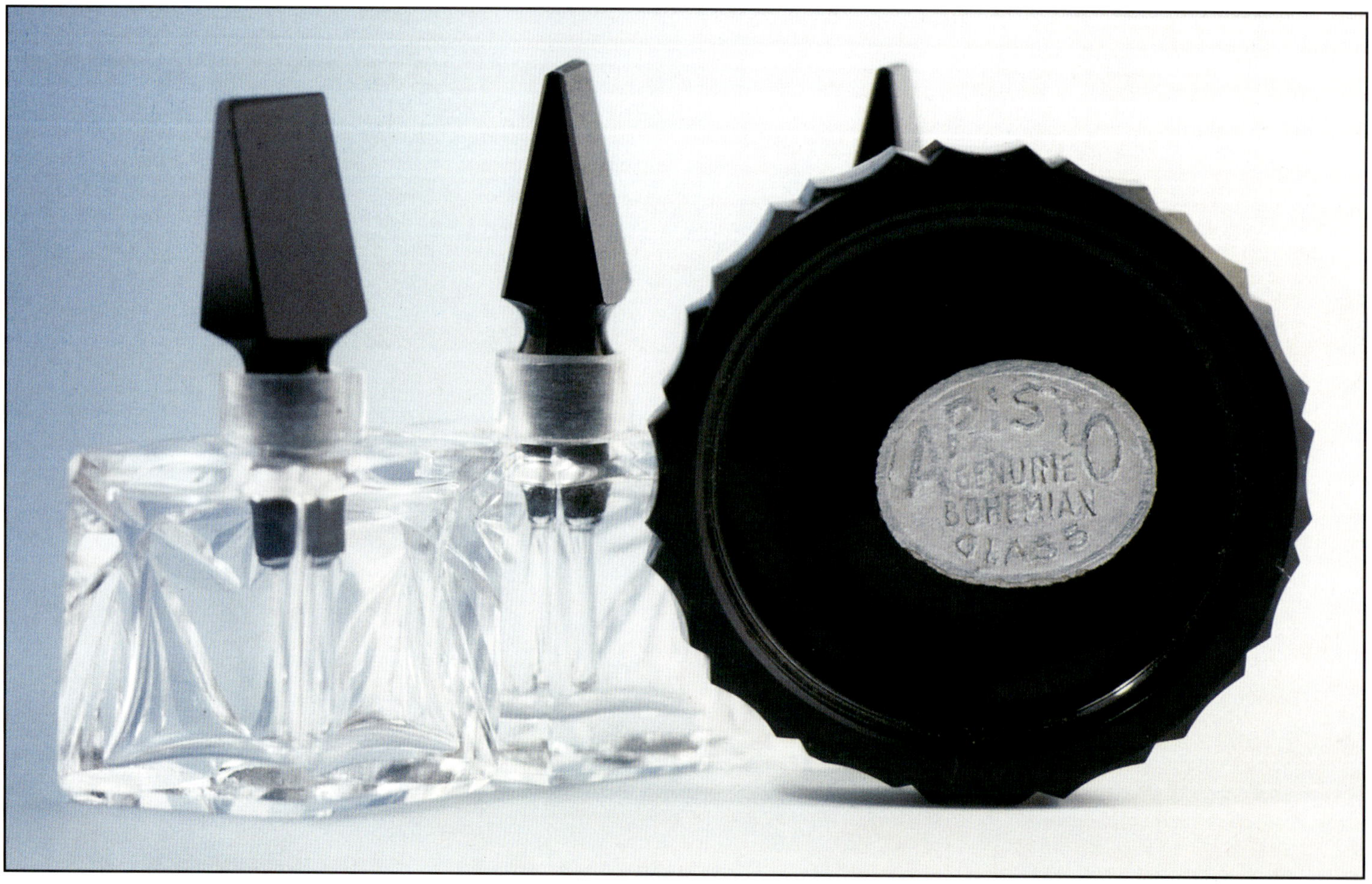

The same set, showing the Aristo sticker in the bottom of the tray.

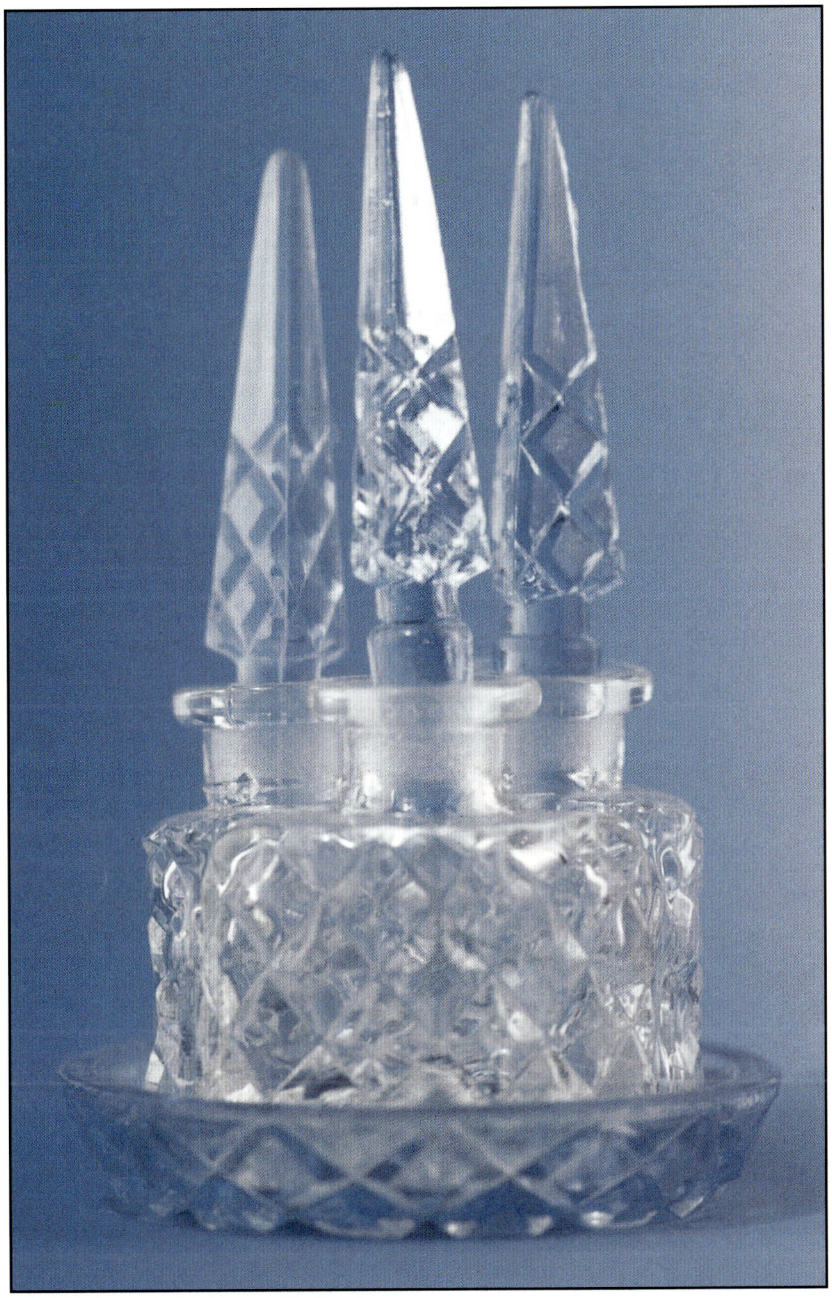

Japanese triplets. These bottles with blue tops fit on a tray the same way as the previous set, but are pressed glass with no hand finish work. 4". $100-150.

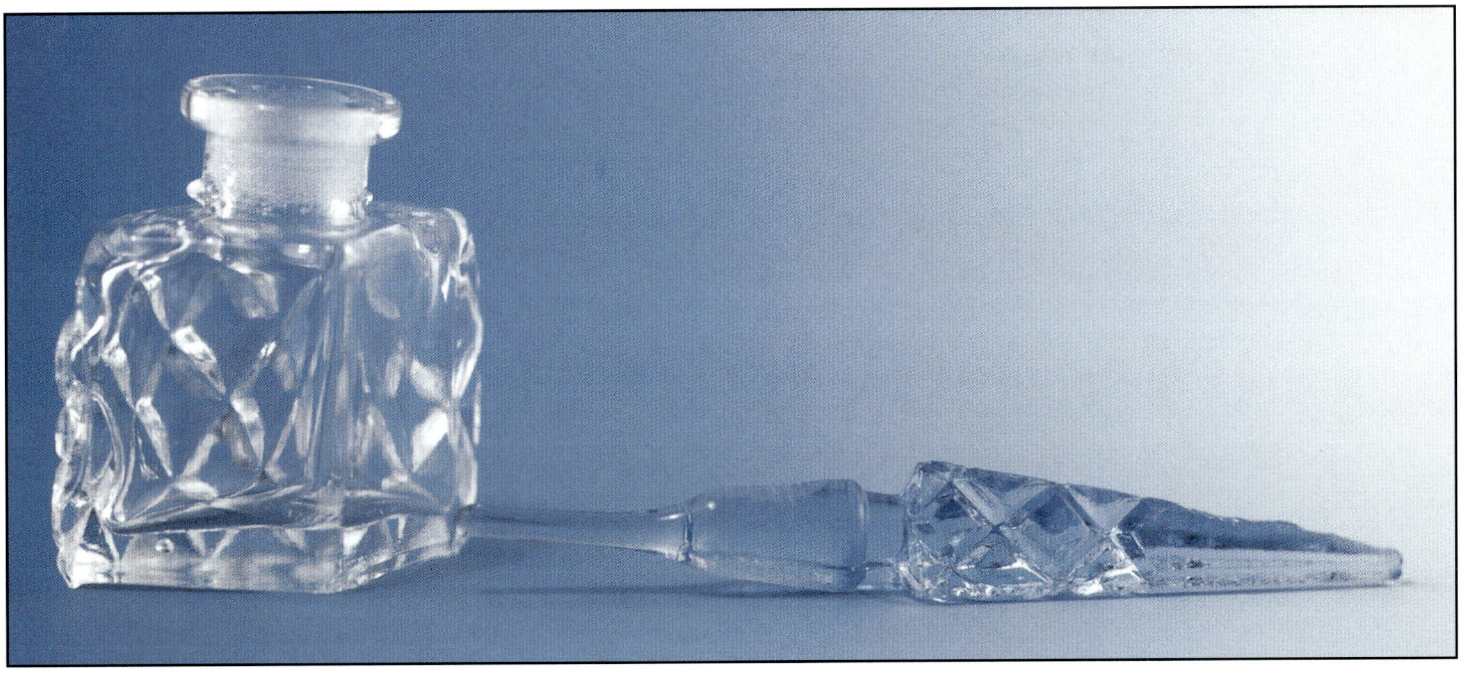

View of one bottle from the Japanese set and one top with stopper.

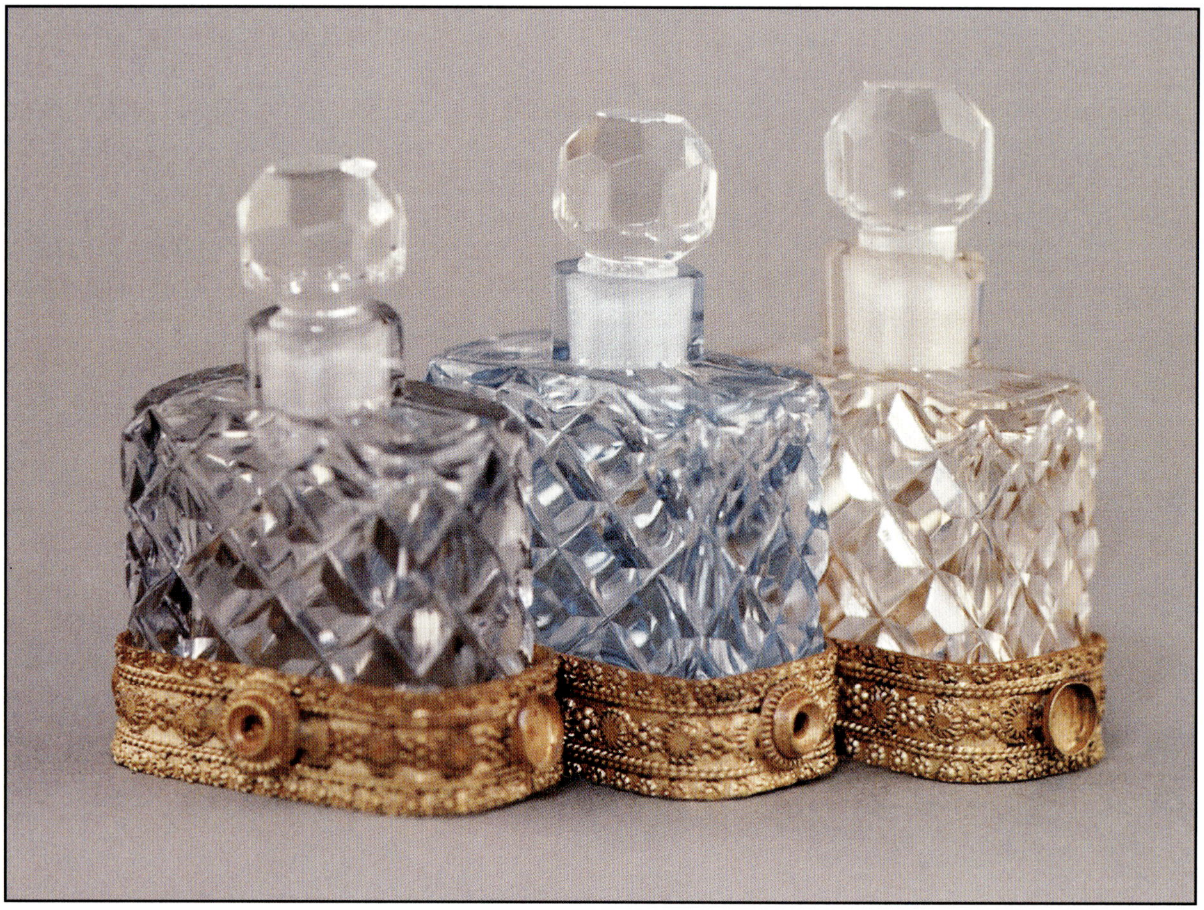

This triplet set in its basket is featured in a 1932 Irice ad. (Jones-North, 1999, p. 90) $150-200.

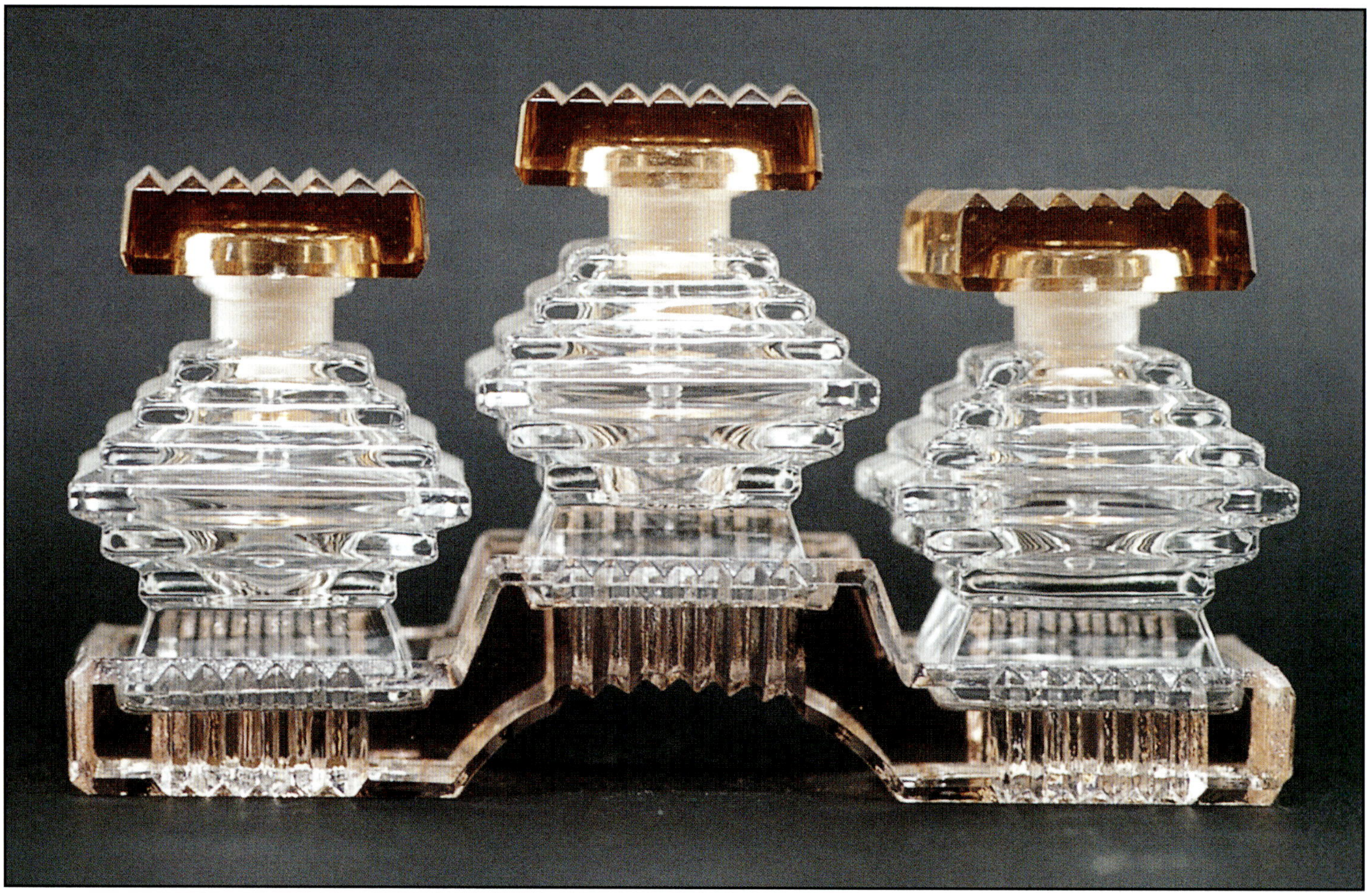

These pink triplets in their stair-stepped pink cut stand are also shown in an Irice ad (Jones-North, 1999, p. 114), for the year 1938. Note the repeating lines in the caps and in the base. 2". *Courtesy of Earline Kopriva*. Set: $300-500.

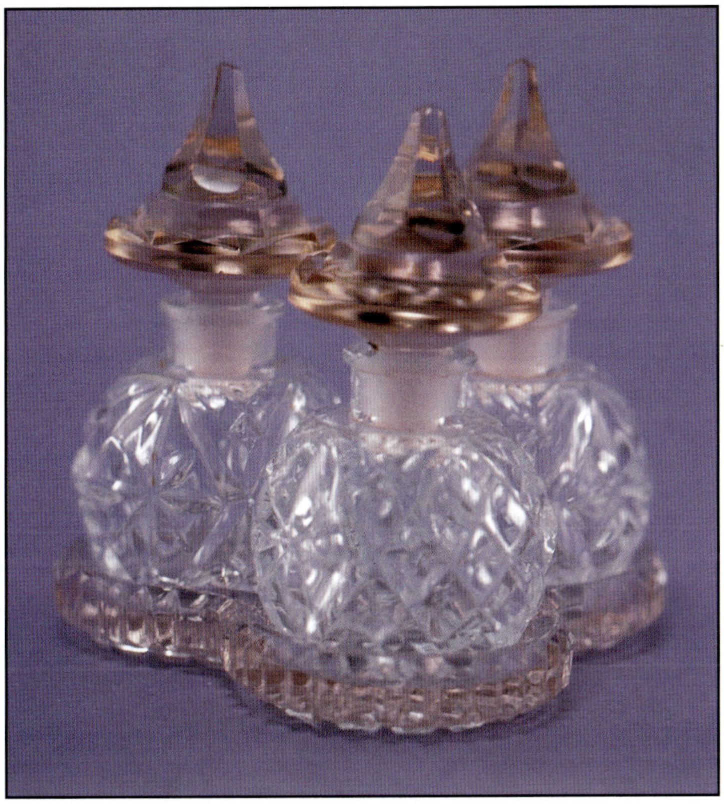

This Irice set has pressed glass bases with a pressed pink tray, but the tops are finely cut in an unusual shape. 2.75". $300-500.

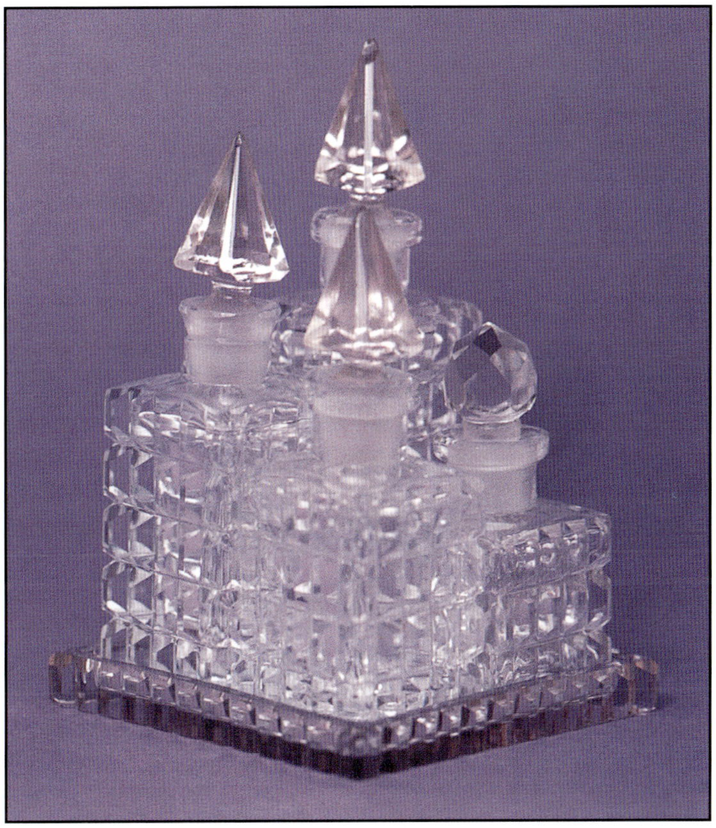

This rare quad set features four squared cut glass bottles of varied heights (2" to 3.5") on a square pink cut glass tray. The matching pink tops are pyramid-shaped. The color is unusual, almost lilac, rather than the traditional orange tinted pink. The smallest bottle does not have its original stopper. $200-300.

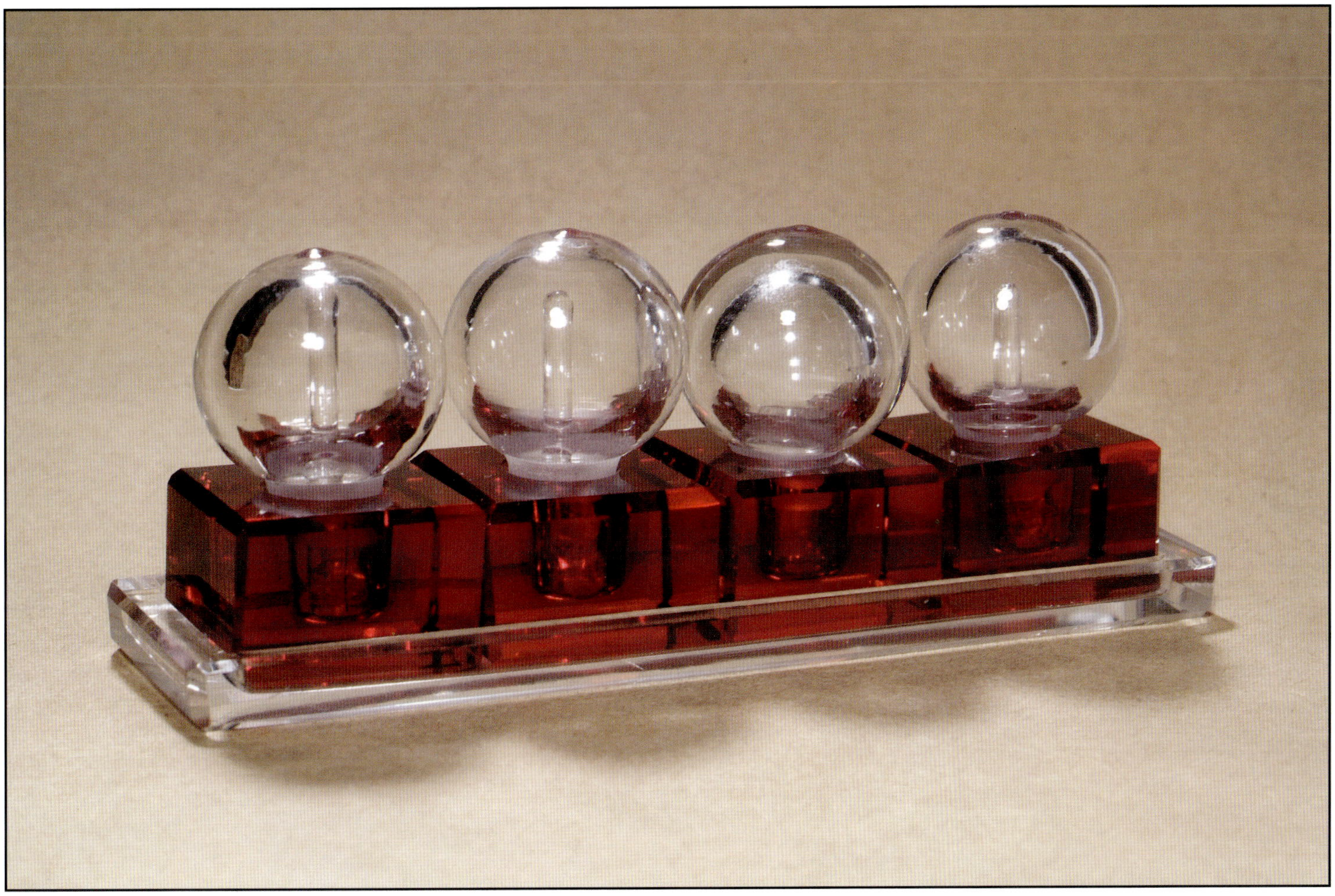

Very rare quad set. Clear bubble-like bottles with ground stoppers fit upside down into red glass blocks, then all fit into a clear glass tray. 1.625" x 1.5"w x 4.4"l *Courtesy of Don Orban. Photos by David Kirk of Kirk Photography.* $500-700.

Part III

Dresser Bottles, Medium and Large

For the next portion of the book, the author is indebted to Earline Kopriva, who has been a patient and generous friend, allowing her collection to be fondled and photographed; and to her husband, Tom, who patiently tolerated the intrusion into their home and their time. Earline is a longtime member of the International Perfume Bottle Association and has been collecting so tenaciously that she is known locally as "that perfume lady."

The medium and large bottles pictured in this section will be familiar to longtime collectors, as they have been the subject of many articles and more than a few books. They are representative of the span and scope of Czech perfume bottles that have long been the target of collectors. Hopefully, the contribution of this chapter will be to show some new items and revisit others in different colors or combinations.

To the avid collector, the author recommends Jones-North, whose *Czechoslovakian Perfume Bottles and Boudoir Accessories Revised Edition* (1999) is the foundation piece on which a library covering this topic should be built.

Cut Glass

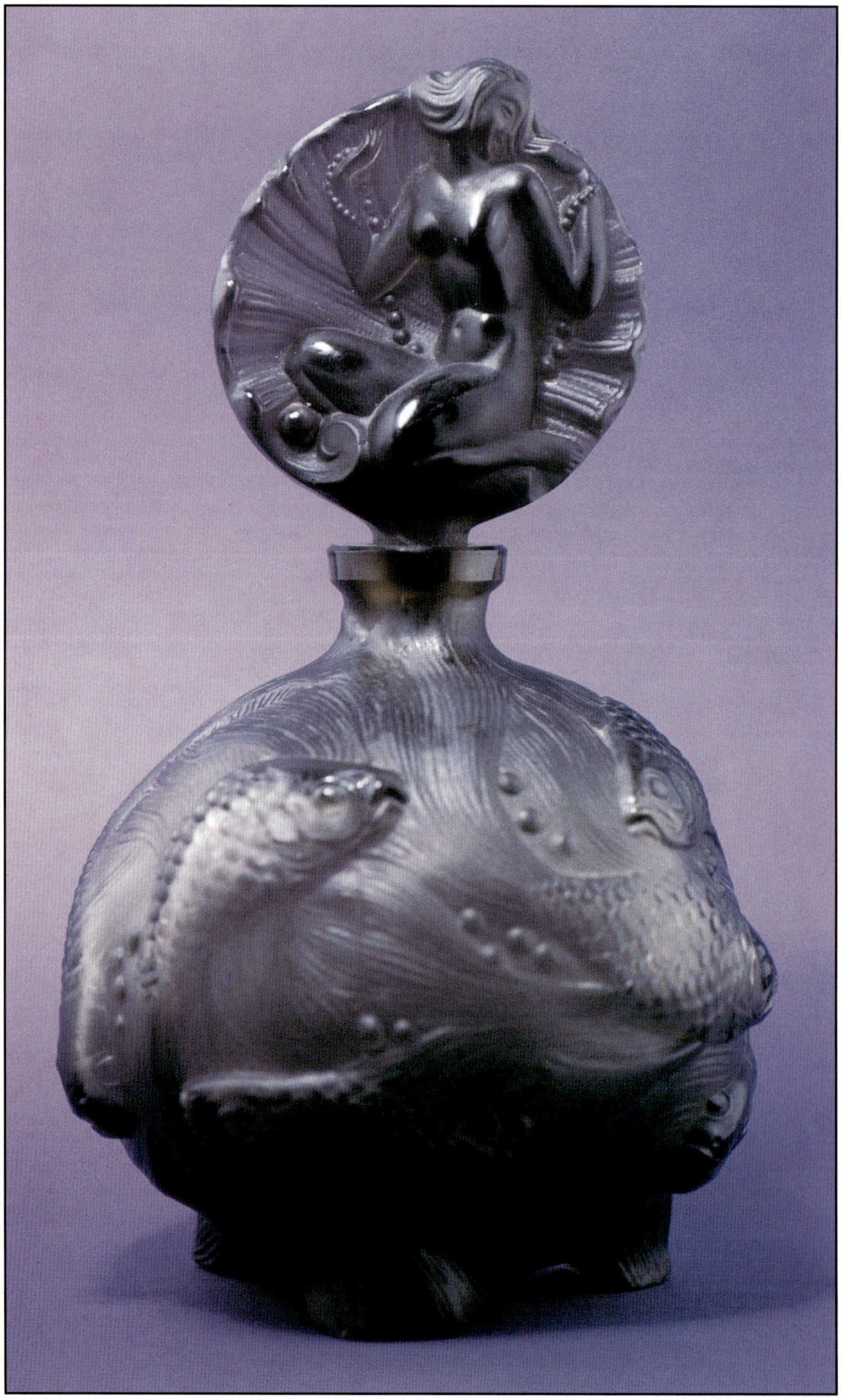

Birth of Venus, a Hoffman bottle in transparent black. 7.125". $2500-3000.

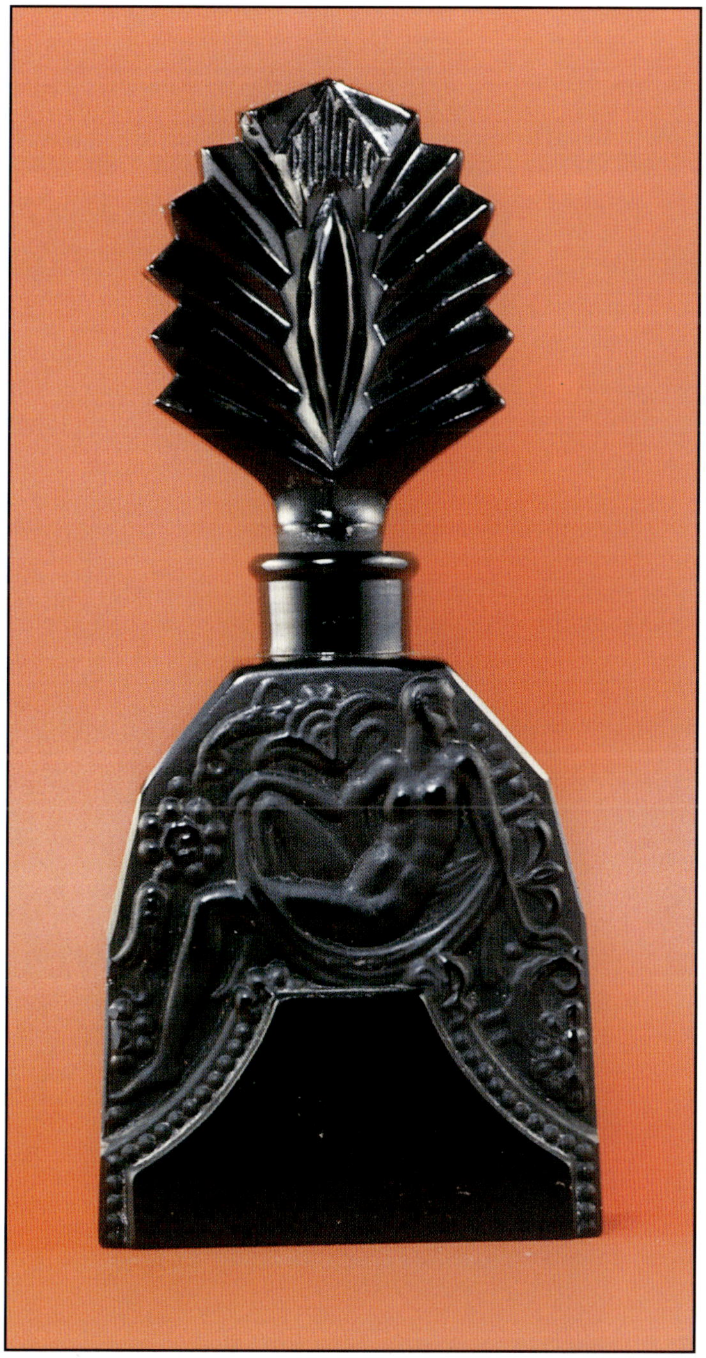

Seated nude in base, opaque black. 6". $1200-1400.

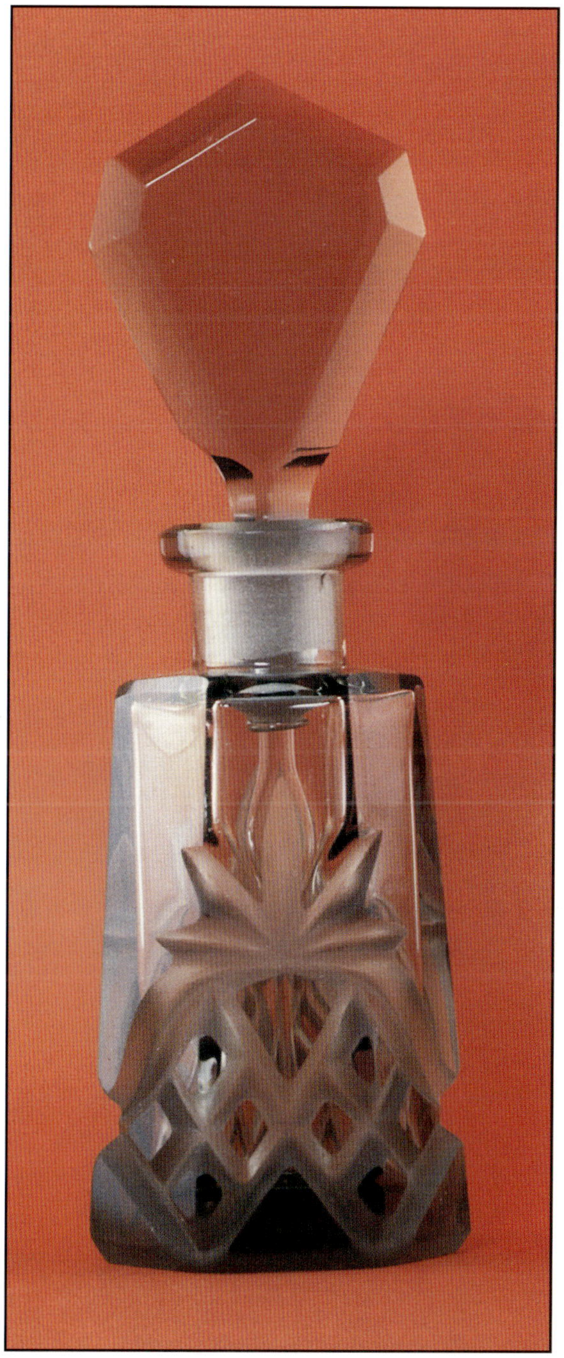

Transparent black, geometric design. 5.5". $150-250.

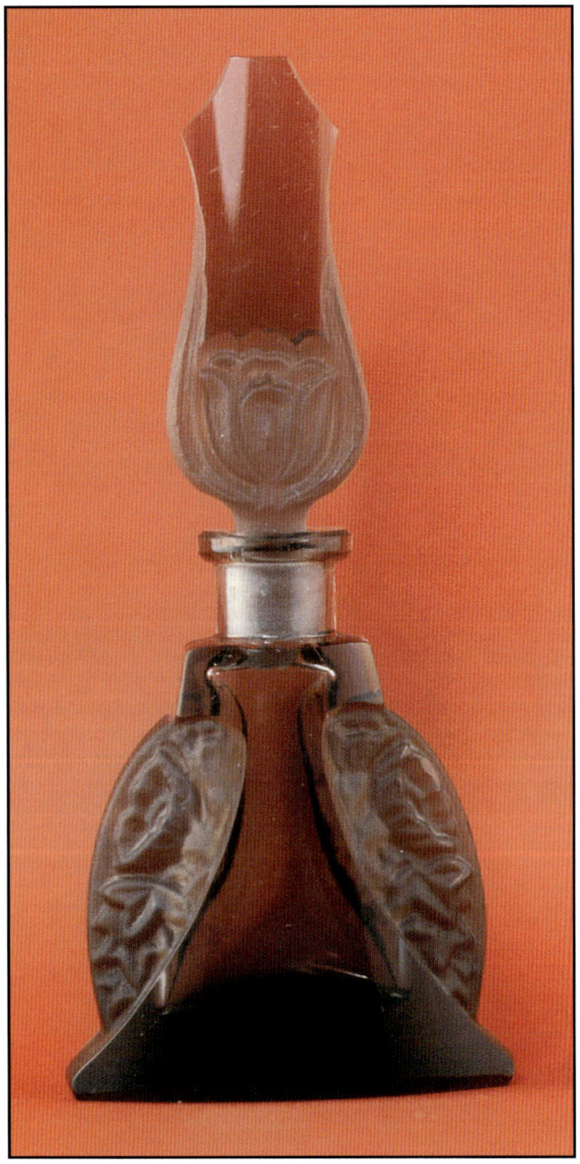

Transparent black, frosted floral detail. 5.625". $250-350.

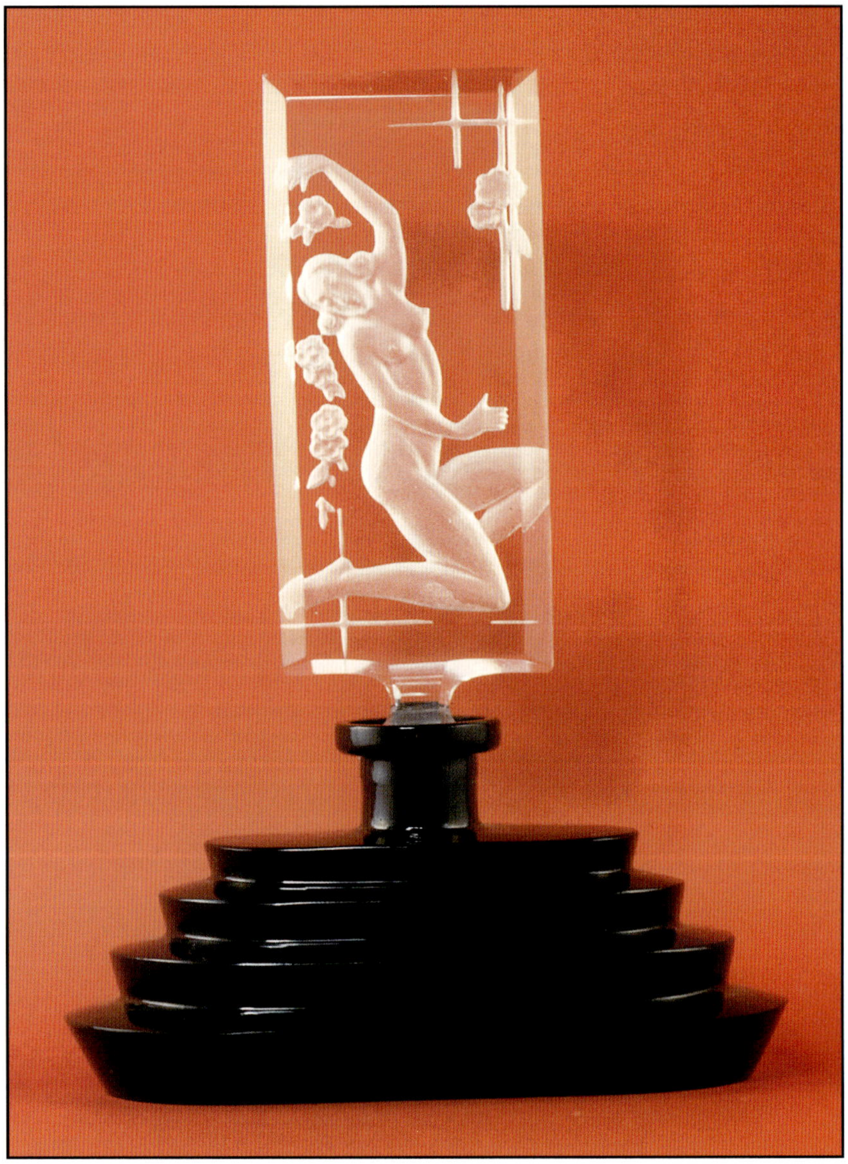

Kneeling nude pitching flowers, opaque black stepped base. 6". $550-750.

Unusual bird figural stopper. Unmarked. 5.25". $300-400.

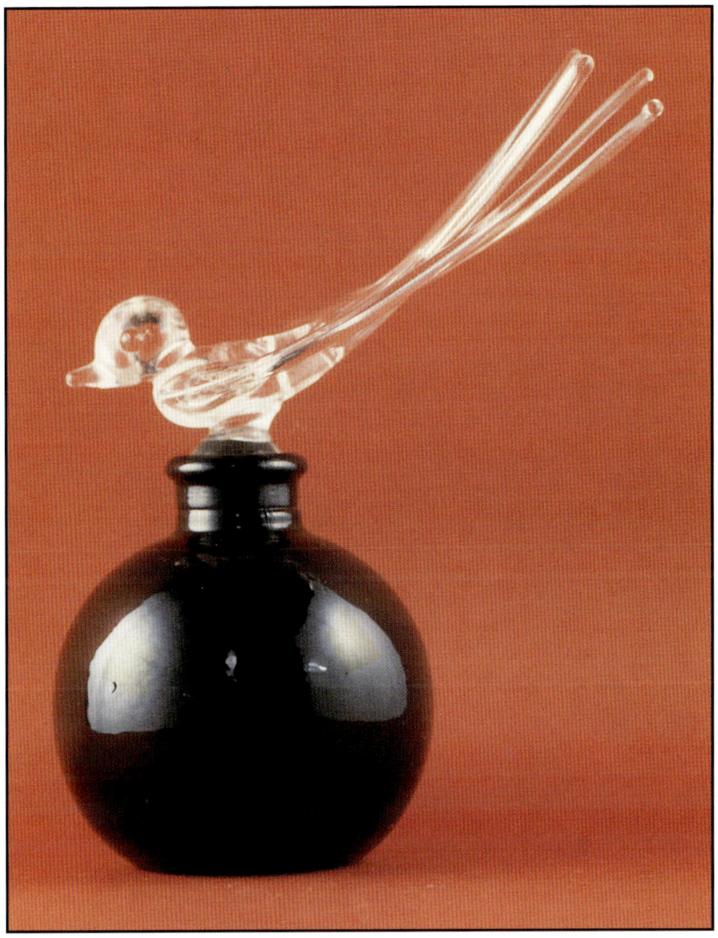

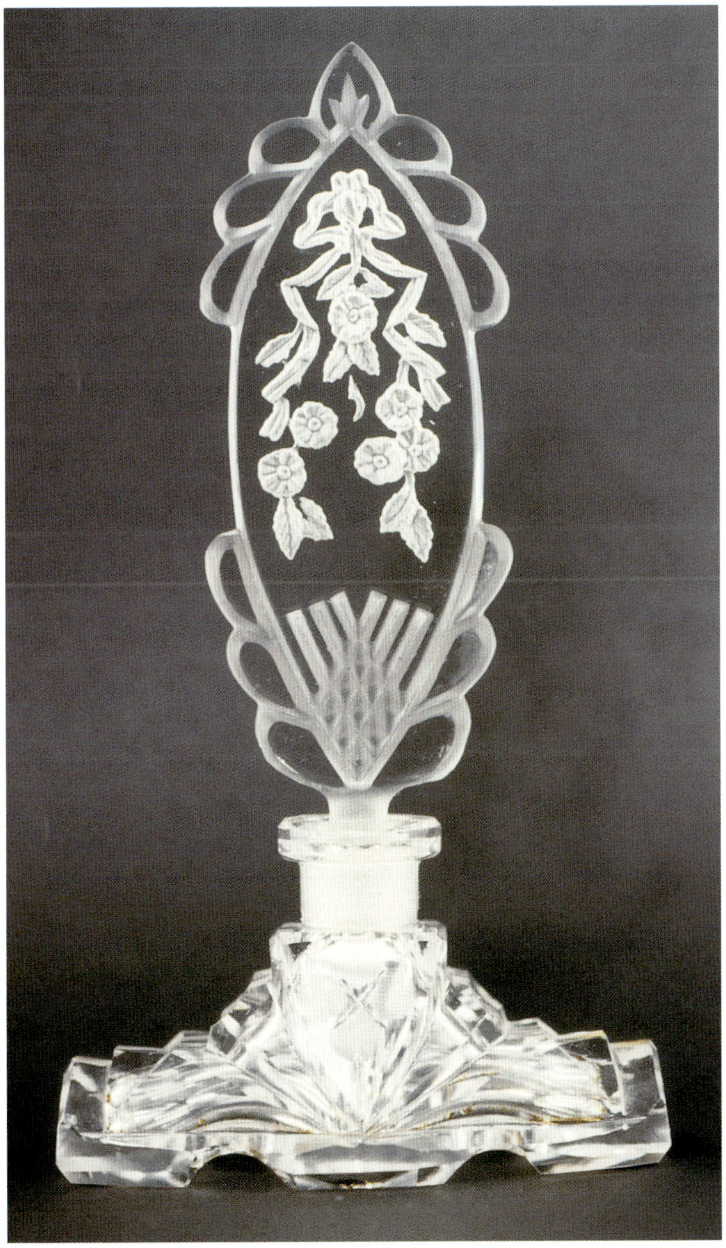

Clear geometric cut bottle with tall, ornate floral stopper. Premier paper label. 6". $250-350.

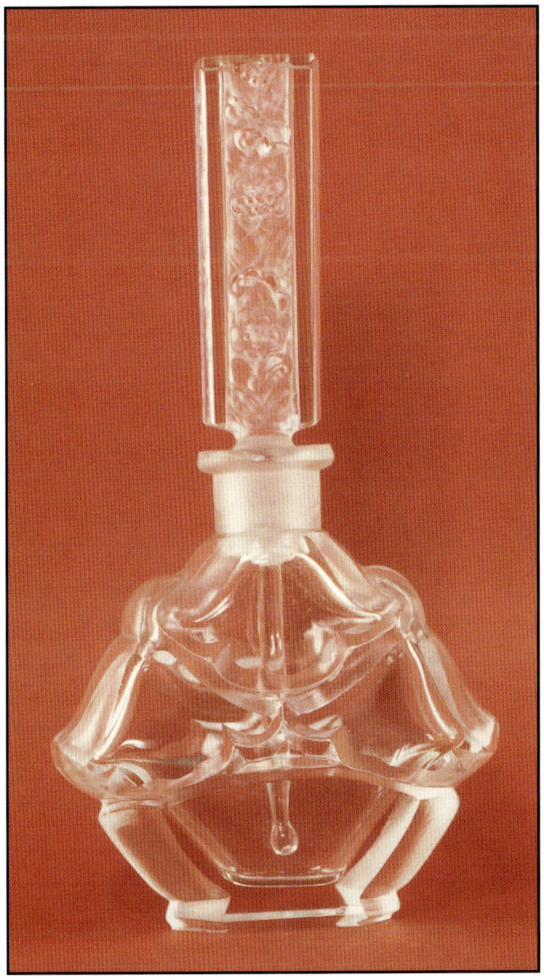

Clear bottle, frosted intaglio detail on stopper. 4.75". $200-300.

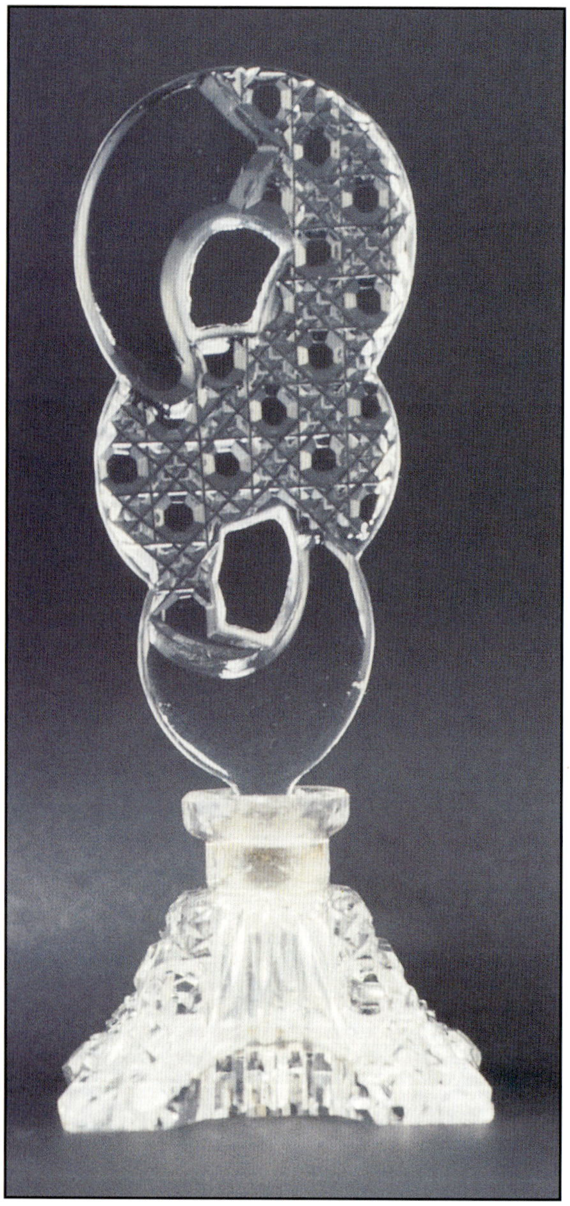

Clear, cut bottle, double pierced stopper with cut design. 5.75". $250-350.

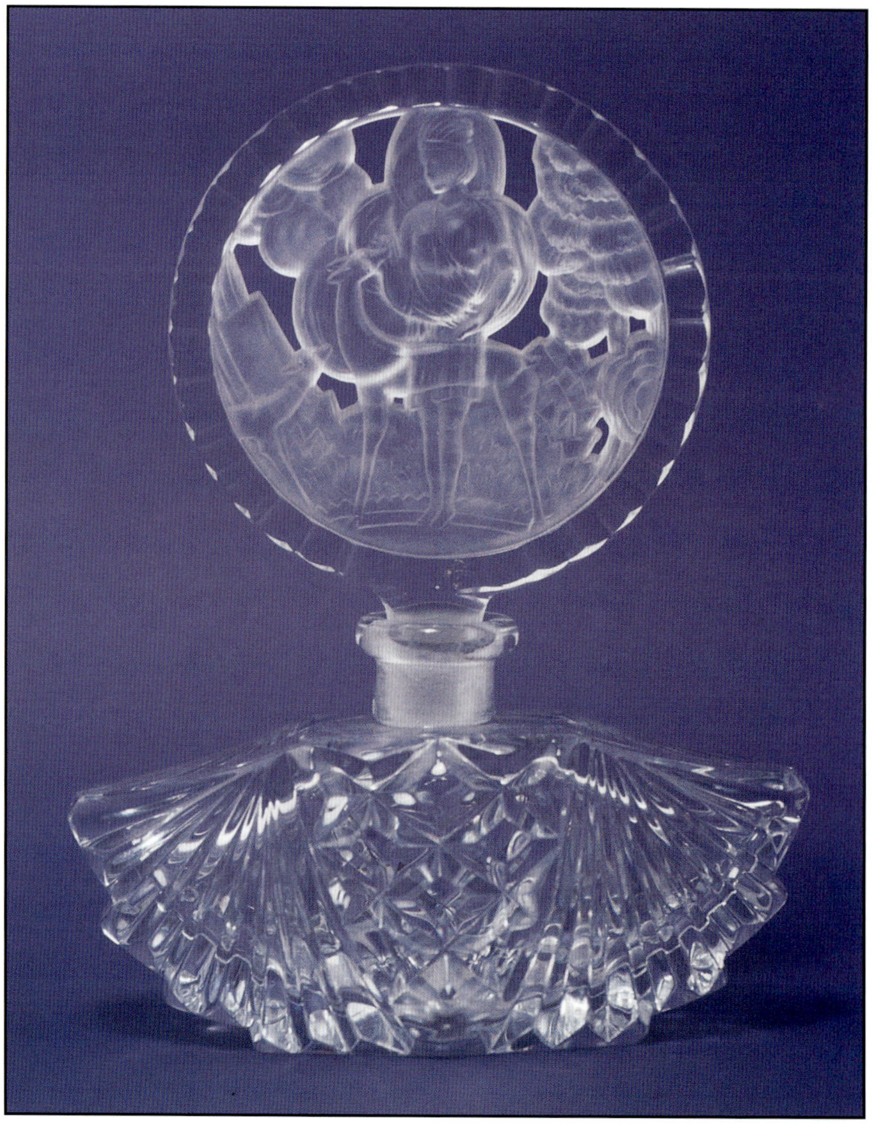

Clear, rocker style bottle with pierced stopper; frosted figural with two deer. 6.25". $750-950.

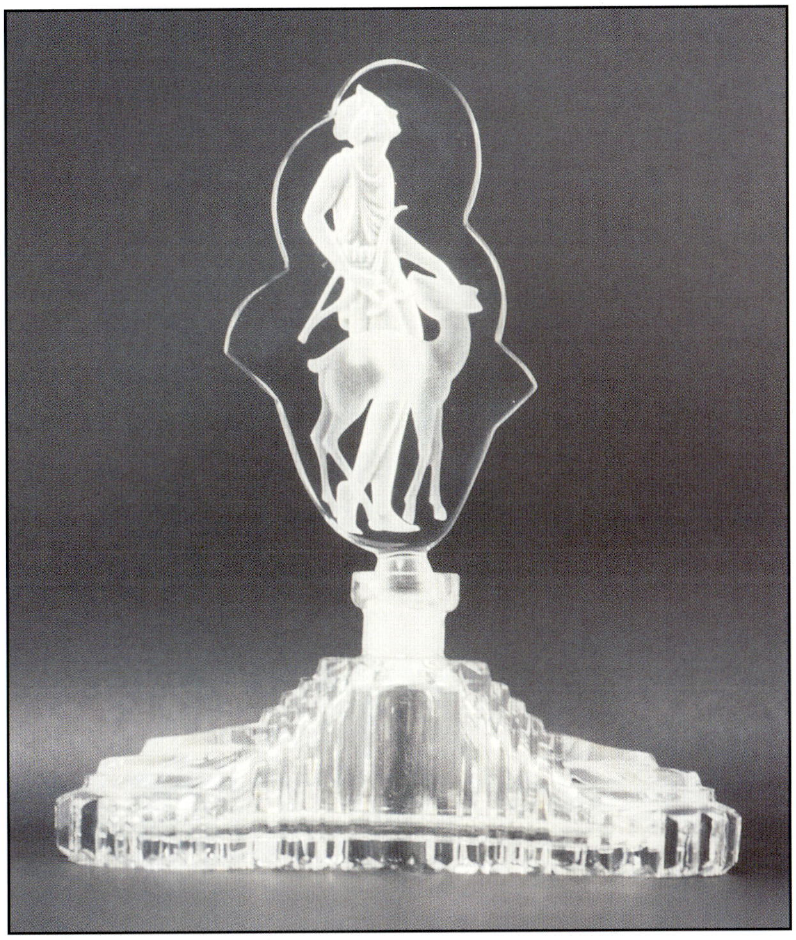

Clear, geometric base; Diana with deer on stopper, double intaglio. 7". $900-1100.

Left: Pierced, floral, Morlee sticker. 5.5". Center: Yellow XOXO top, Irice sticker. 6". Right: Clear, geometric base and top. 5.75". $200-300 each.

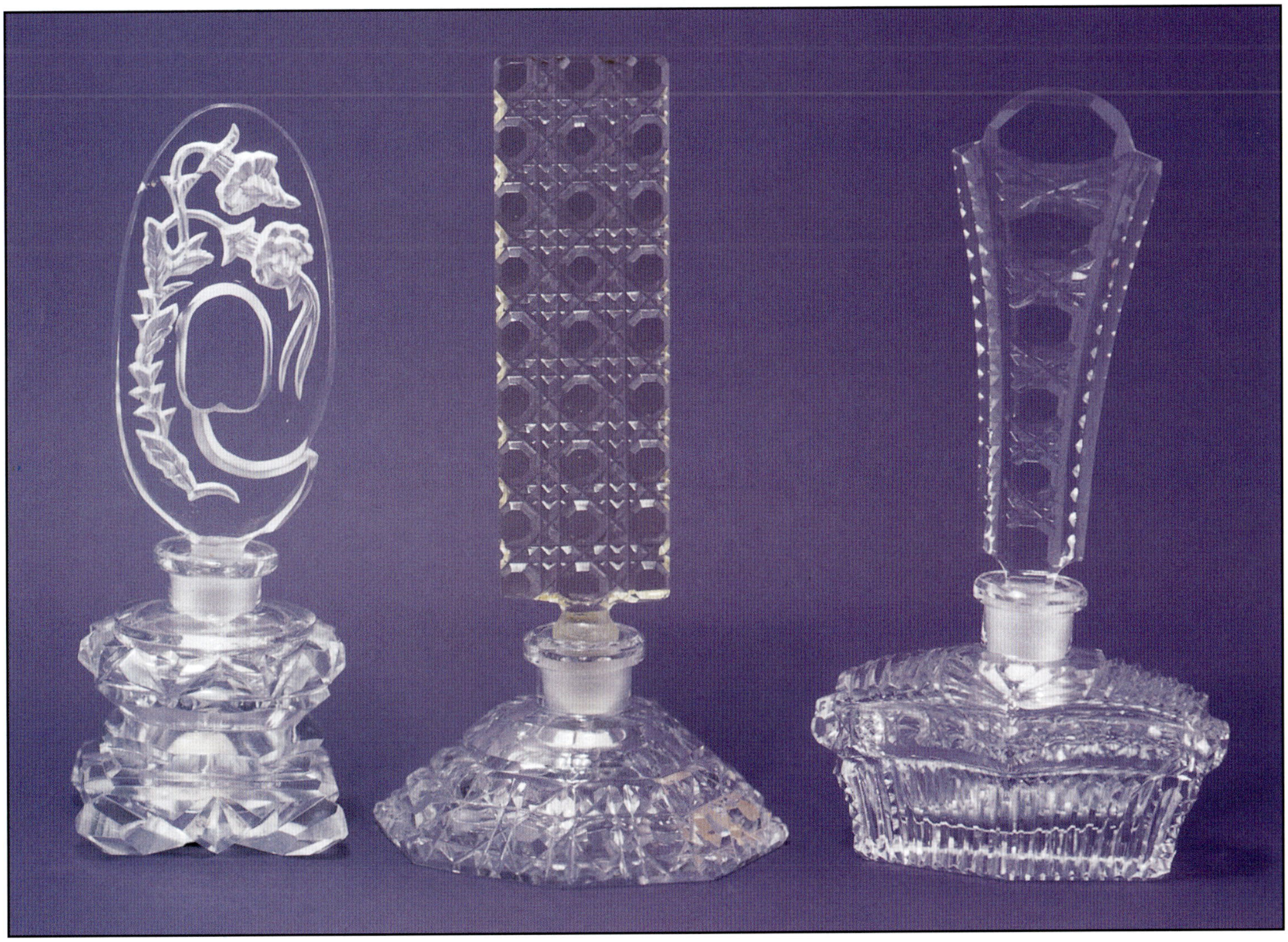

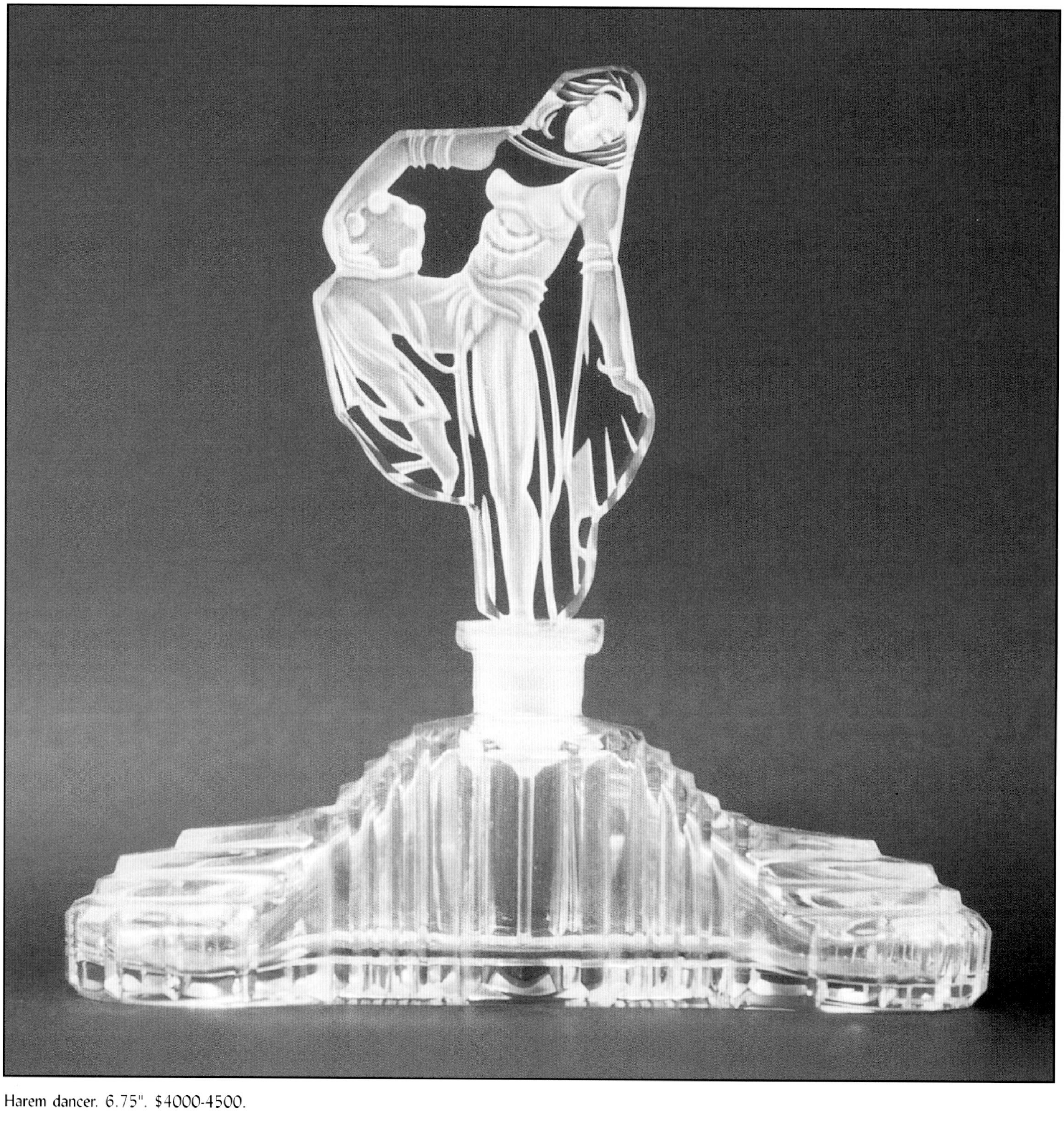

Harem dancer. 6.75". $4000-4500.

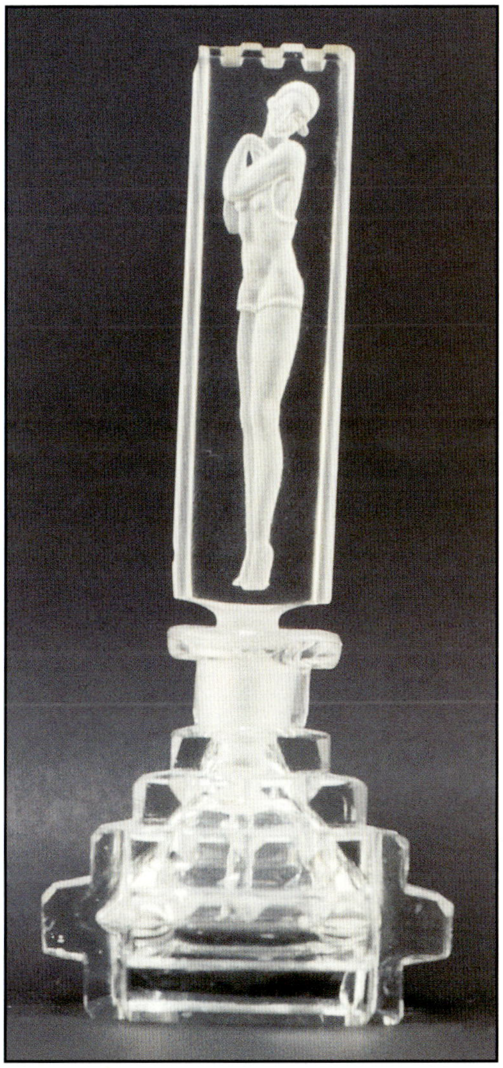

Bathing beauty, clear, cut glass. 6.25". $350-500.

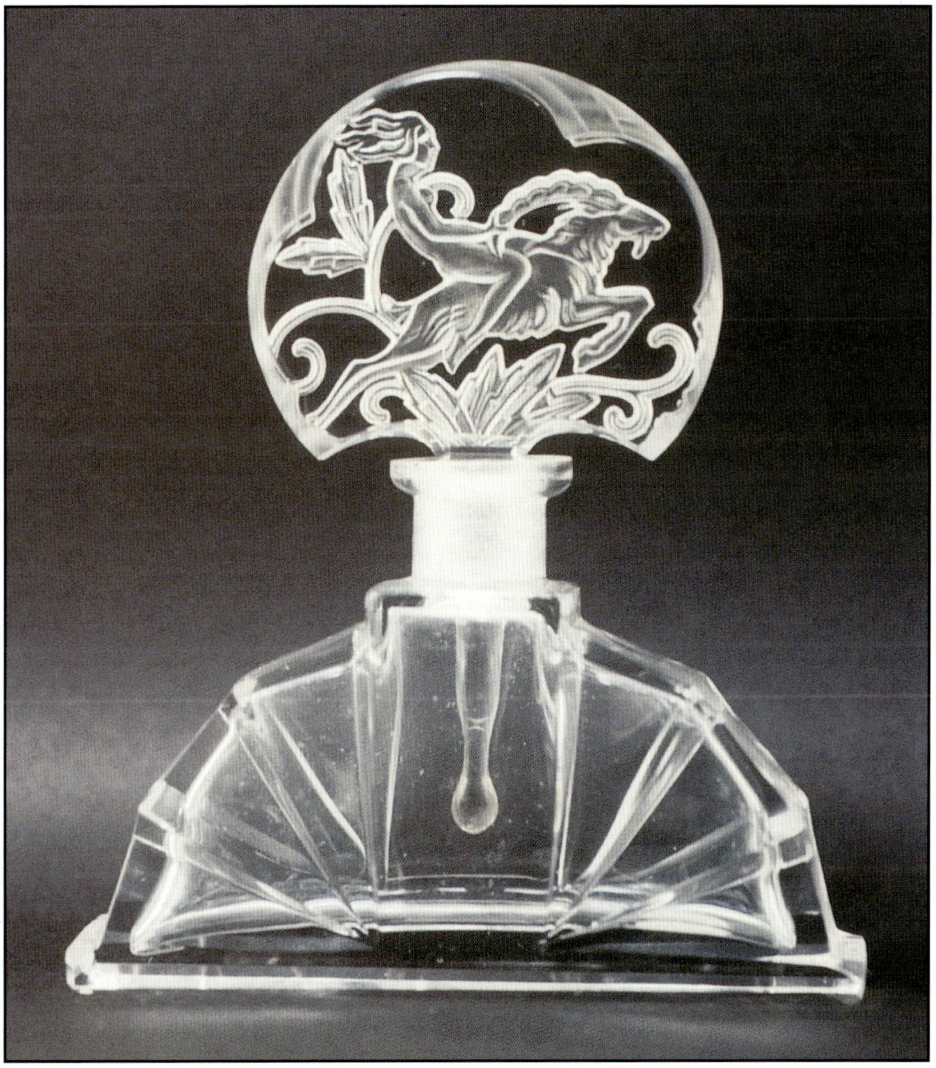

Nude on a goat. Clear, cut glass. 5.75". $500-700.

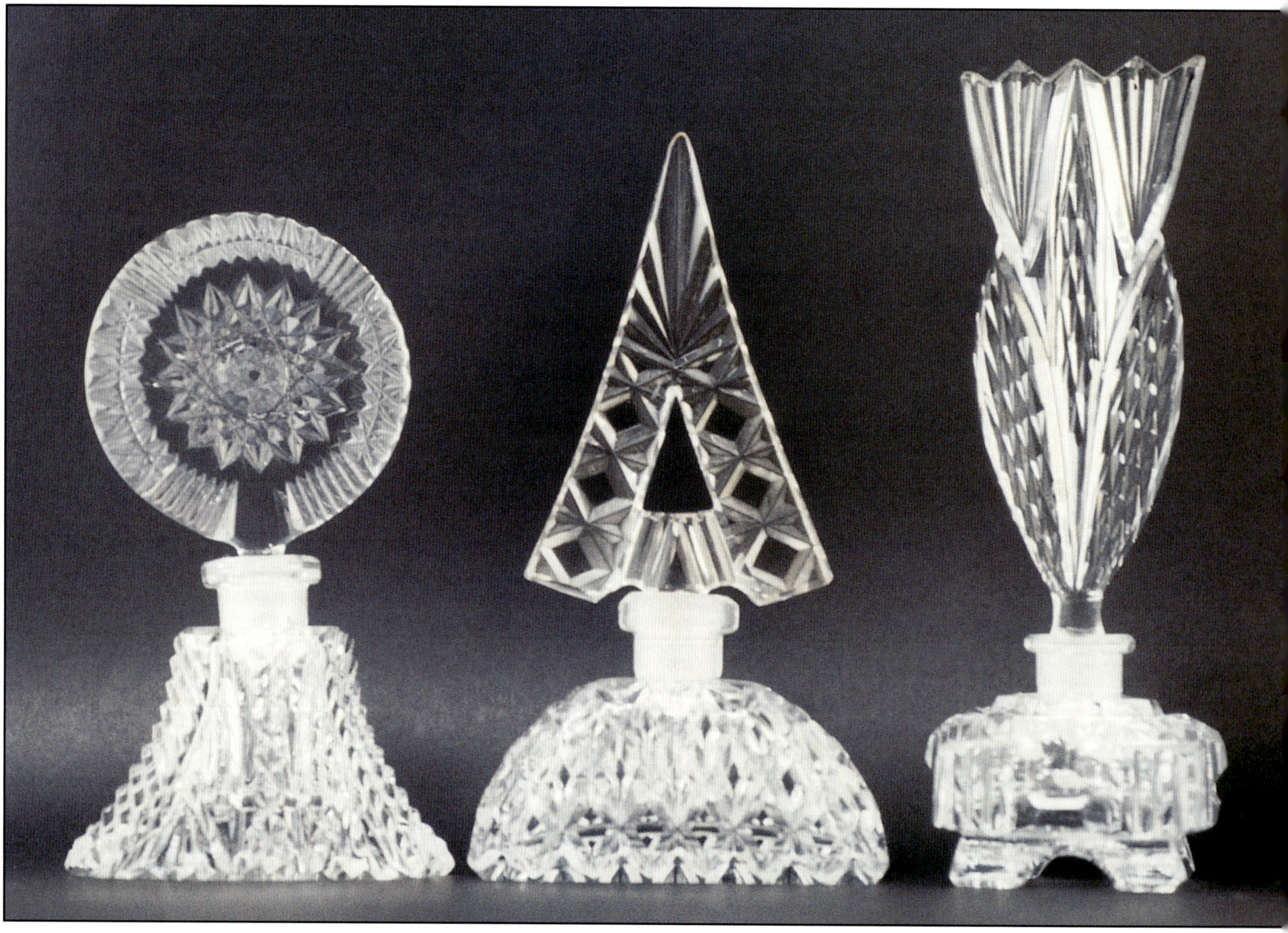

Left: Clear starburst, geometric cuts. 5.2". Center: Clear base; yellow, triangular pierced top. 6". Right: Clear, cut, footed base; tall, cut top. 6.5". $250-350 each.

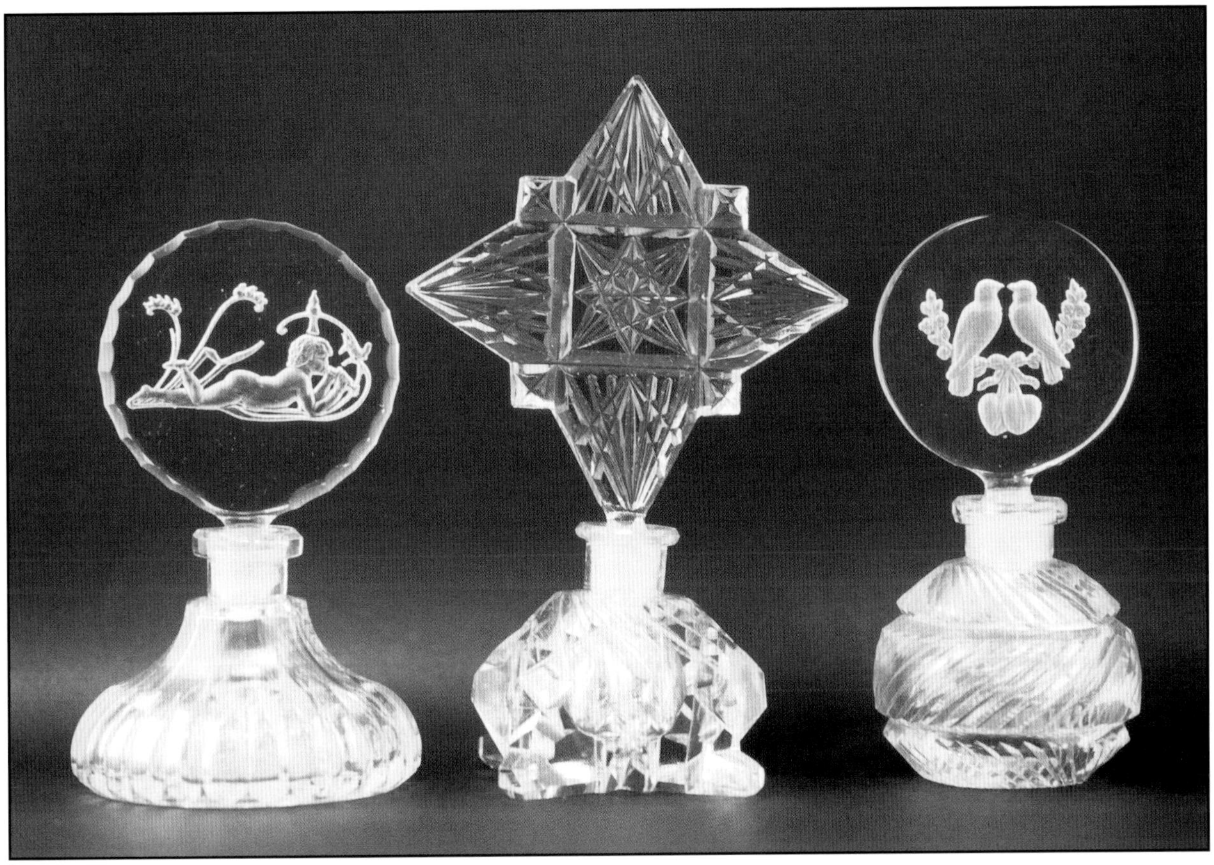

Left: Clear, child playing to birds. 4.375". $400-600. Center: Clear "Super Star." 6". $300-500. Right: Clear, lovebirds. 4.75". $350-550.

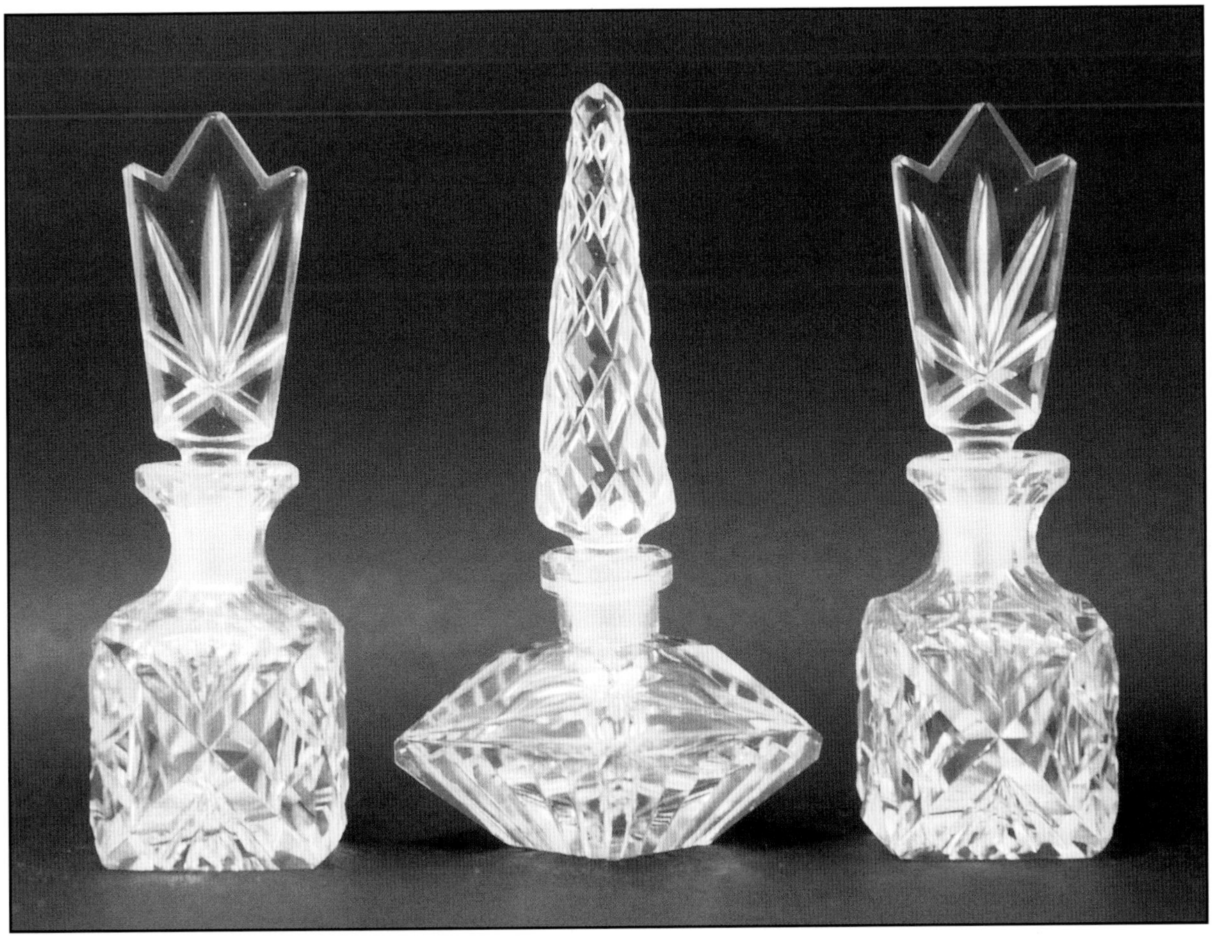

Matched small bottles, 3.75". Center has spire top. 4". $100-150 each.

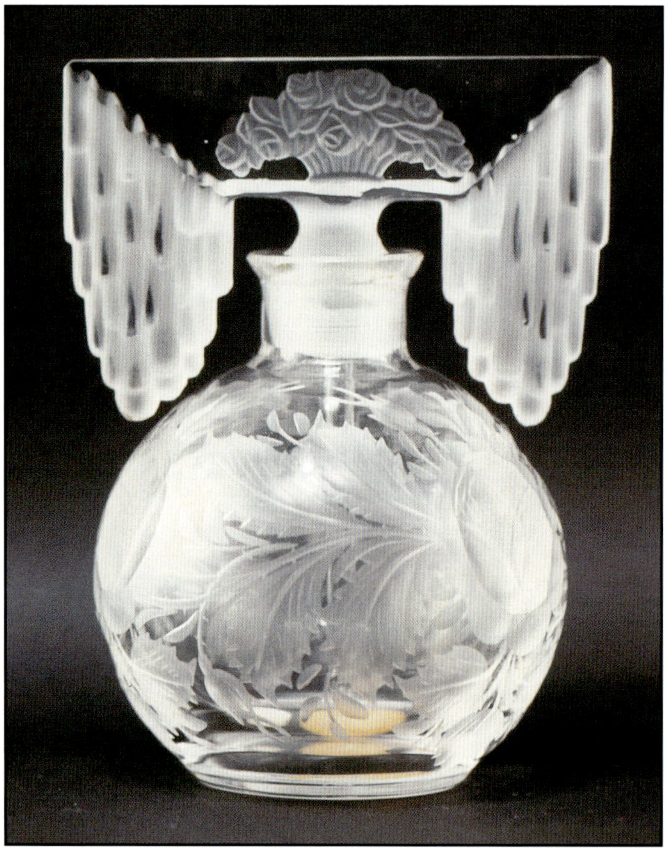

Clear, cut and intaglio roses, tiara stopper. 4.375". $700-900.

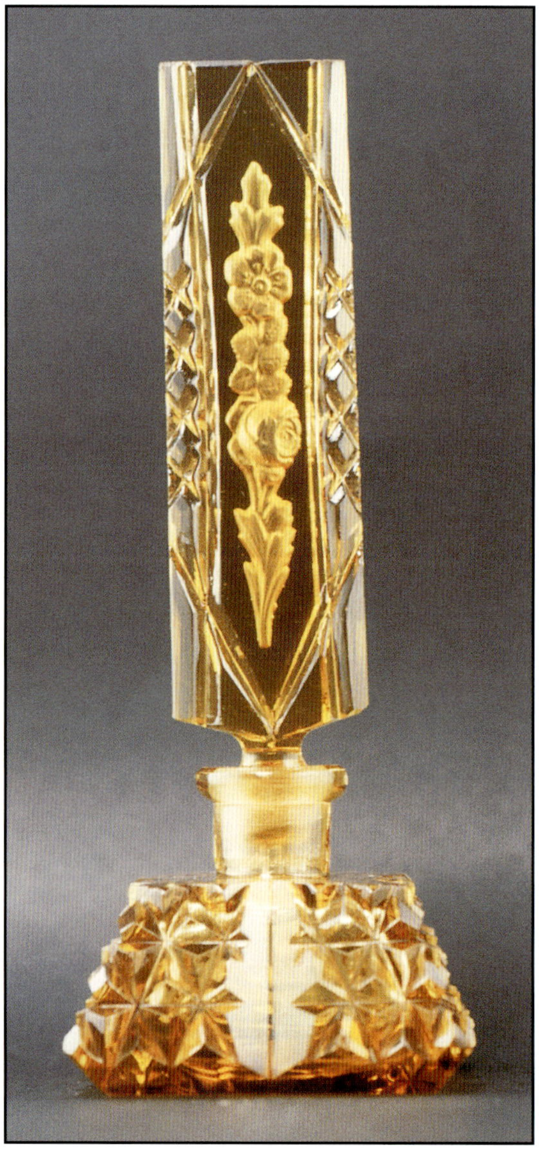

Amber roses above a geometric amber cut base. 5.5". $300-400.

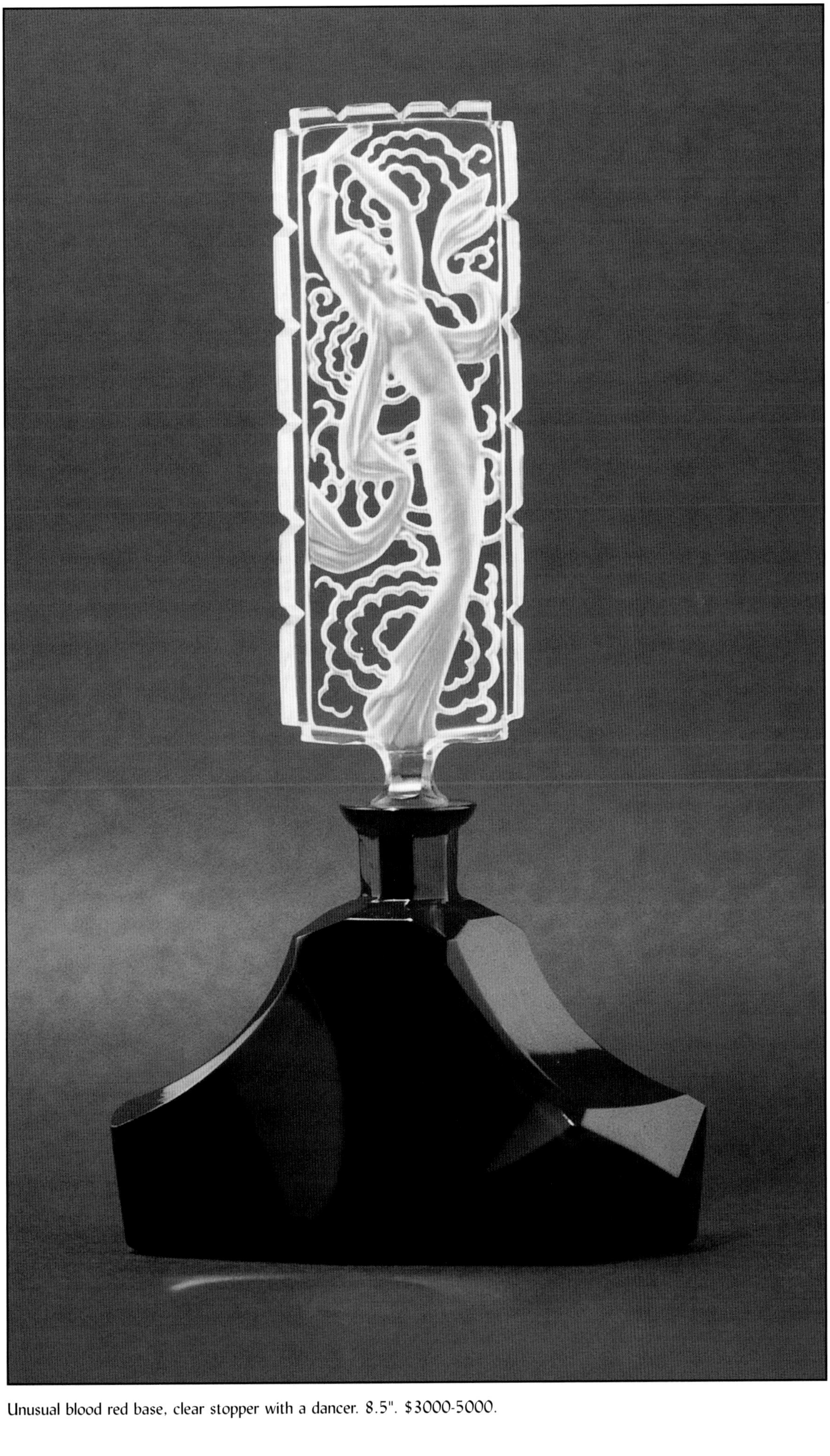

Unusual blood red base, clear stopper with a dancer. 8.5". $3000-5000.

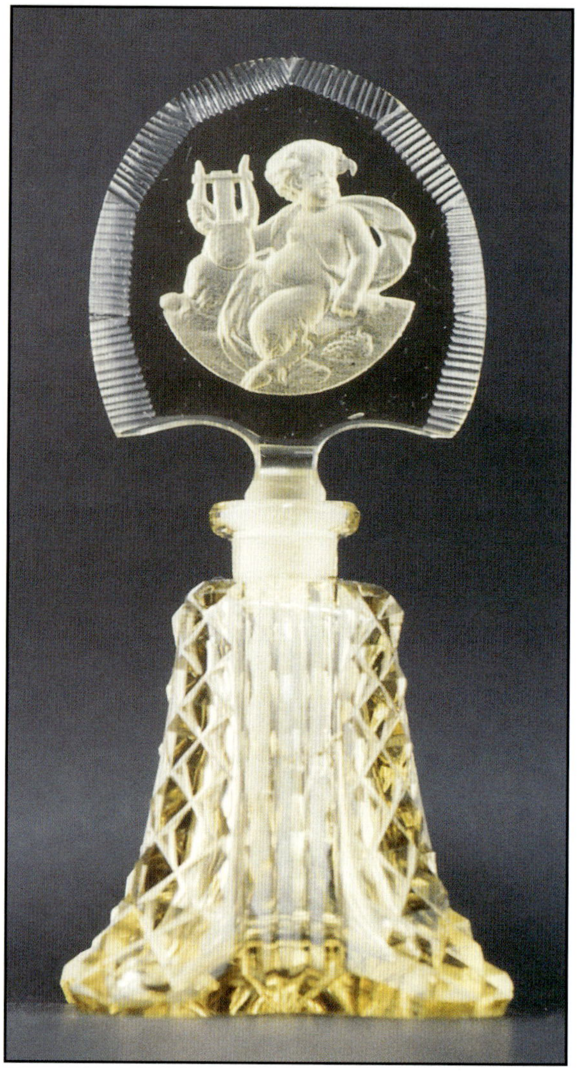

Yellow cut glass base; clear, cut top with figure of Bacchus holding a lyre. 5.5". $350-550.

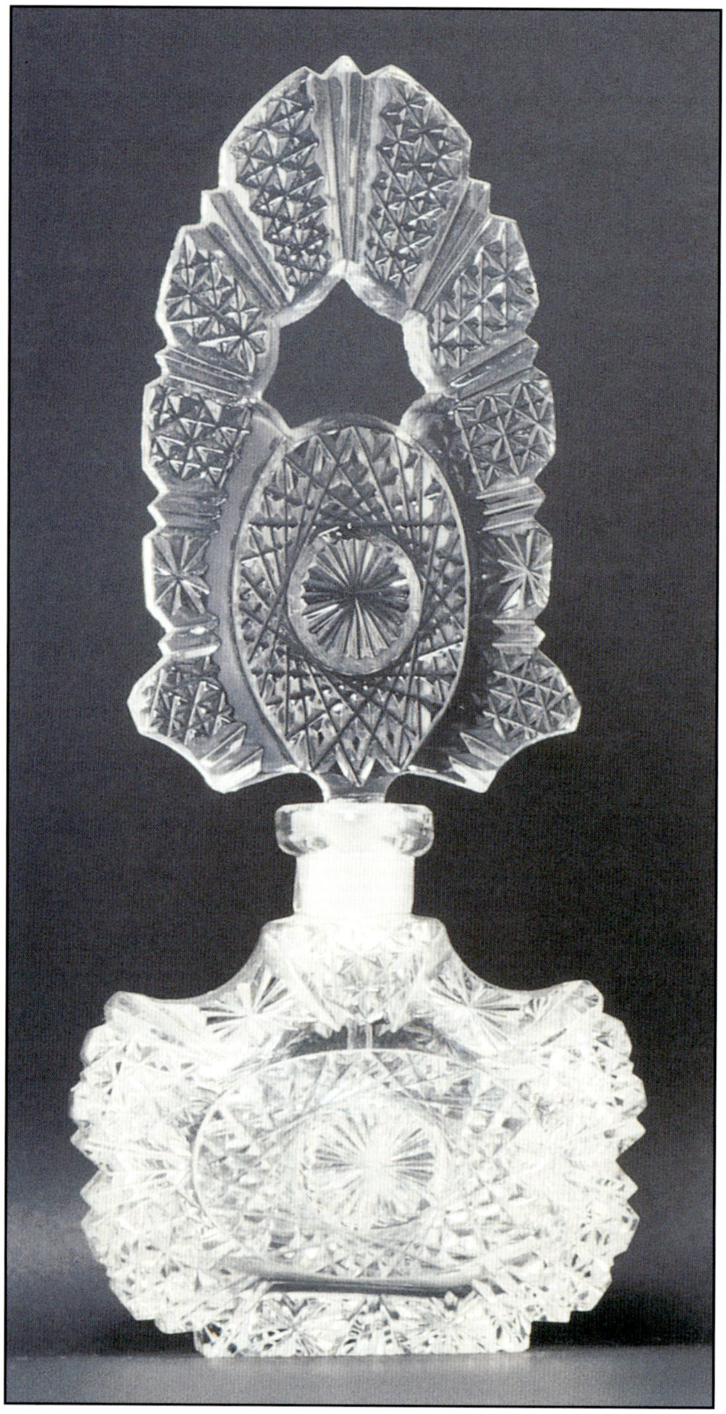

Elaborate, clear, cut base and top with radiating circles. 7.5". $300-500.

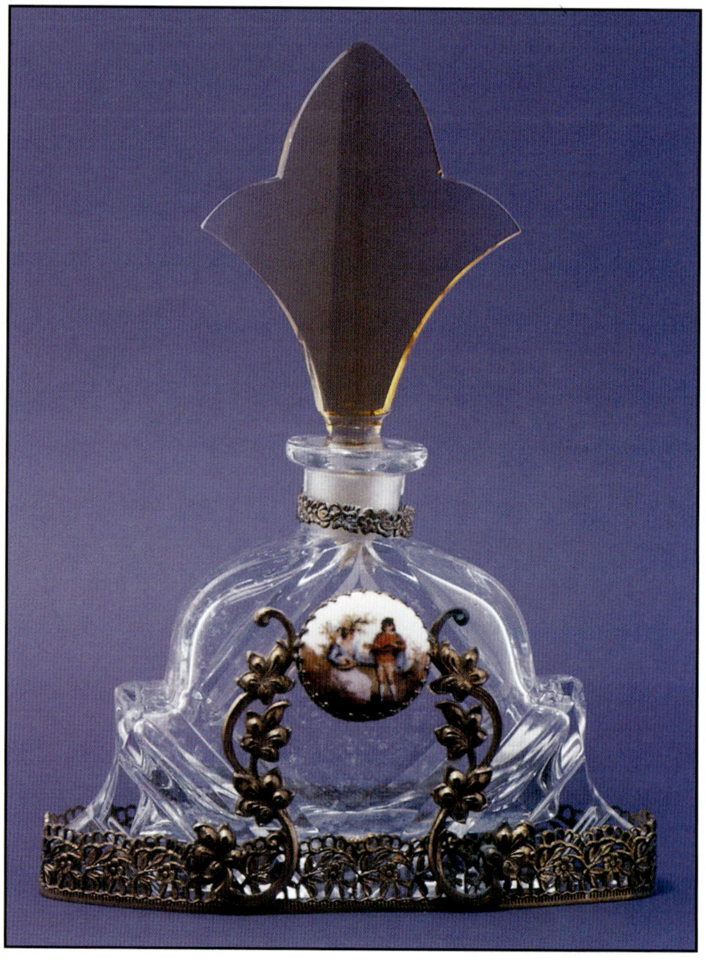

Clear, cut, jeweled base with cameo, amber top. 6.5". $600-800

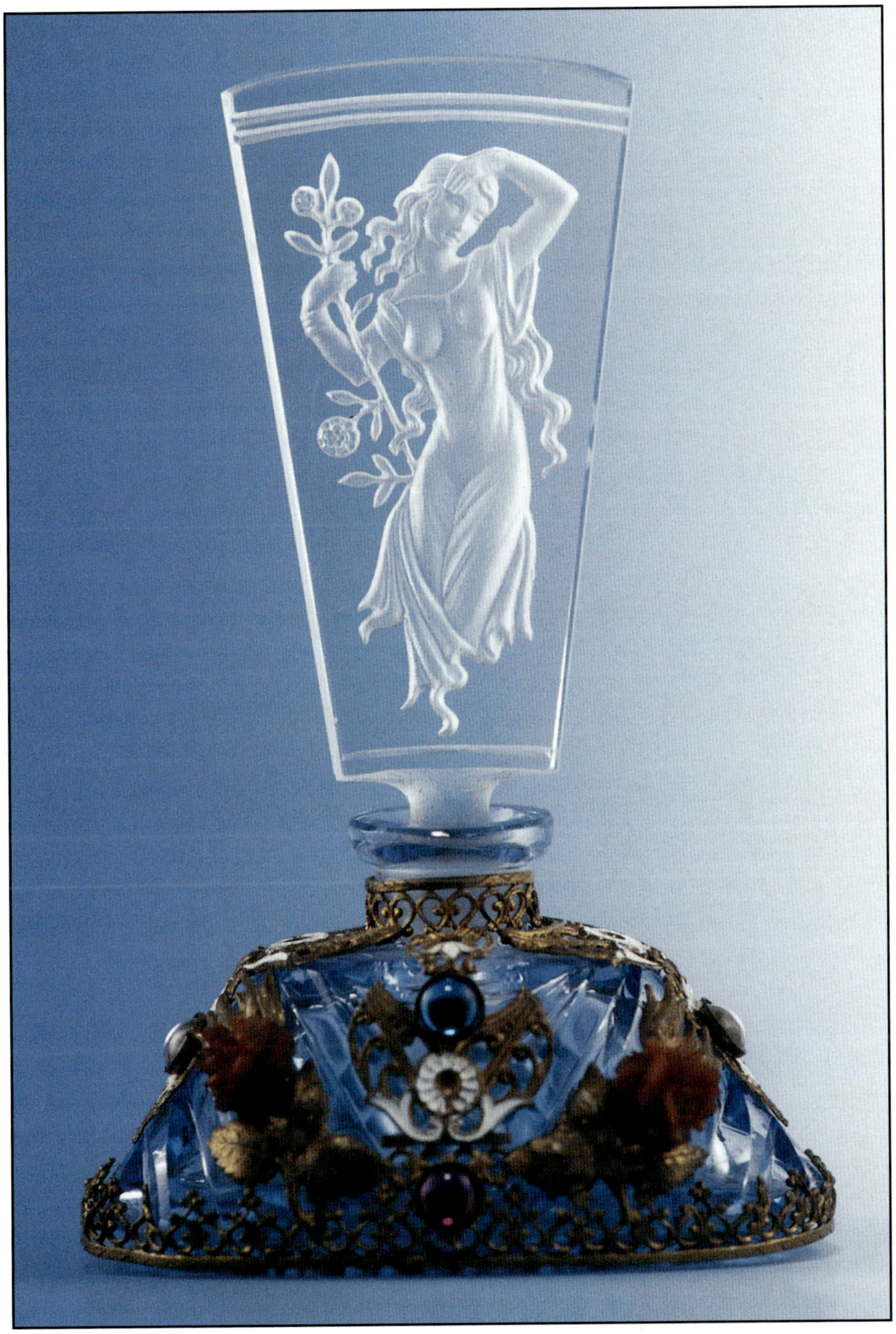

Blue, cut glass, jeweled filigree; figural stopper of a peering woman with a rose. 5.5". $1000-1200.

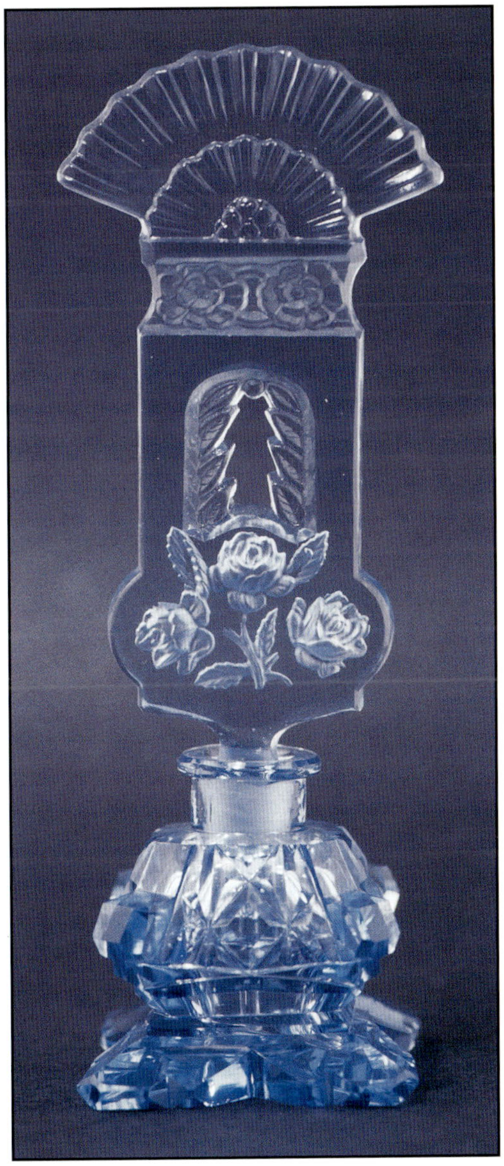

Blue cut glass base and tall, pierced, blue top. 6". $400-500.

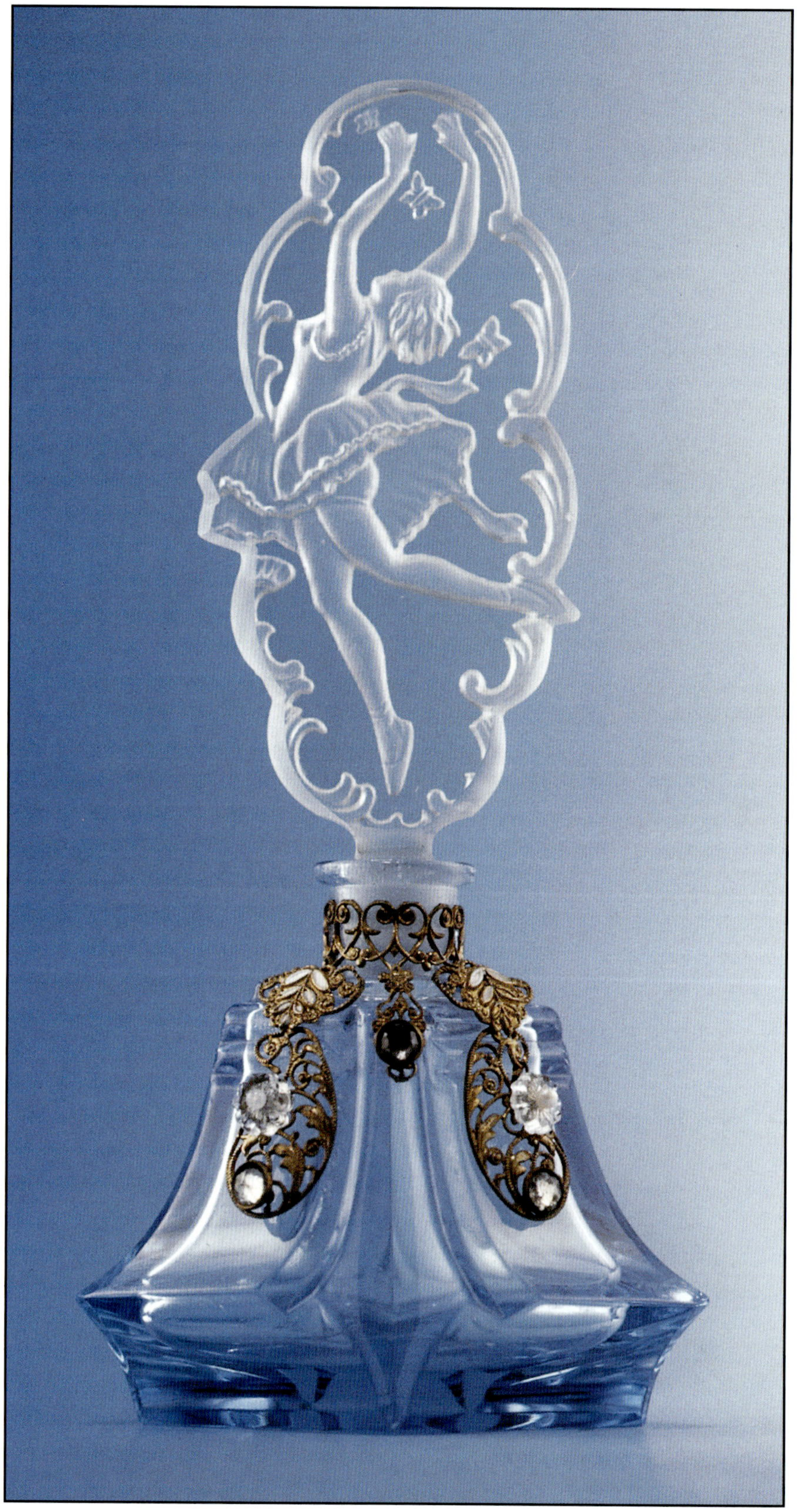

Blue cut glass, jeweled filigree; clear, figural stopper, girl with three butterflies. 7.375". $4000-$5000.

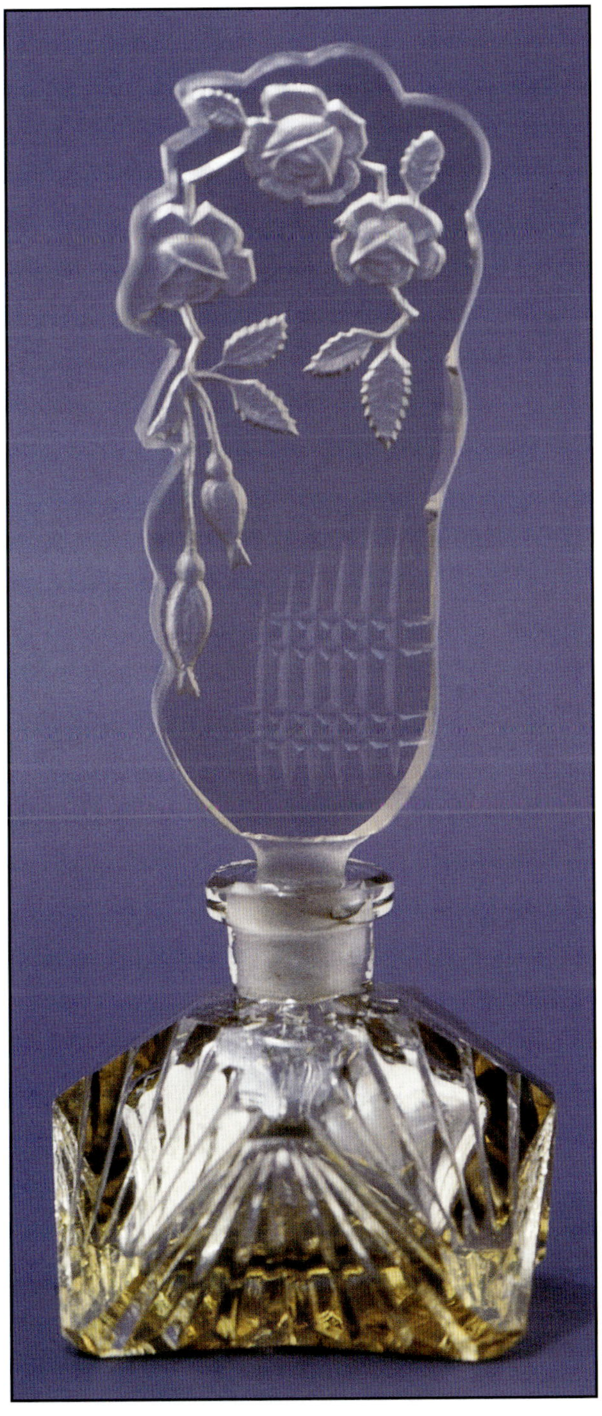

Yellow cut glass, intaglio and cut yellow stopper. 6". $400-500.

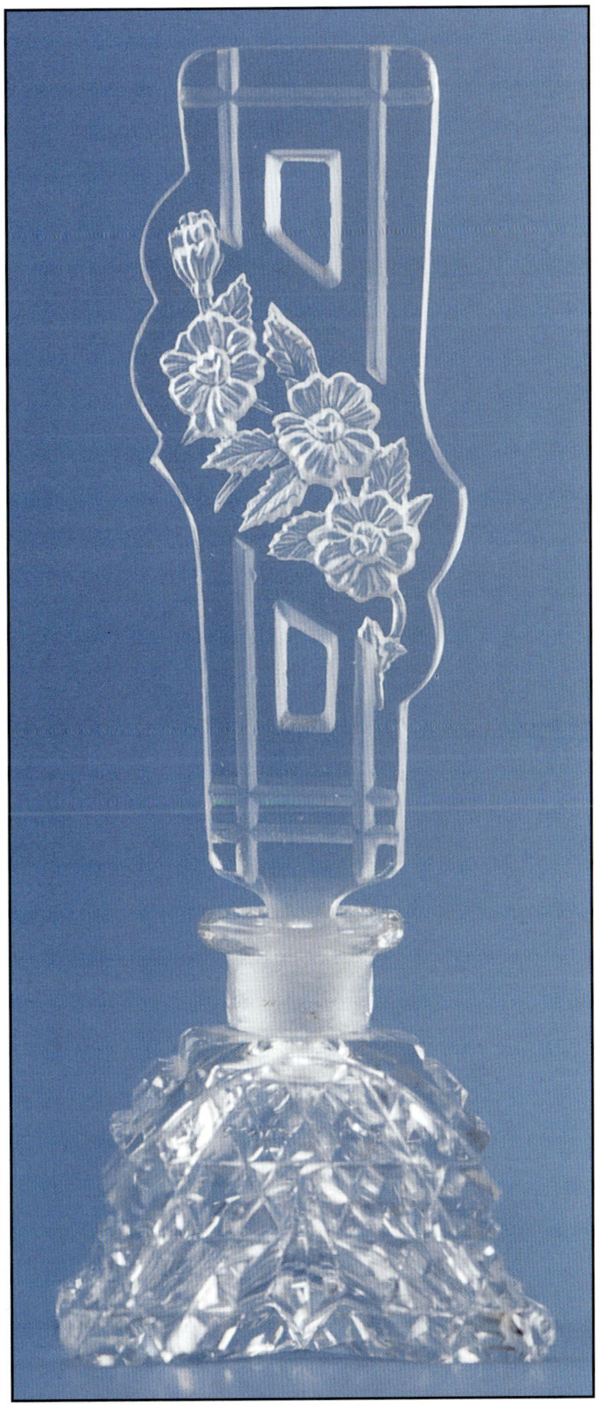

Clear, cut glass, tall, elaborate cut with intaglio roses, double pierced stopper. 5.75". $400-500.

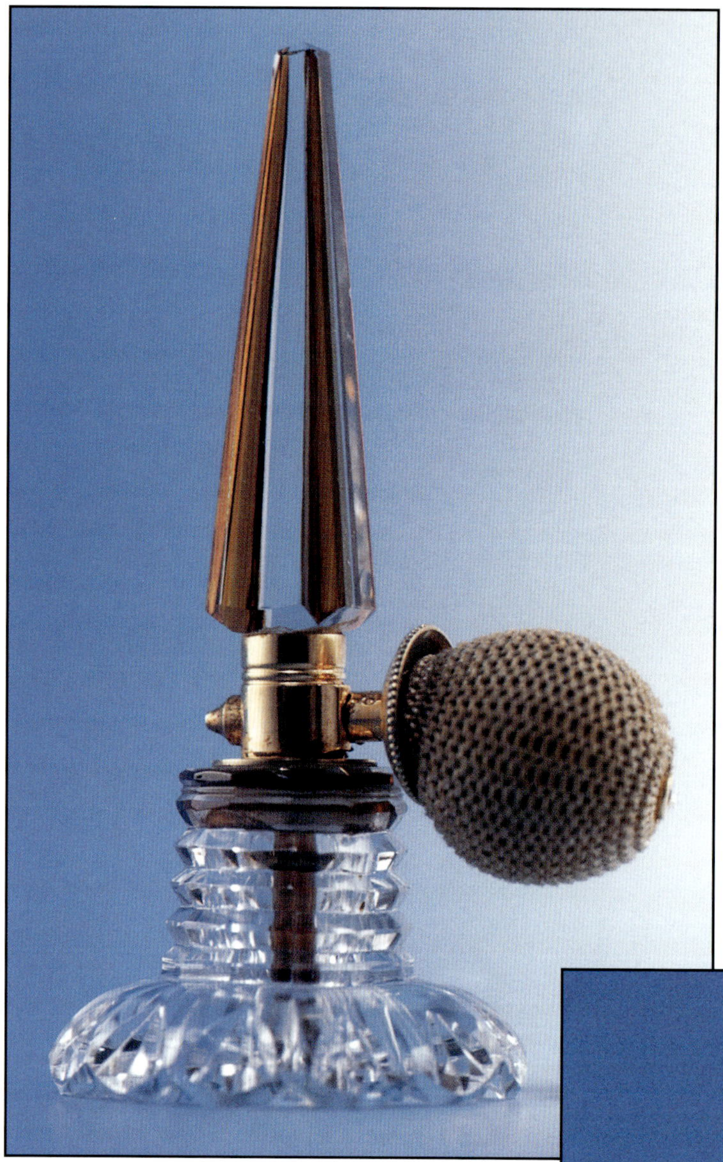

Cut glass atomizer, clear with yellow stained spire. 5.5". $200-300.

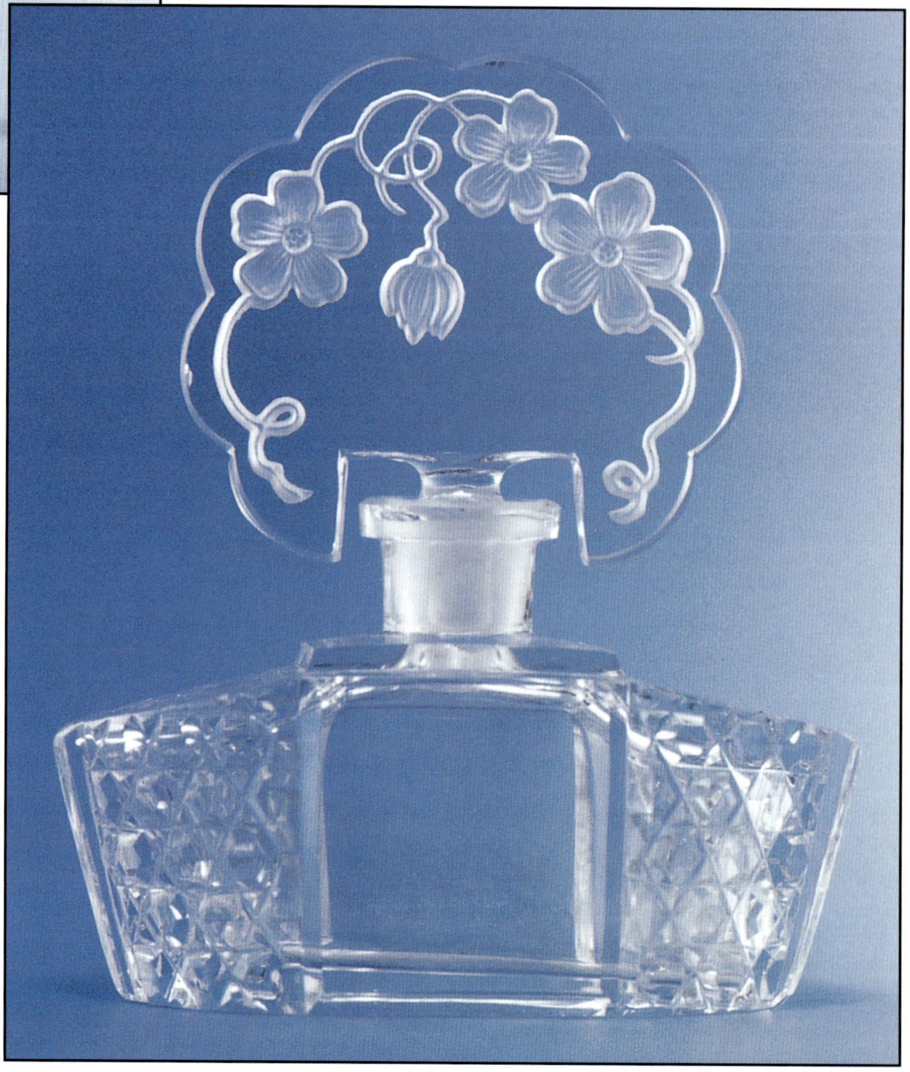

Clear, frosted intaglio roses in bottle and "cloud" top. 5.5". $250-300.

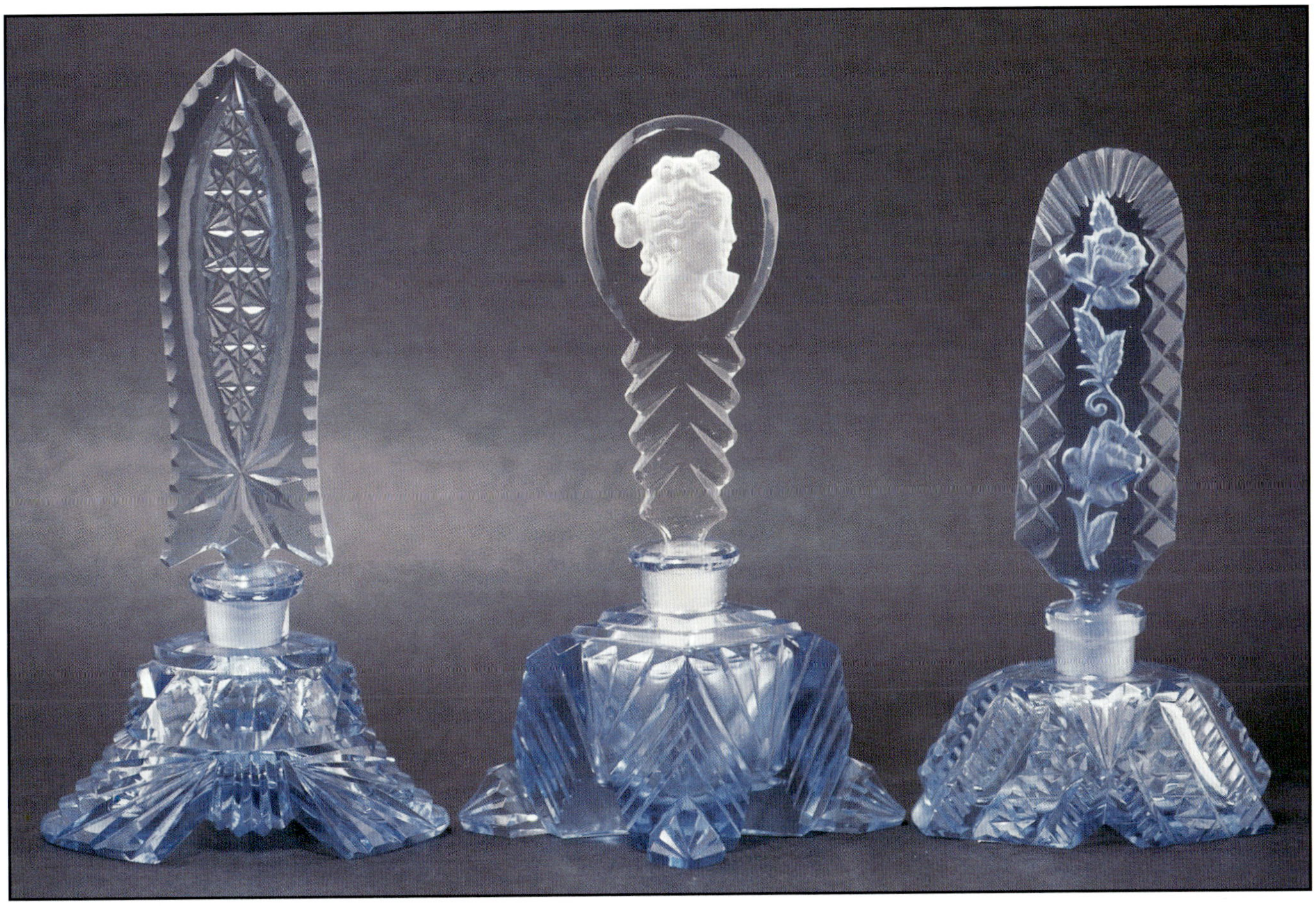

Three blue cut glass bottles. Left: Geometric cuts, 6.375". Center: Cameo girl in stopper. 6". Right: Floral stopper, lighter blue. 5.625". $300-450 each.

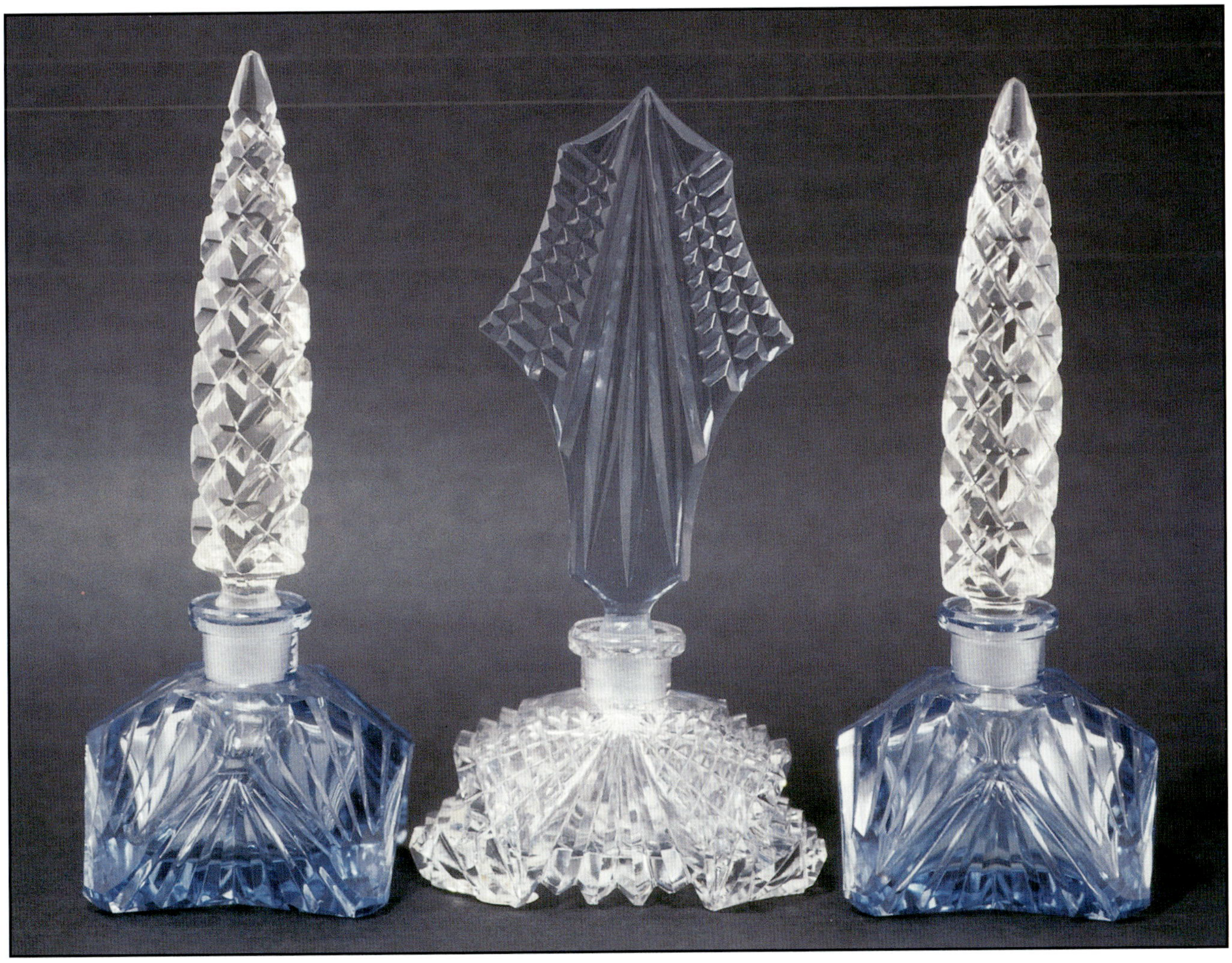

Blue and clear crystal. Left and right: matched Morlee pair. 6.25". Center: Irice, 6". $300-450 each.

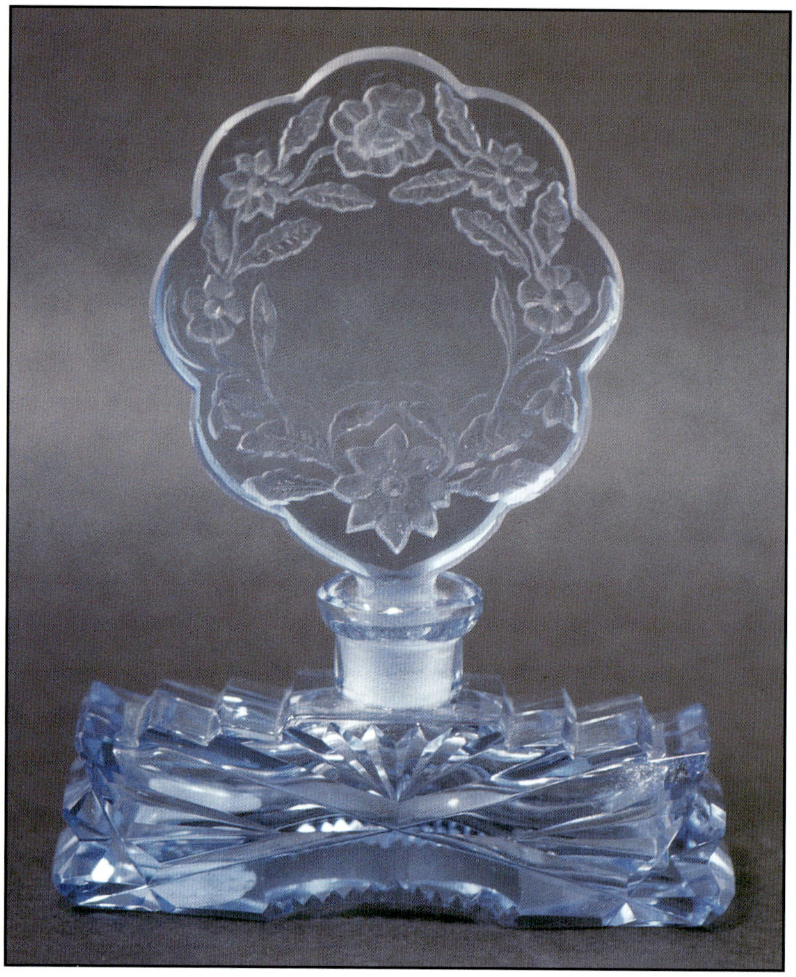

Blue, rectangular, cut base; blue floral wreath stopper. 5". $350-450.

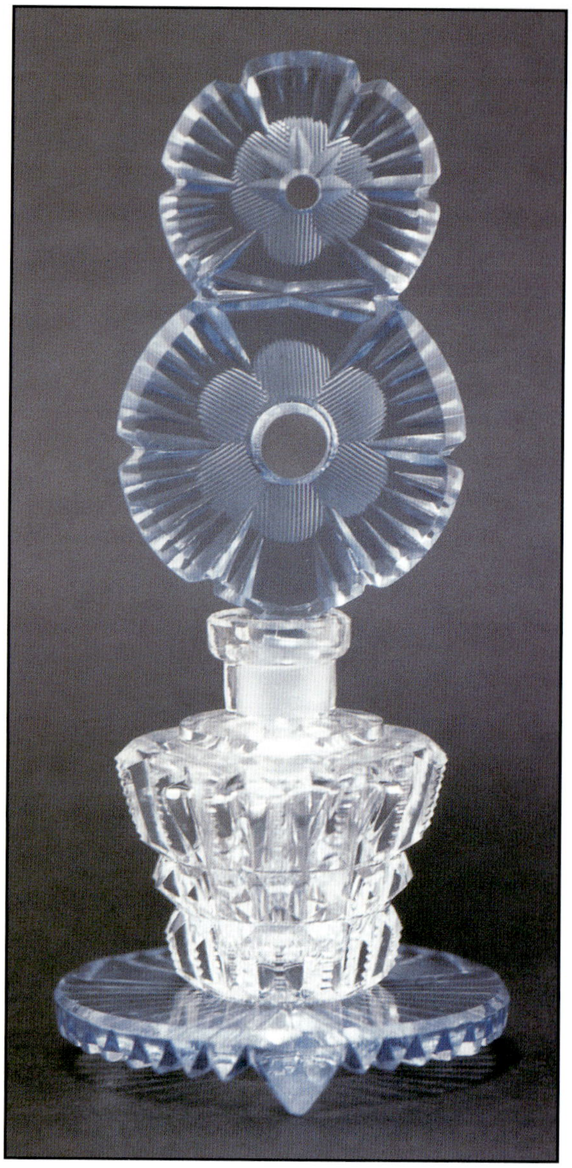

Blue, clear, three part bottle. 5.75". $300-450.

Same bottle, showing separate parts.

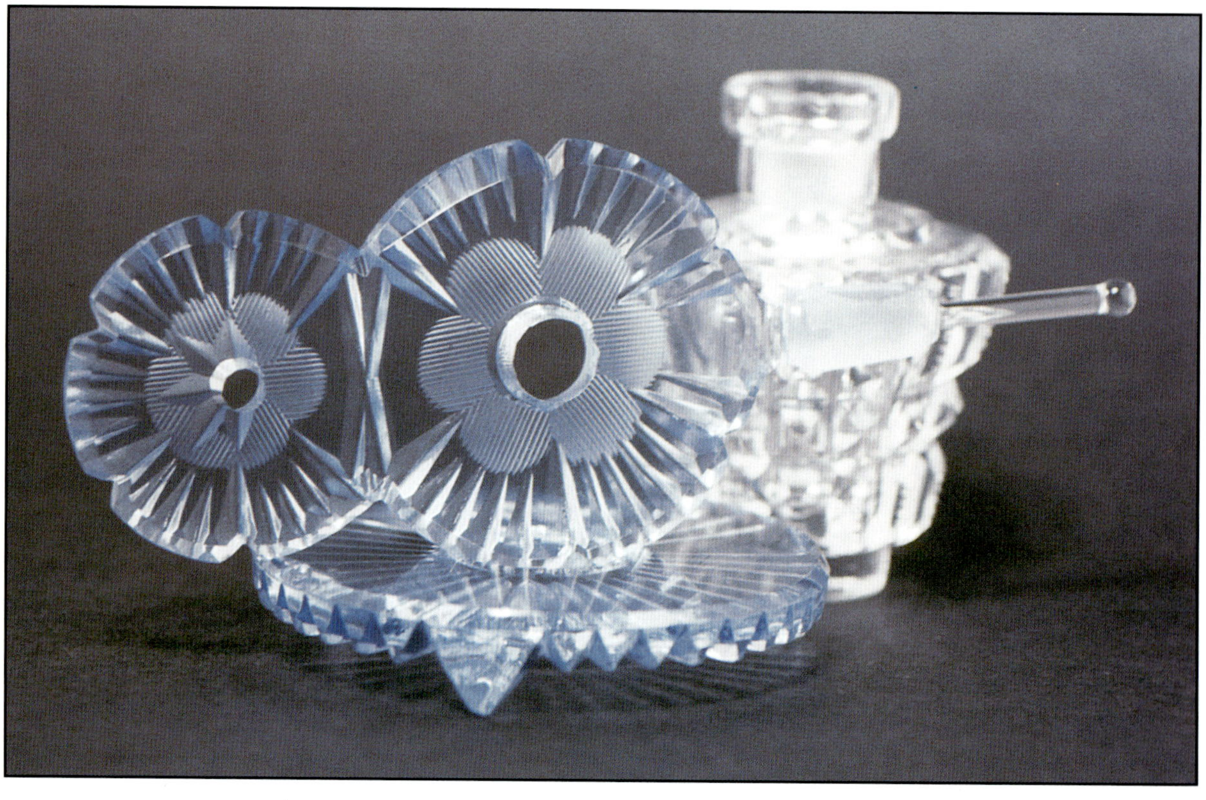

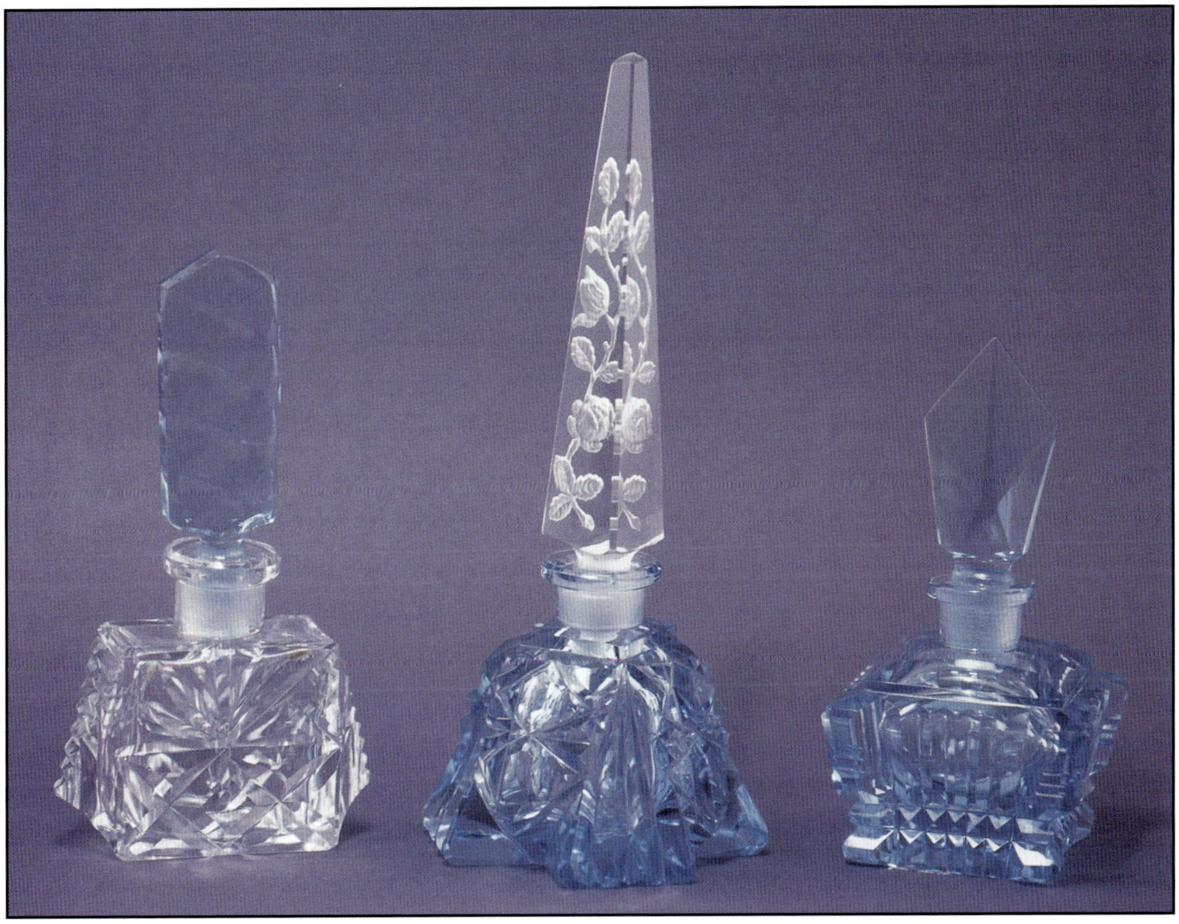

Three blue and crystal bottles. Left: Clear base, geometric cuts, blue stopper. 4.75". Center: Blue cut base, clear triangular spire with intaglio flowers cut into the back side. 6.25". Right: Blue faceted top on blue geometric base. 4.25". $200-300 each.

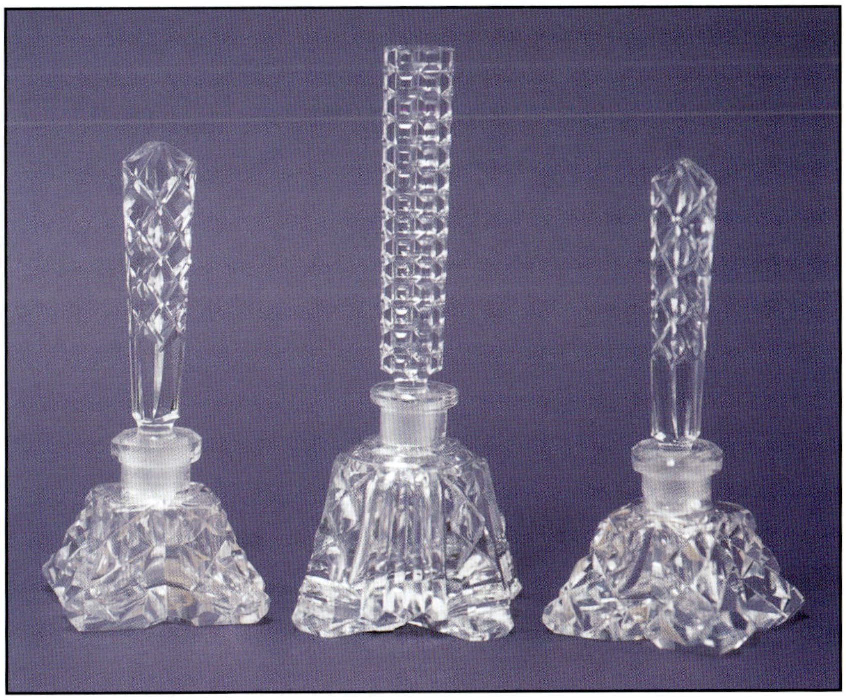

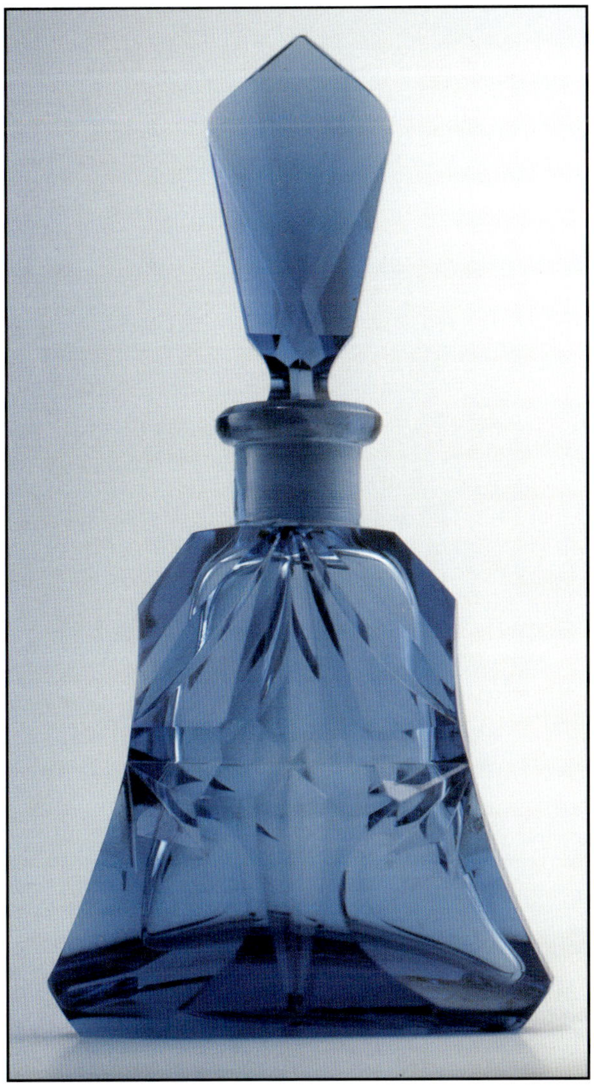

Left and right: Matched pair, Aristo, 4". $150-200 each. Center: Clear, geometric cut. 4.75". $200-250.

Cobalt blue bottle and top, geometric cuts, faceted top. 5.25". $650-750.

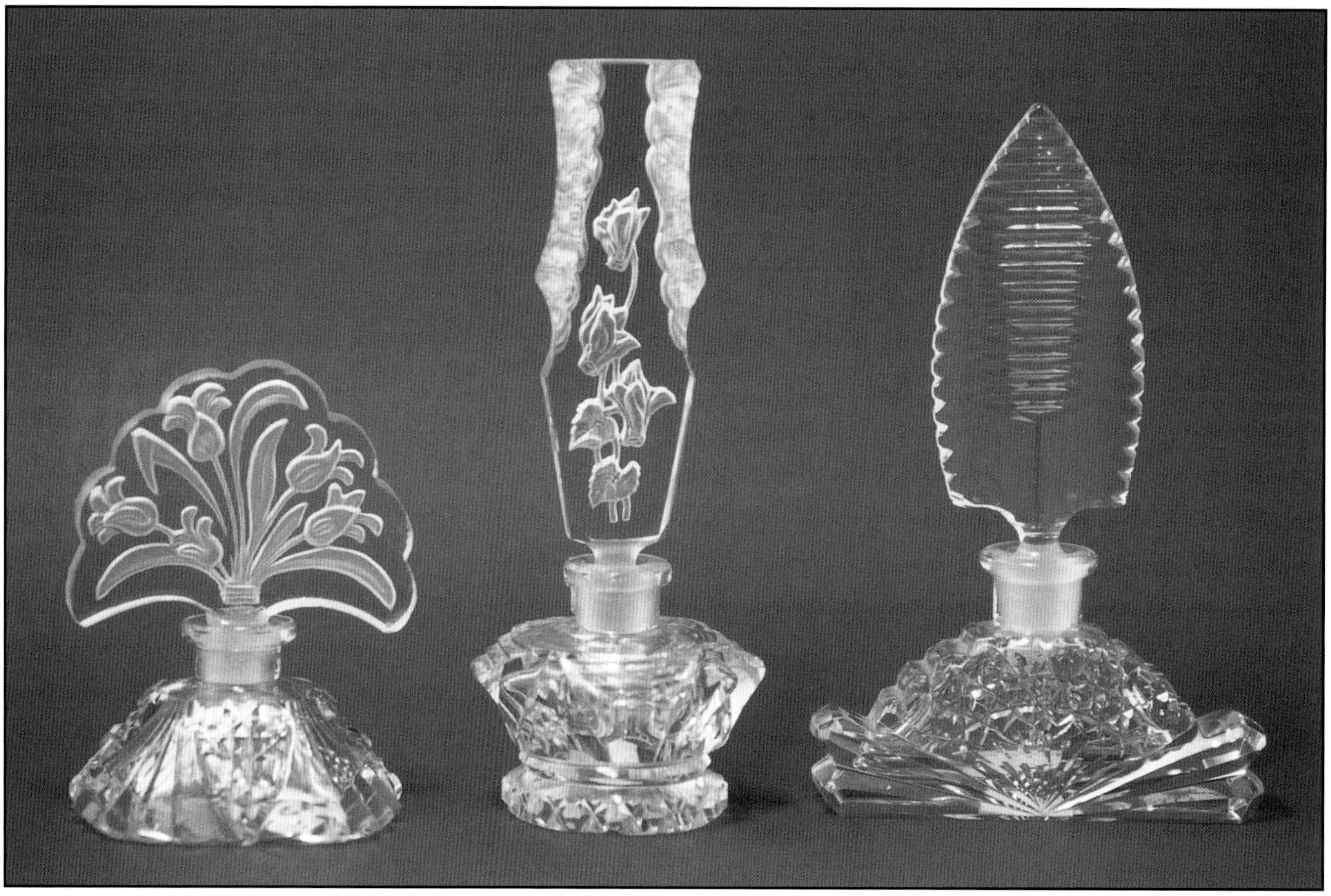

Left: Clear, cut base, intaglio floral spray top. 3.875". $300-400. Center: Clear, cut base, intaglio and frosted stopper. 6.25". $500-600. Right: Clear, cut base, tall, geometric cut stopper. 6". $250-350.

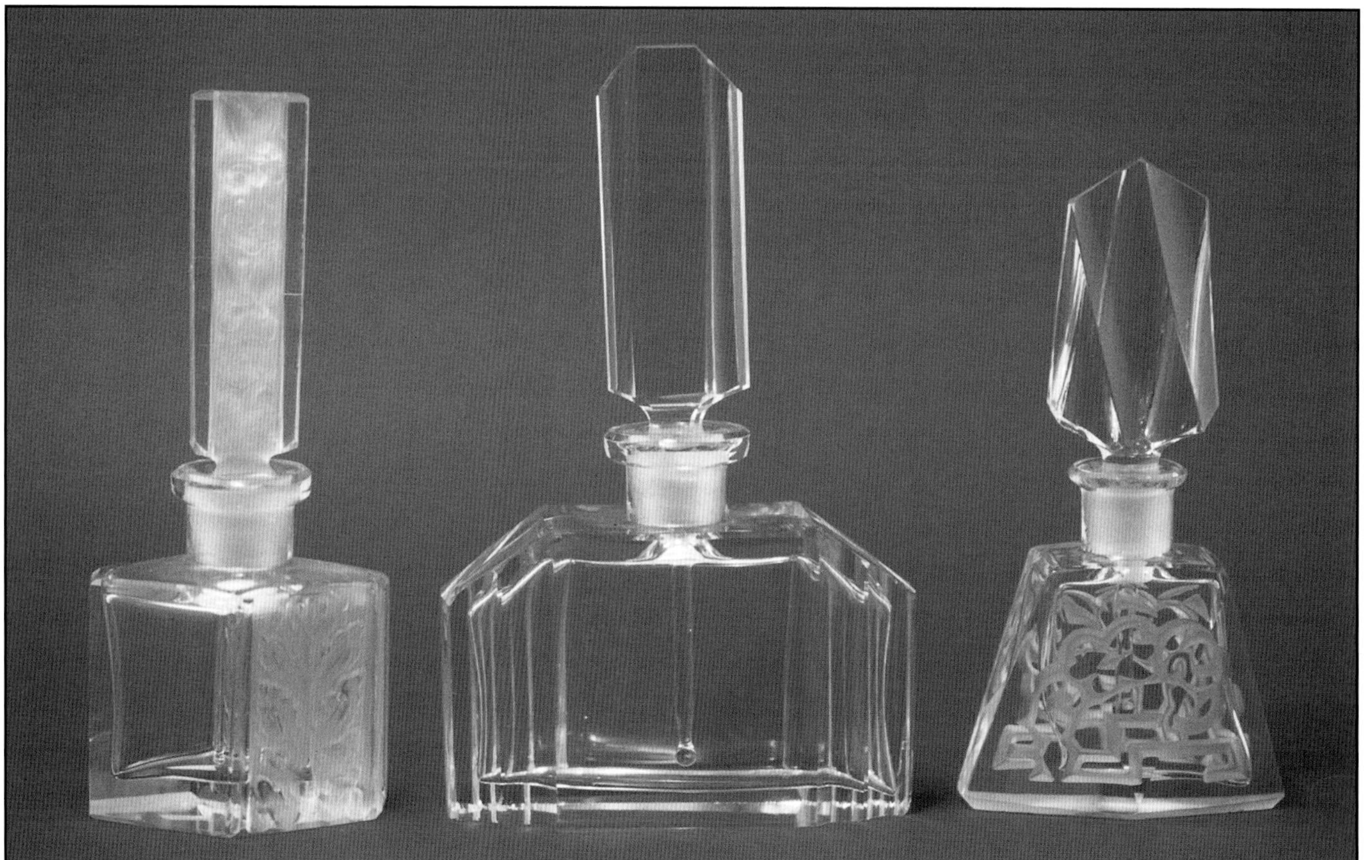

Left: Clear, cut and frosted bottle and top. 5". $250-350. Center: Clear, simple cuts. 5.5". $200-300. Right: Clear, intaglio base, geometric cut stopper. 4.5". $150-250.

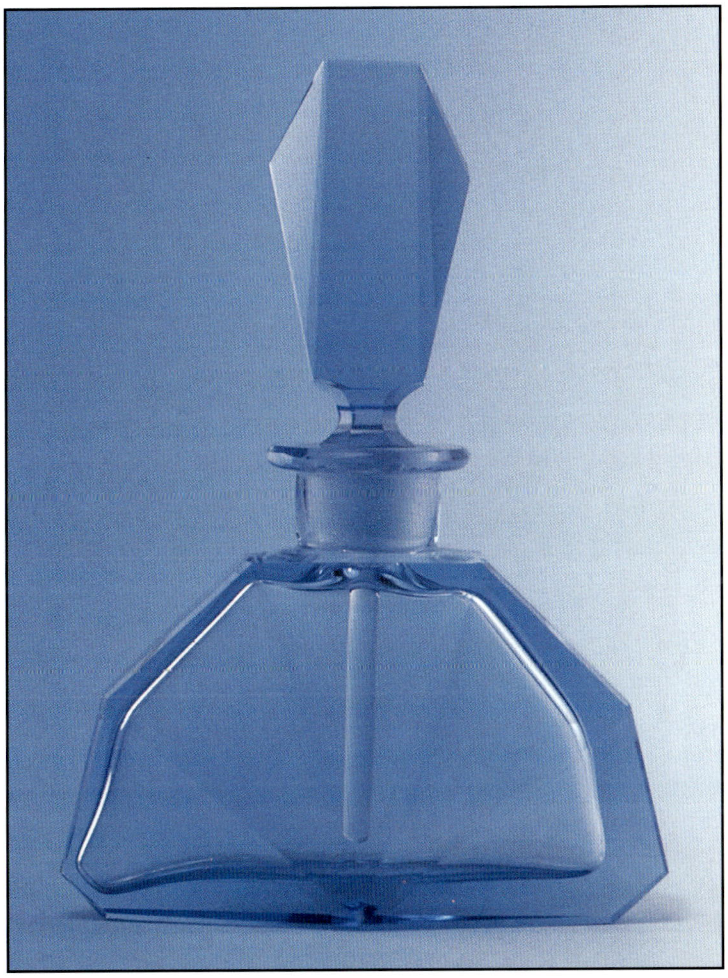

Simple cut, cobalt blue. 3.75". $400-500.

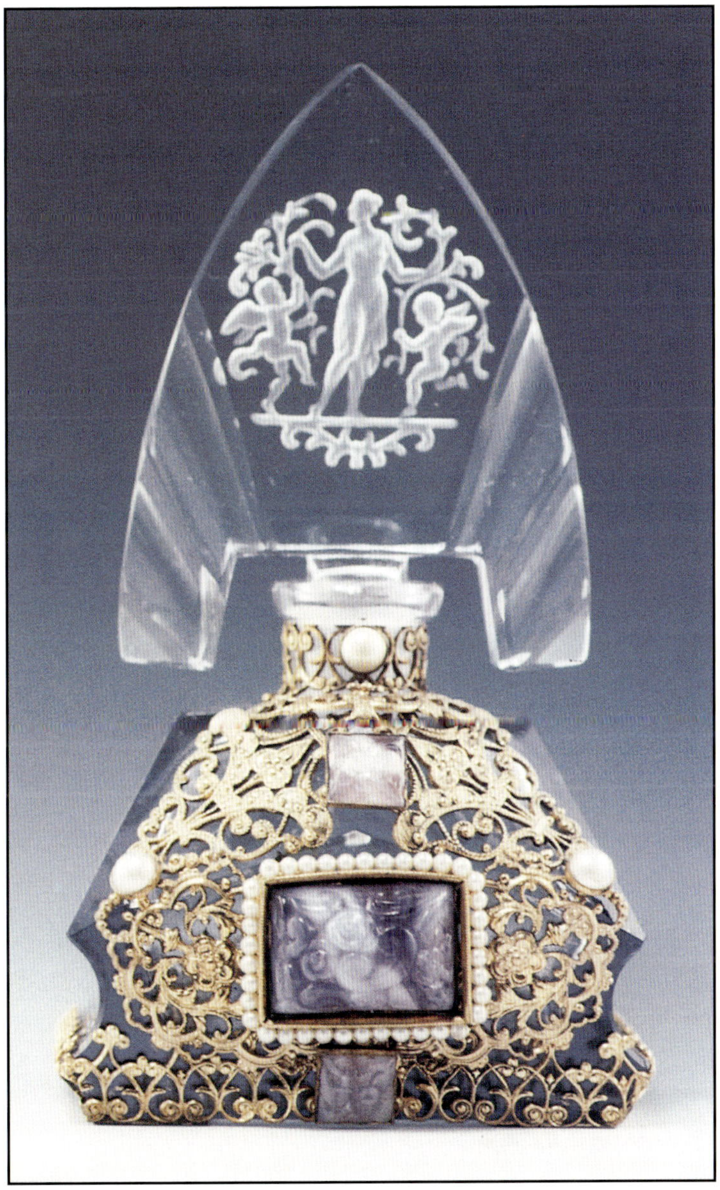

Amethyst cut, jeweled base; figural, tiara top. 6". $600-900.

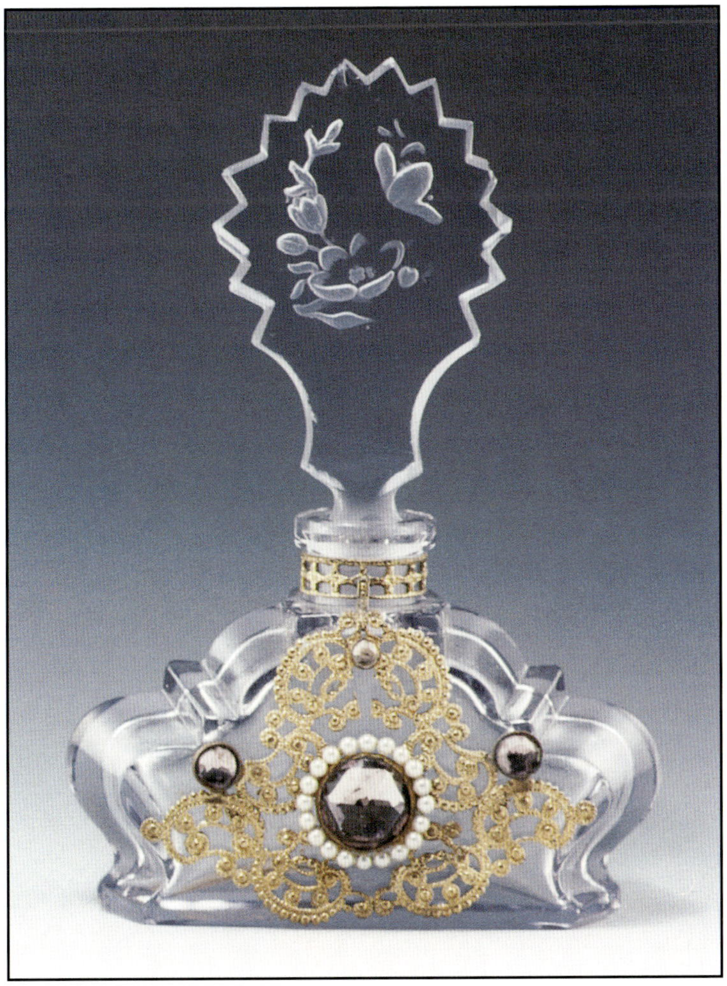

Amethyst cut, jeweled base; butterfly and flower intaglio top. 5.5". $550-650.

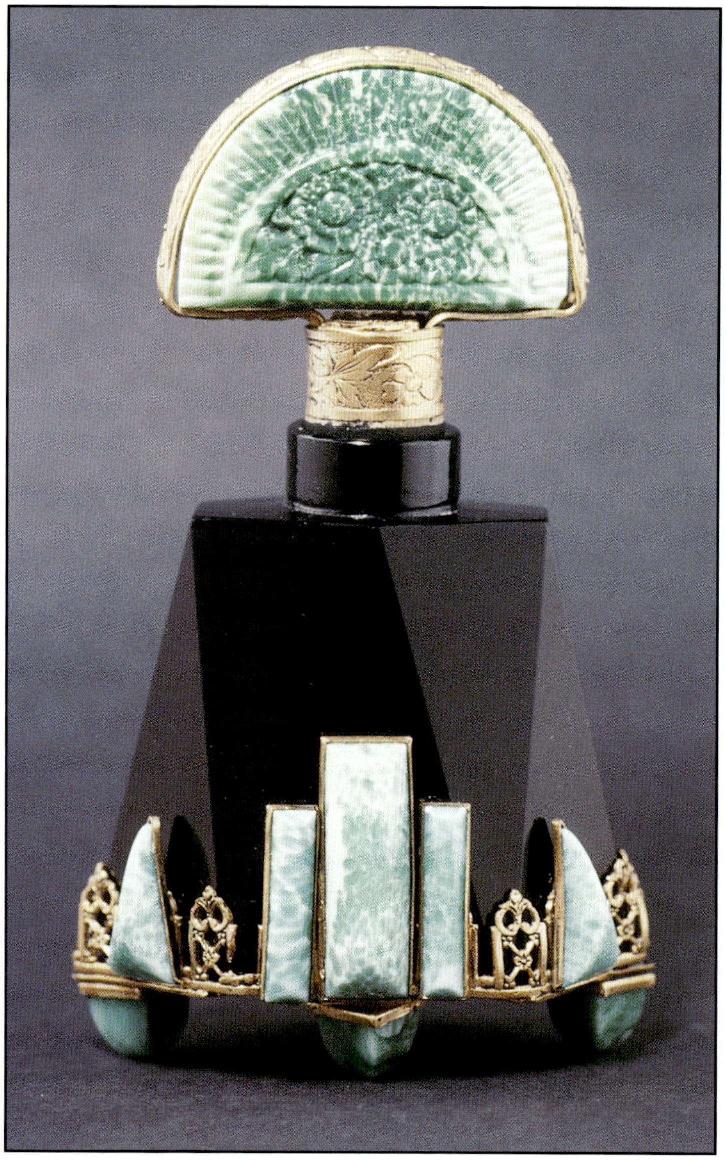

Opaque black cut base with filigree and opaque green gem ornamentation, gold and green stopper. This bottle was used commercially by Fournier. (Leach, 1997, p. 126) 4.75". $1200-1500.

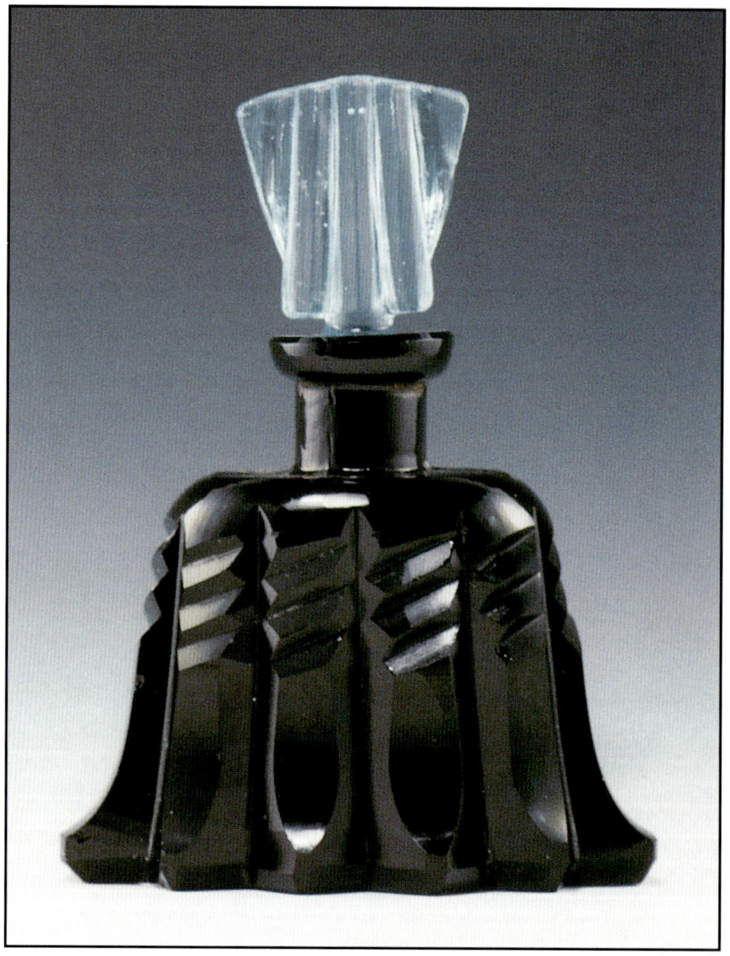

Opaque black, cut base, teal top, Irice. 3.75". $350-450.

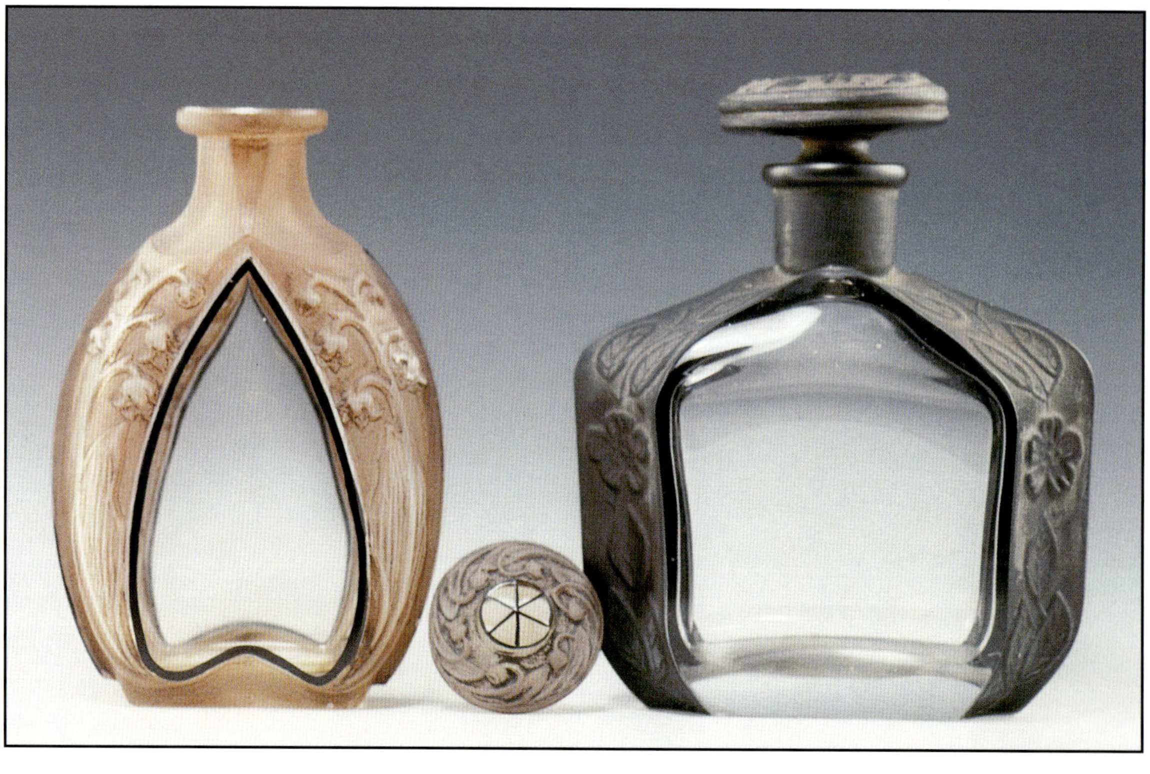

Two clear bottles with applied patina. Left: Brown patina with black accents, heart shaped window. Note stopper detail. 4.375". $700-900. Right: Black applied patina, clear window. 4". $700-900.

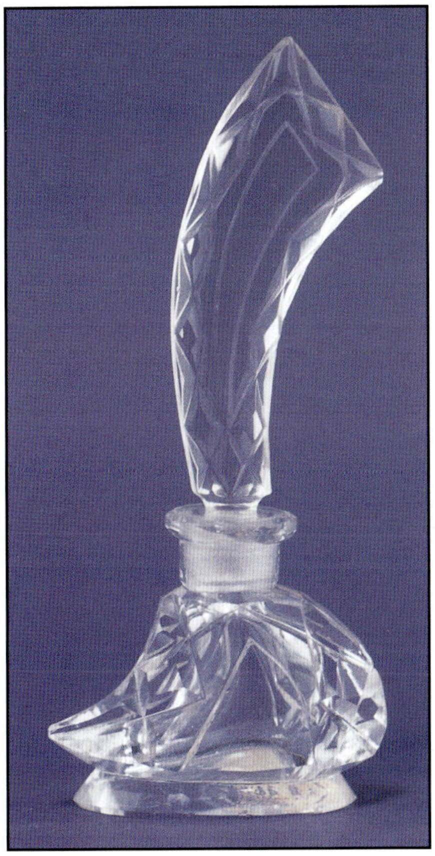

An odd duck. Clear cut, asymmetrical base and top. 5.75". $175-275.

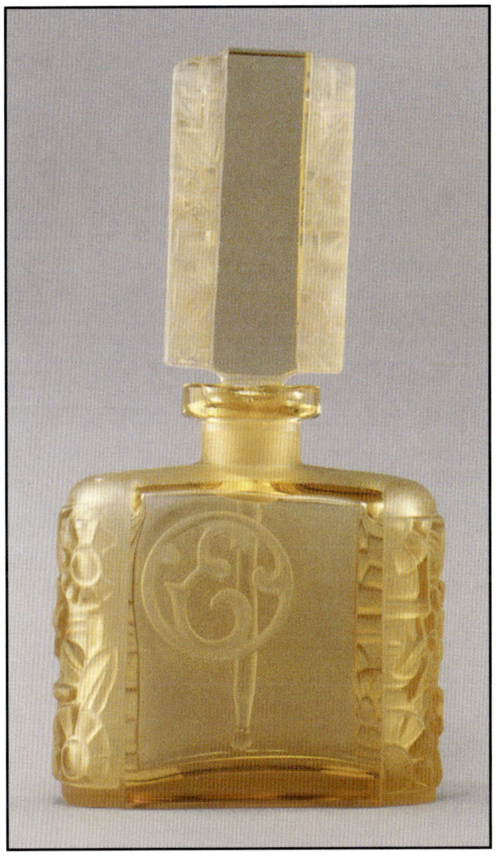

Yellow cut glass, frosted, intaglio, with the initial "E". 5.5". $350-450.

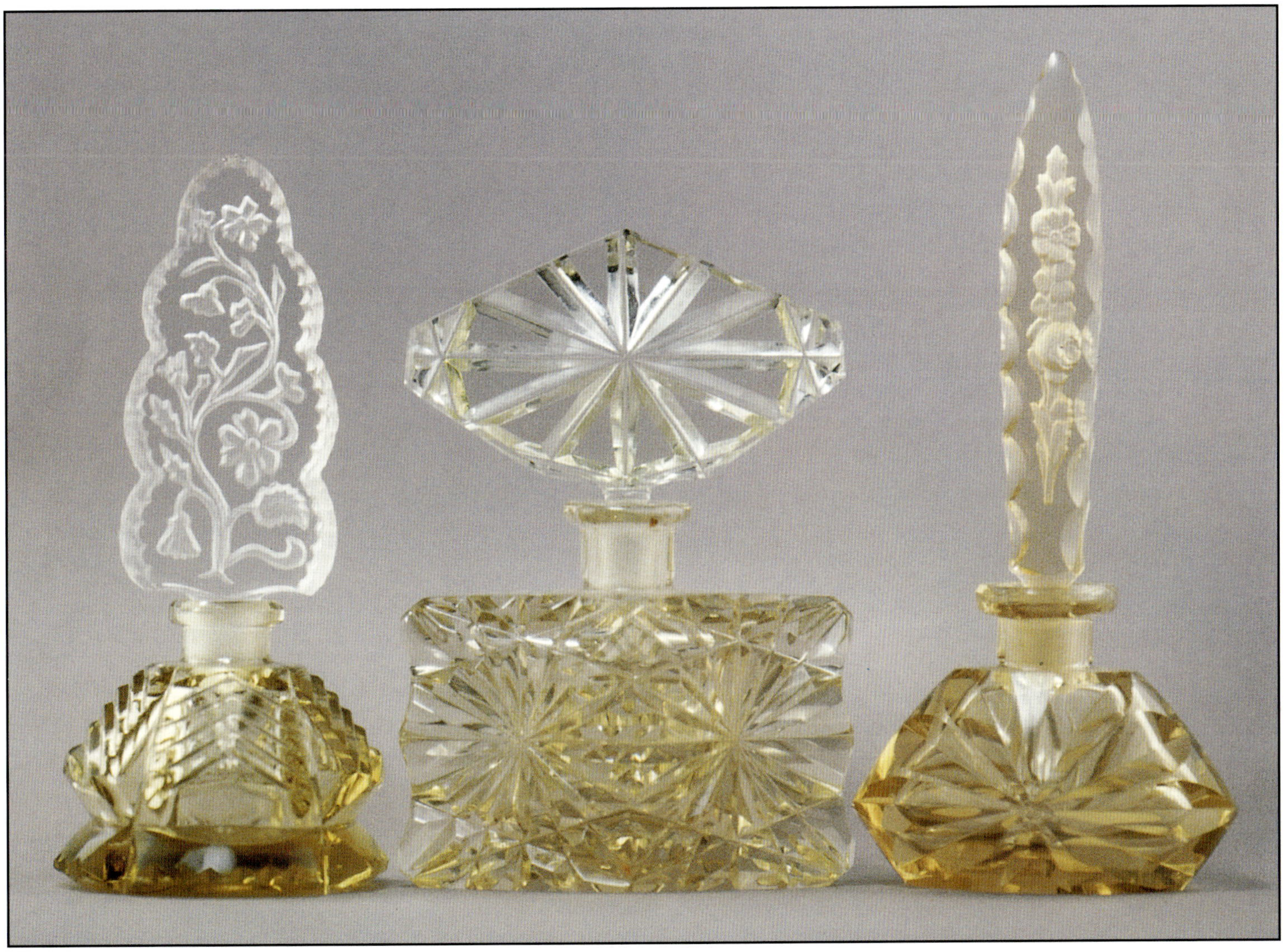

Left: Yellow cut glass base, clear floral intaglio top. 5.75". Center: Lemony (lighter) cut glass base and top. 5". Right: Yellow cut glass base and top, intaglio rose vine. 6.25". $350-450 each.

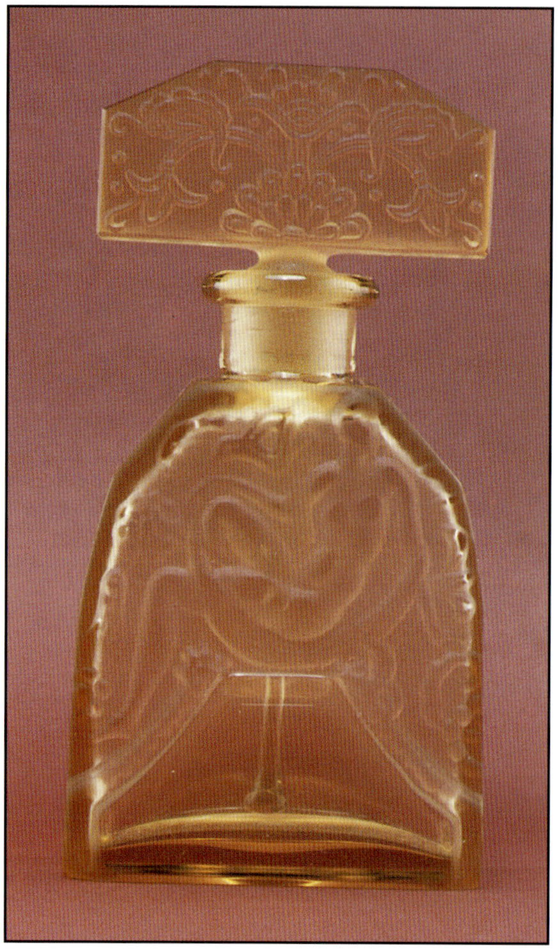

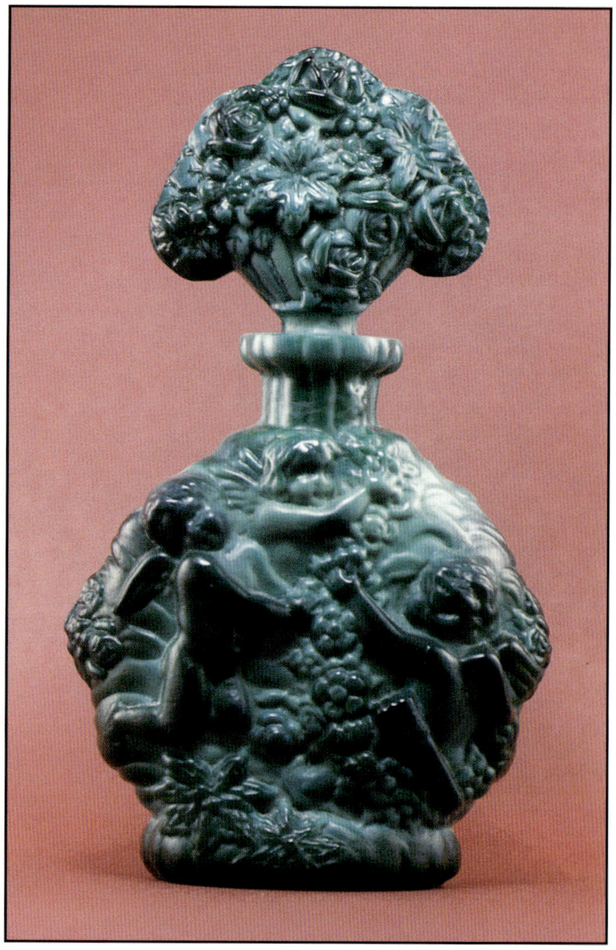

Right:
Bottles in this style were used commercially by Max Factor. Yellow cut glass, seated nude in base, floral intaglio top. 4.875". $1200-1500.

Far right:
Malachite glass base with cherubs, molded top. 6.75". $450-550.

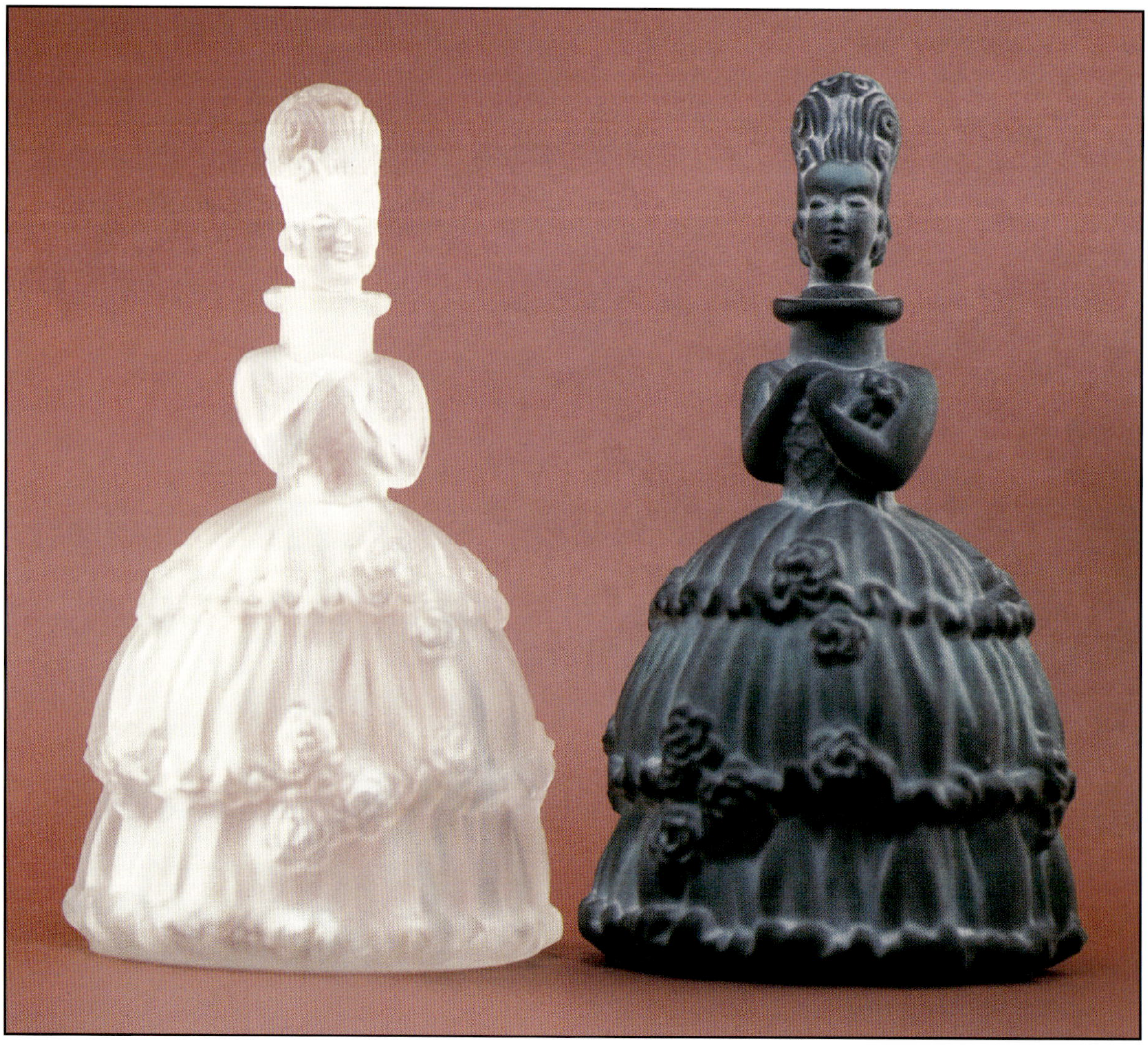

Mmes. Pompadour. Left: clear and frosted. 6". $150-250. Right: Malachite, frosted. 6.25". $250-350.

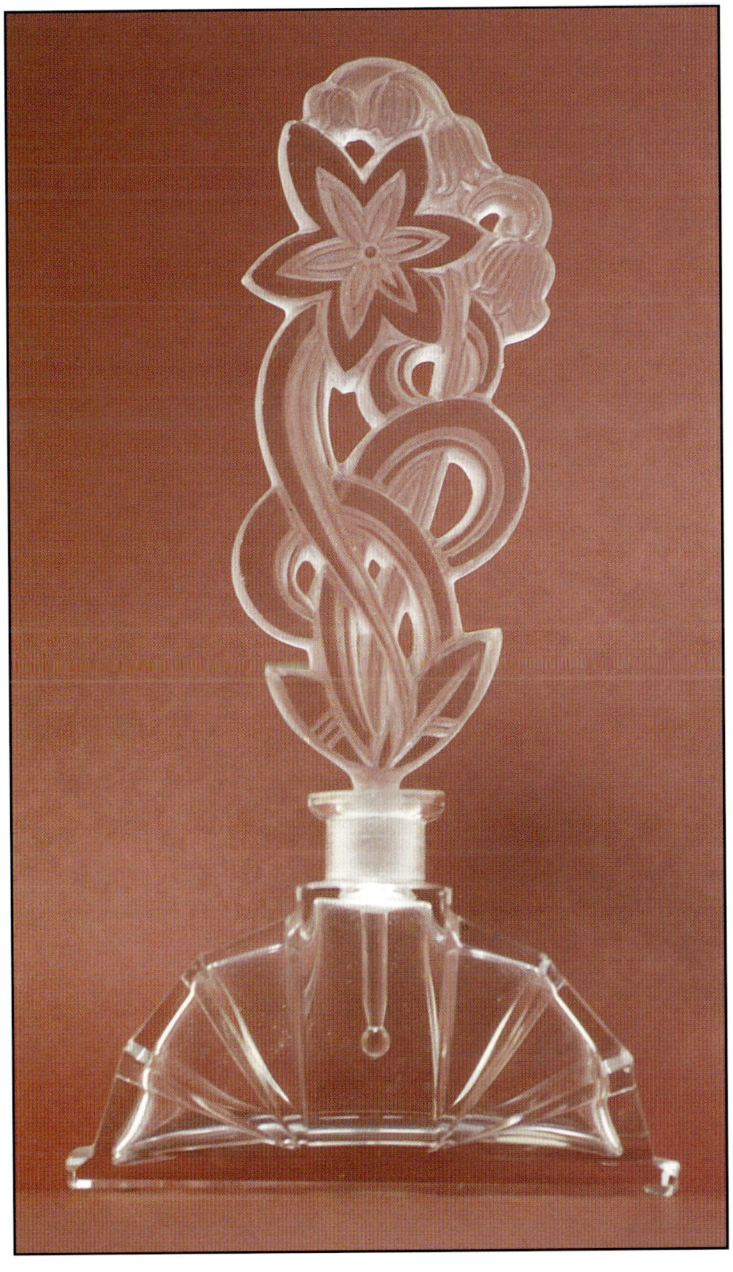

Rocket star. Fireworks stopper over simple cut glass base. 8". $500-600.

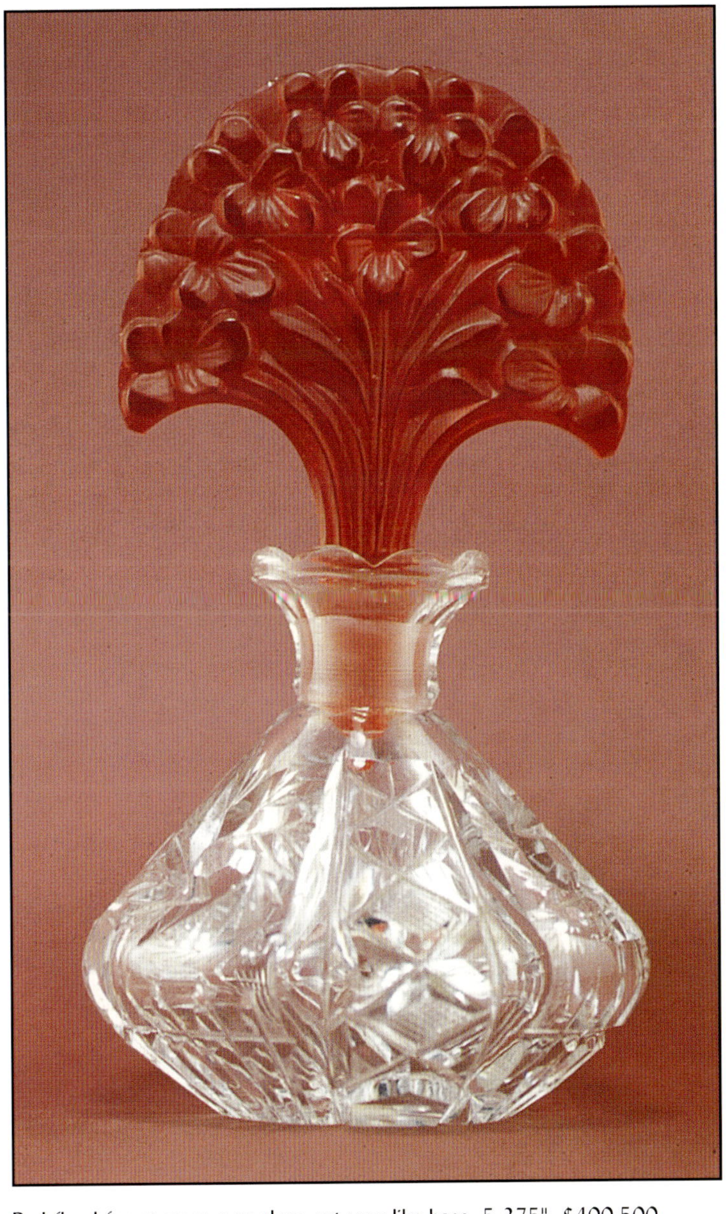

Red floral fan stopper over clear, cut vase-like base. 5.375". $400-500.

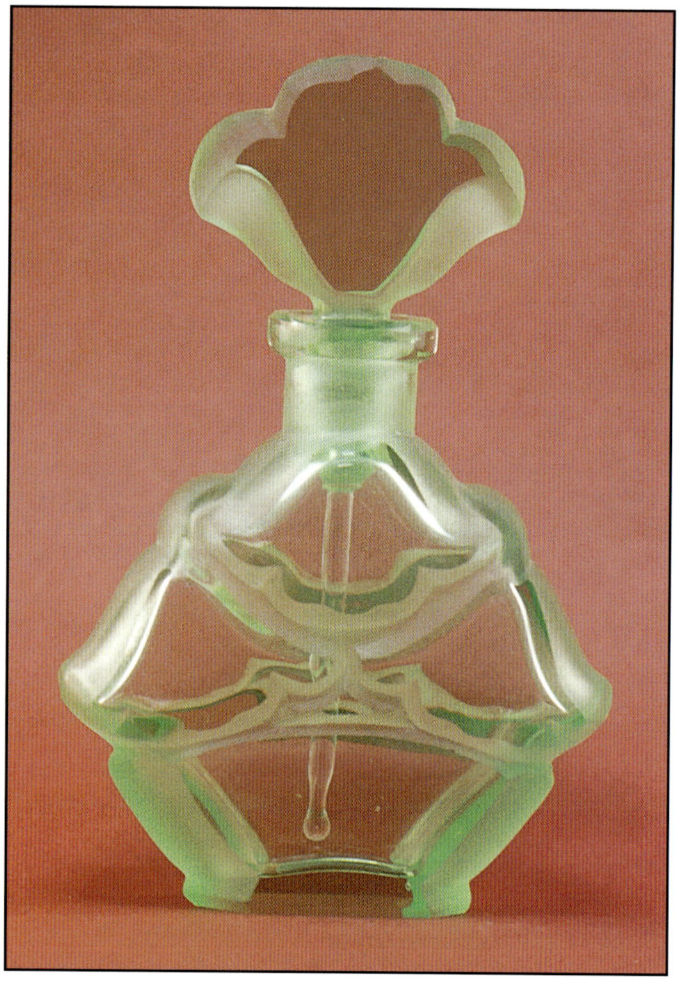

Green cut glass base and stopper with frosted detail. 4.75". $250-350.

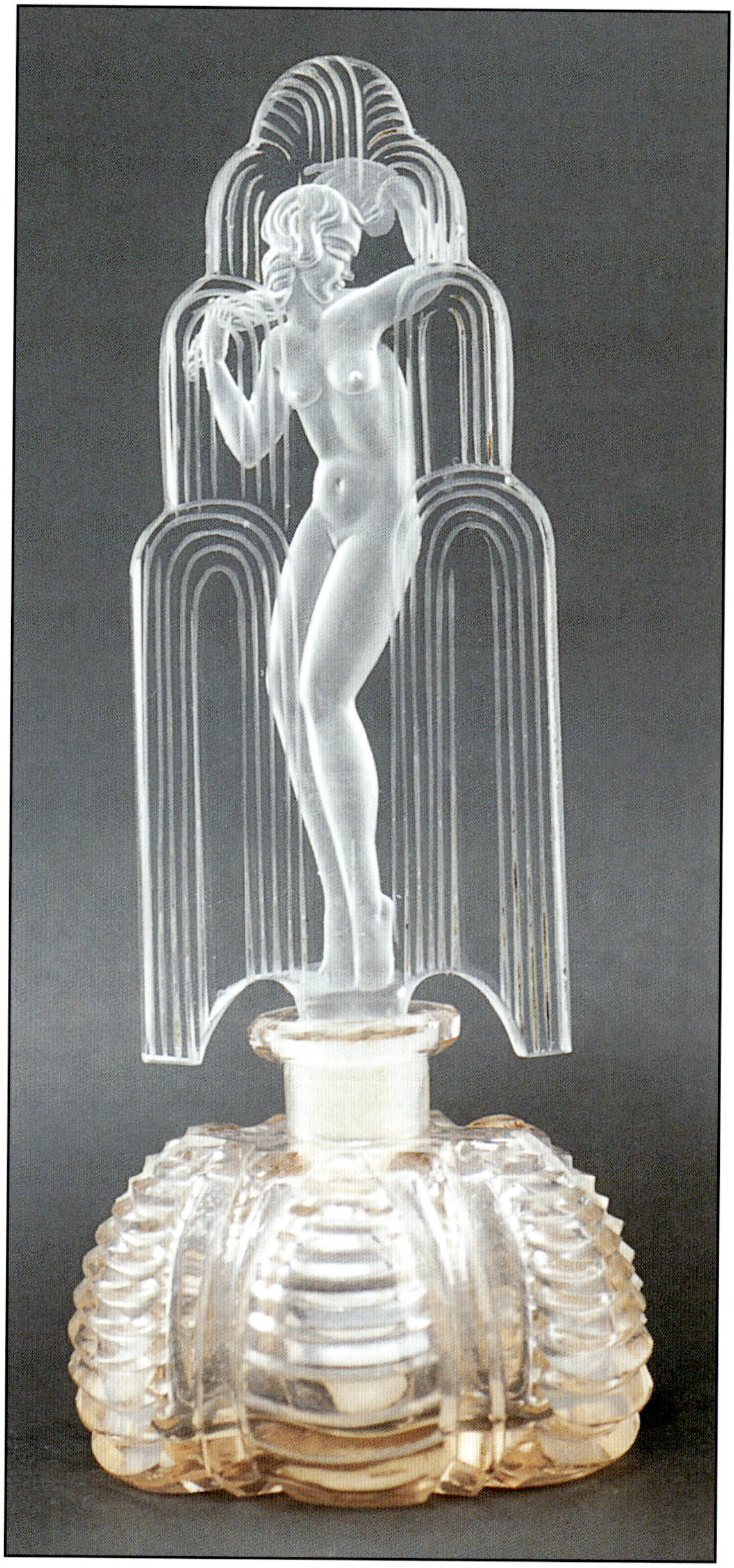

Waterfall nude stopper over pink cut glass base. 7". $2500-3000.

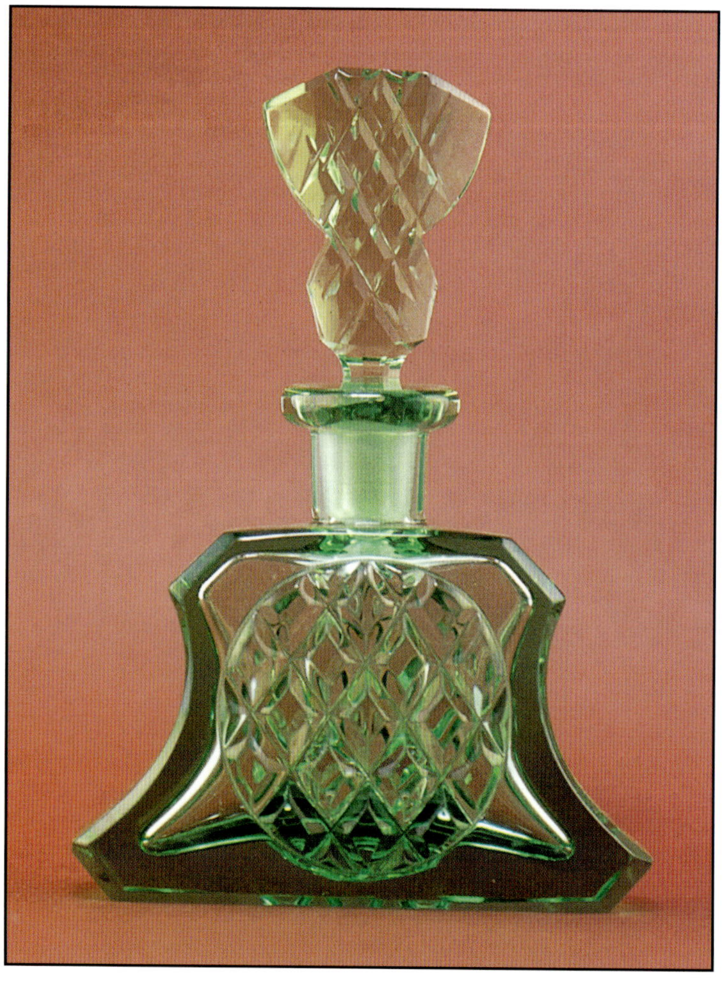

Green geometric cut glass and stopper. 5.125". $200-300.

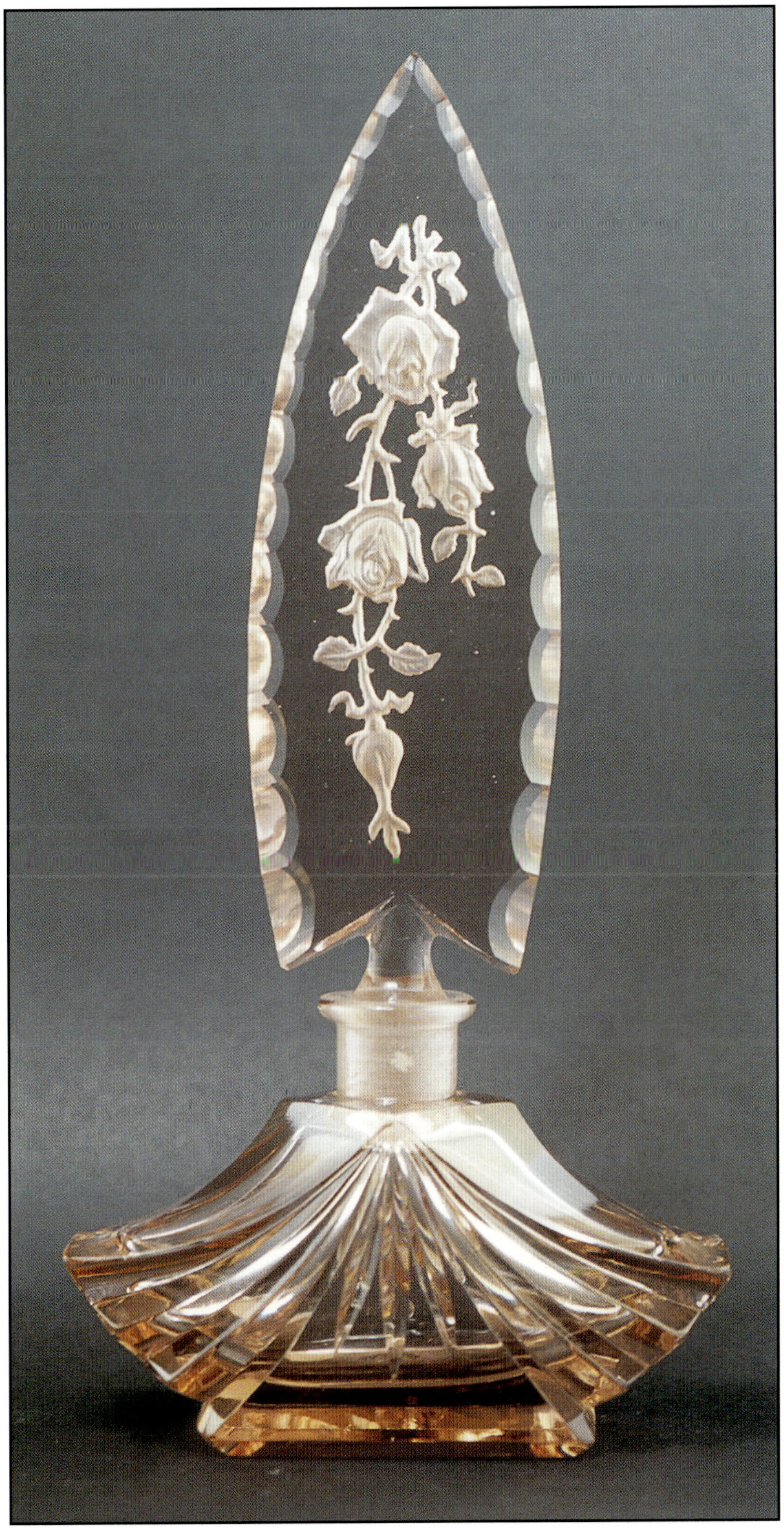

Pink cut glass base and stopper with downward vine of roses. Exceptionally large at 9.125". $700-900.

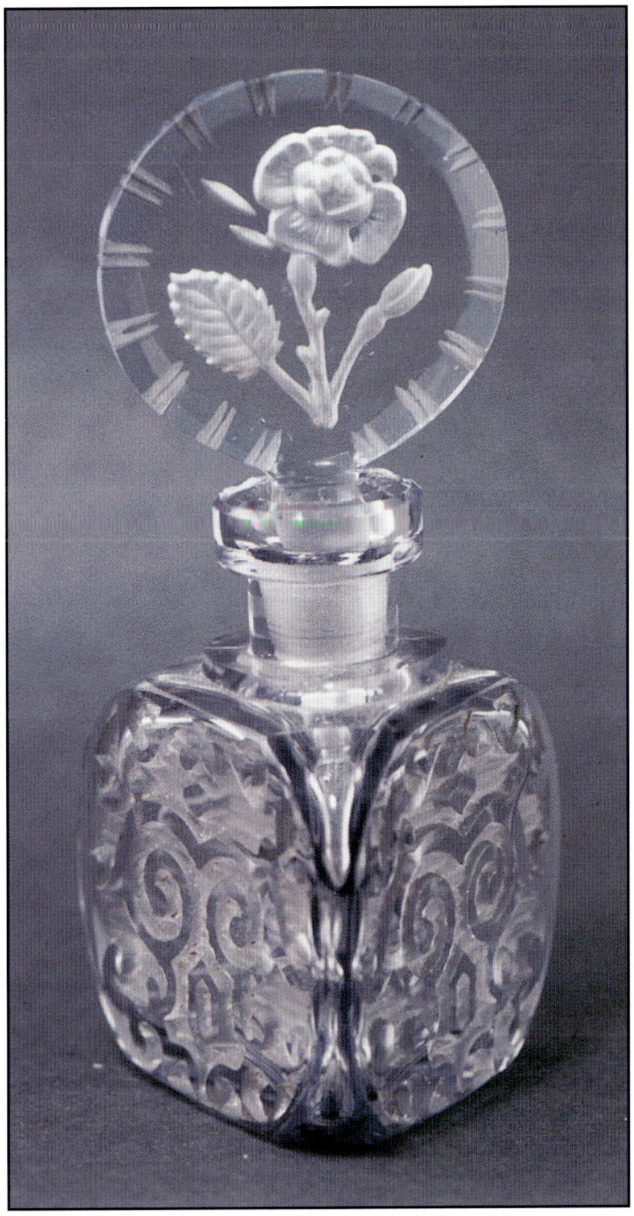

Amethyst, cut glass, three-sided bottle; amethyst, single rose intaglio top. Irice sticker. 5". $450-550.

Left: Amethyst cut glass (lighter, bluer color), elaborate cut and intaglio roses top. 6.5". $350-450. Center: Squared amethyst cut base, faceted amethyst top. 4.75". $200-300. Right: Amethyst cut glass base, top, clear, feather edged, daffodil bouquet. 6.5". $300-400.

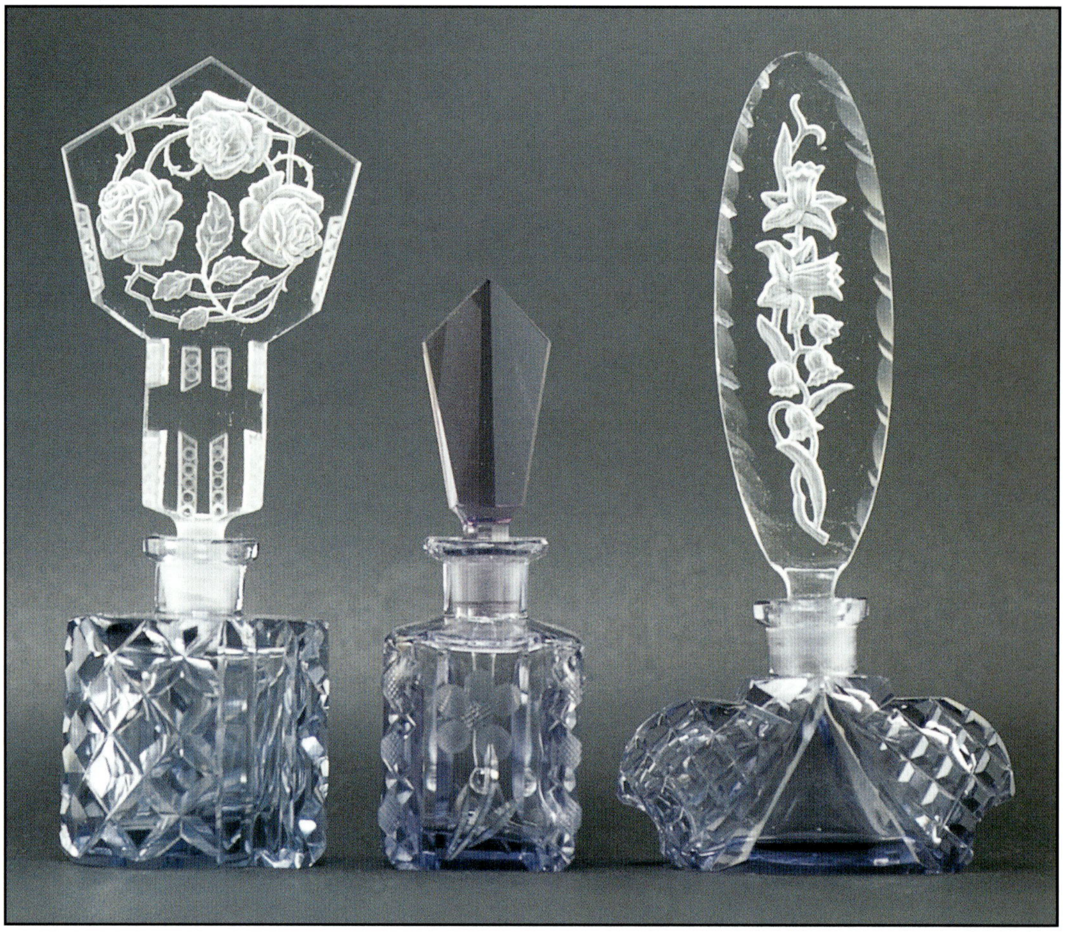

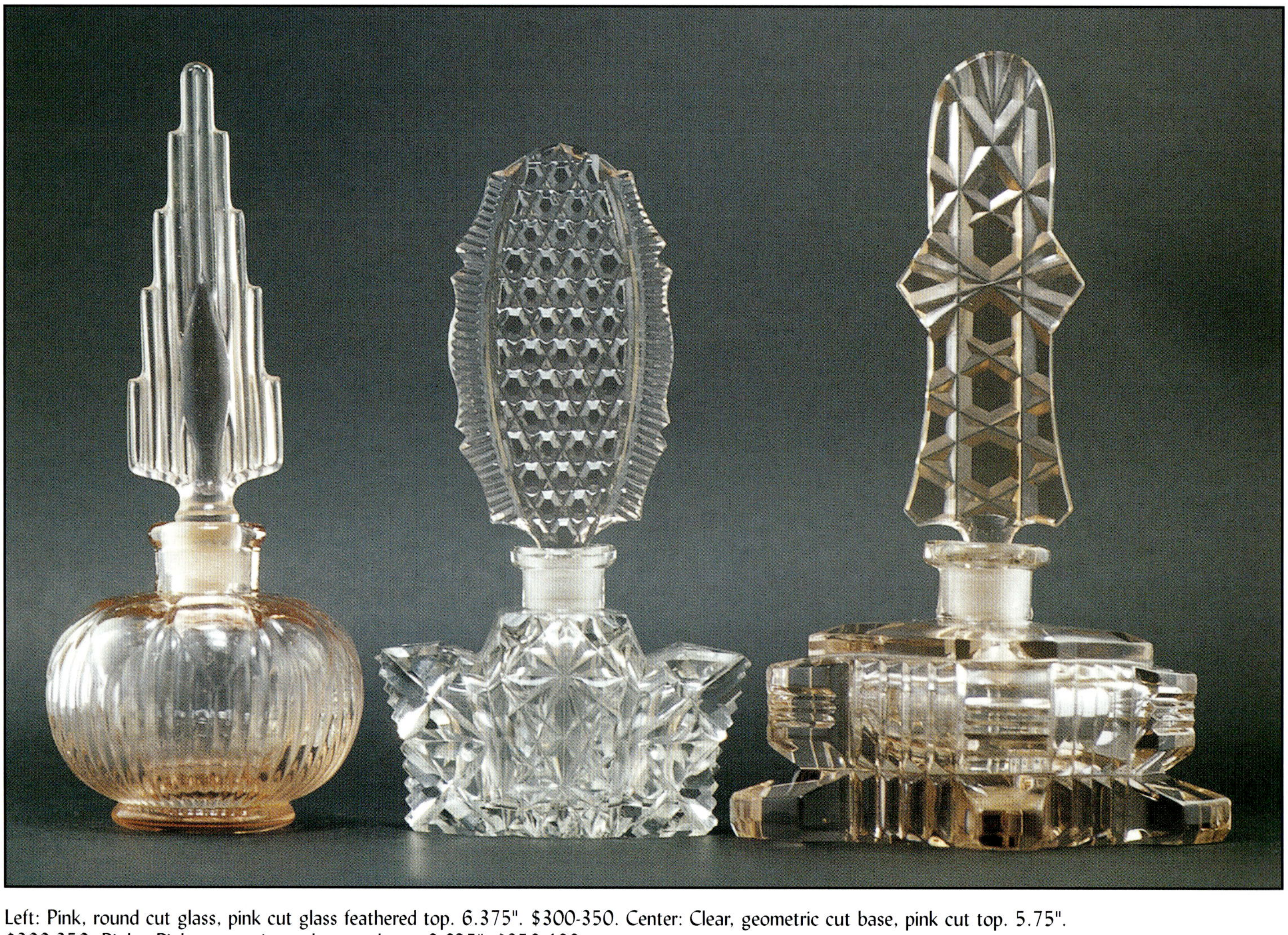

Left: Pink, round cut glass, pink cut glass feathered top. 6.375". $300-350. Center: Clear, geometric cut base, pink cut top. 5.75". $300-350. Right: Pink geometric cut base and top. 6.625". $350-400.

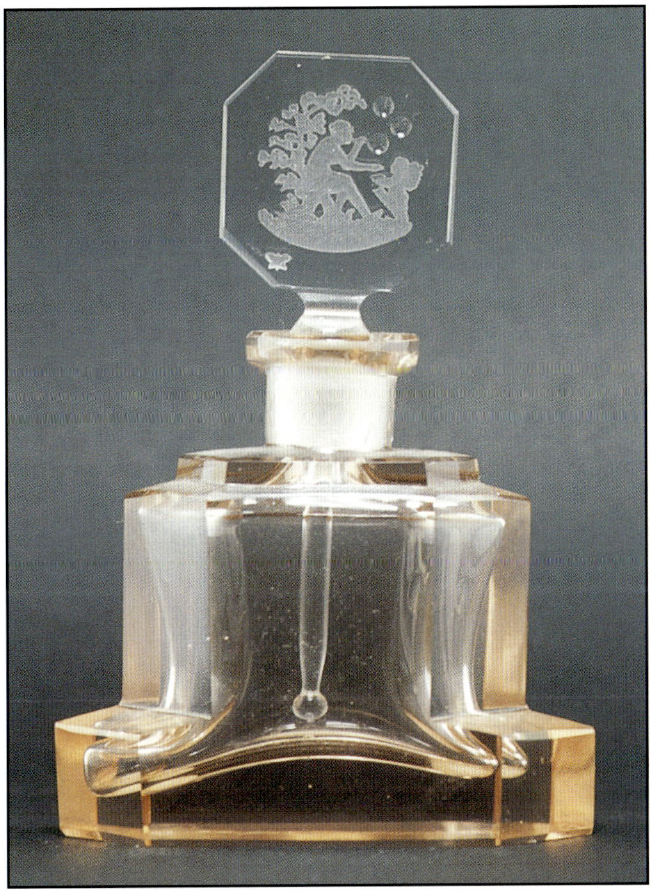

Hoffman bubble blower. Pink, cut base. 4.375". $750-900.

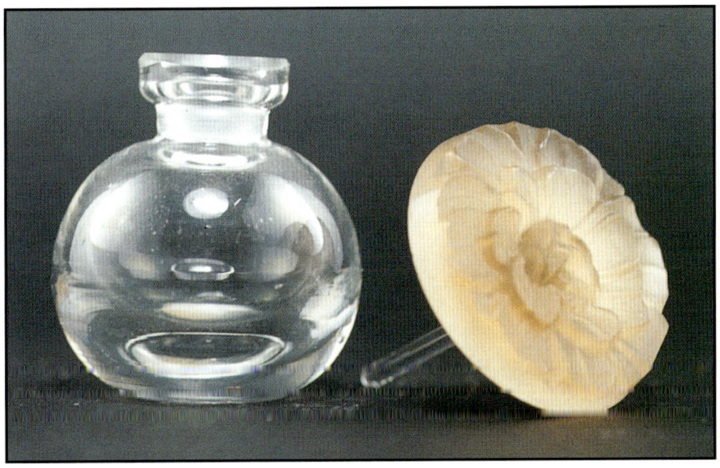

Clear crystal, round base. Flat, pink Narcissus top. 2". $150-200.

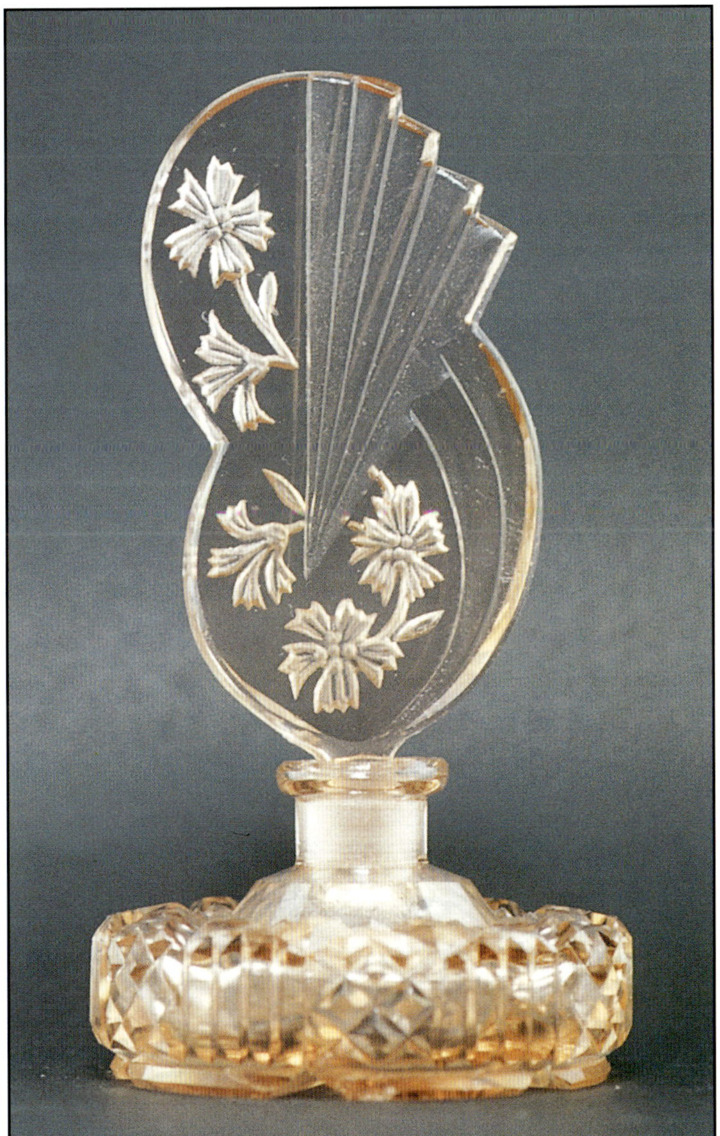

Pink cut glass base and top with floral intaglio, cuts. 5.25". $250-300.

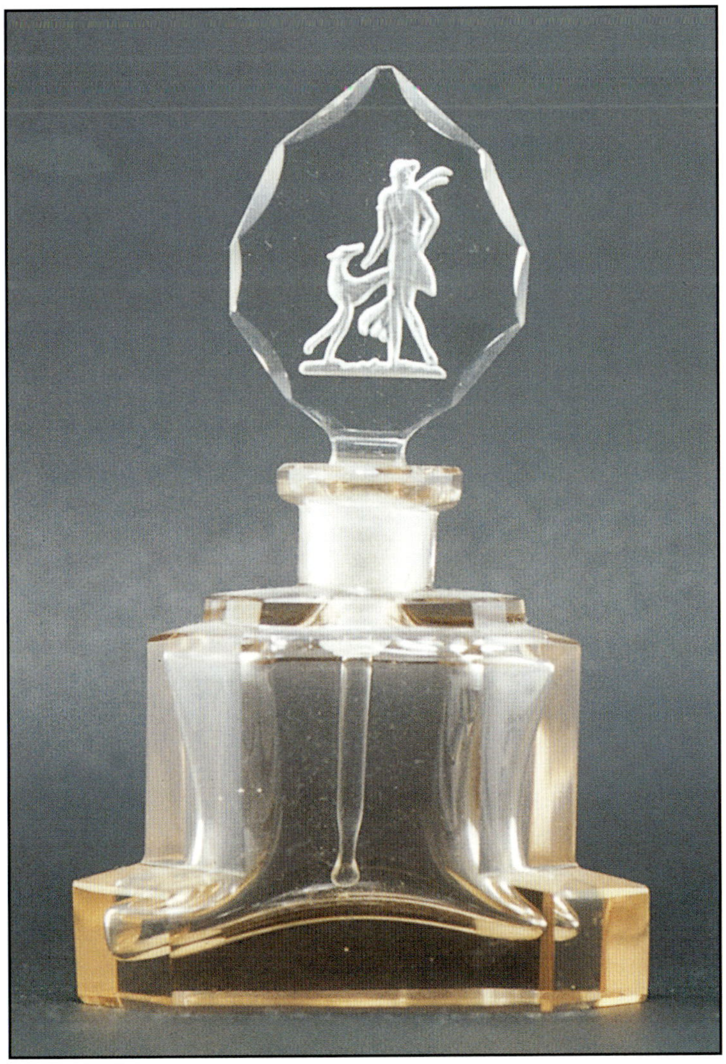

Clear, cut, pink base; top, clear, woman and a greyhound. 4.875". $550-650.

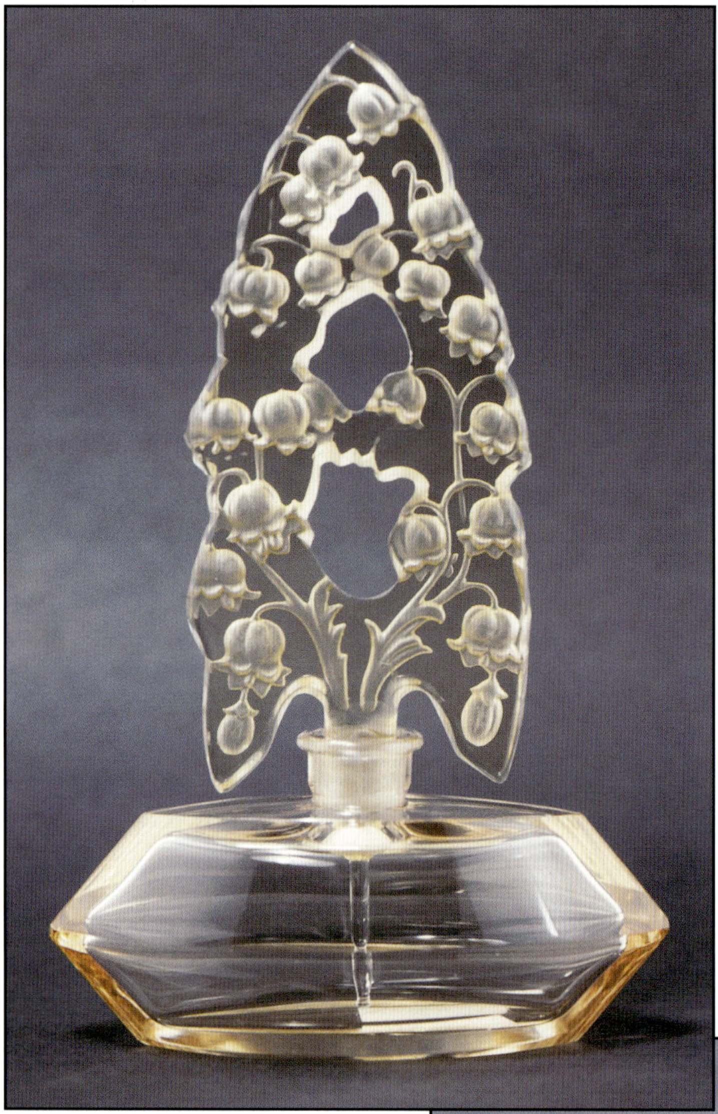

Amber cut glass base with triple pierced amber lily-of-the-valley top. 7". $600-800.

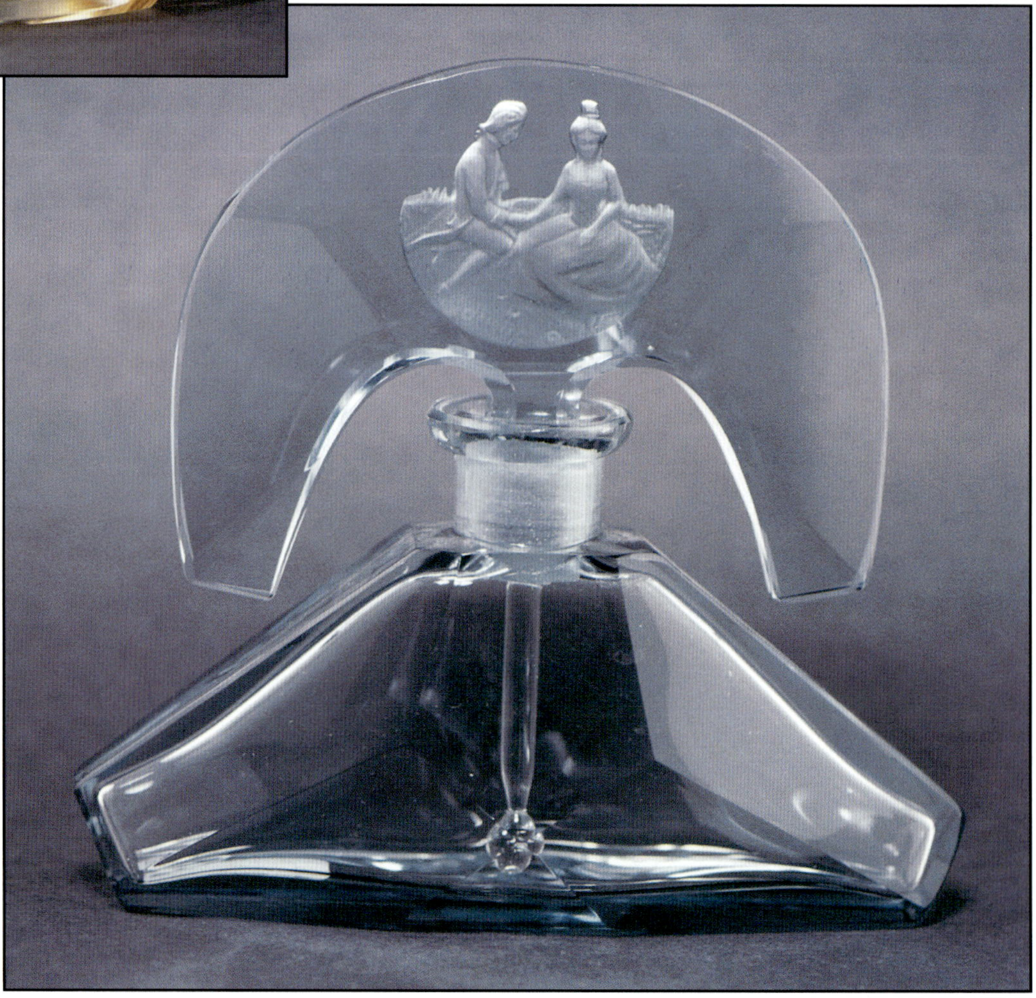

Smoke colored bottle and tiara stopper featuring a courting couple. 4.625". $1000- 1200.

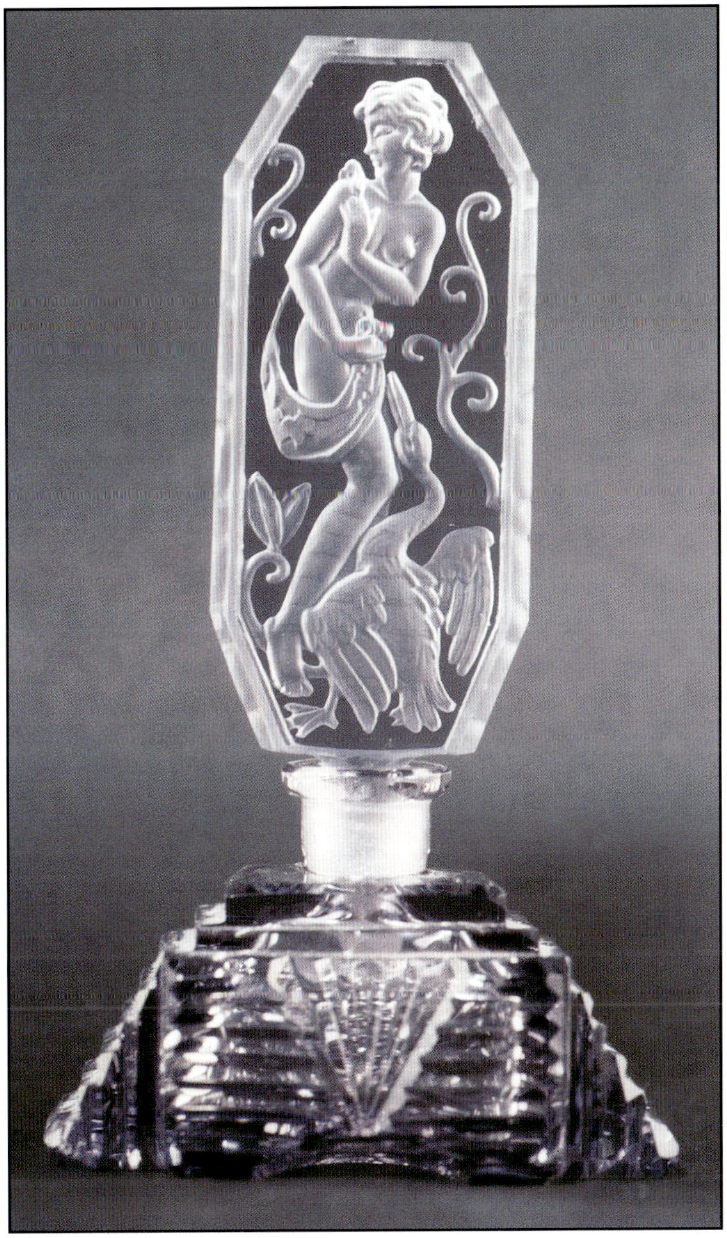

Leda and the Swan. Amethyst cut glass base and amethyst intaglio top. 5.75". $200-300 (repaired plug). If mint, $450-700.

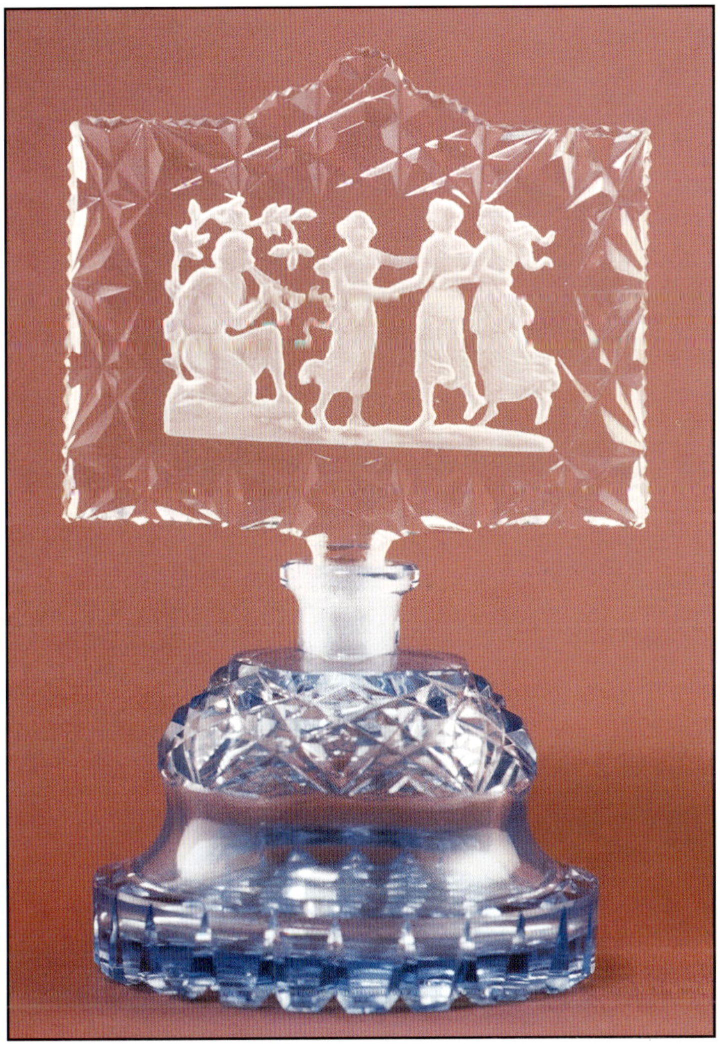

Classical scene of a musician and dancers above a bell-shaped, blue, cut glass base. 6.25". $500-700.

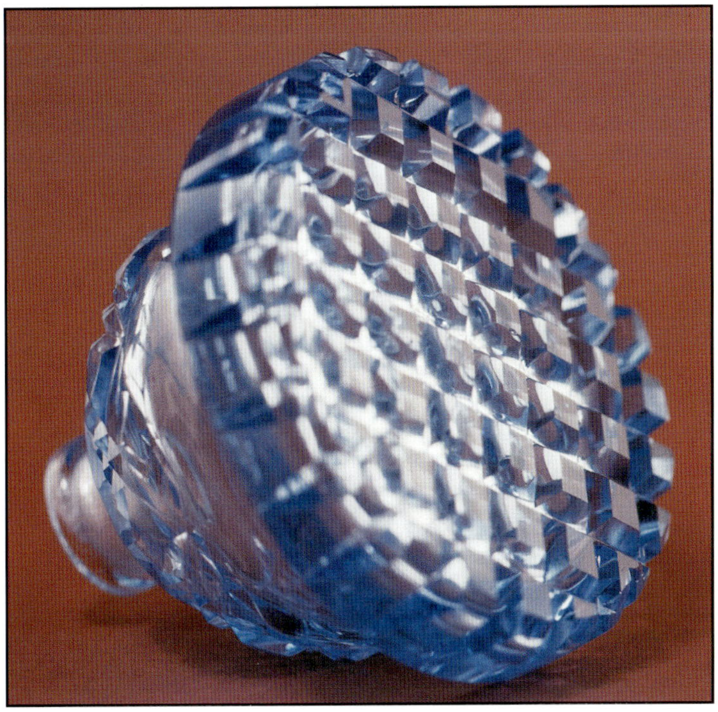

View of the previous bottle, showing cut detail in the underside of the base.

Three transparent black bottles. Left: smaller cut glass smoke bottle with cut and beveled top. 3.75". $100-150. Center: Stately version of similar design. 5.5". $200-250. Right: Geometric, wheel-cut starburst design; beveled stopper with two circle designs. 4". $250-300.

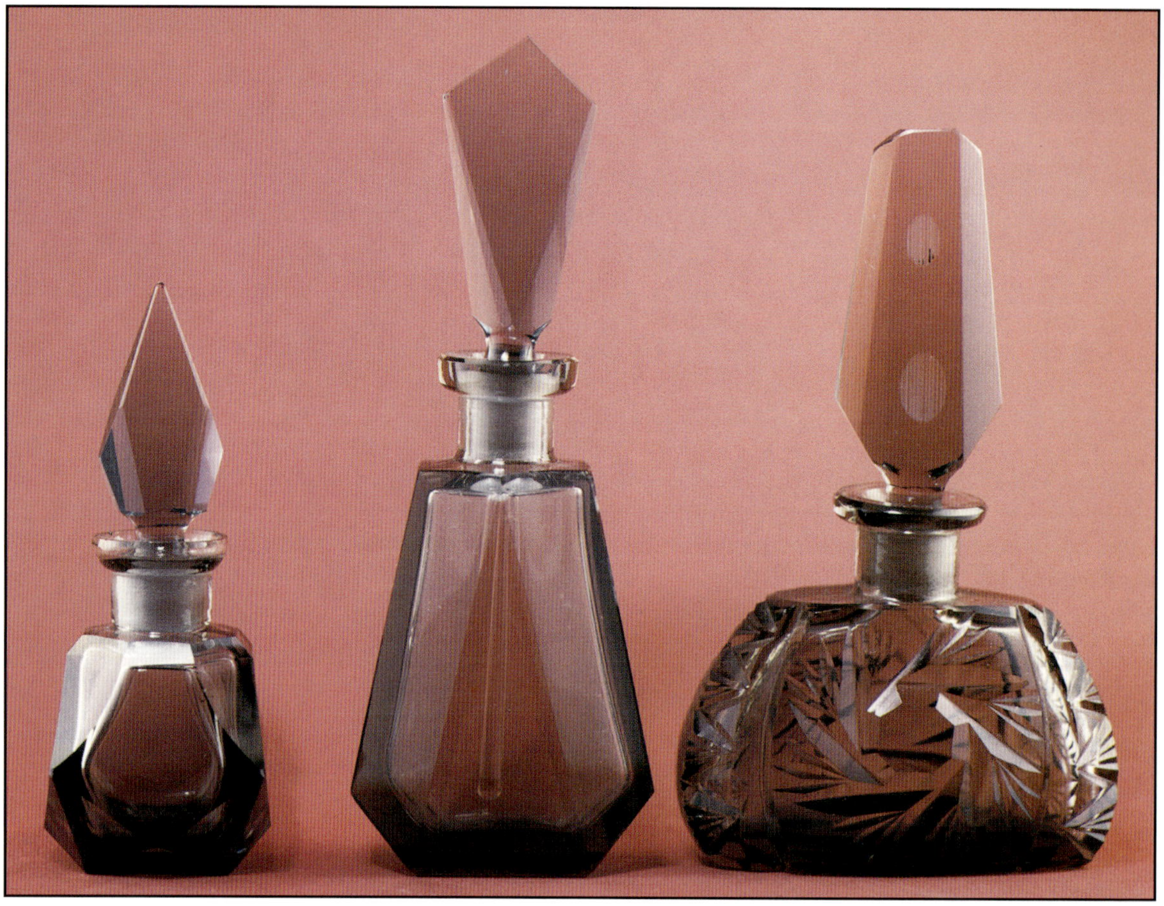

Right:
Clear, cut glass base with opaque black arrowhead shaped stopper. Paper Aristo sticker. 4". $150-200.

Far right:
Opaque black base, acid marked and labeled with an Aristo sticker on the back. The filigree features enamel work and pearls and an opaque red carved rose. The floral intaglio stopper is light pink. 5". $350-450.

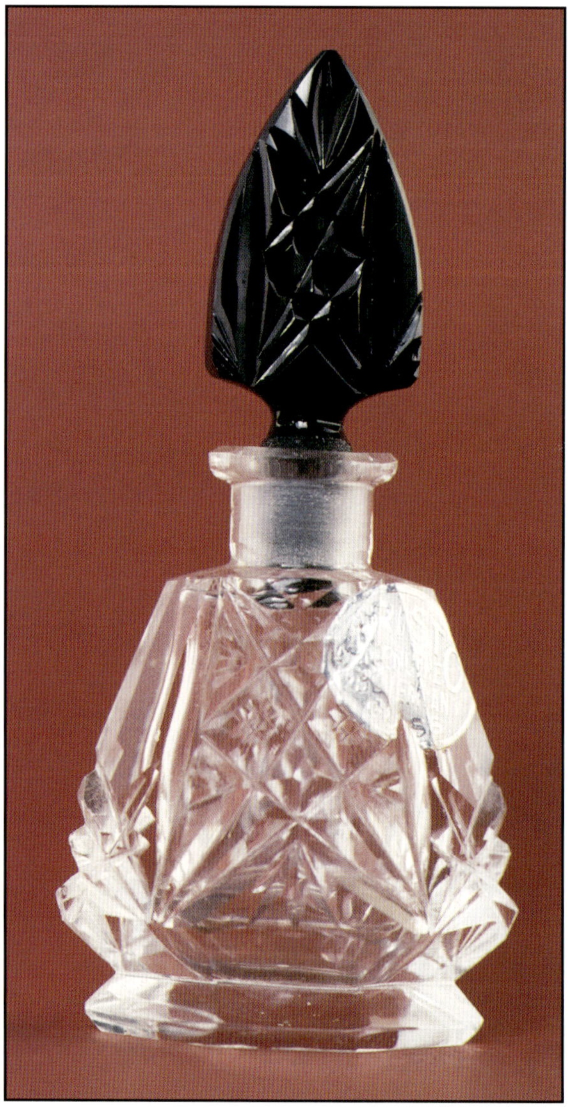

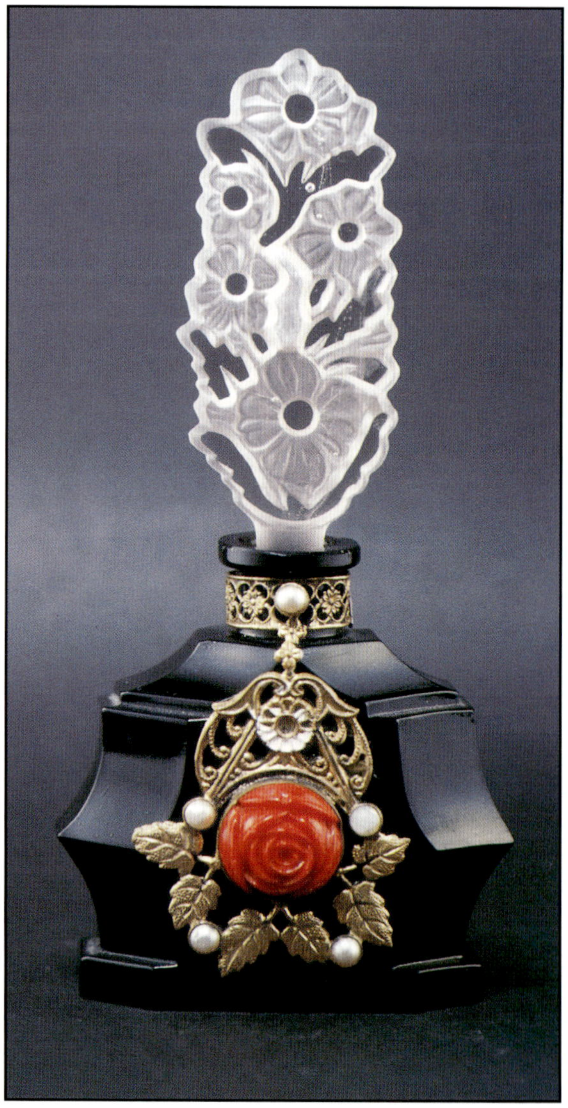

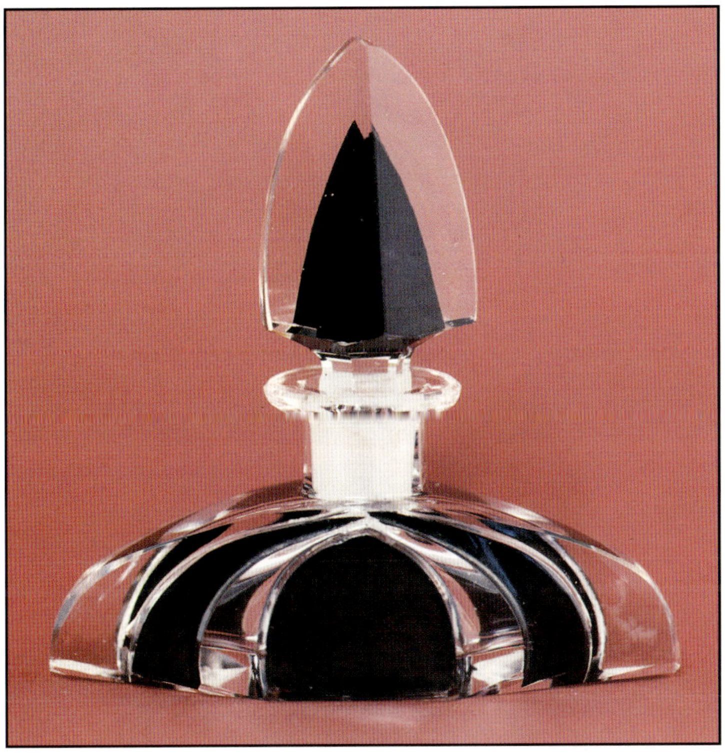

Black and clear art deco bottle. 3.5". $250-350.

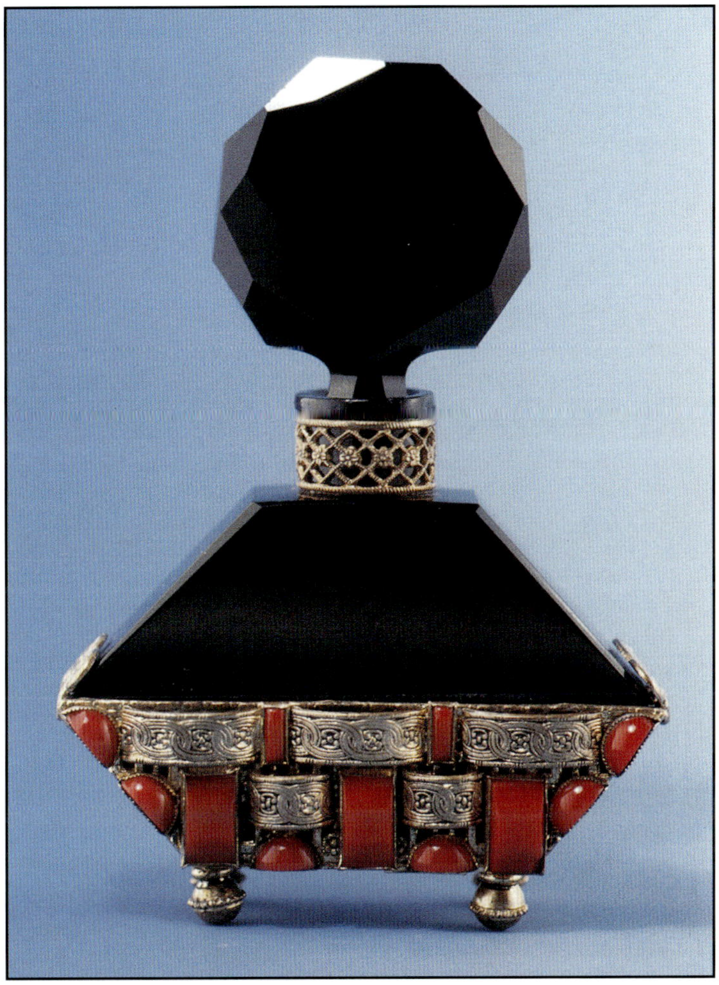

Opaque black bottle with ormolu filigree in a three-dimensional woven pattern with opaque red stones. Black stopper is cut to scallop the edges. Metal tag. 4". $650-850.

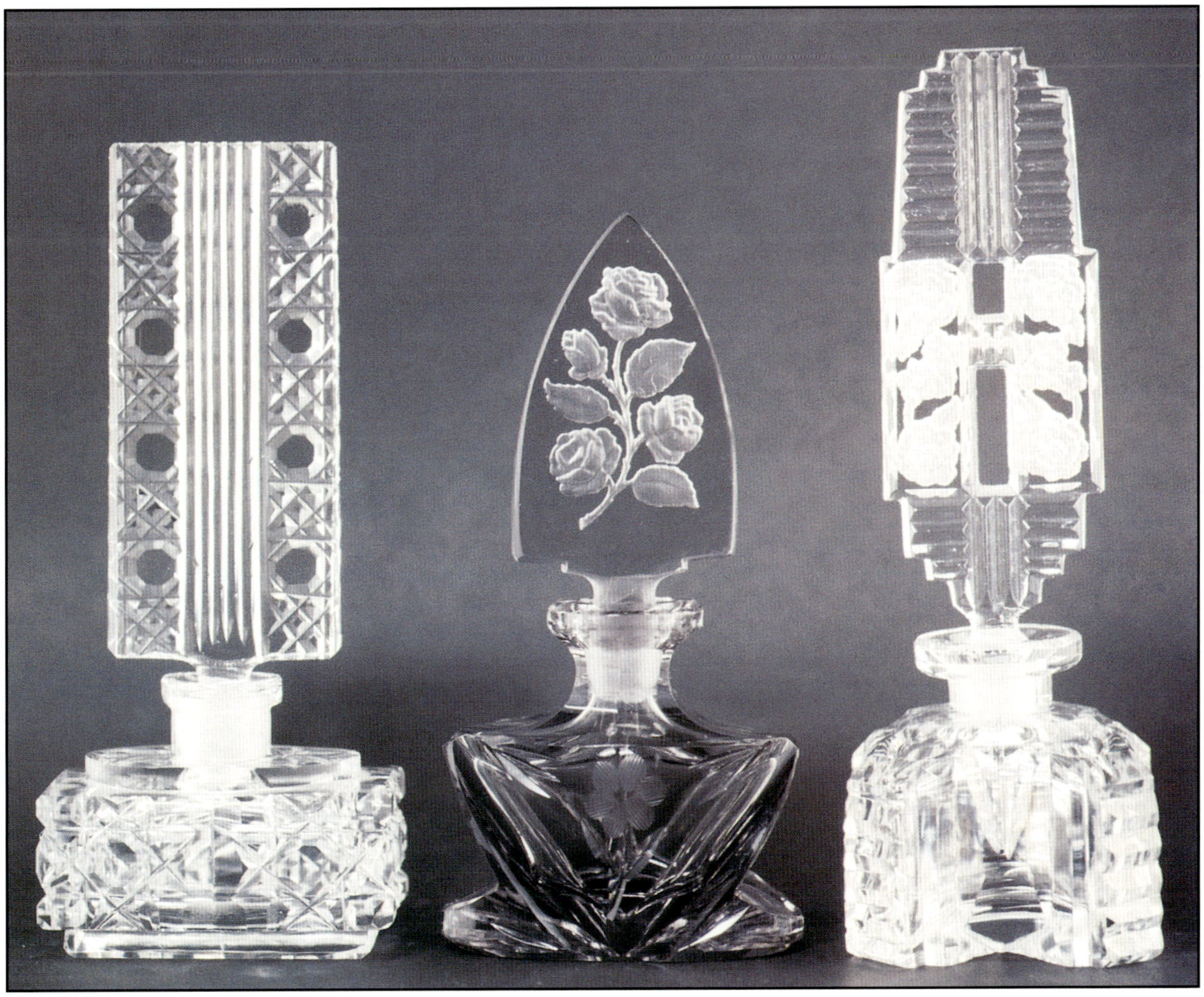

Left: clear base with tall cut yellow stopper, XOXO pattern in both the base and the stopper. 5.5". $250-300. Center: Amethyst cut base, amethyst stopper with intaglio roses. 5". $250-300. Right: Cut glass base with clear cut double pierced stopper. 6.25". $250-300.

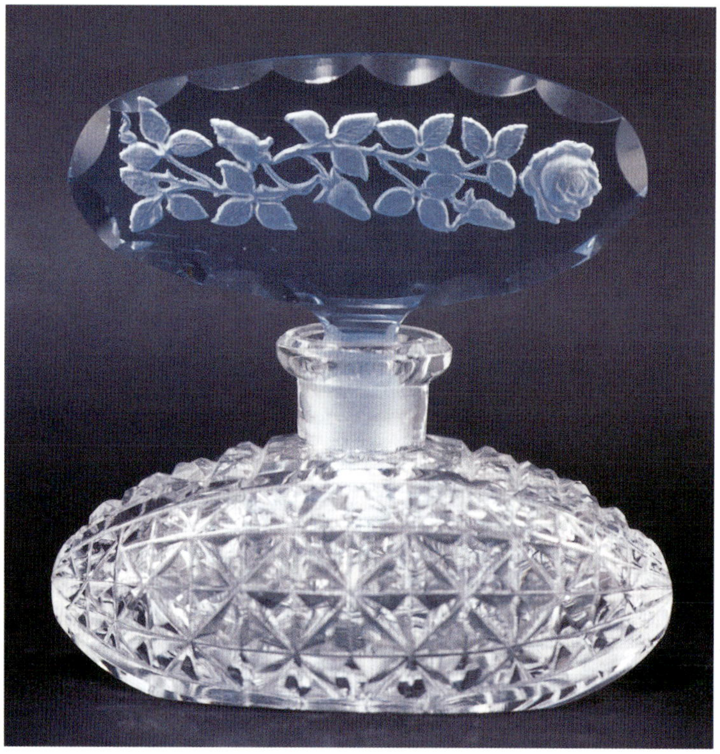

Oval bottle in clear cut glass with a blue oval floral intaglio stopper. 3.5". $400-500.

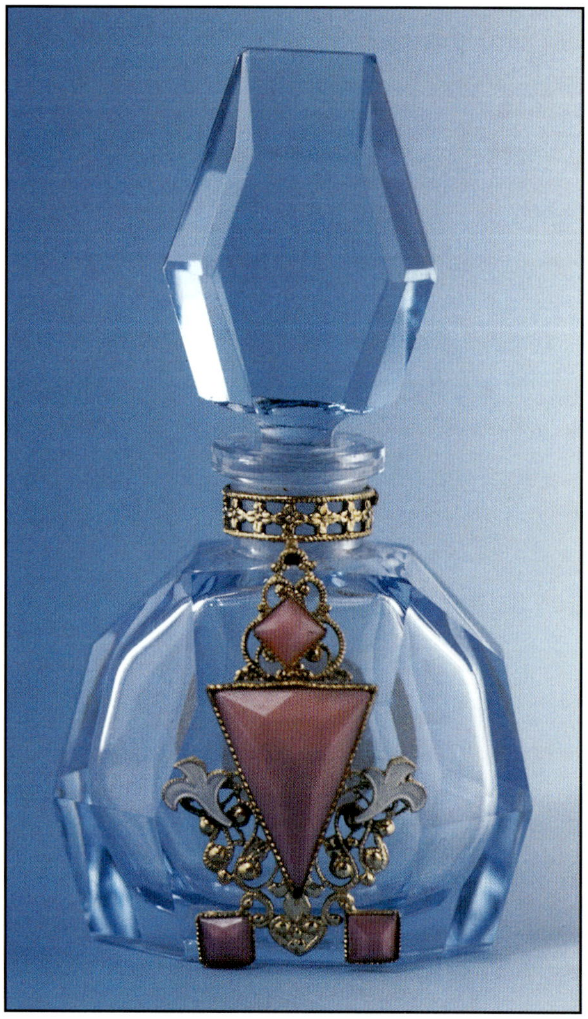

Blue cut glass bottle and stopper. Filigree is set with opaque pink stones. Metal tag in neck of the filigree, Aristo paper sticker on the back. 4". $350-450.

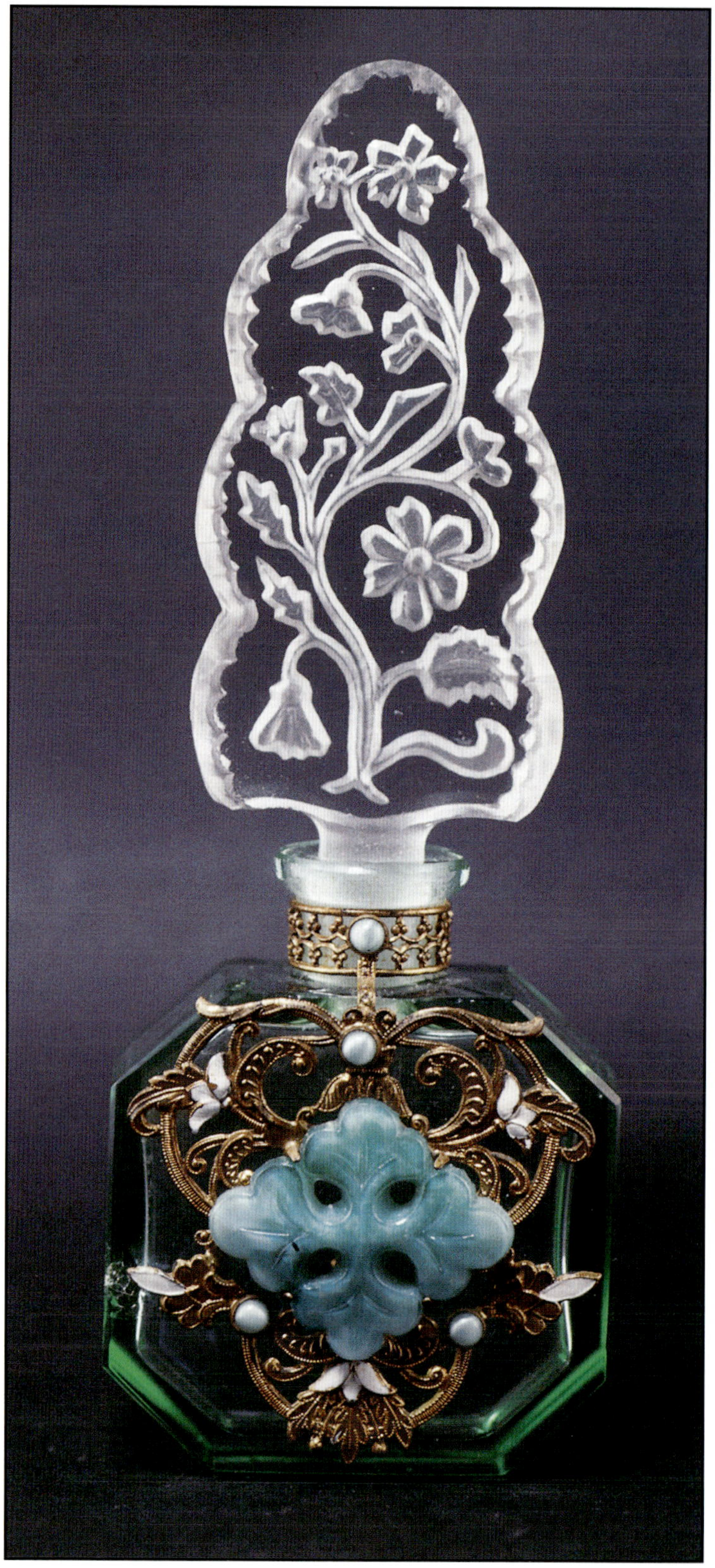

Green cut base with jeweled filigree featuring green cabochons and a green pierced medallion. Metal tag. Clear, cut glass; floral intaglio stopper. 5.875". $400-500.

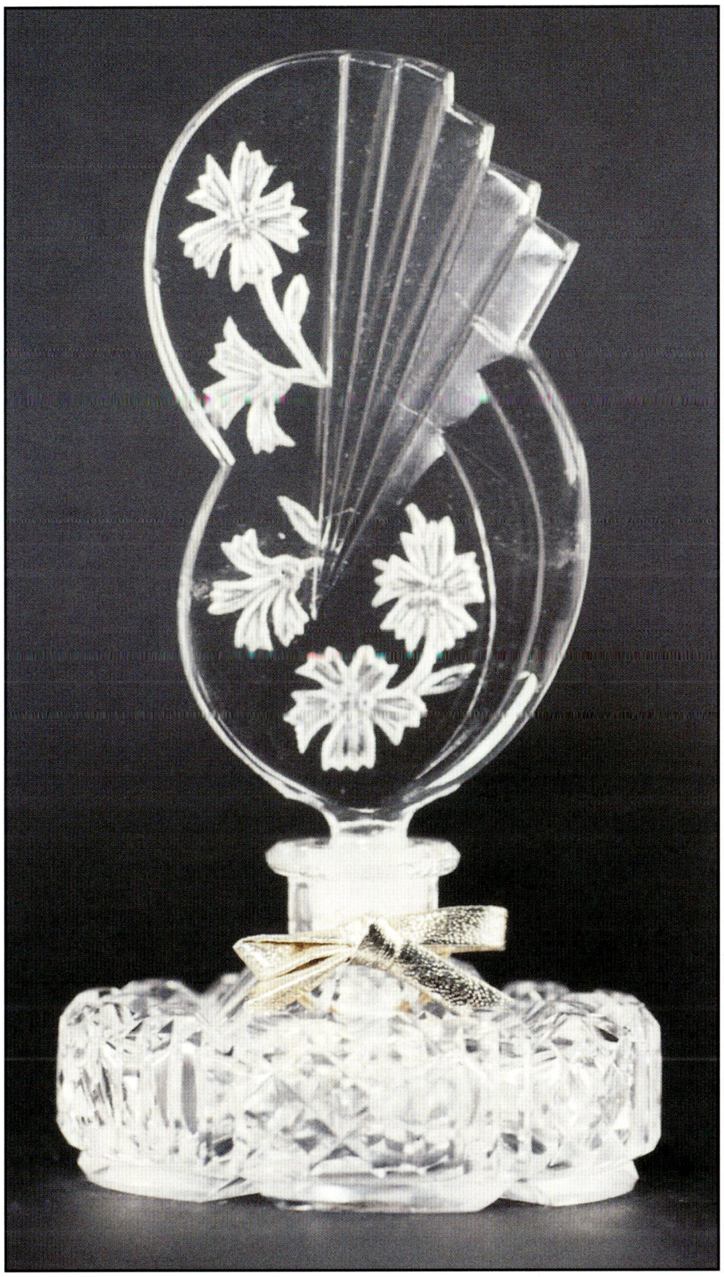

Cut glass base with a whimsical cut and intaglio top. 5.25". $100-200.

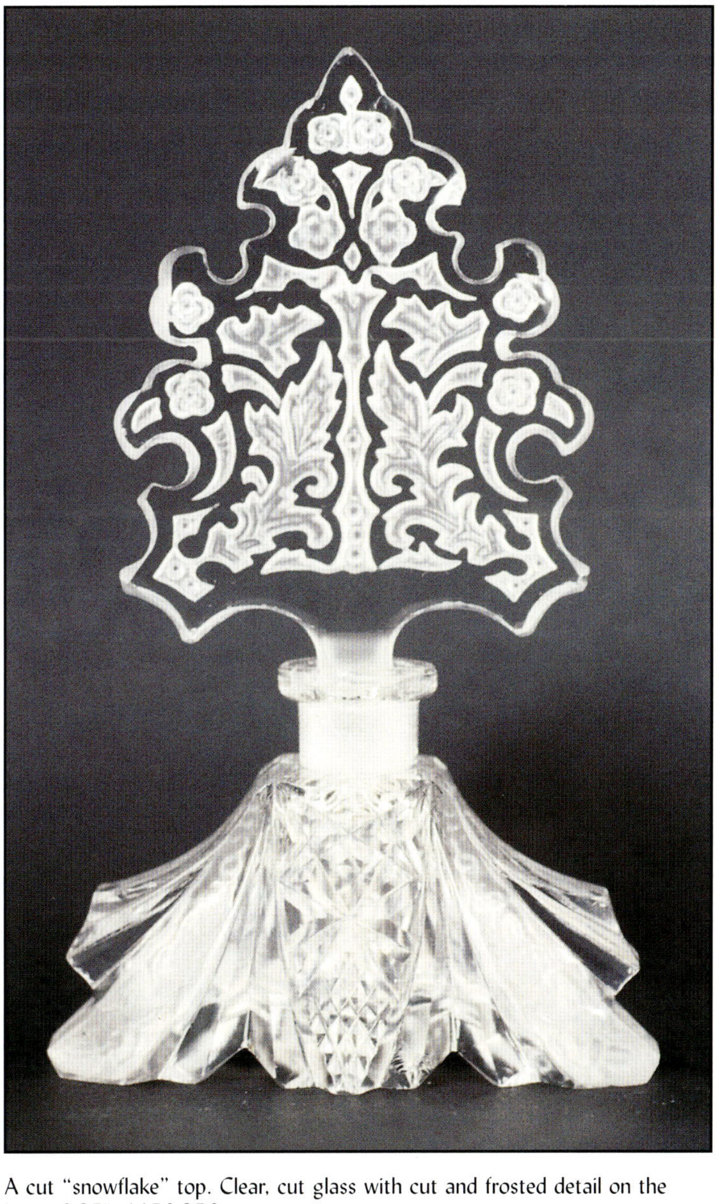

A cut "snowflake" top. Clear, cut glass with cut and frosted detail on the base. 6.25". $150-250.

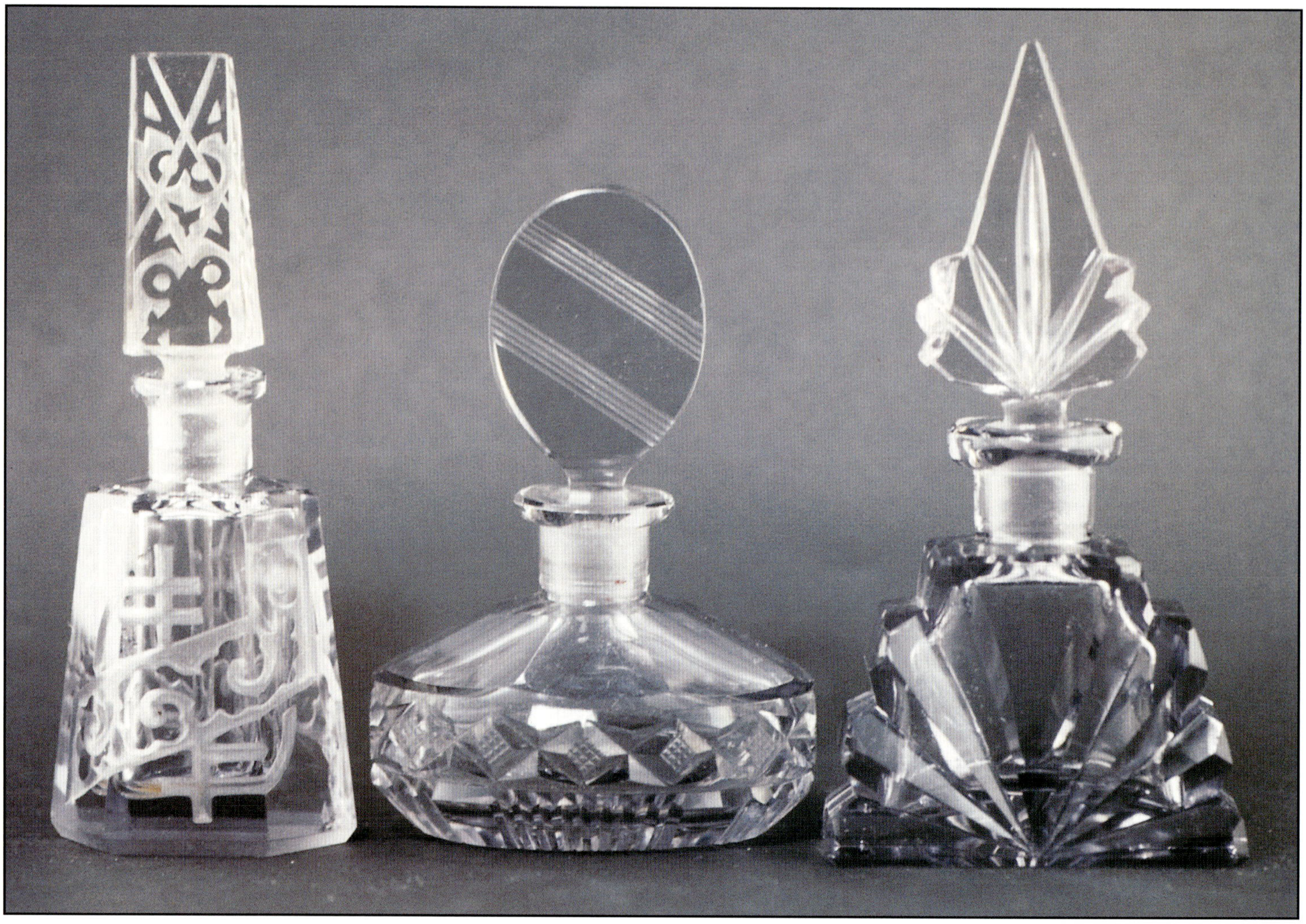

Three amethyst bottles. Left: Six sided facet-cut bottle with a "router-looking" design. 4.625". Center: Oblong bottle with cut design. 3.75". Right: Geometric cuts in the top, accenting the cuts in the base. 4.5". $200-300 each.

Right:
Yellow cut base and stopper. This bottle has an Irice paper label on the bottom. 4.5". $250-350.

Far right:
This cut glass bottle with gold ormolu and amethyst faceted gems is marked Austria in the metalwork. 3.75". $350-450.

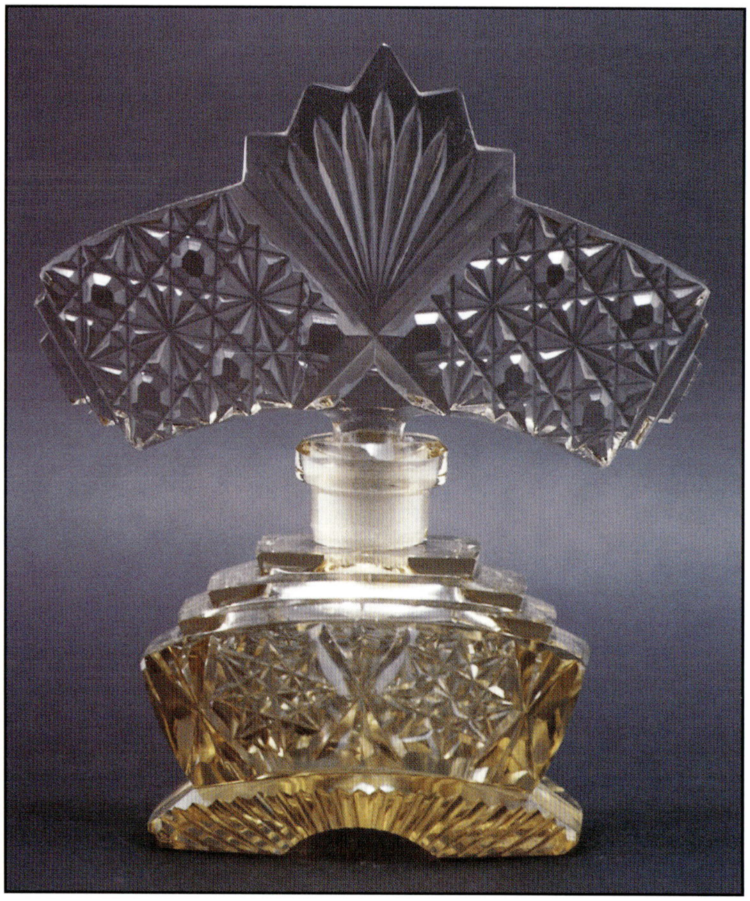

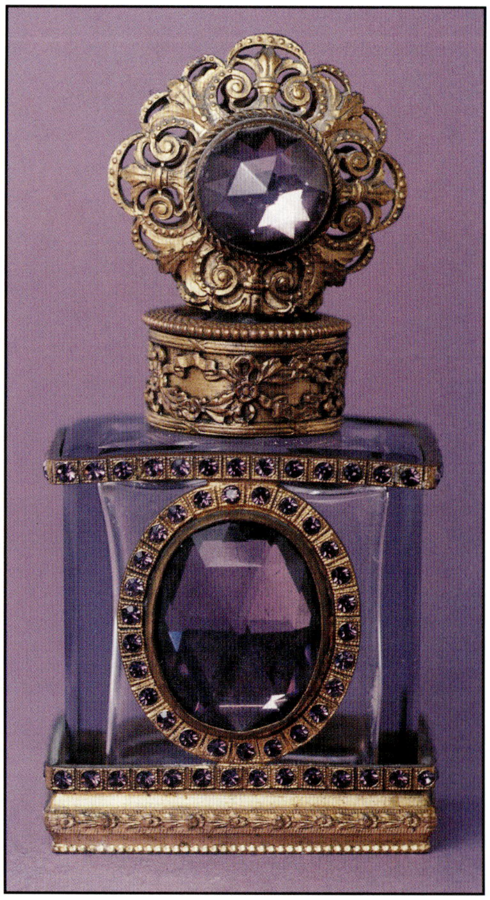

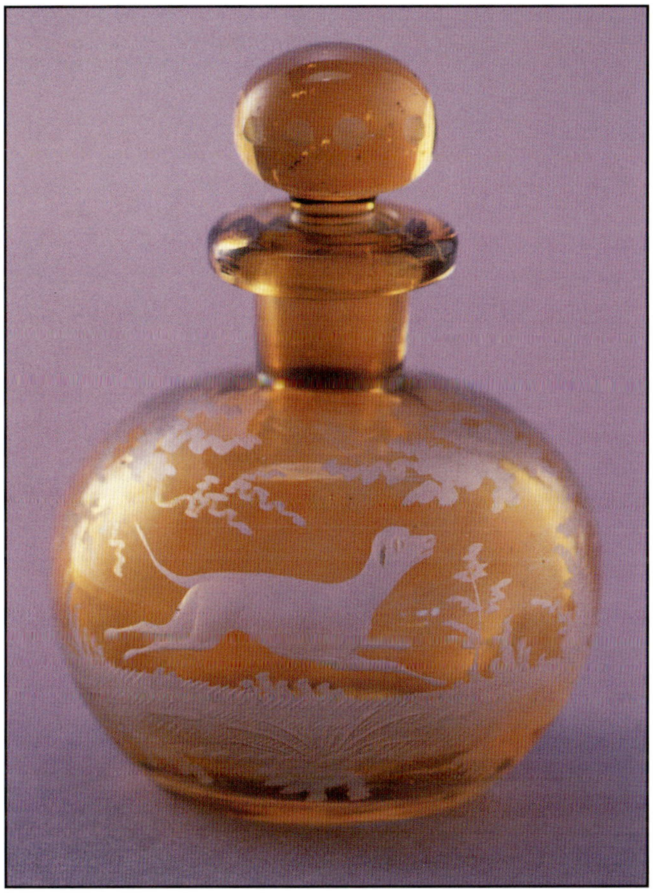

Unmarked Bohemian perfume with a hunting dog and forest scene etched through yellow surface stain. 3.5". $200-300.

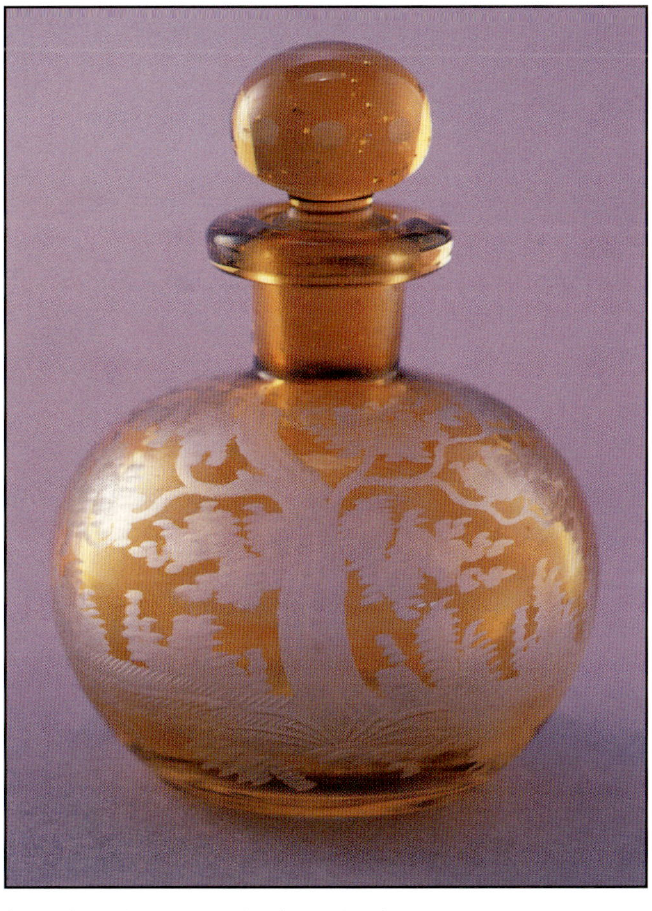

A tree from the reverse side of same bottle.

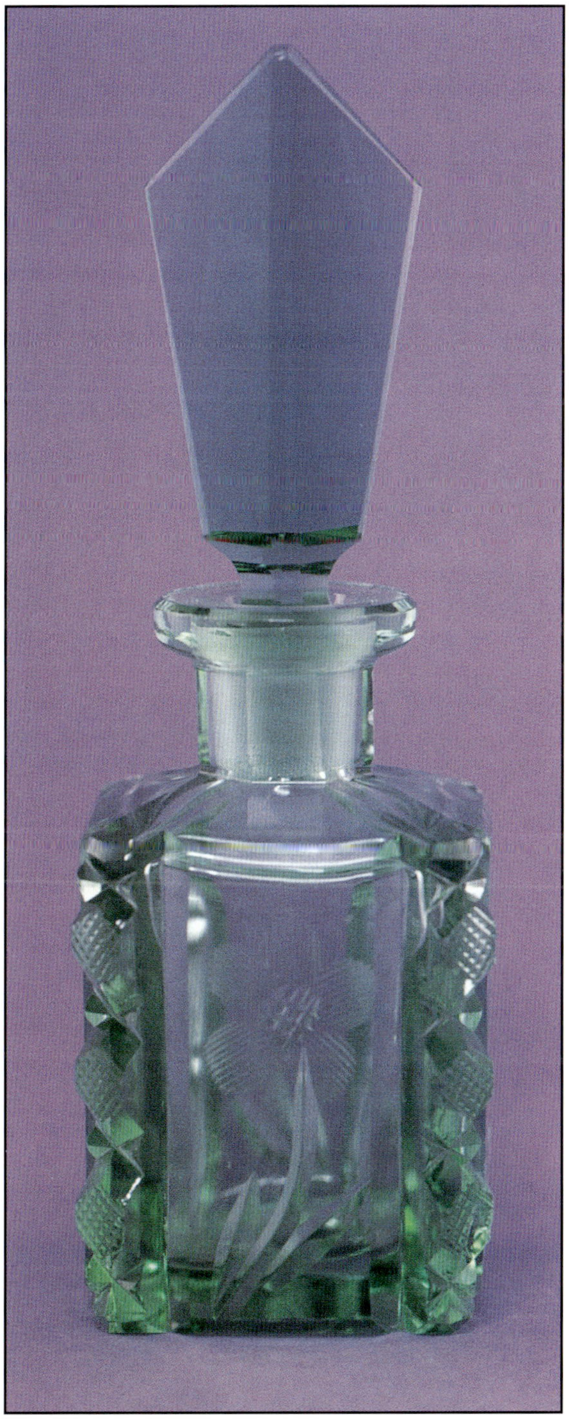

Square cut green glass with etched flower design and beveled green stopper. 4.75". $125-175

Atomizers

Spectacular in their own right are the atomizer bottles. Often they were part of a dresser set that could have included a tray and a companion bottle with a stopper and dauber. Atomizers are sometimes passed over by collectors because of damaged or missing squeeze bulbs. The bulbs, however, can be replaced, and restoring the bottle can be its own reward. Since most collectors use the bottles for display only, worn or missing bulbs have become less of a distraction and more of an authentication of the age of the item. This sampling of atomizer and companion bottles shows the diversity of design and grace of this romantic vanity accessory.

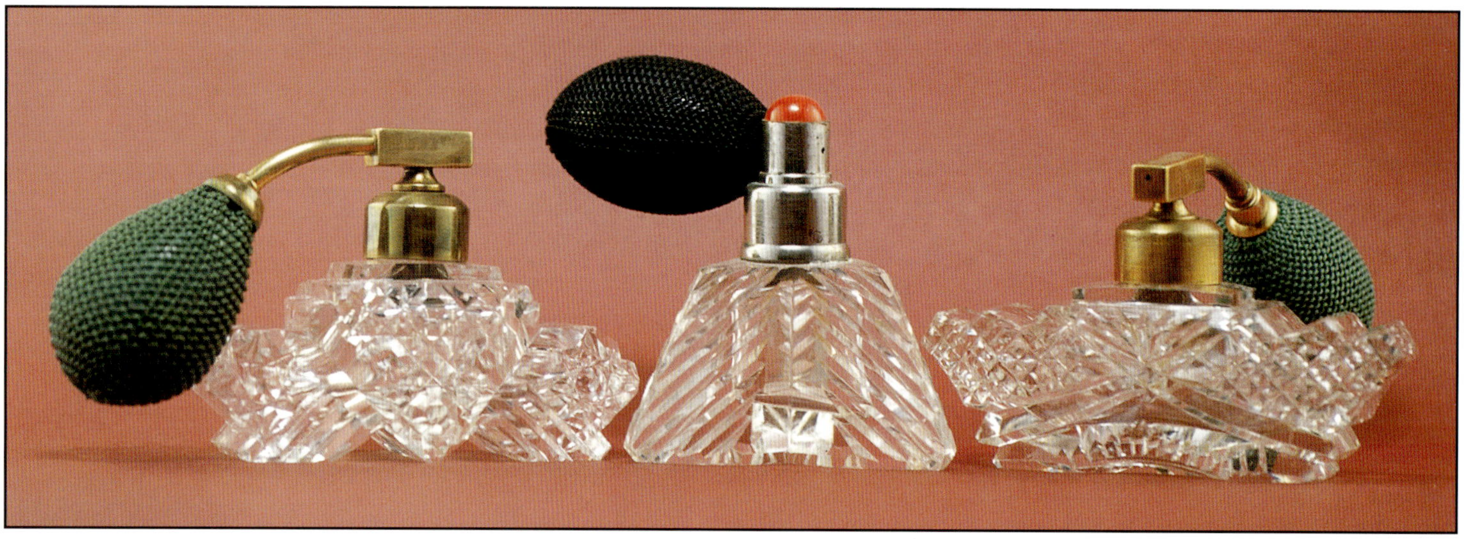

Three cut glass atomizers. Left: 2.5". Center: 2.75". Right: 2.25". $100-150 each.

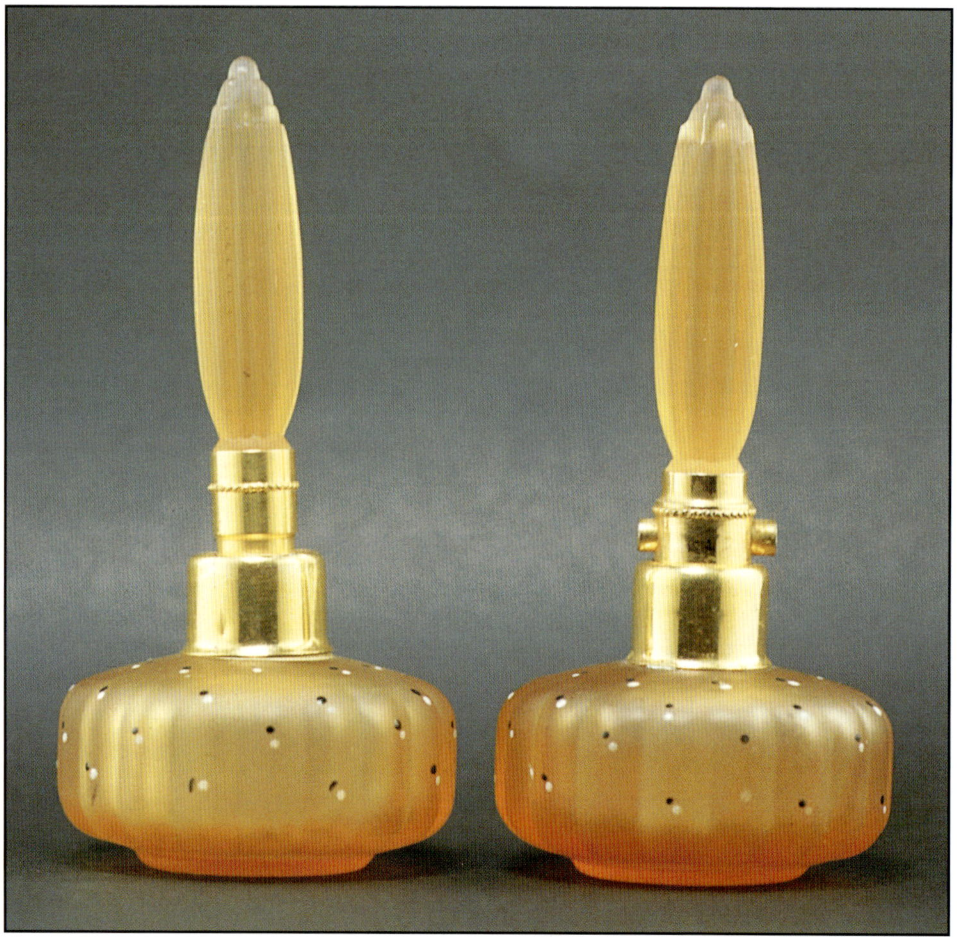

Yellow pair, atomizer and dresser bottle, satin glass with black and white enamel. 4.375". $300-400 the pair.

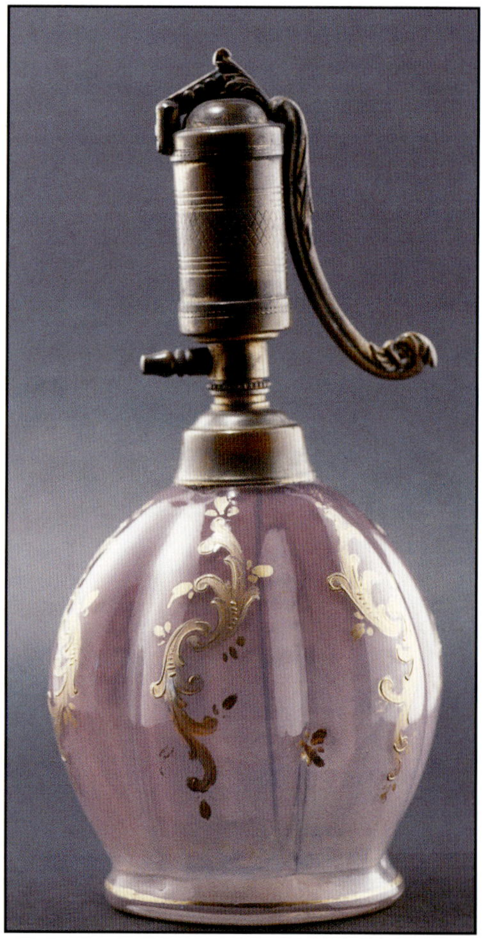

Purple pump, atomizer bottle with gold detailing. 8". $300-500.

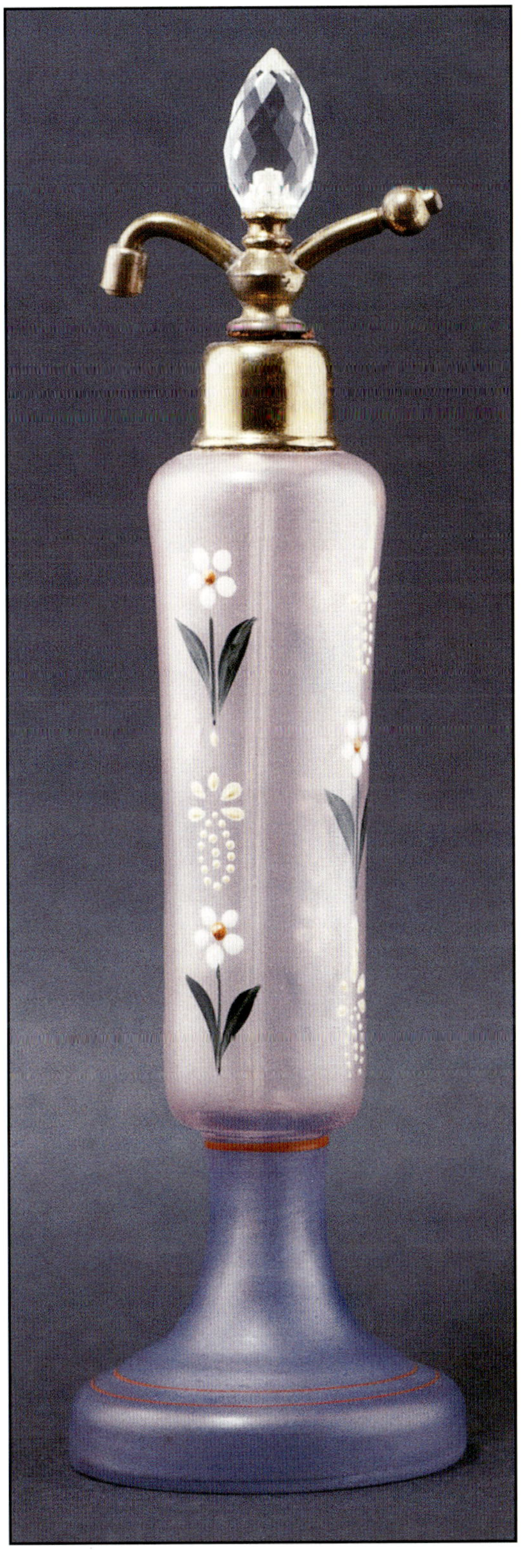

Lavender atomizer with enameled dot flowers, prism finial. 9". $150-250.

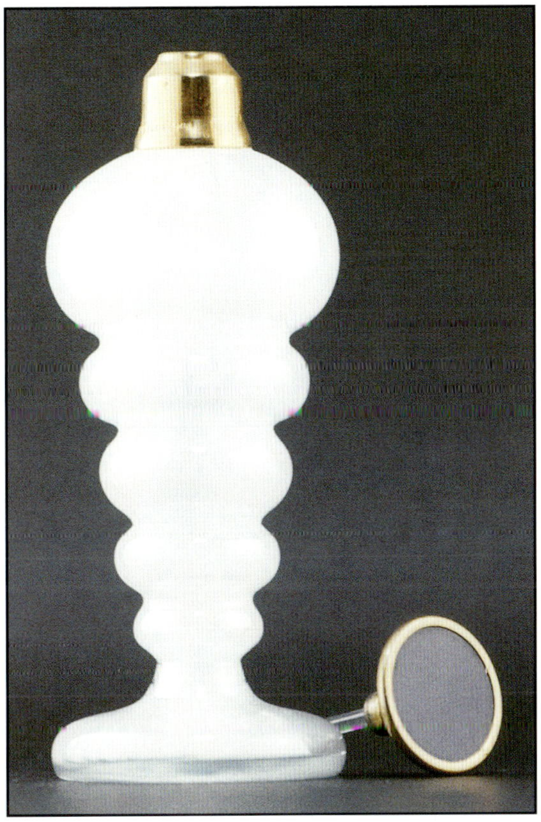

Iridescent white blown bottle with a navy blue wafer stopper. 5.25". $100-200.

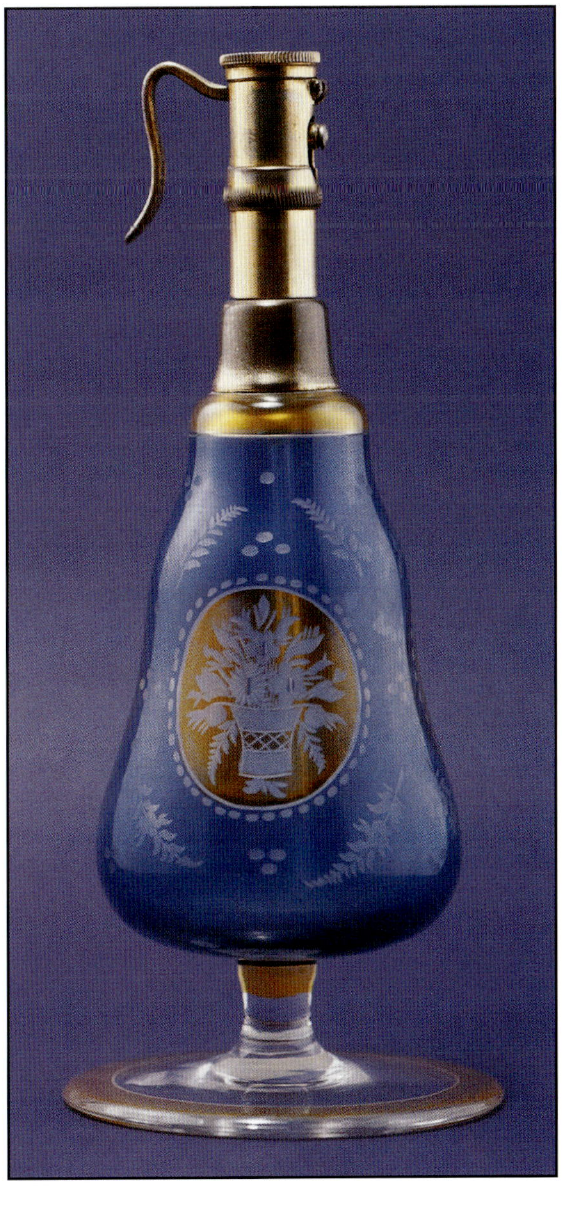

Blue atomizer with a clear window featuring an etched flower basket. 7.75". $300-500.

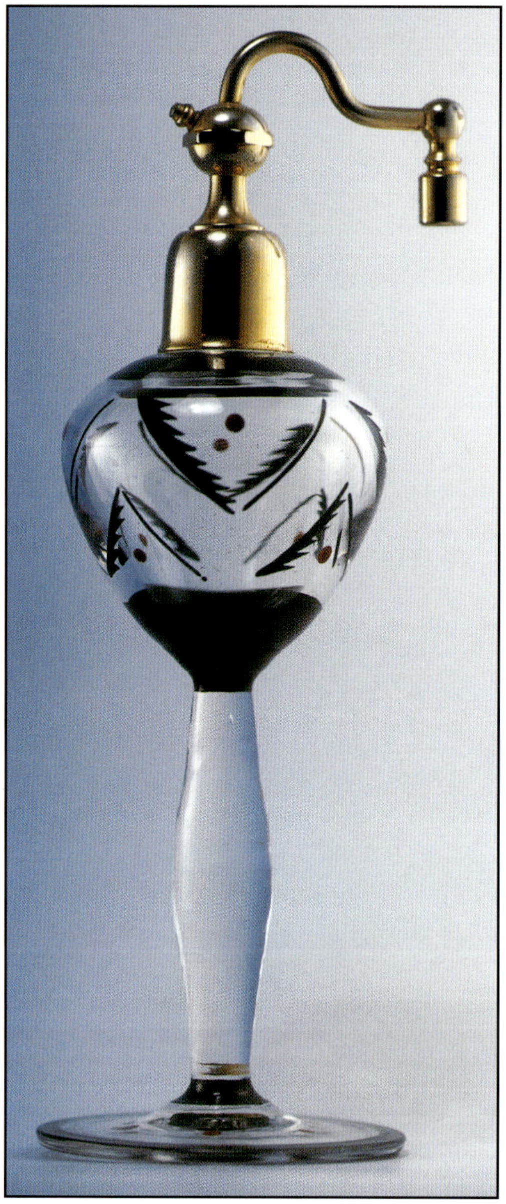

Art deco atomizer with black "feathers" and red enameled dots on clear. 7.375". $150-250.

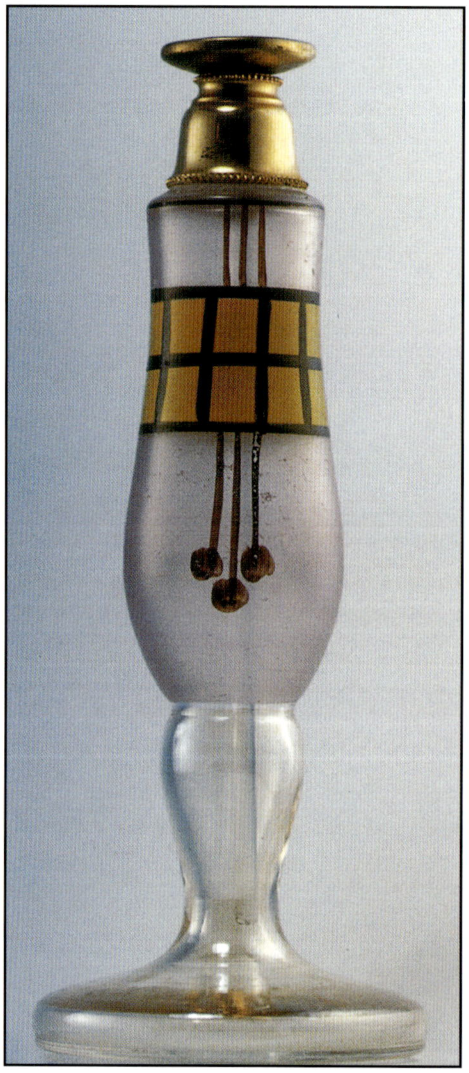

Tall frosted and enameled lavender dresser bottle. 6.625". $200-300.

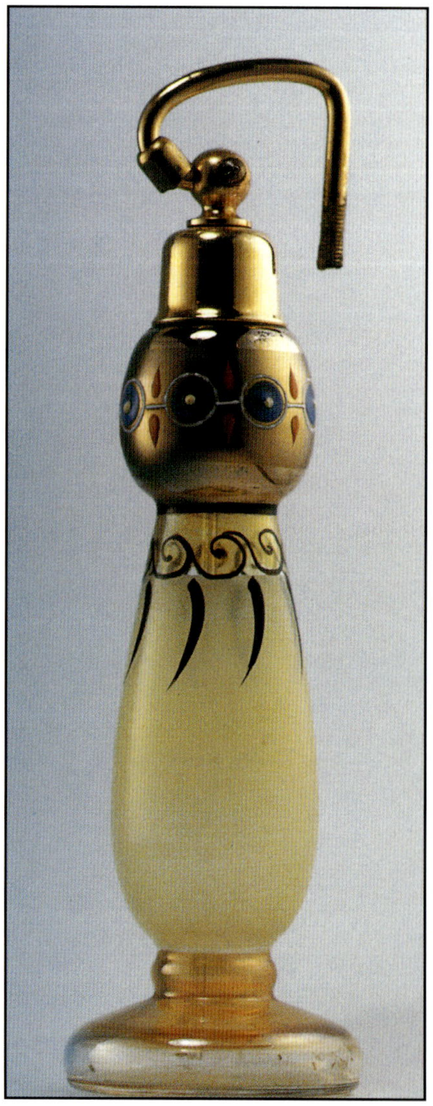

Tall, frosted yellow atomizer with gilding and enameled decoration in black, blue, and red. $150-250.

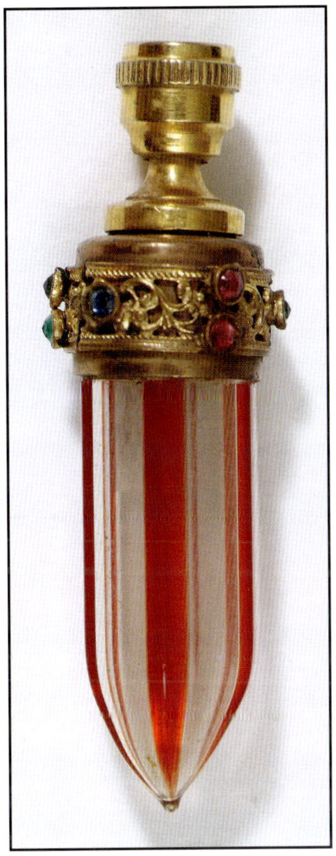

Tiny clear hexagonal bottle with red edges. Jeweled band at neck, shaker top. Marked. Very unusual. 2.125". *Courtesy of Don Orban. Photo by David Kirk of Kirk Photography.* $300-400

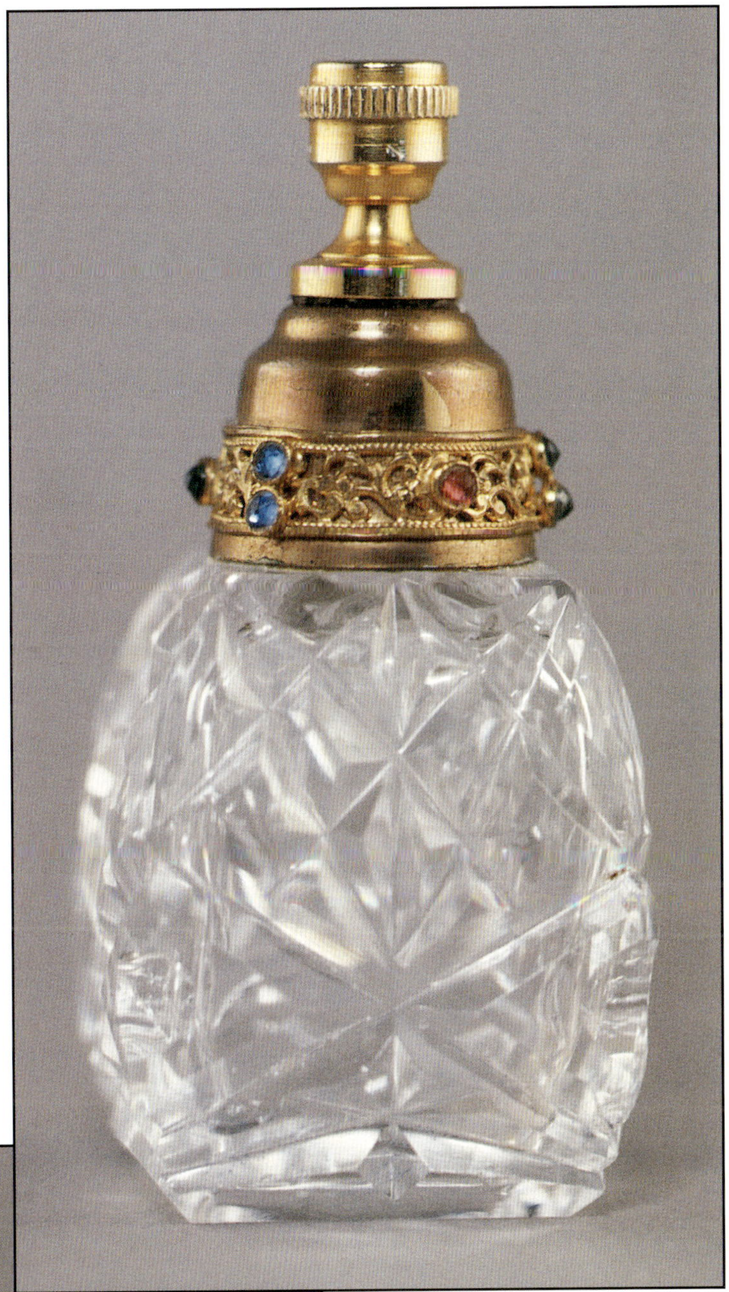

Not an atomizer, but a "shaker" bottle with a top portion that opens separately, allowing perfume to be sprinkled out of the tiny holes at the top. The base is cut glass; the top features jeweled filigree. $300-400.

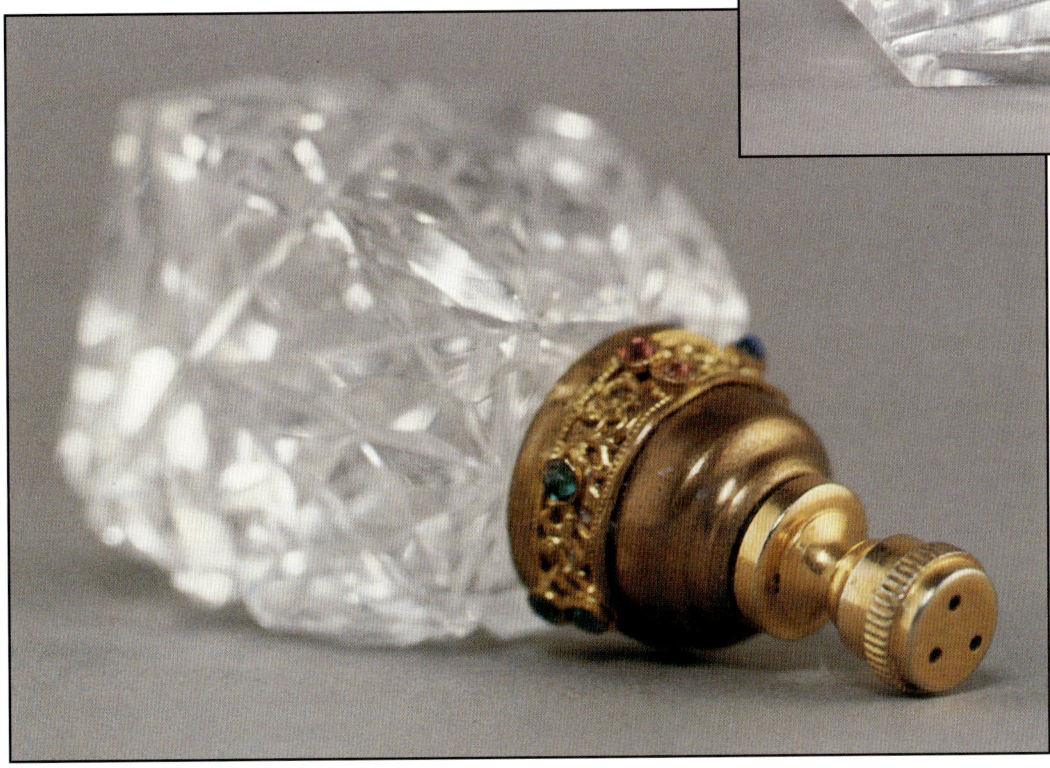

Another view, showing the shaker top. The bottle is filled by unscrewing the whole neck portion from the collar piece.

Cased, Blown and Pressed Bottles

Not all Czechoslovakian dresser bottles were made of cut glass. Layered or cased bottles were produced and decorated with paint, gilding, jeweled metal work, and enameling. Bottles were blown and pressed. Their versatility is an enduring compliment to the craftsmanship of the men and women who produced and refined them.

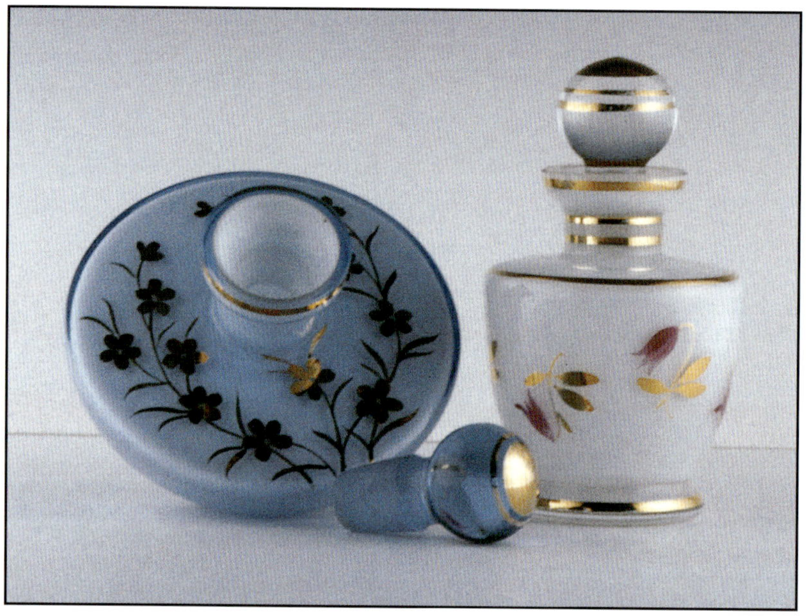

Two Irice cased bottles. Left: Transparent blue over opaque white, this bottle has a transparent blue stopper. Both bottle and stopper have applied gilded decoration. 3.125". Right: This bottle is clear over opaque white with gold and purple floral design and additional gold trim on both the bottle and clear stopper. 2.5". Both bottles have Irice paper labels on the bottom. $50-100 each.

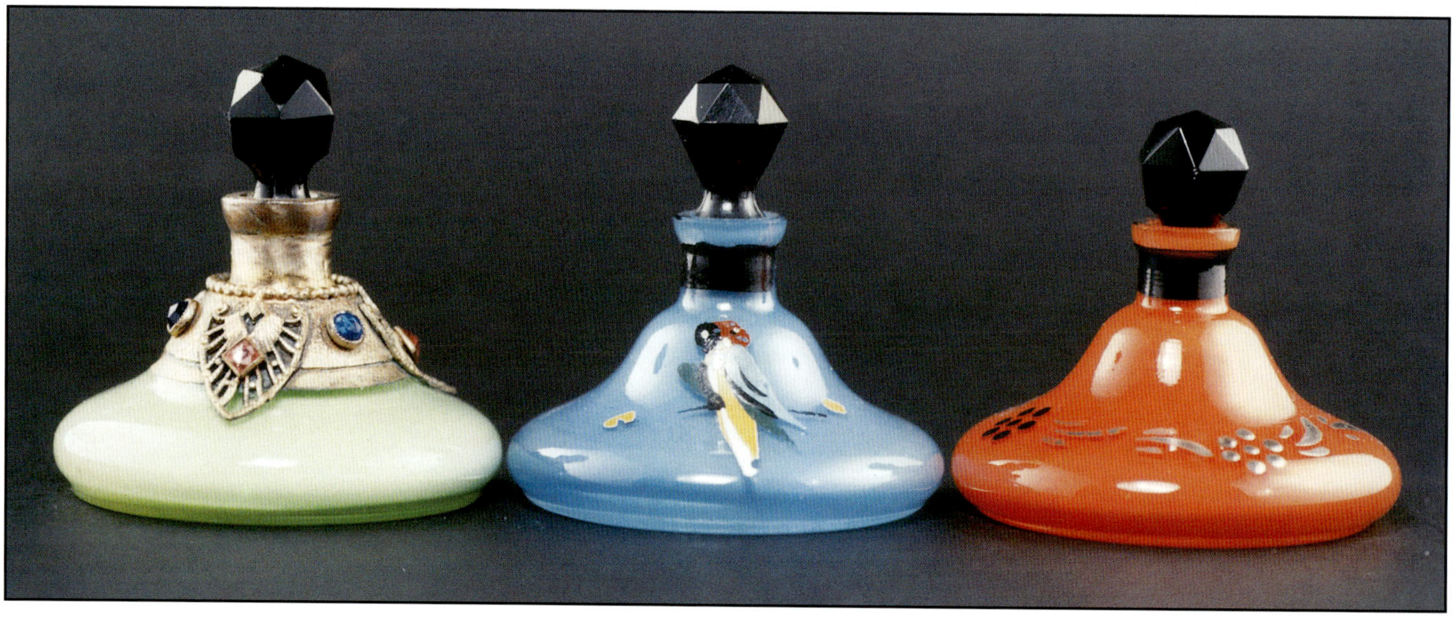

Three cased bottles. Left: Clear over green, this bottle has a collar of filigree with blue and pink stones. Gilt has been added to the neck and the area below the metal. The stopper is opaque black and faceted. The piece is marked E &JR Czechoslovakia. 2.5". $250-350. Center: Clear over blue, this cased bottle has a painted parrot and painted black trim at the neck. The stopper is faceted, opaque black glass. The bottle is also acid marked as above. 2.875". $250-350. Right: Clear over red cased glass, this bottle has, in addition to the same acid mark as the two previous, a paper label that reads: "E &JB Sterling Silver Deposit." It has both silver and black detailing and an opaque black, faceted top. 2.25". $250-350.

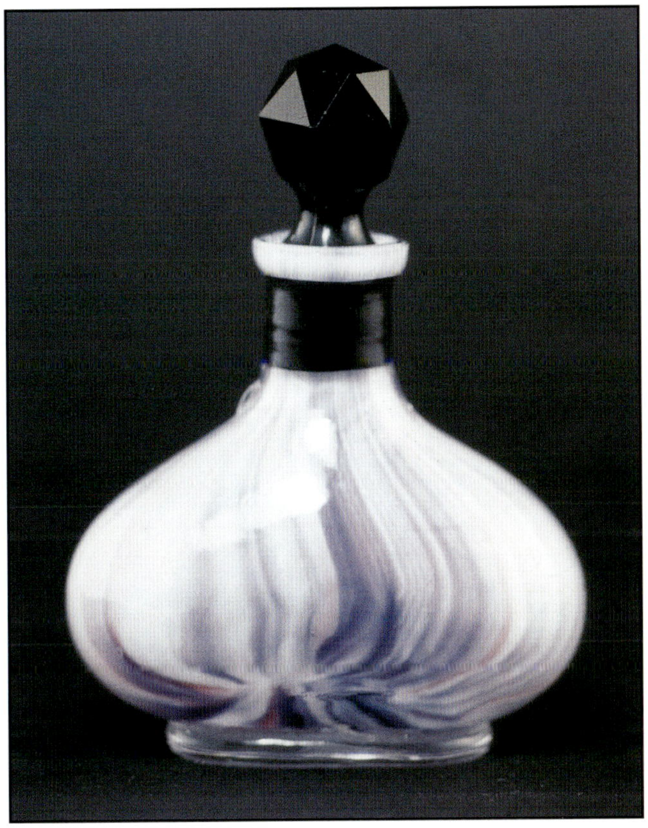

Variegated purple stripes lie under clear casing on this intriguing bottle, which rests on a clear footing. The black band at the neck was applied. It has a black, faceted stopper and is acid marked. 2.875". $100-200.

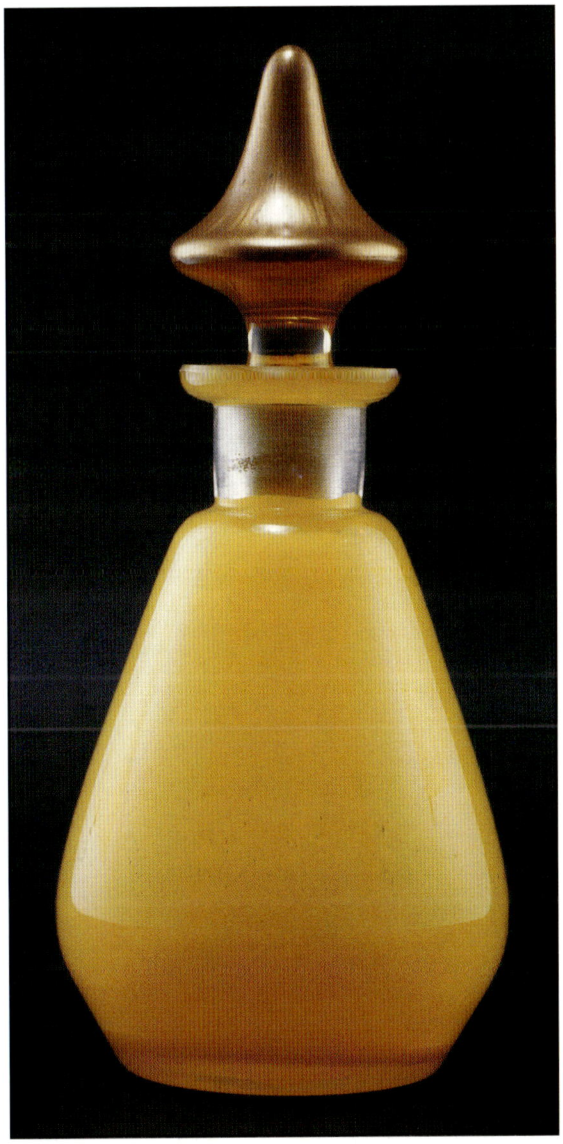

Clear over bright yellow, the stopper for this bottle is Vaseline glass. The "pagoda" top has been painted gold. Acid marked. 5.5". $100-150.

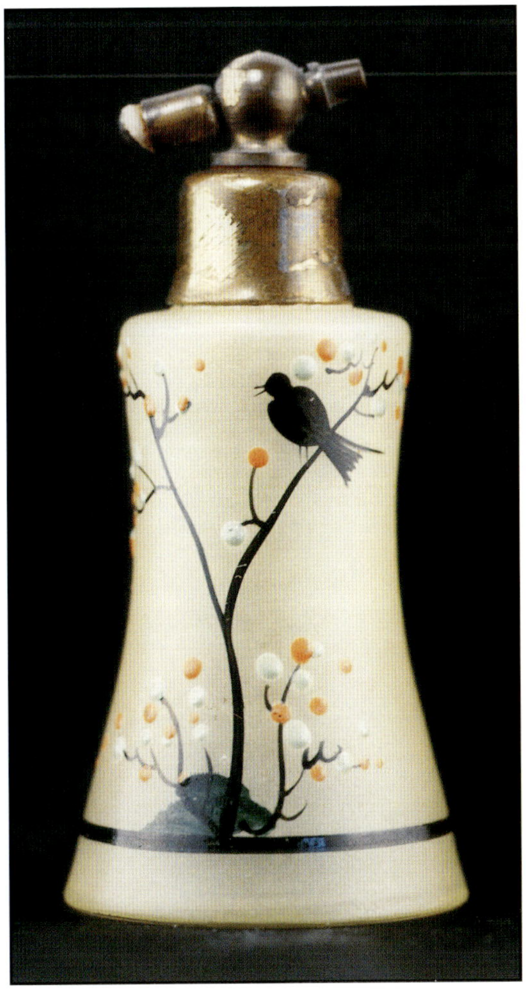

Yellow frosted atomizer bottle with applied enameled bird and bush in black with green leaves and orange berries. Marked in the metal top. 3.625". $75-125.

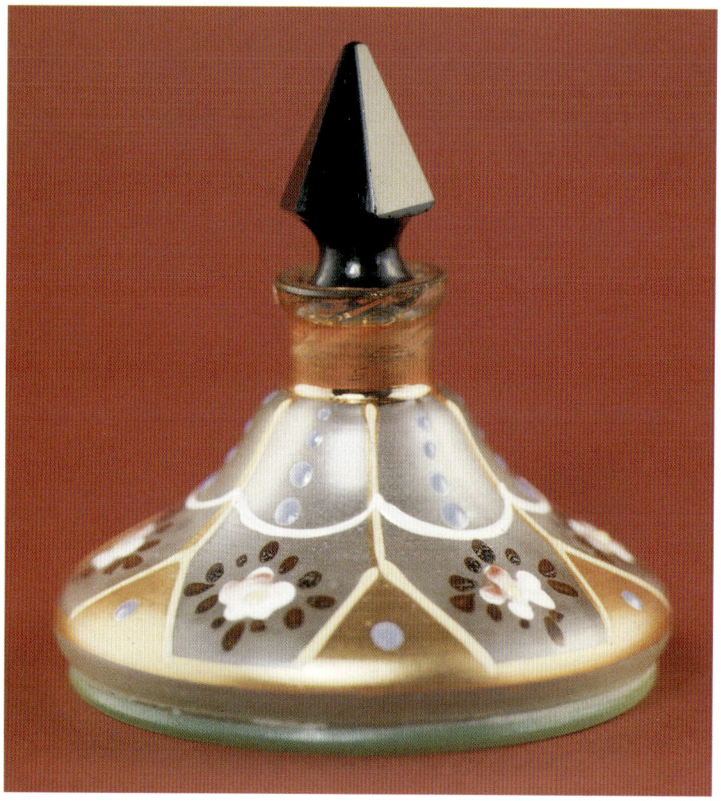

Frosted Vaseline glass with gilt and enameling in gold, yellow, pink, white, and brown. The stopper is opaque black and is faceted to a point. 2.5". $300-400.

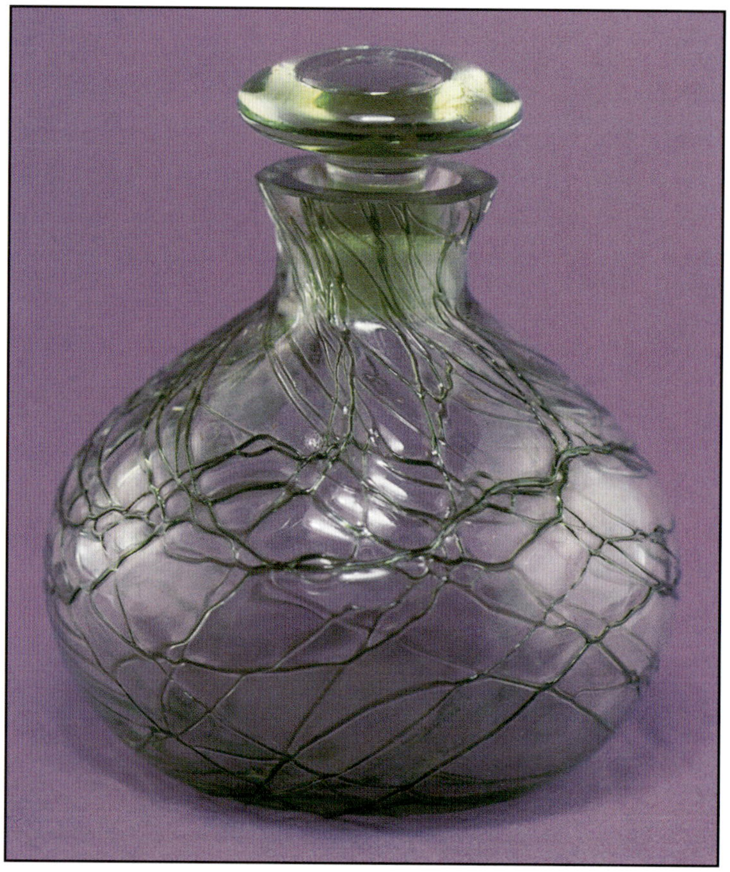

Green crystal blown bottle with a button style stopper and green threading. Acid marked in base. 4.25". $75-125

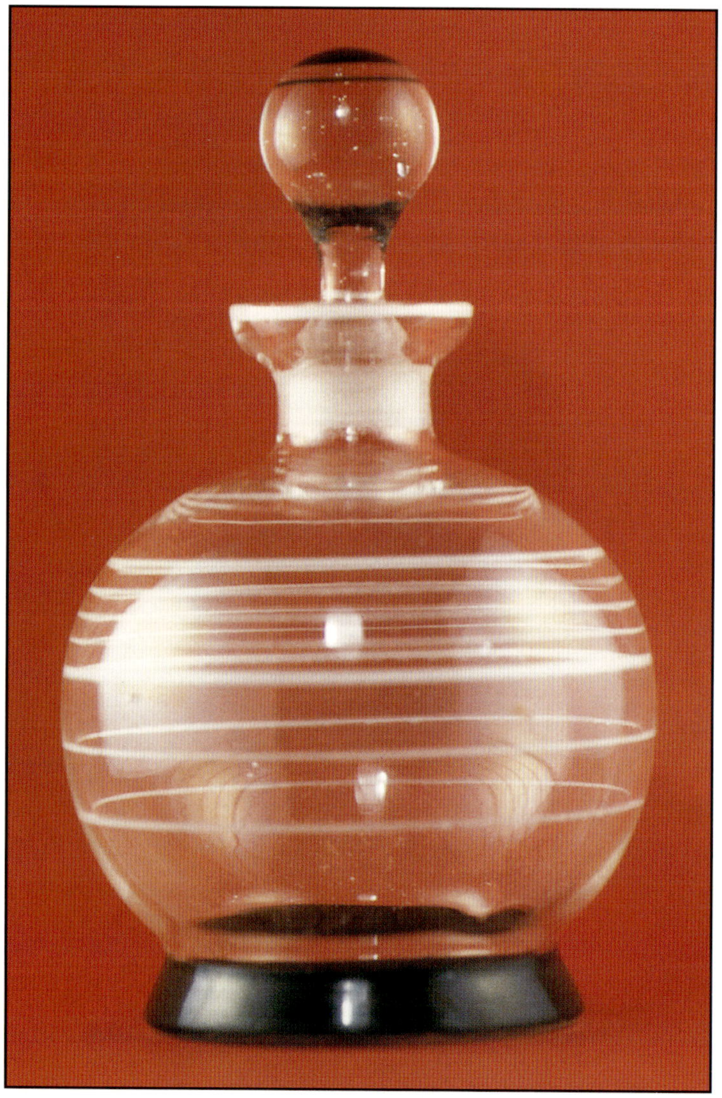

Blown striped bottle with a black band at the base and a clear top. $75-125.

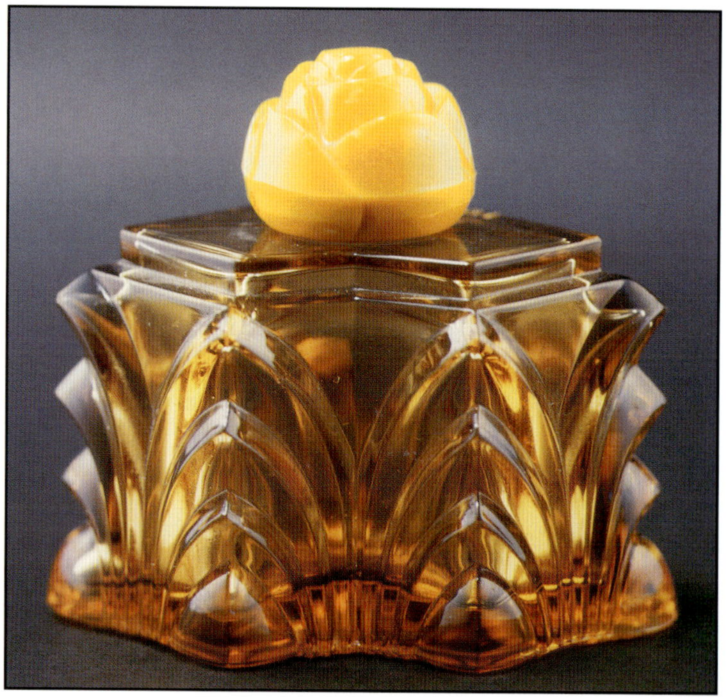

This pressed amber bottle has an elaborate pattern and a yellow, hard plastic rose-shaped cap. "Czechoslovakia" embossed in the base. 3.75". $35-50.

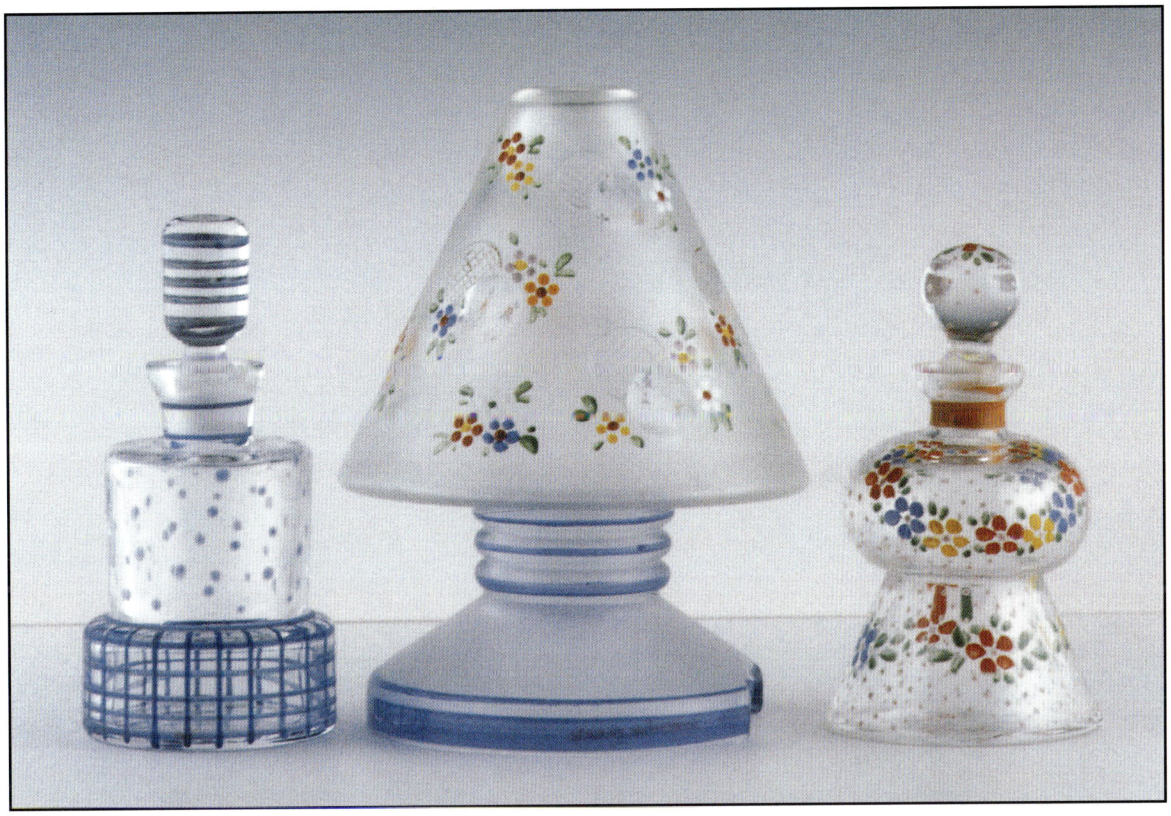

Left: Clear bottle with blue enameled stripes and dots. 3.625". $75-125. Center: Perfume lamp in clear with colorful enameled dots forming flowers. 4.5". $100-150. Right: Clear, snow woman shaped bottle with dots forming red, blue and yellow floral garlands with green dot leaves. 3.375". $75-125.

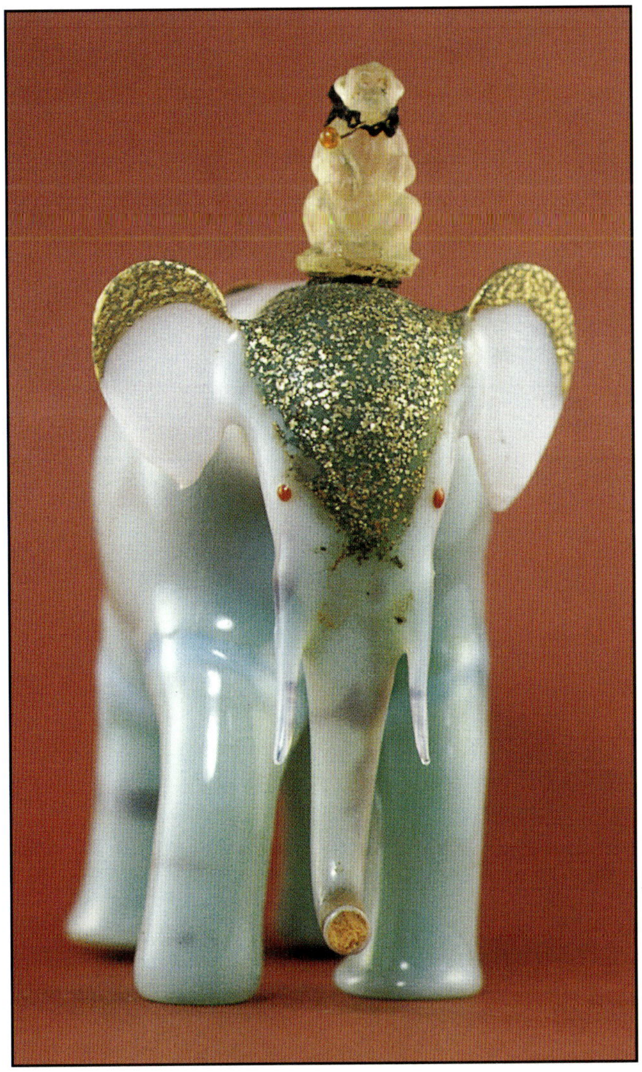

Oncoming blown elephant in soft blue translucent glass carries a Czech glass monkey on his back. He glitters with gold decorating his forehead and upper ears. His eyes are applied red glass. The stopper is a cork at the end of his trunk. 4.5". Value unknown.

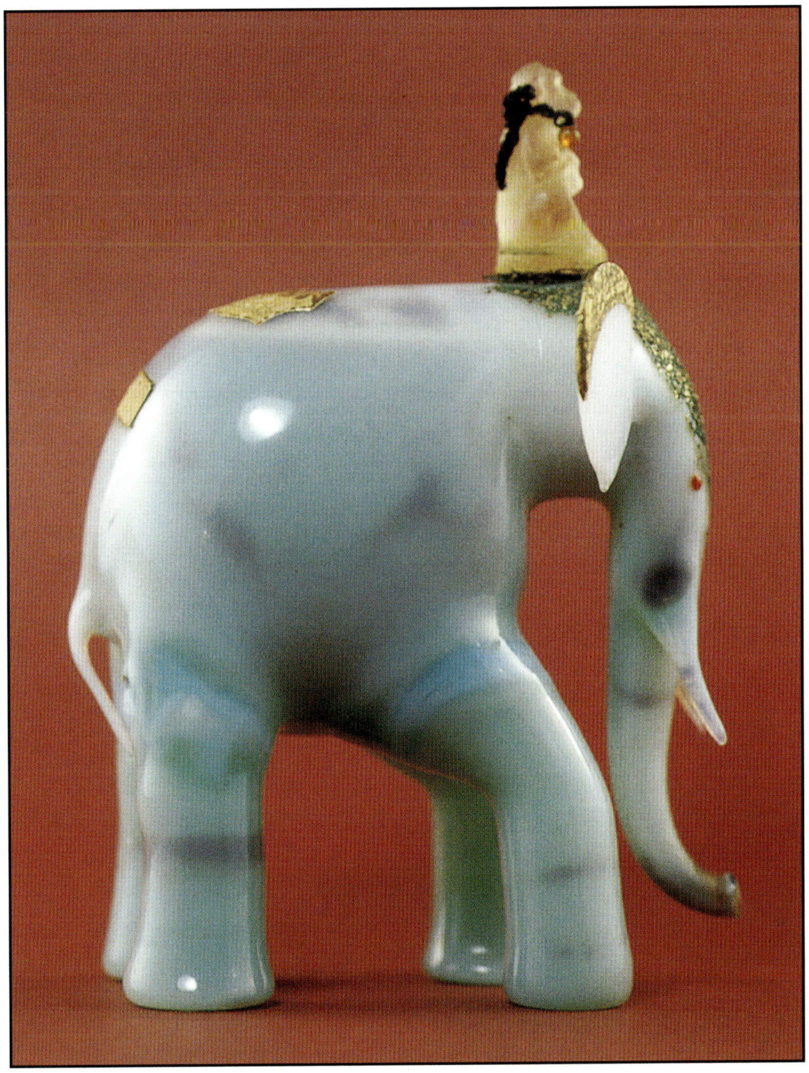

Side view of elephant and monkey.

Hoffman, Schlevogt, Ingrid

The Heinrich Hoffman (1875-1939) name quickly becomes a familiar one to collectors of Czechoslovakian perfumes. Bottles of his design are prized for their rich quality and beauty. He is credited for creating intaglio cutting (negative molding with a frosted finish) and for the nude dauber. His creations often feature classical scenes and painstaking finish work. His trademark is an open-winged butterfly. Hoffman lived in Paris, but his designs were produced in Gablonz, Czechoslovakia.

Hoffman hired Henry G. Curt Schlevogt, who, like himself, was the son of a glassmaker. Curt Schlevogt worked with molds and developed an opaque, stone-like glass. Married to Hoffman's daughter, Charlotte, Schlevogt returned to his father's company in 1930 when Charlotte died giving birth to their daughter, Ingrid. Continuing to work with the opaque glass and with molds that he had developed or were given to him by his father-in-law, Curt Schlevogt introduced the Ingrid line of glass vanity products in 1934 at the Leipzig exposition. The line was popular and included dresser sets with powder boxes, stoppered perfume and atomizer bottles, as well as vases, cups, lamps, hand mirrors, trays, ring and trinket boxes, and purse bottles. (Note: For pictures of original catalog advertising pages, see: Nový, 2002, p. 164; and Truitt V.I., 1995, p. 128-129)

Production was reduced and altered under the Nazi occupation during World War II. When the war ended, Schlevogt was charged with political crimes and sent to prison. His second wife, Margaret (Goldi) Scheibler Schlevogt, and his daughter, Ingrid, fled the country, taking little with them. Released in 1948, Schlevogt spent most of his remaining life, from 1950 until his death in 1984, in Paris, where his daughter still lives. (Note: an excellent and more detailed account of the Hoffman-Schlevogt story can be found in Jones-North, 1999 revised edition, addenda by Ken Leach, pp. 136-139)

Original Ingrid pieces, many of which bear the Ingrid name in an acid mark, were made primarily between 1934 and 1938. Some items in the green malachite glass were produced in the 1950s, after the industry had been nationalized. (See Jones-North, 1999, pp. 83-88) These were not acid marked, but were marked with a paper tag. Some items were made in pastel clear and frosted glass from Ingrid molds in the 1950s.

Purse bottles made in 1934 through 1938 were made in opaque black (jet or onyx), opaque green (malachite or jade), and opaque blue (lapis or turquoise) glass. Donna Sims, in her article featured in Monson and Baer's *The Beauty of Perfume*, May 1996, shows classic opaque Schlevogt and Hoffman bottles in fourteen colors and color combinations. Of the purse bottle colors, green is the most common. Black and lapis are more rare, and other colors are very unusual.

Items in the following photos are not limited to perfume bottles, but include some other vanity table art. Some of these pieces would have been parts of dresser sets that would have included perfume bottles and atomizers.

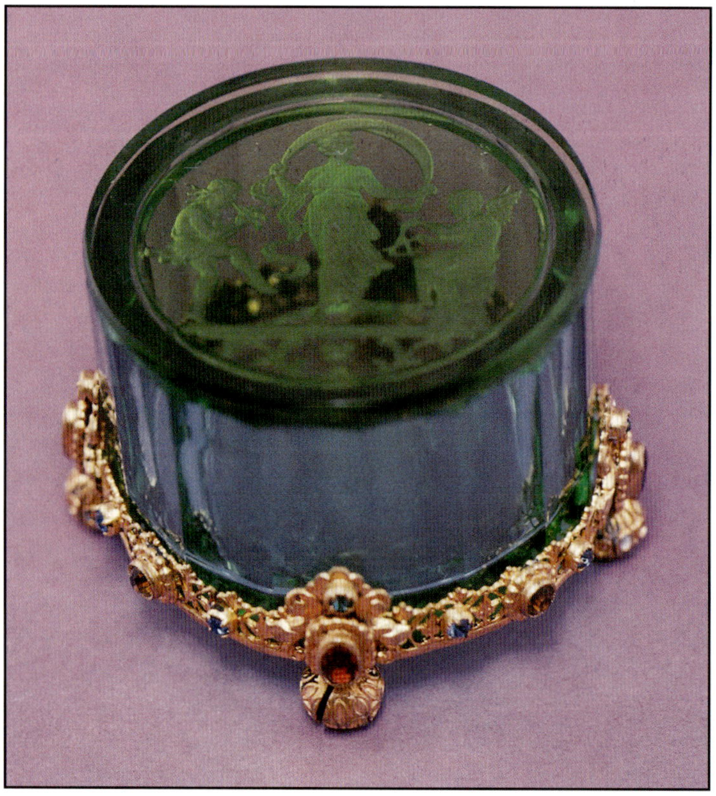

Green, cut glass Hoffman trinket box on a jeweled, footed stand. Intaglio top features a woman with a scarf, two musicians. Hoffman butterfly mark. 1.75" high, 2" diameter. $500-600.

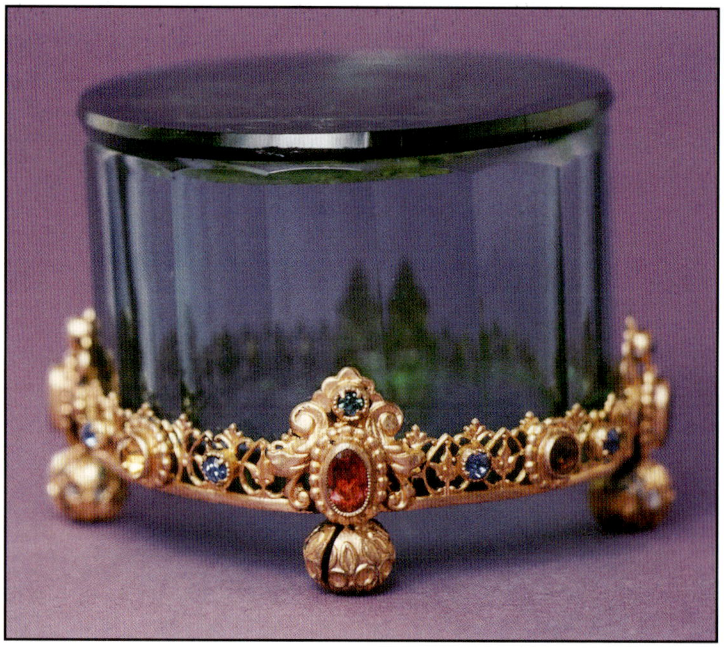

Hoffman box showing jeweled detail.

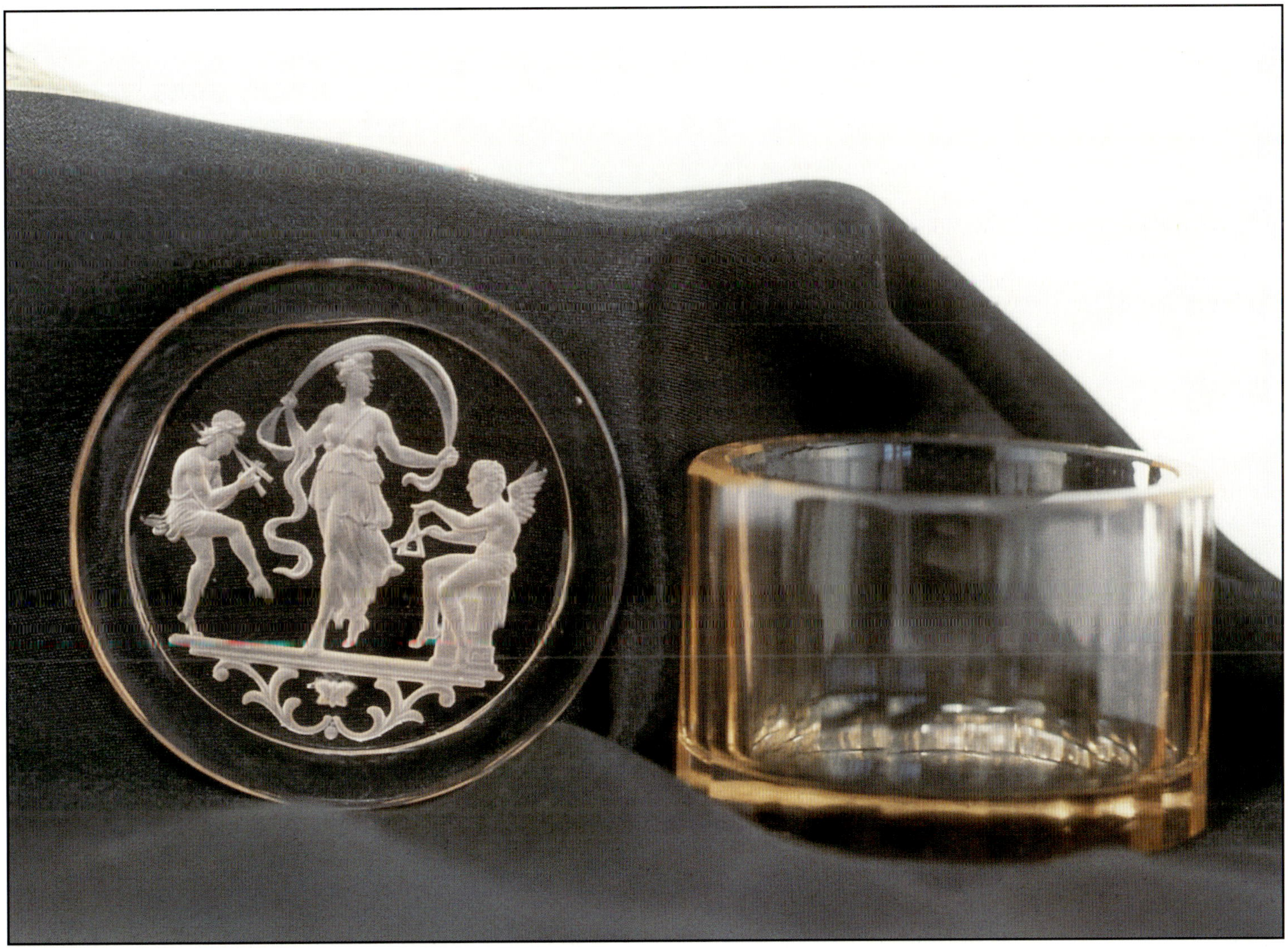

Hoffman box in pink, showing detail of top and Hoffman butterfly mark. 2.375". $200-400.

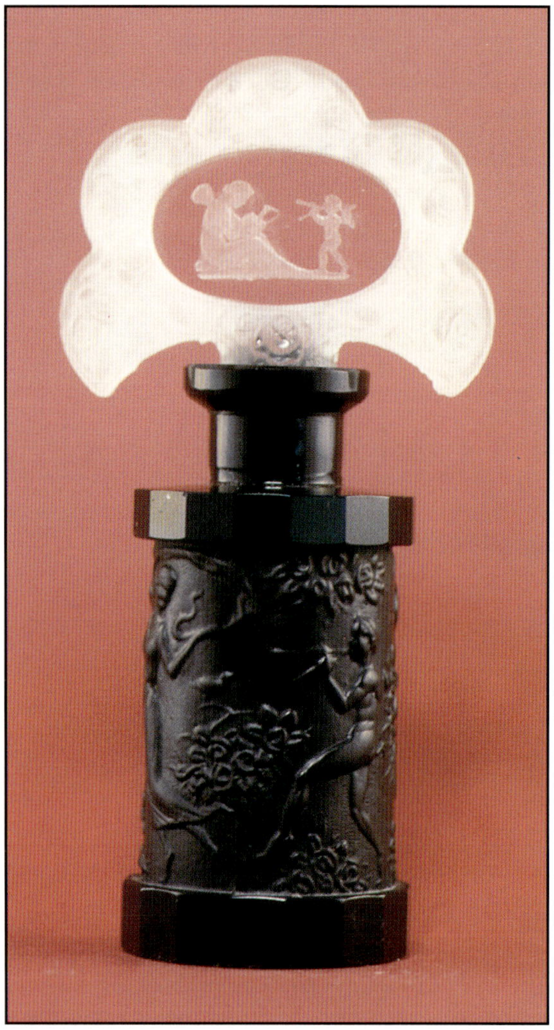

Right:
Hoffman opaque black bottle with classical scene of a piper and three women dancing with scarves. Window in the clear and frosted stopper is filled with an intaglio scene. 4.5". $550-750.

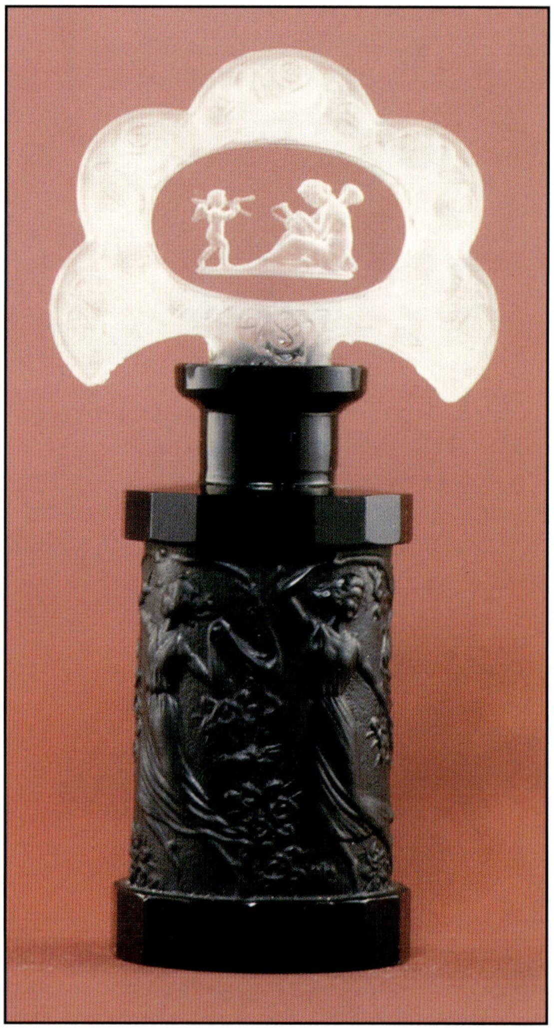

Far right:
Same bottle, showing more of the molded scene. The Hoffman butterfly is seen just in front of the second dancer's foot.

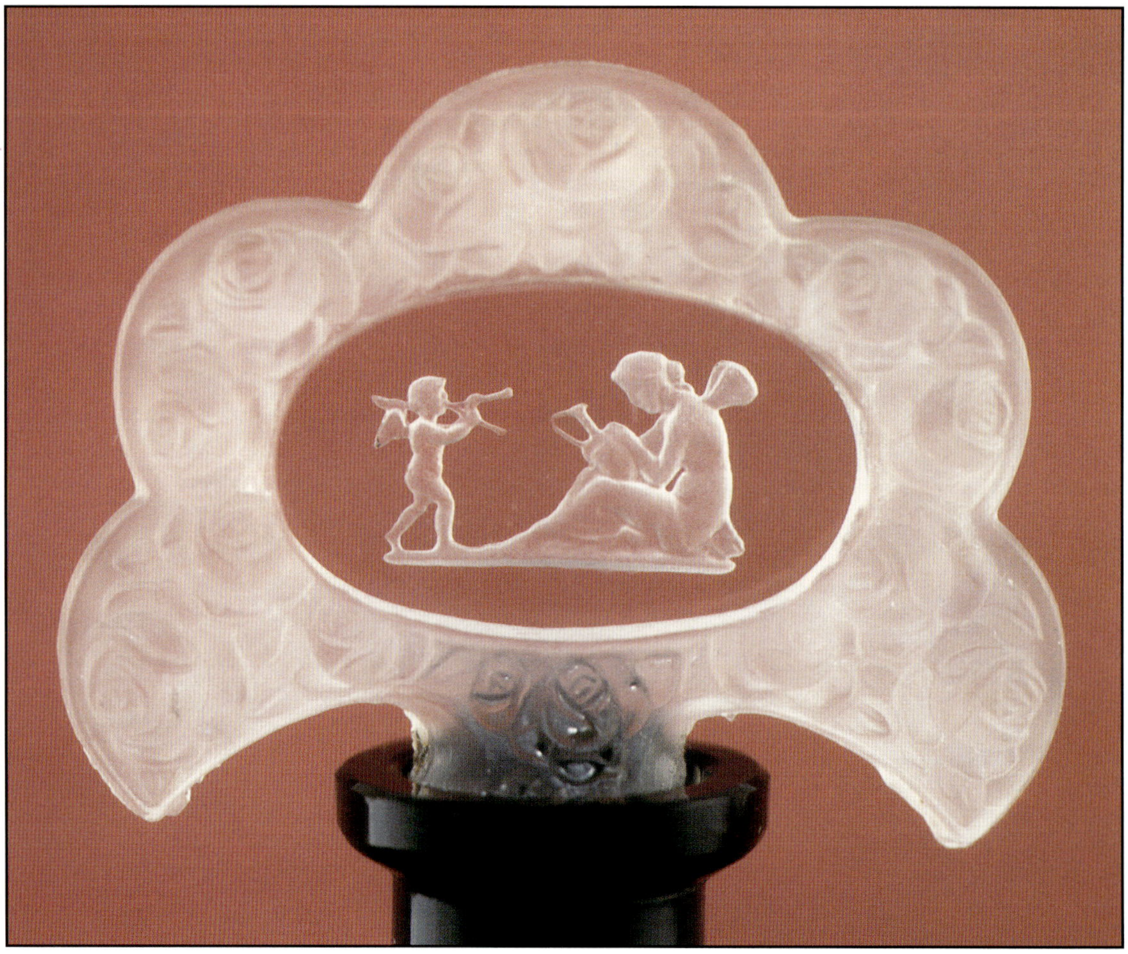

Detail of the stopper, with intaglio scene of a seated nude and a cherub playing pipes. Cloud outline formed of roses.

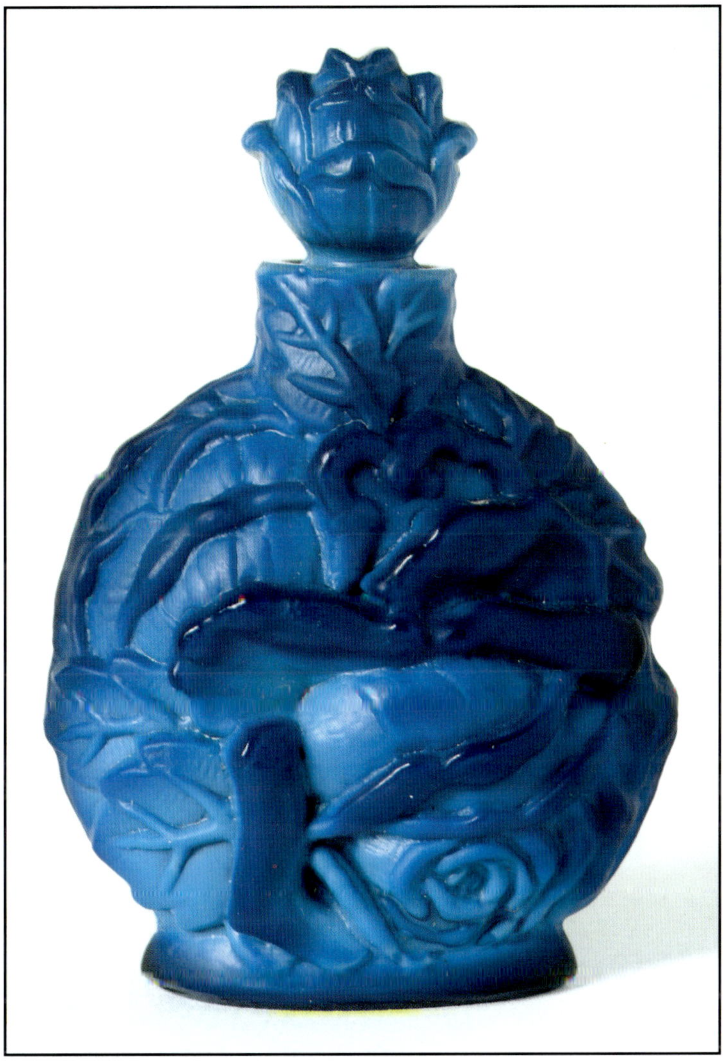

Lapis glass mini bottle with large rose blossoms and leaves molded in high relief. Stopper is rosebud with glass dauber. 2.375". *Courtesy Don Orban. Photo by David Kirk of Kirk Photography*. $175-200.

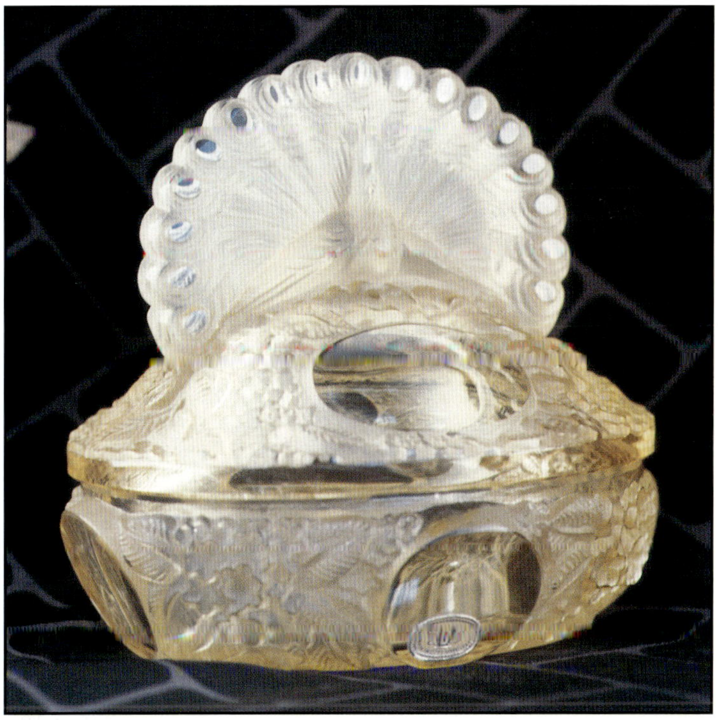

Frosted and cut yellow Ingrid powder box. The spread tail of the peacock forms the handle for the lid. 4.75". $300-500.

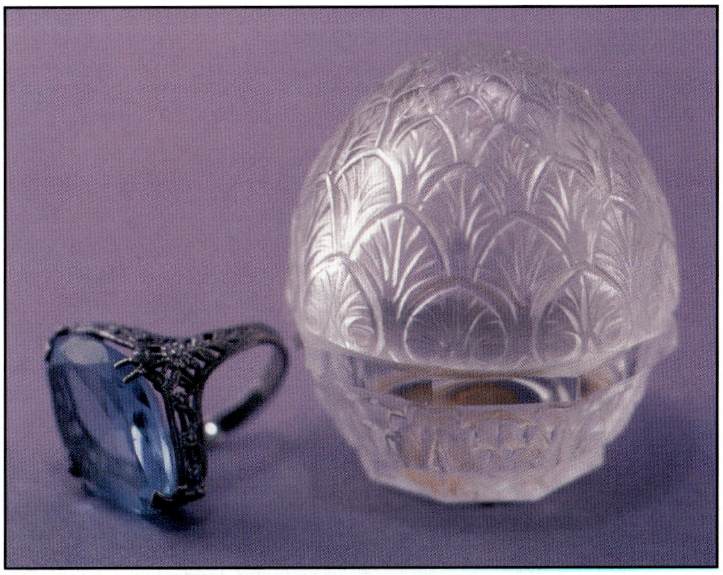

Ingrid ring box with artichoke pattern in the top. 1.75". $300-500. Shown with Czech ring of silver and blue crystal. $40-50.

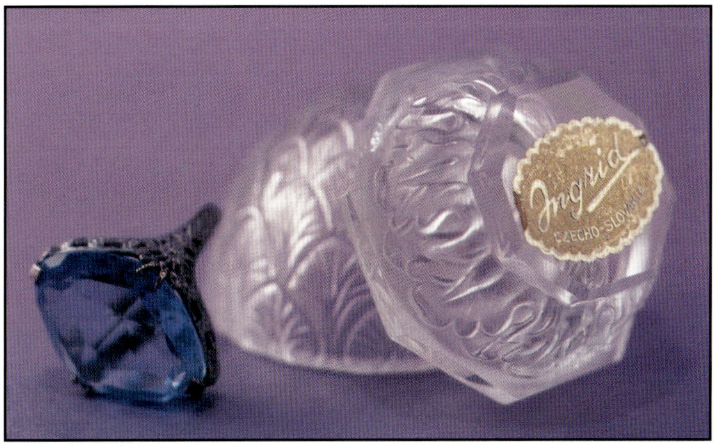

Bottom view of the ring box, showing Ingrid label.

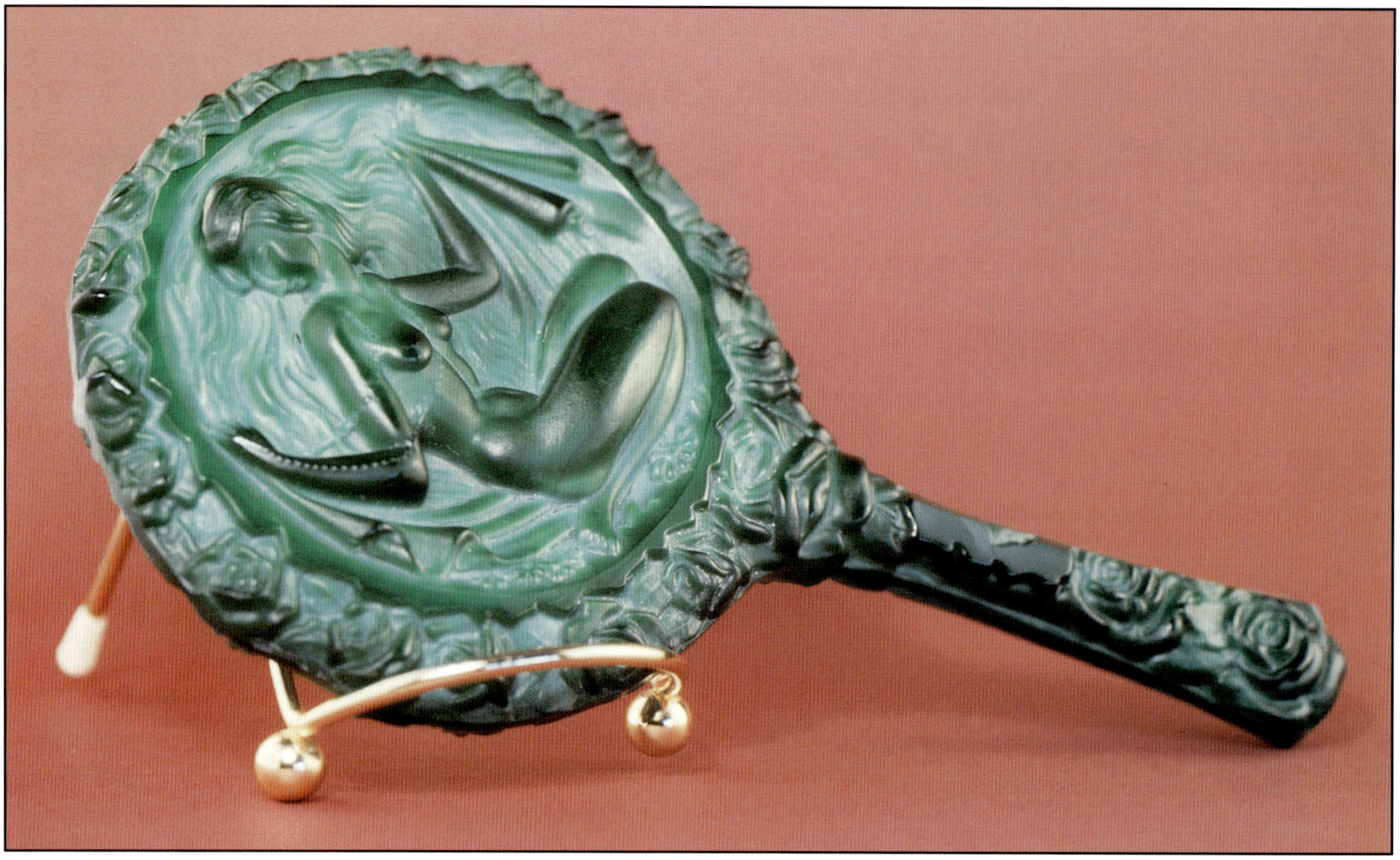

Ingrid malachite glass mirror with sitting nude. Floral edging. 7.25" x 4.125" $300-500.

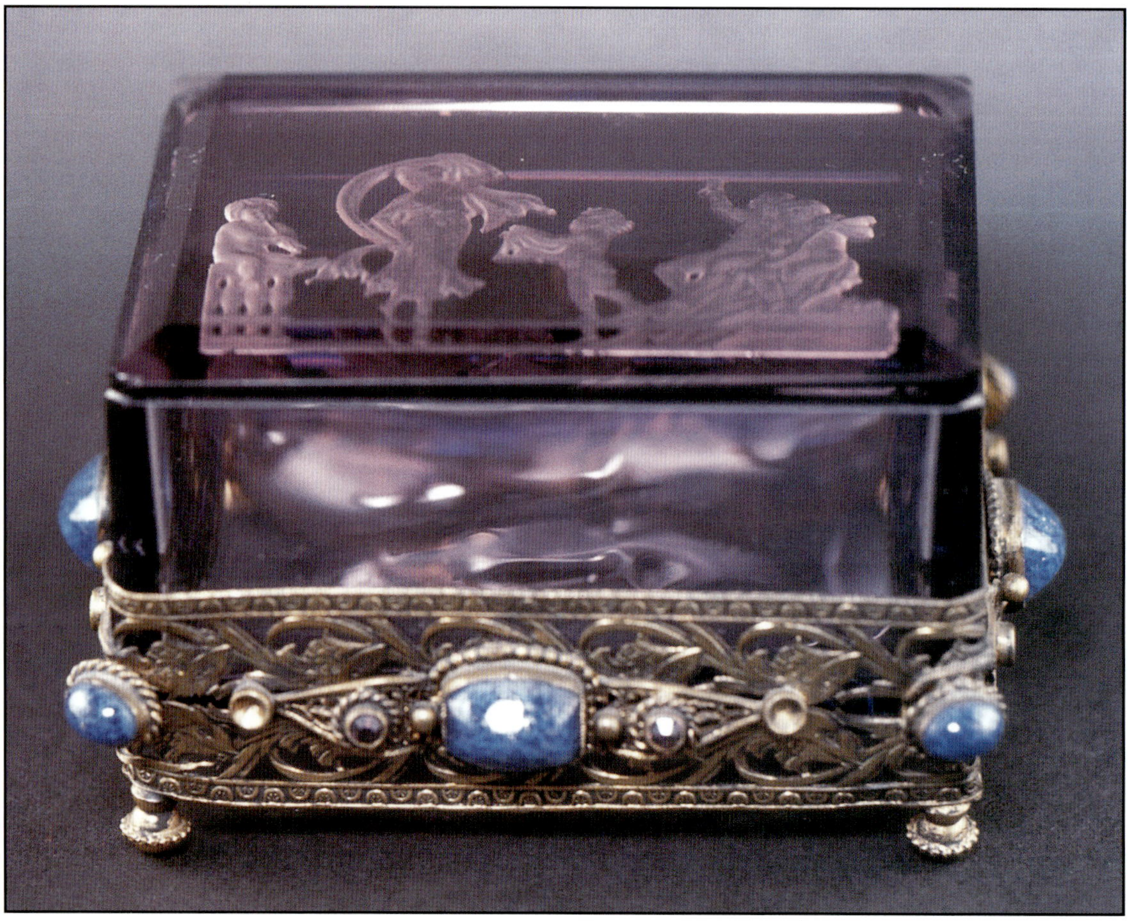

Jeweled amethyst box with cut intaglio top. The scene is of a dancing woman and figures of cherubs and musicians. Unmarked. 2.375" x 3.75". $500-600.

Commercial Czech

Although most Czech perfume bottles were sold empty, some were sold to perfumers, where they were filled, labeled, packaged, and sold commercially. We know about many of the finer quality cut glass, jeweled, or intaglio design bottles from Ken Leach (Leach, 1997, p. 124-127), but we know less about other perfumers who filled Czech bottles.

"Triomphe" appeared with red and green tops and in containers with a range of quality. The red topped bottle shown here is made of cut glass and has an acid mark in the base. The paper label reads: "Parfum Triomphe Compounded in Grasse, France," while the label on the pressed and frosted green topped bottle reads: "Triomphe Parfume, Carrel Ltd. Distributing, Chicago, Illinois." The second bottle is smaller and of lesser quality.

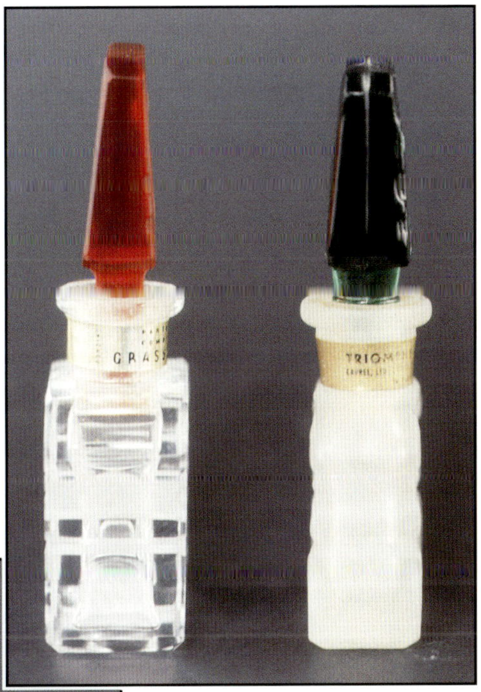

Side view, showing differences in width and finish quality.

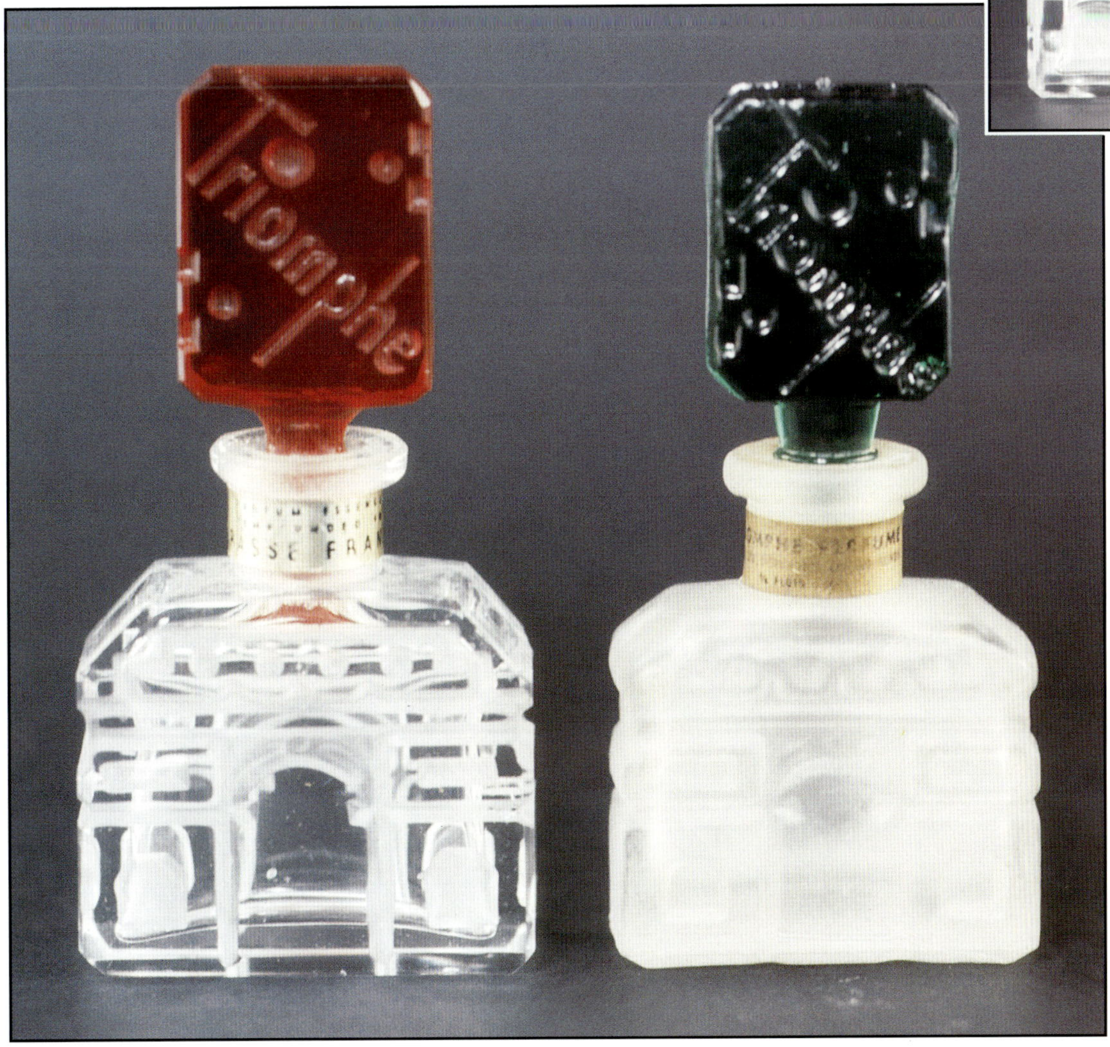

Two Triomphe bottles. Left: Cut glass with cut red top and frosted detail, paper label and acid mark. 2.875". $150-200. Right: Pressed frosted bottle with label and green pressed top. 2.75". $125-175.

Juerelle used Czech bottles with some perfumes, as did de Raymond. One of the pictures below shows three tiny purple crystal cube bottles that were sold empty, along with a boxed de Jonge set of floral scents and a red-capped Charvai "Lilac" that all are startlingly similar.

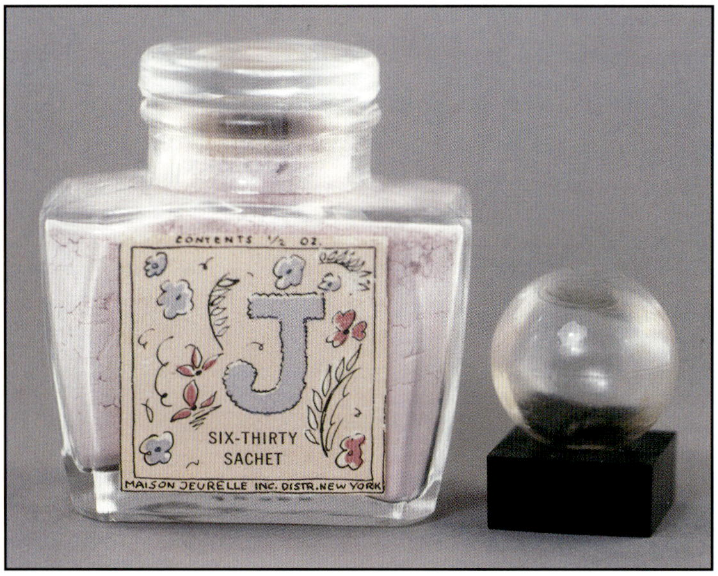

Two Juerelle products. Left: "Six-Thirty Sachet." 2.375". Right: Maison Juerelle "Le Secret." 1.25". Juerelle used finer cut glass bottles with the perfumer's name cut into the stopper.

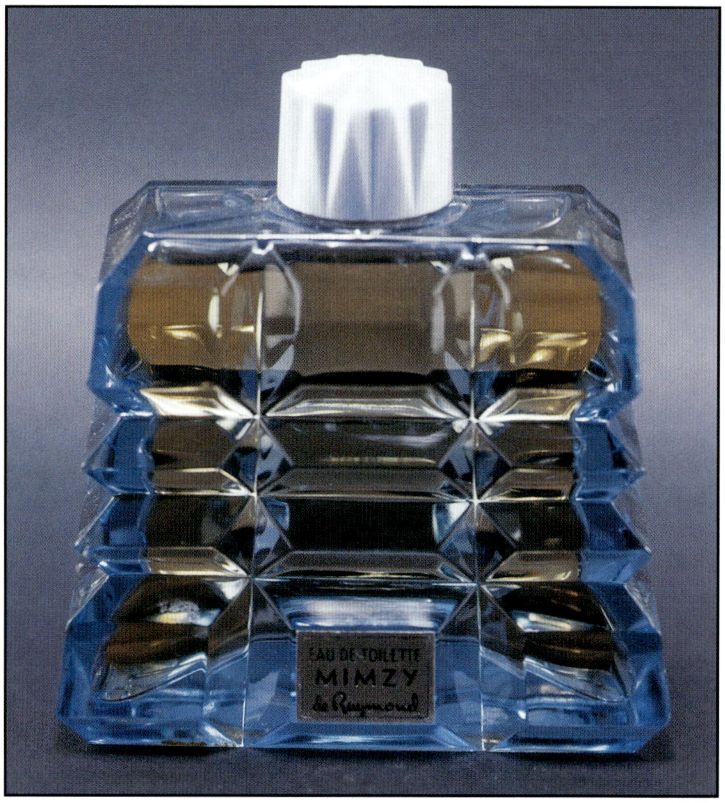

This pressed glass bottle with a white plastic cap held "Mimsy" for de Raymond. 3.875". $35-55.

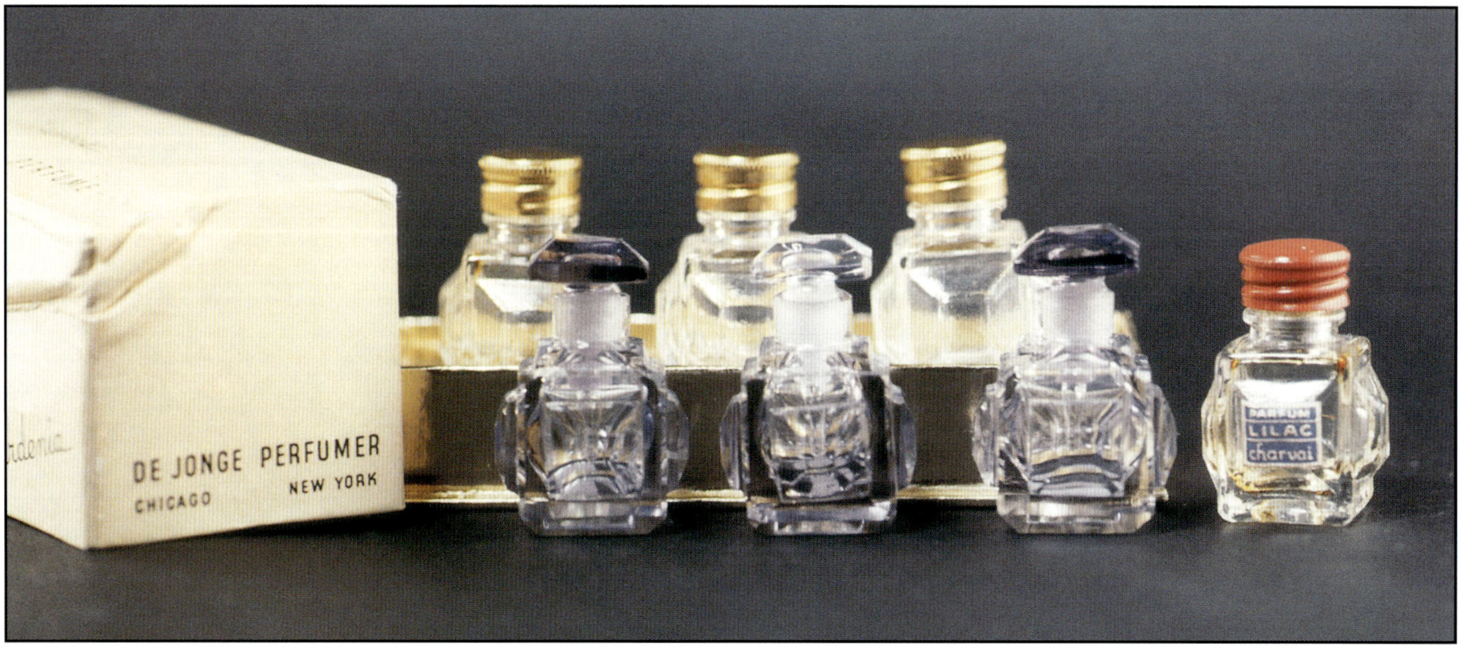

Three cut glass dresser minis shown with similar commercial pressed bottles—a boxed trio of floral scents by de Jonge Perfumer and a red capped bottle from the same mold, "Lilac," by Charvai. 1.375". $10-55.

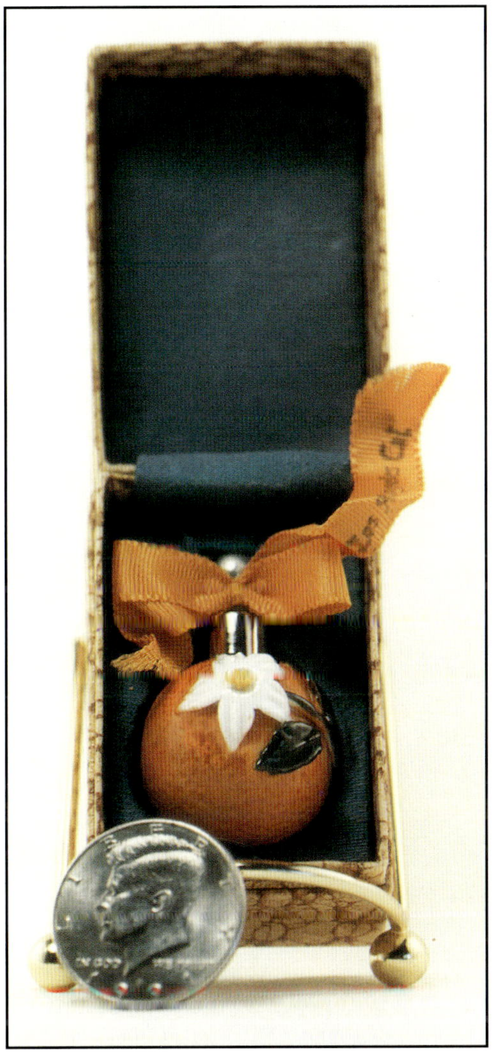

This Czech blown bottle with applied glass decoration and a mercury dauber bears a decorative ribbon that reads, "Los Angeles." 2". $150-200.

Bottles were also produced for the tourist trade, like the orange bottle pictured here in its box. Though the box and bottle are marked Czechoslovakia, the ribbon at the neck of the bottle reads "Los Angeles." The bottle was probably filled with a locally produced orange blossom perfume.

Perfumers who used Czech bottles for some of their scents included Baldwin (Otesa), Charmante (Helen of Troy), Duvelle (Le Gui-Mistletoe), F. Wolfe & Sohn (Velchen), and Weil (Zibiline). Dralle, a German company, packaged perfumes in some caged purse bottles. It is possible to find these occasionally, still in their boxes. Tiny glass perfume bottles from Czechoslovakia also were used on bracelets or were used by various perfumers for sample sizes.

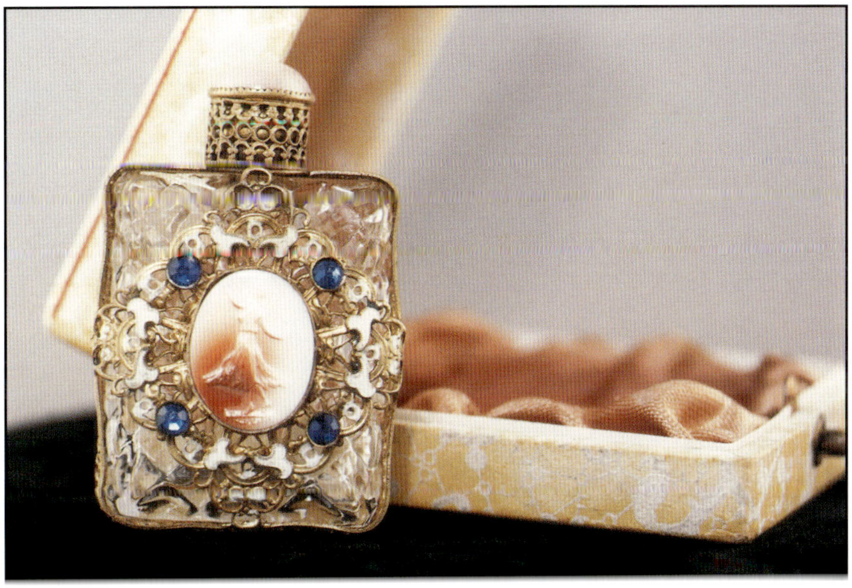

A typical presentation for Dralle perfumes, Hamburg, Germany.

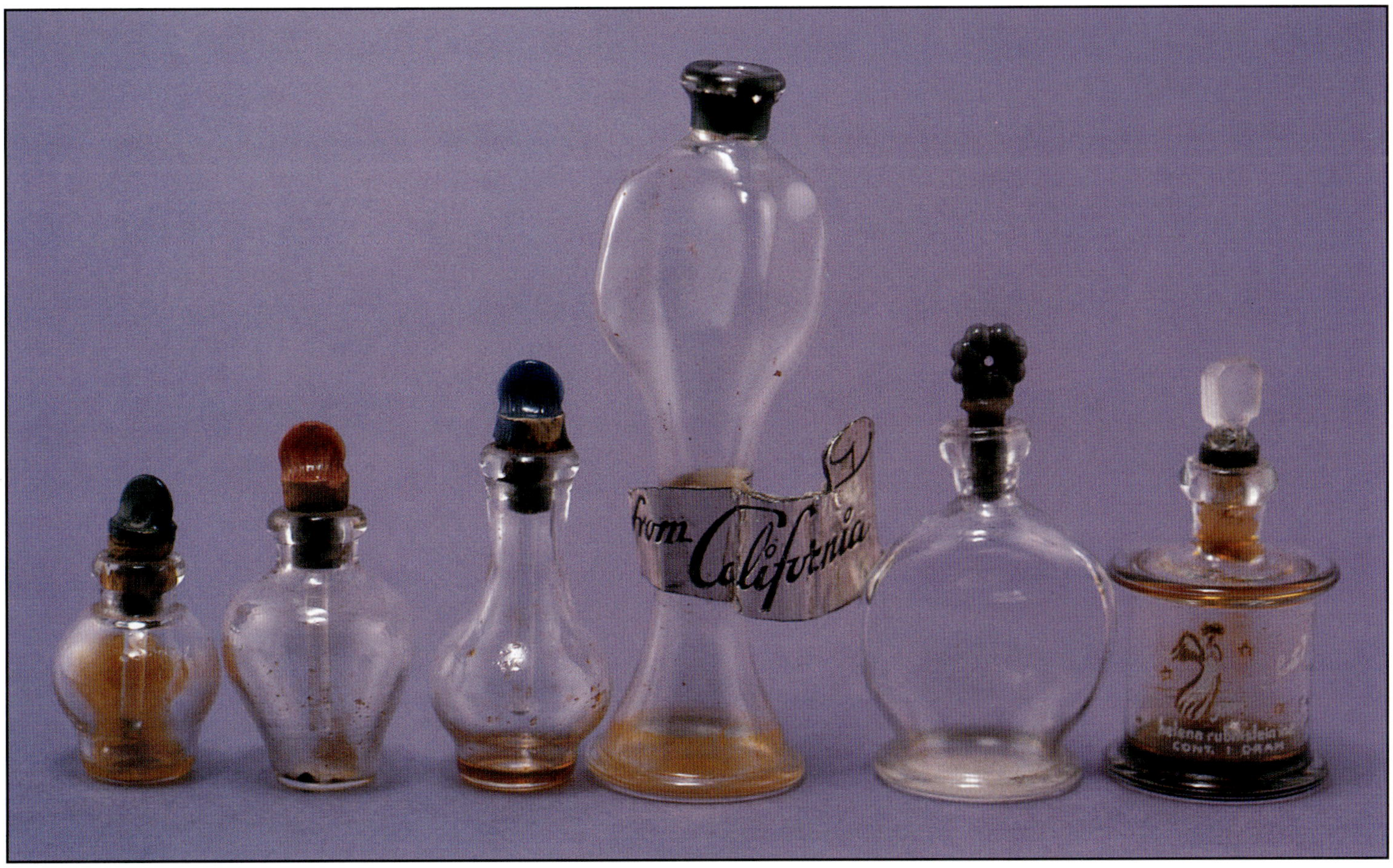

A grouping of tiny blown bottles used to decorate bracelets or as sample bottles. On the far right is a sample for Helena Rubenstein's "Heaven Sent." Sizes range from 1.125" to 2.75". Heaven Sent, $100-200; others, under $50.

Corday used intaglio glass tops for their perfume solids for Toujours Moi and Fame. Though not marked Czechoslovakia, the assumption that the intaglio portion is Czech would certainly be defensible. The three pictured are various scenes of cupid and a woman. The scene in the green solid includes what appears to be the Hoffman butterfly. The blackface solid container is made of plastic, but is marked Czechoslovakia in the bottom.

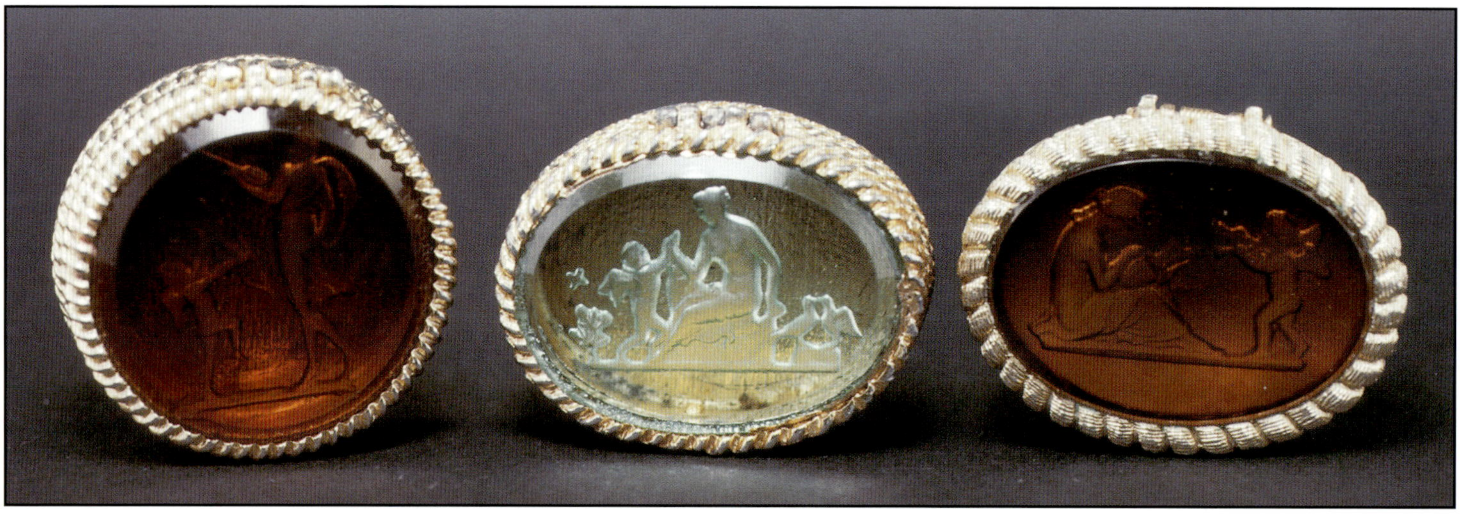

Solid scent boxes. The right and left were used by Corday for "Fame" and "Toujours Moi." Center, green intaglio, is unmarked. Round, 1.5". Oblong, 1.625". $50-100 each.

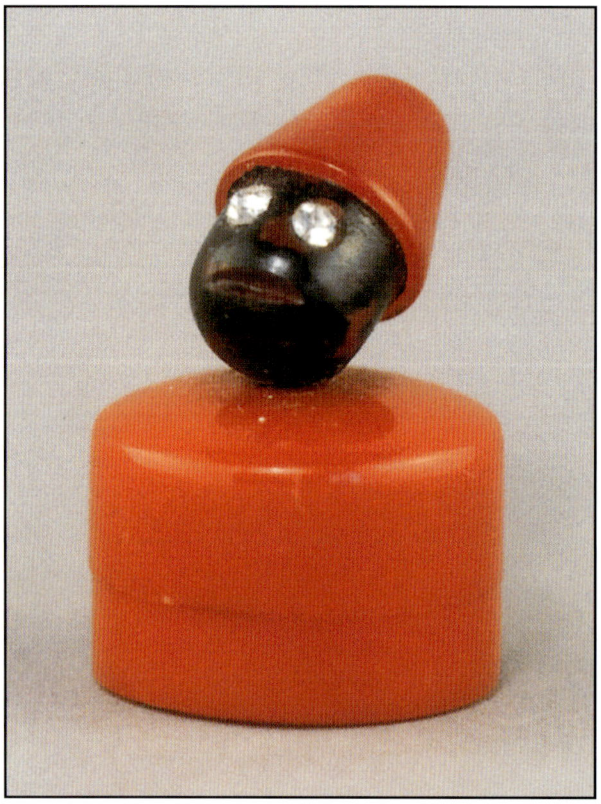

Blackface perfume solid for an unknown scent. The container is red plastic, marked. 1.125". $75-100.

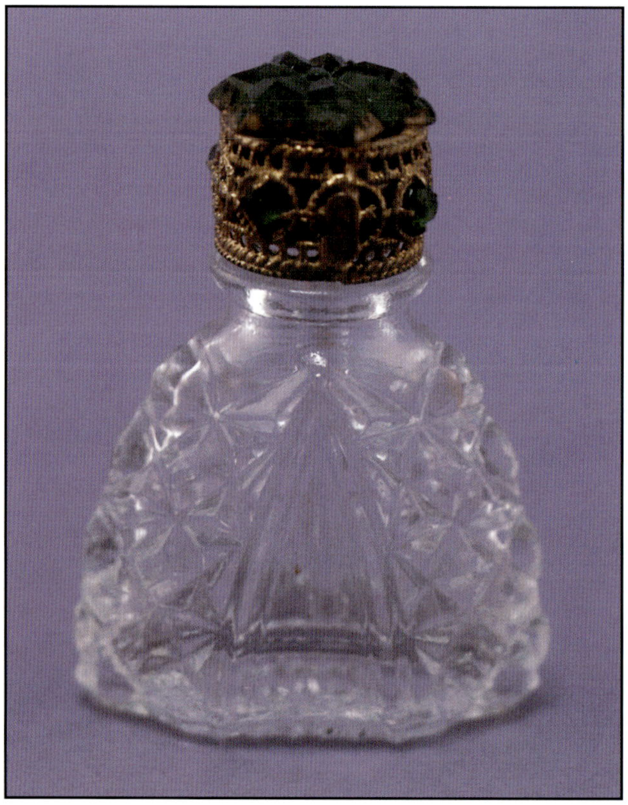

Small pressed purse bottle with a green flat flower cap had a smooth area in the center front for the label of an unknown perfumer. 1.875". $75-100.

Glassexports

In the West, little was known of Czechoslovakian glass production after the industry nationalized in the late 1940s. Recently, with the opening of the country to the West, information is emerging about an industry that many thought had been a casualty of World War II and its aftermath. A hardbound product catalog entitled No. I *Glassexport, Section 14, Praha, Czechoslovakia* shows that a variety of glass products were sold in the late 1940s and early '50s. This catalog shows many glass kitchen and table accessories such as salt and pepper shakers, cruets, liquor decanter sets with glasses, bridge sets, candy dishes, trinket boxes, ashtrays, and open salts with intaglio designs. It also features perfume bottles and dresser sets, including bottles, powder boxes, atomizers, and trays.

The catalog is printed in black and white, and has no date or text other than the item numbers. It appears that the glass was available in clear only. Some items appear to have been pressed glass, and not cut. Though a "hands on" examination might well show that and other differences between the finish detailing of these bottles and those produced prior to World War II, the fact remains that some of the popular designs were being manufactured into the next decade and possibly longer.

A selection of pages from the catalog is reproduced here. These pages show some of the traditional figural and other designs. Many of the styles are heavier and less ornate, which could have signaled a change in taste, a need to produce items with less time-consuming handwork, a lack of skilled workers in the trade, or all of the above.

Shown just before the catalog pages are two bottles similar in style to items in the catalog. These are not marked.

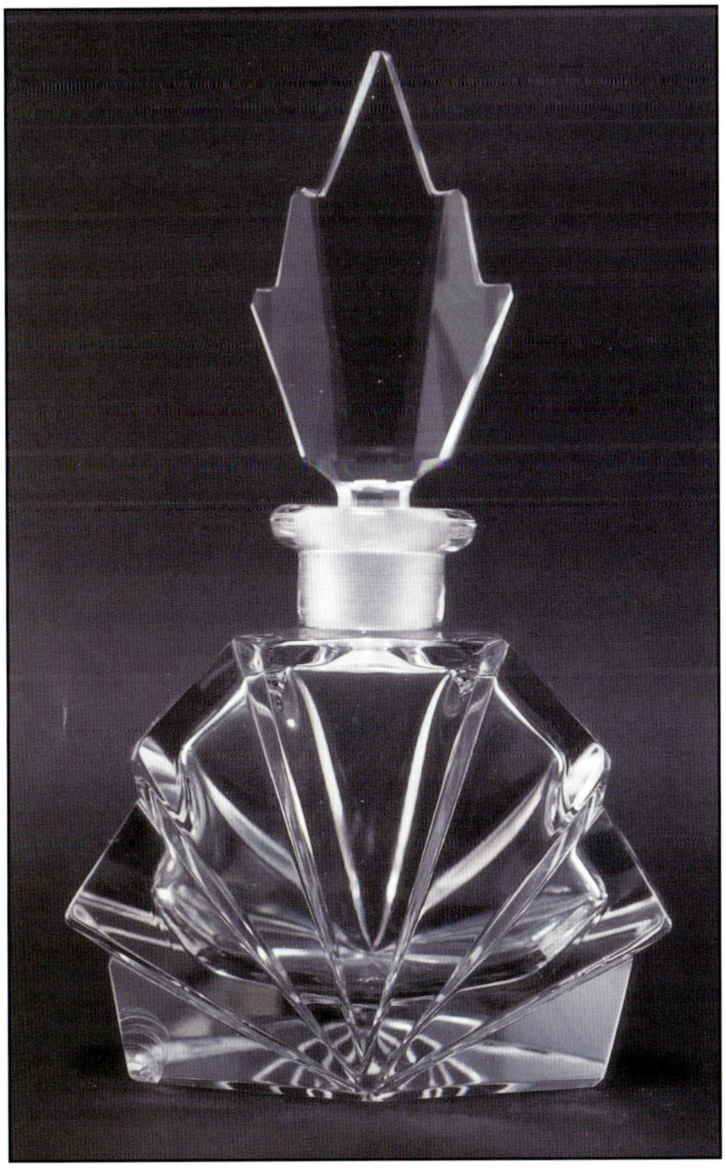

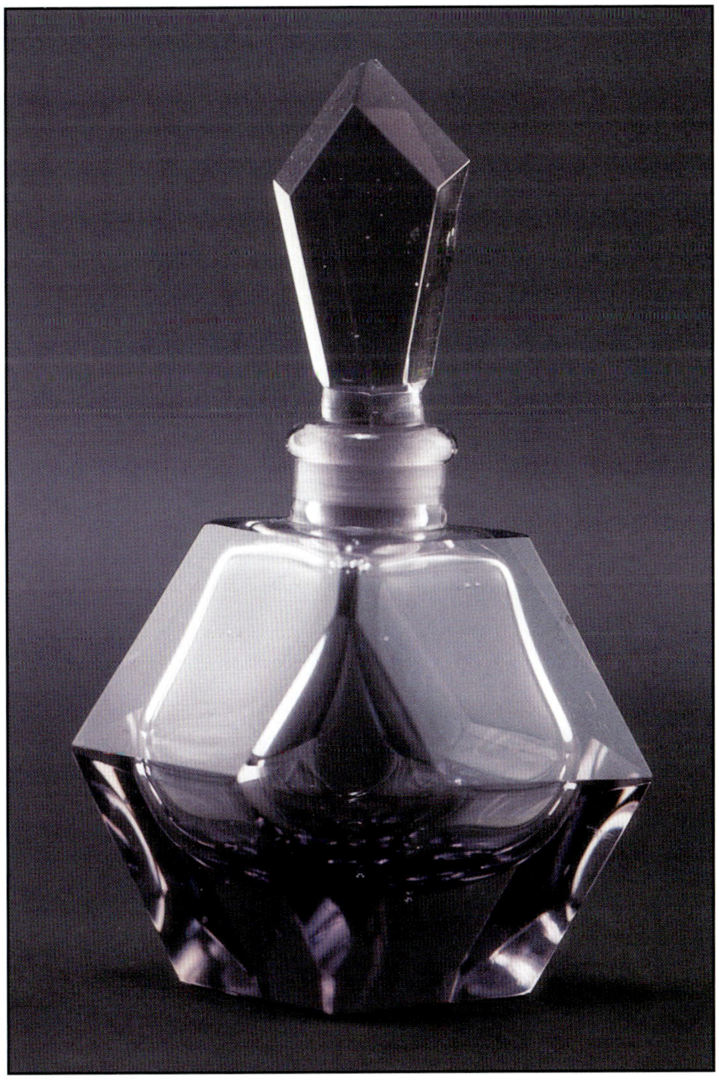

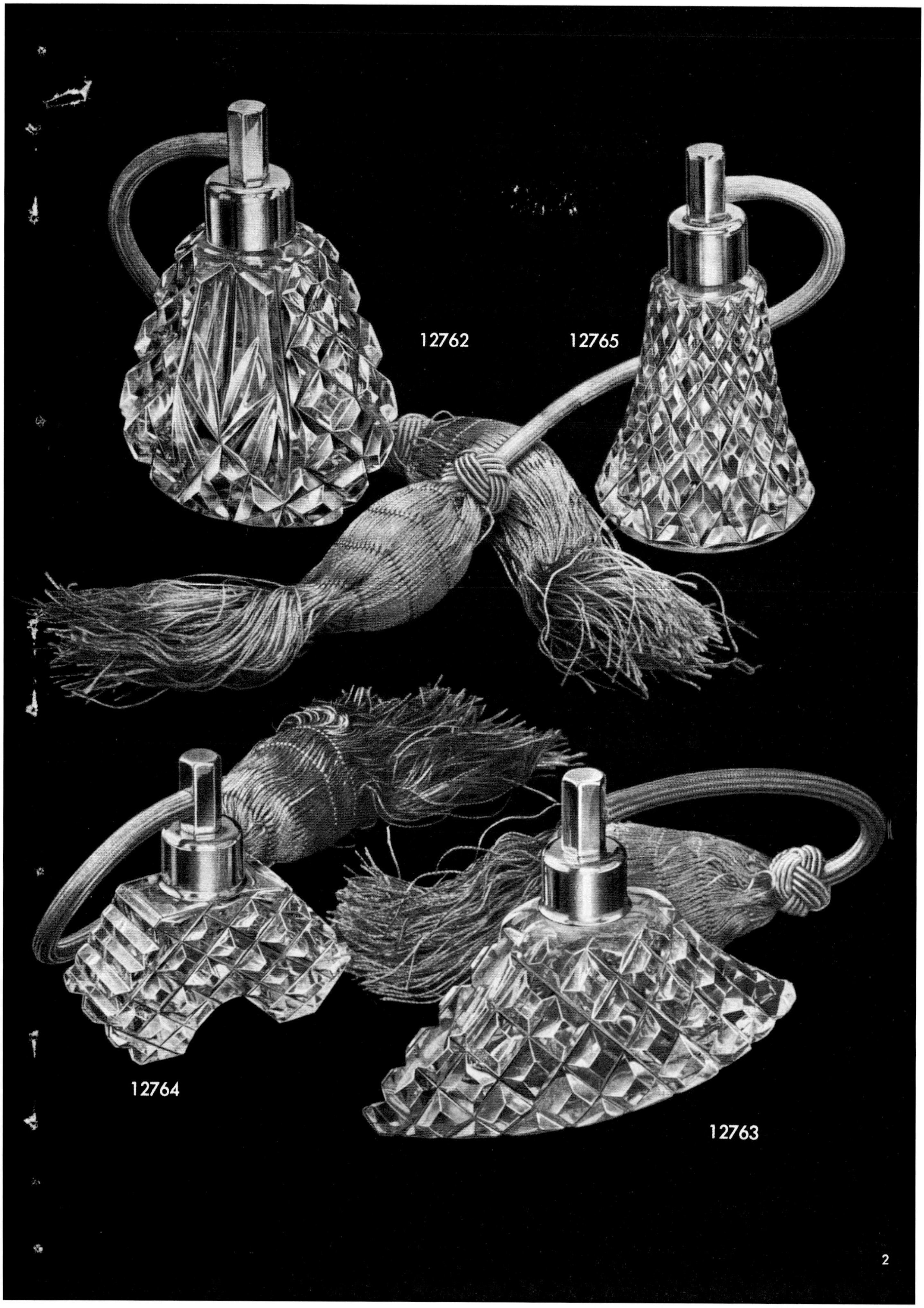
12762
12765
12764
12763
2

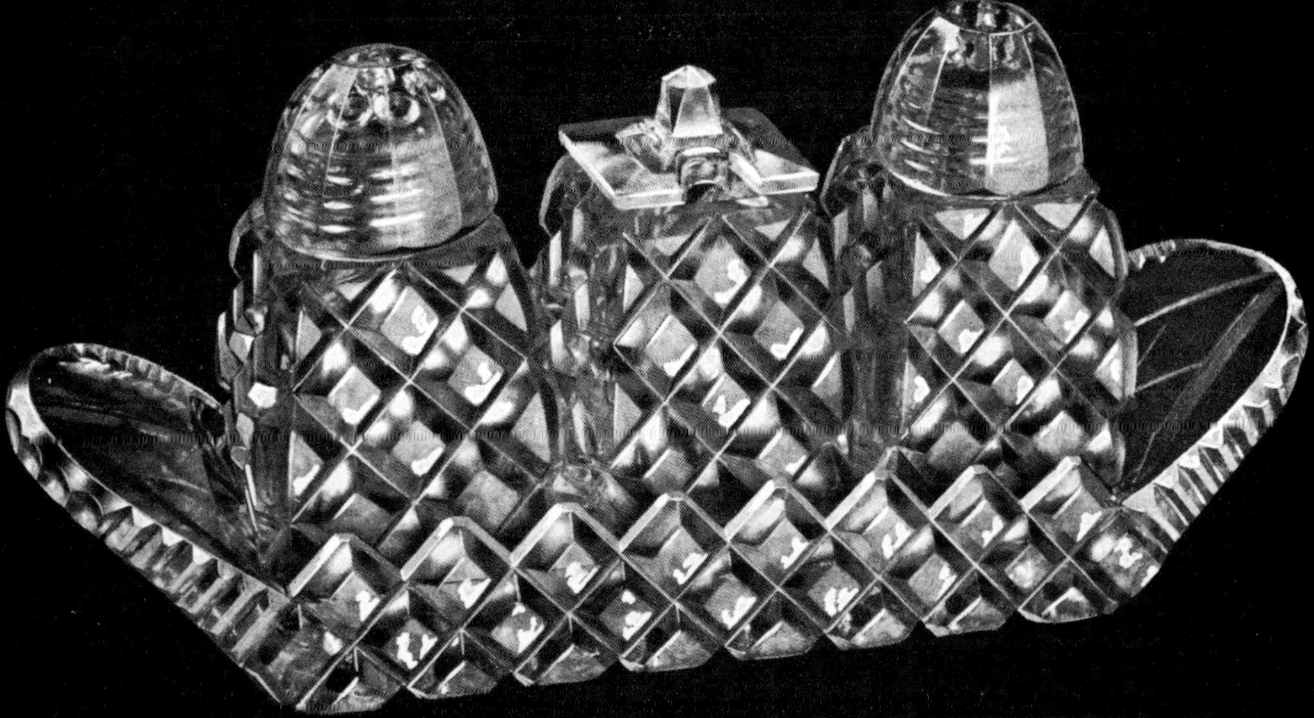

40152

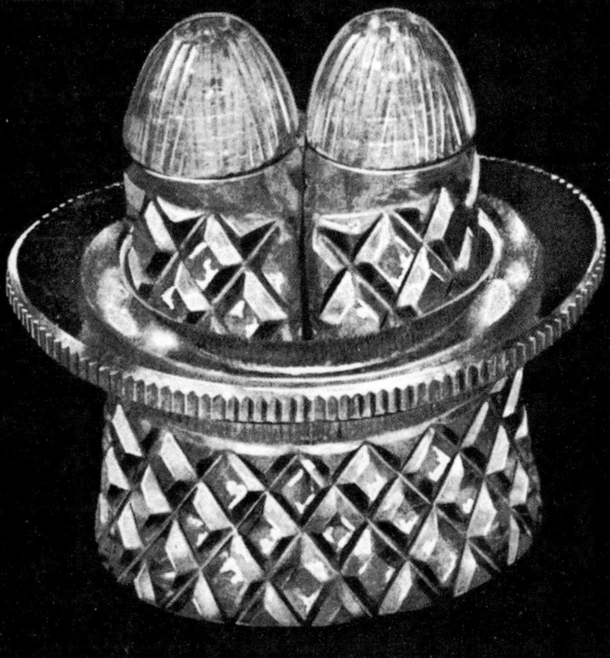

40177

14

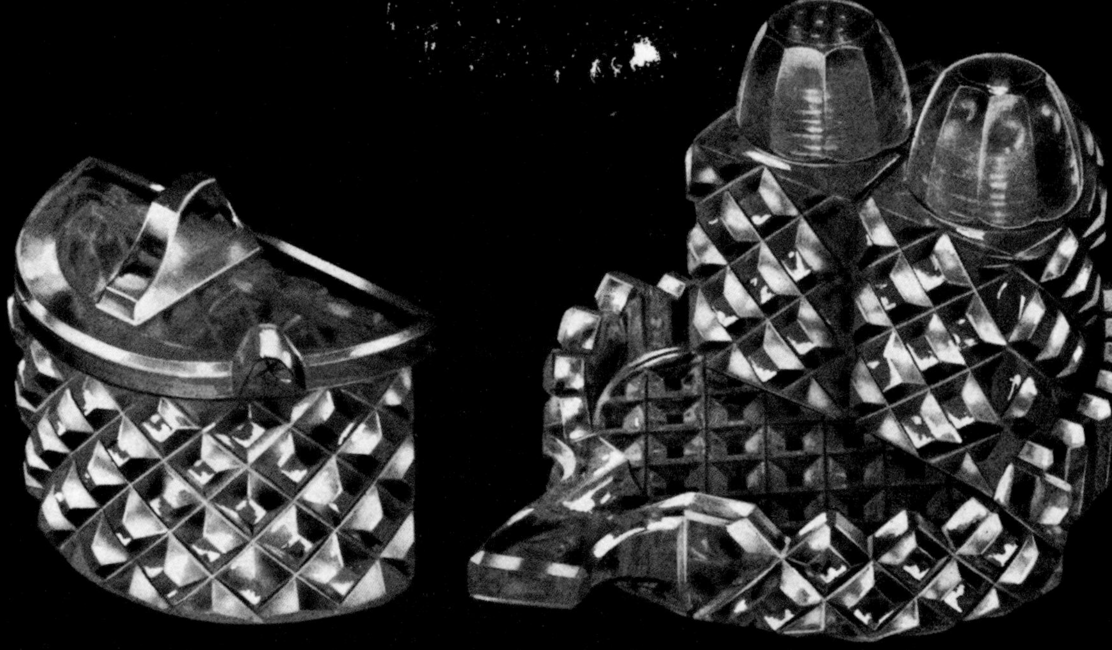

41032

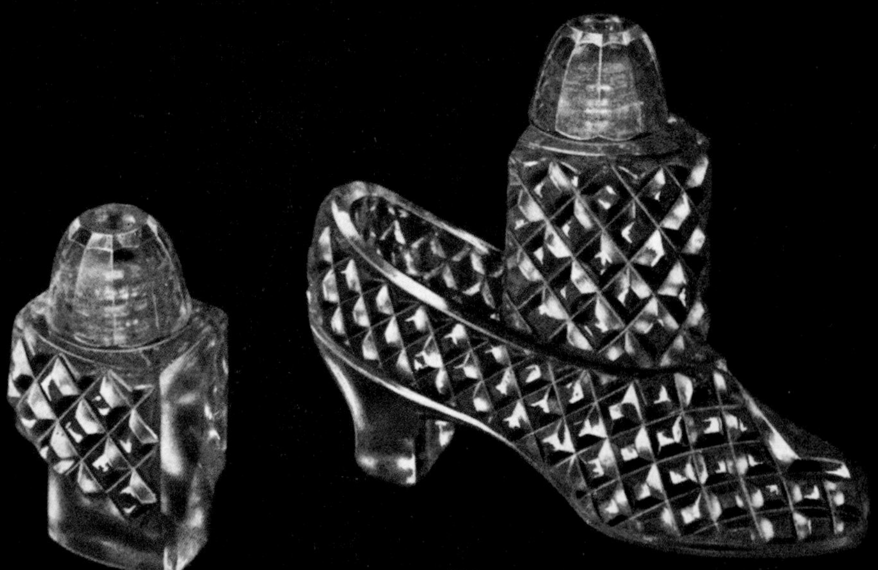

40225

15

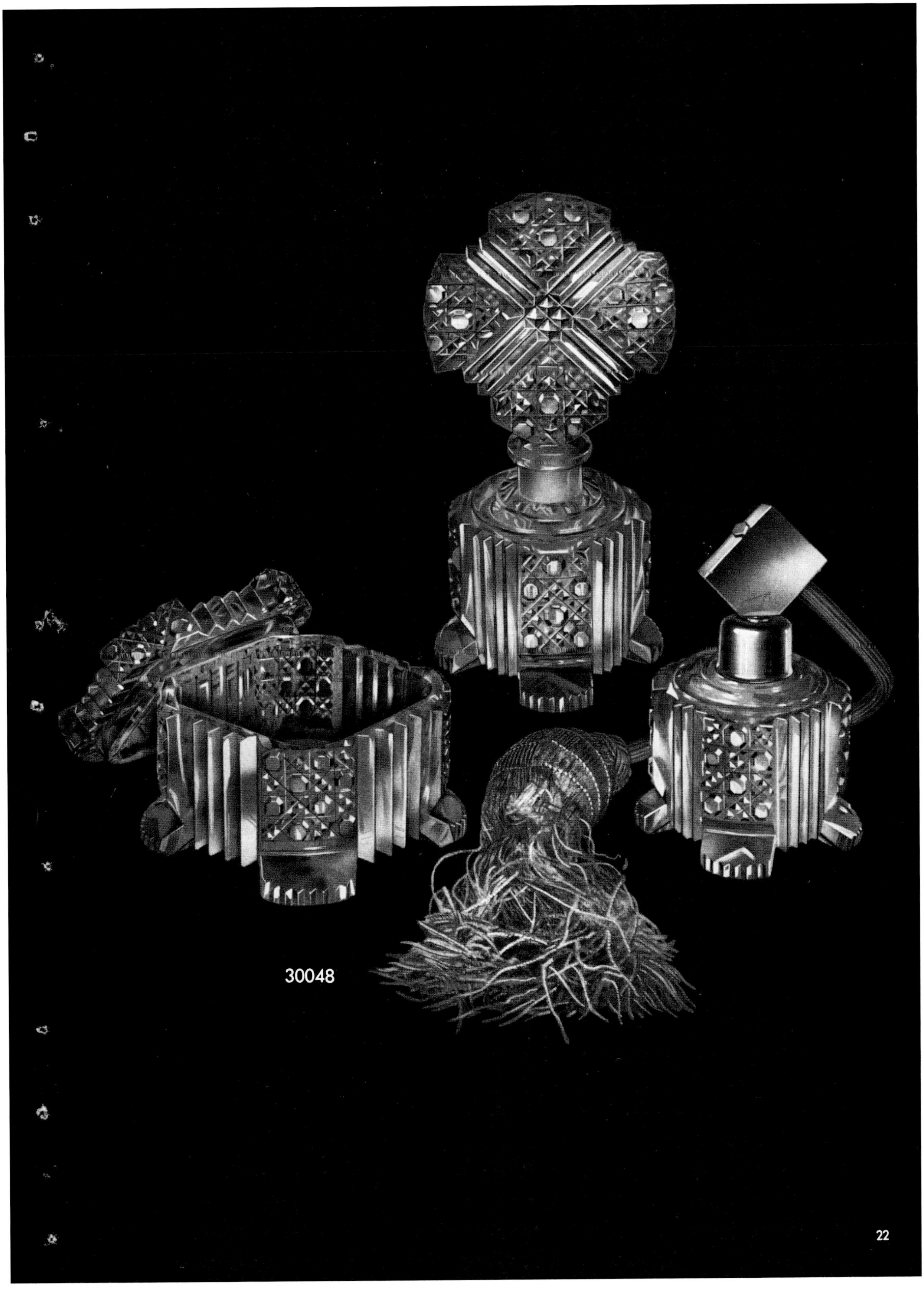

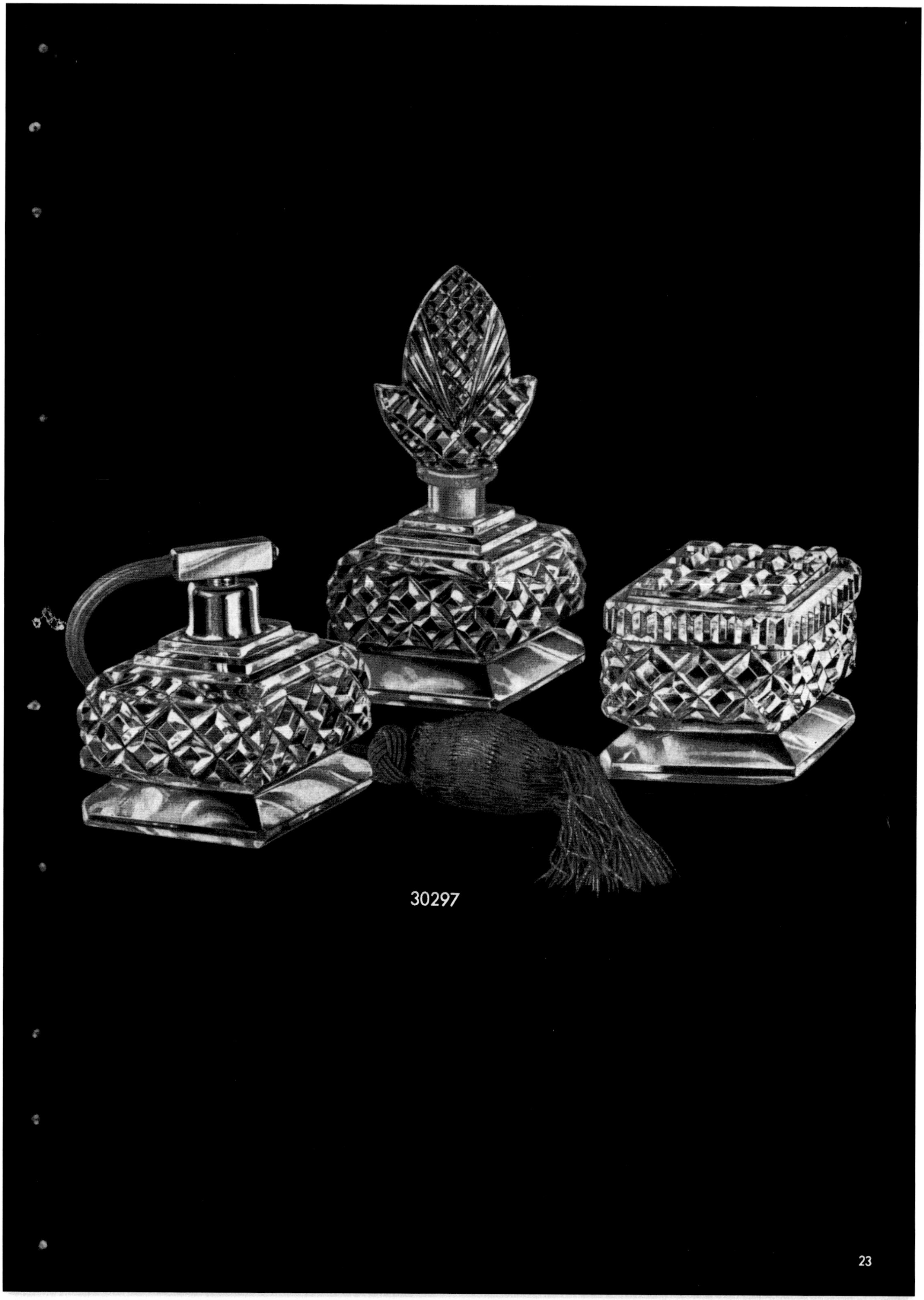

30297

23

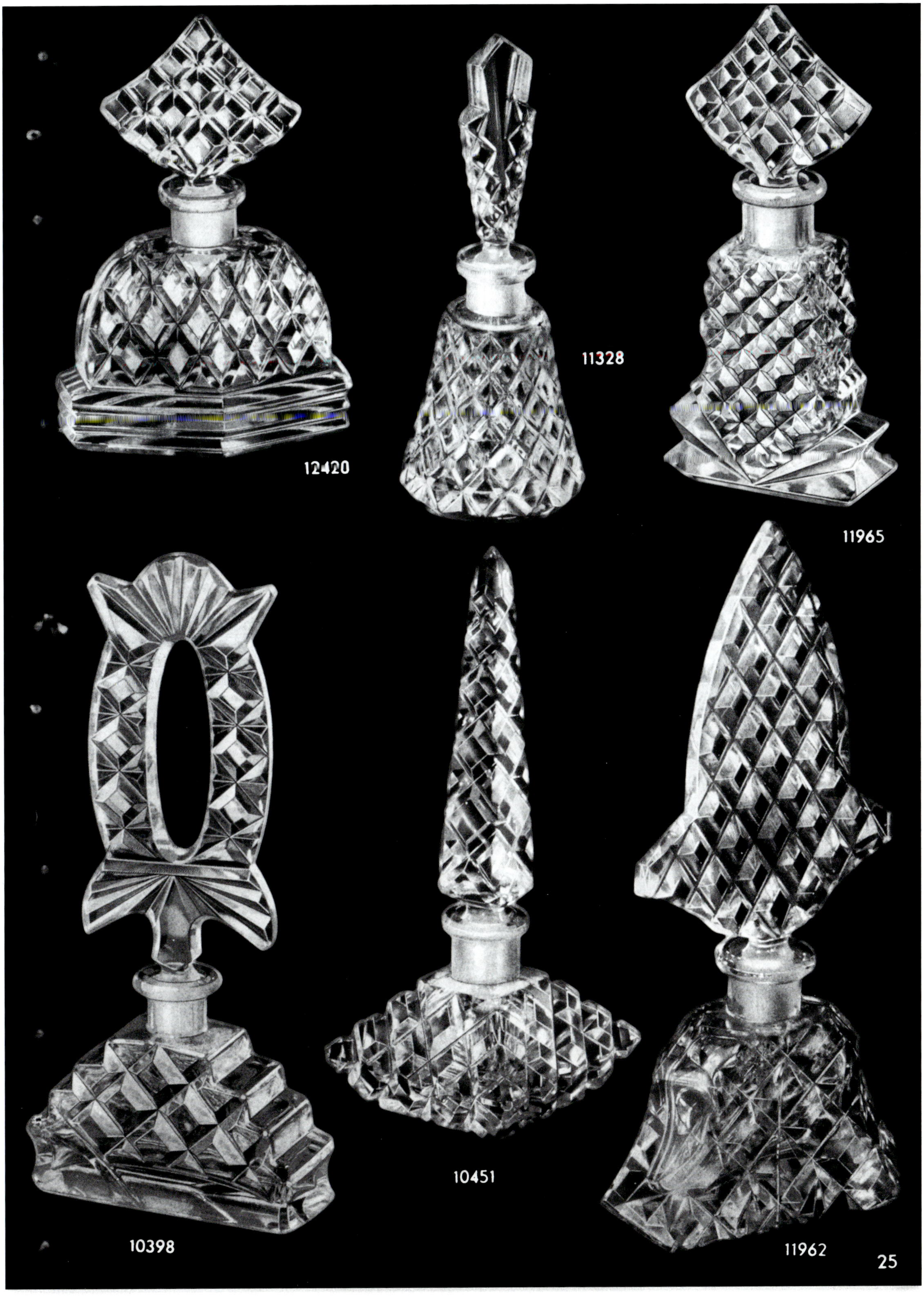
11328
12420
11965
10451
10398
11962
25

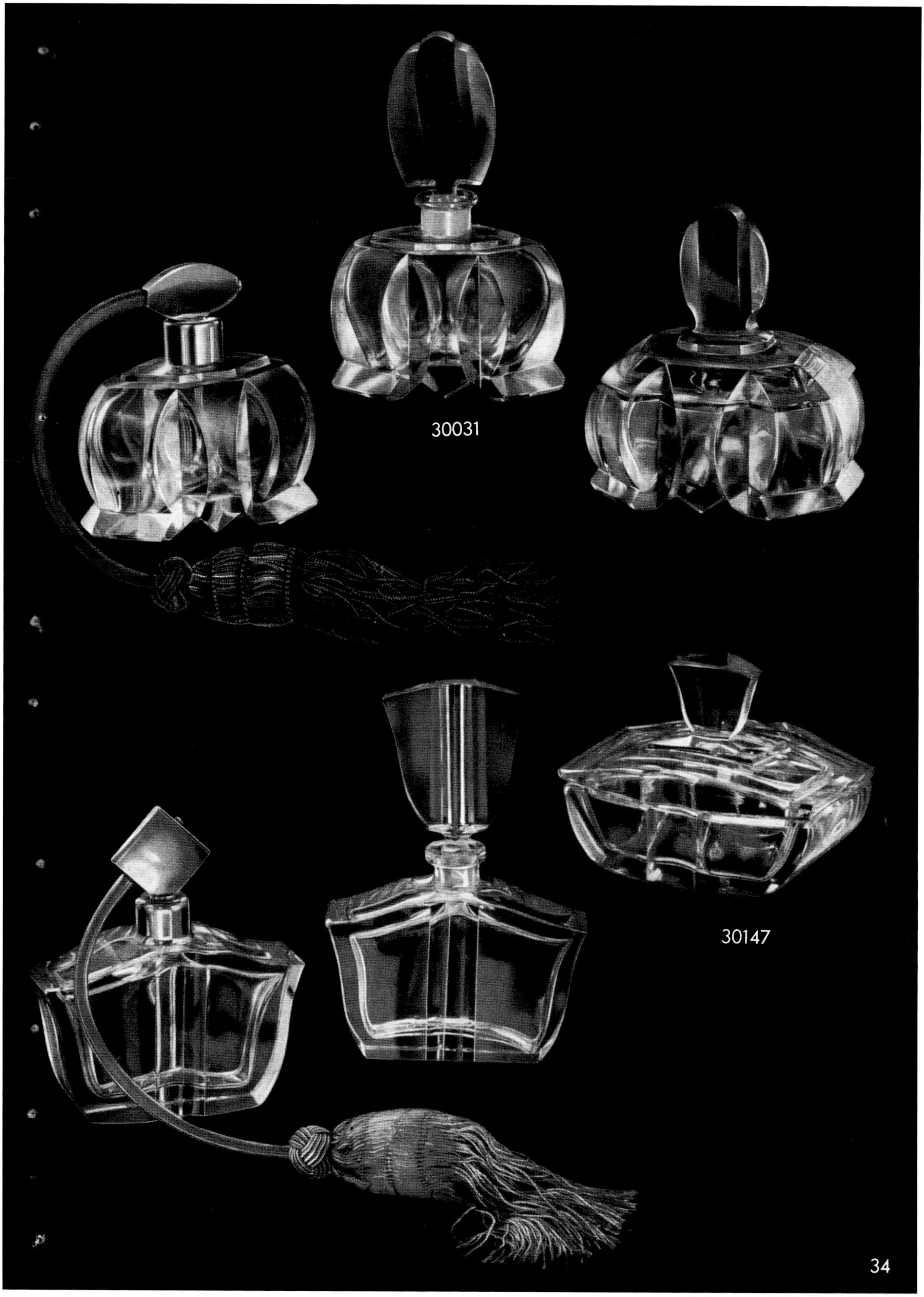
30031
30147
34

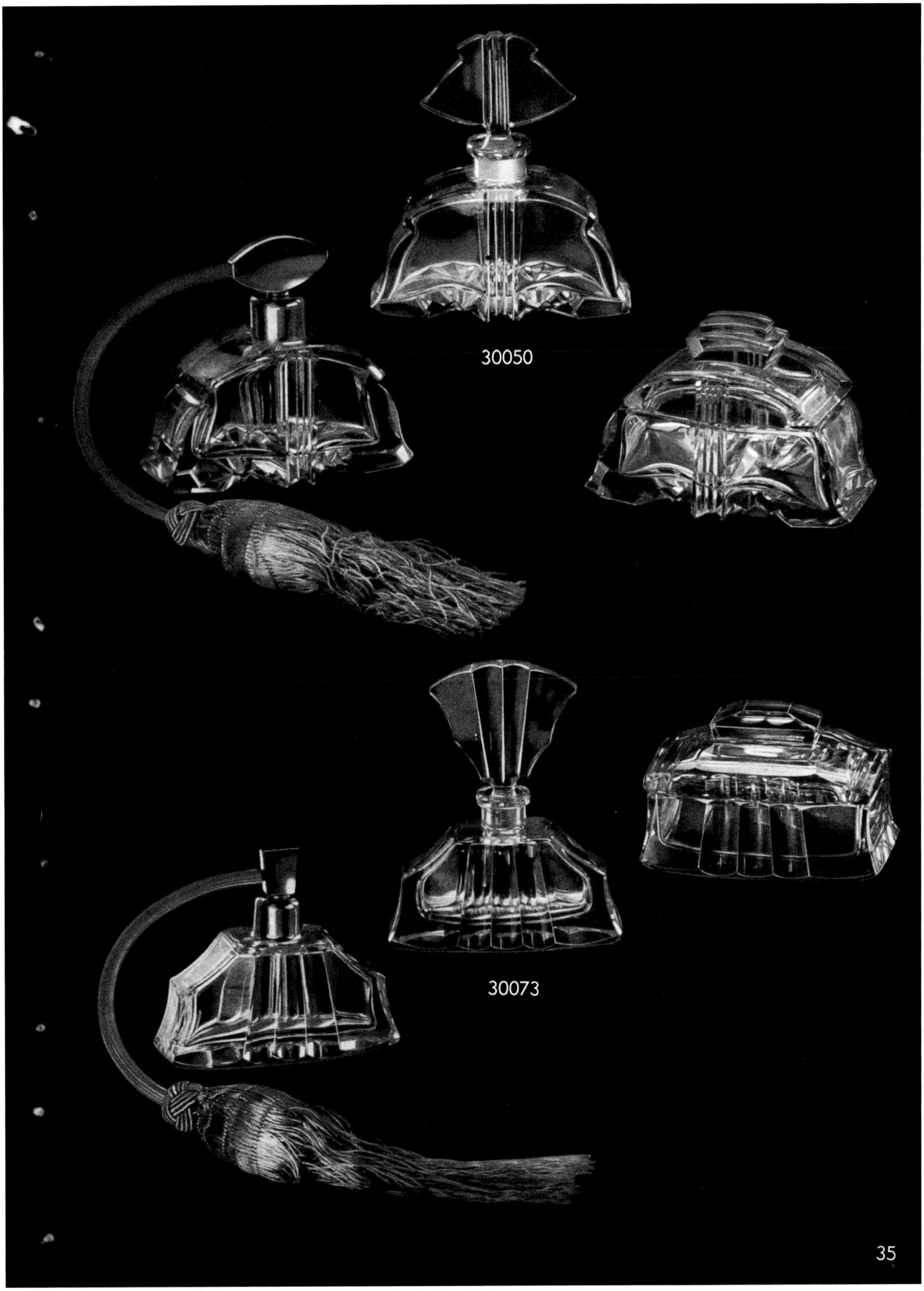

30050

30073

35

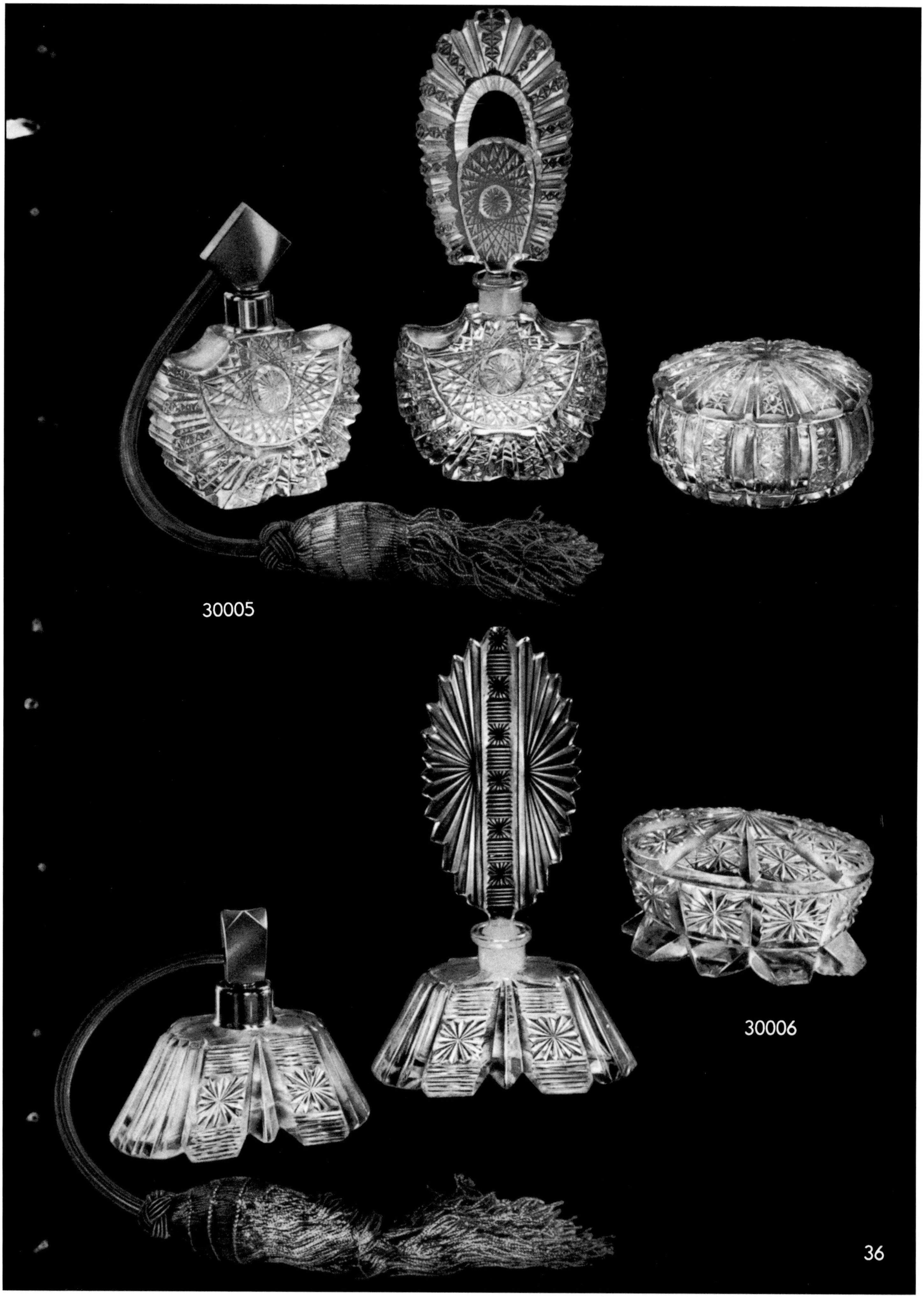
30005
30006
36

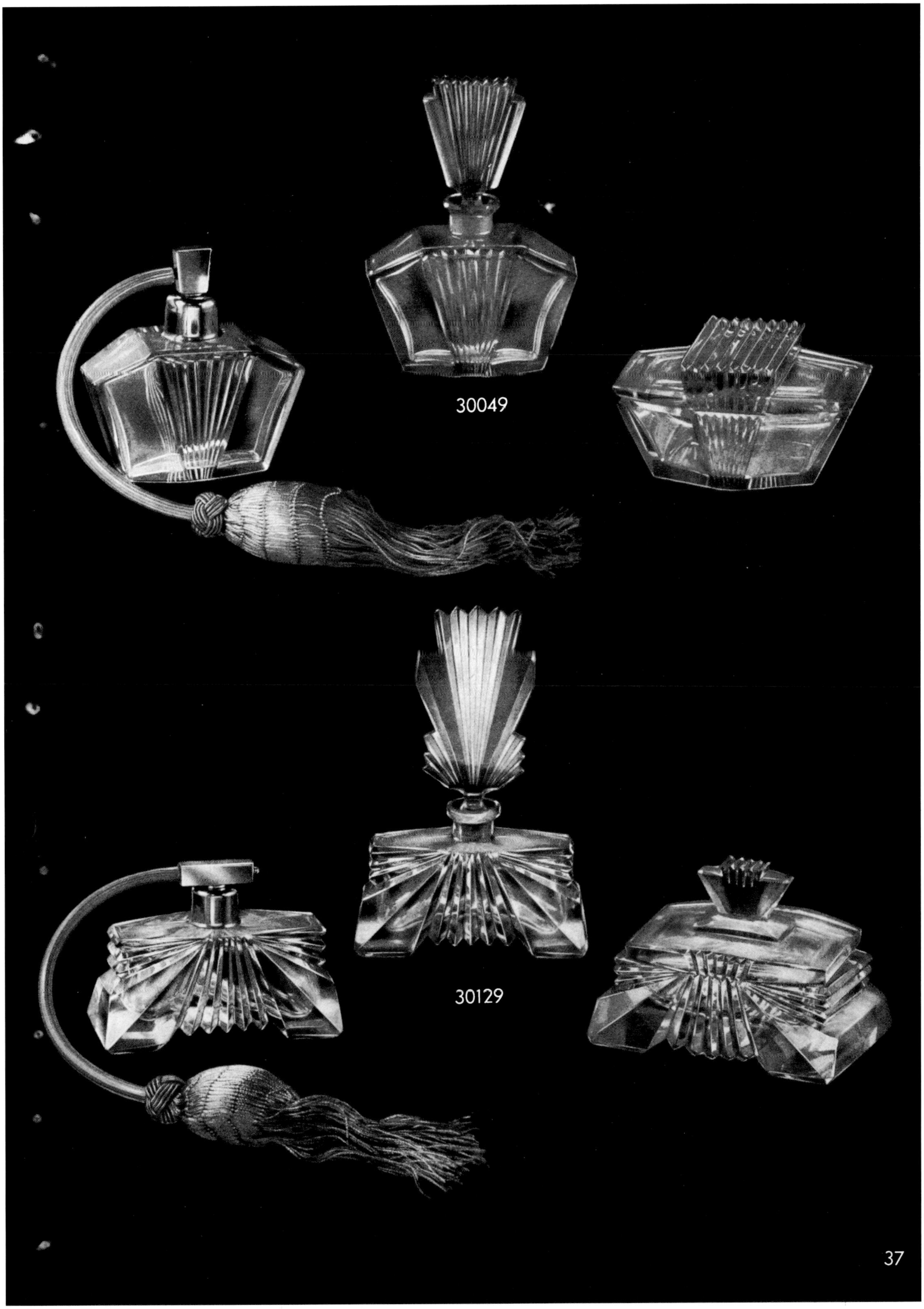
30049
30129
37

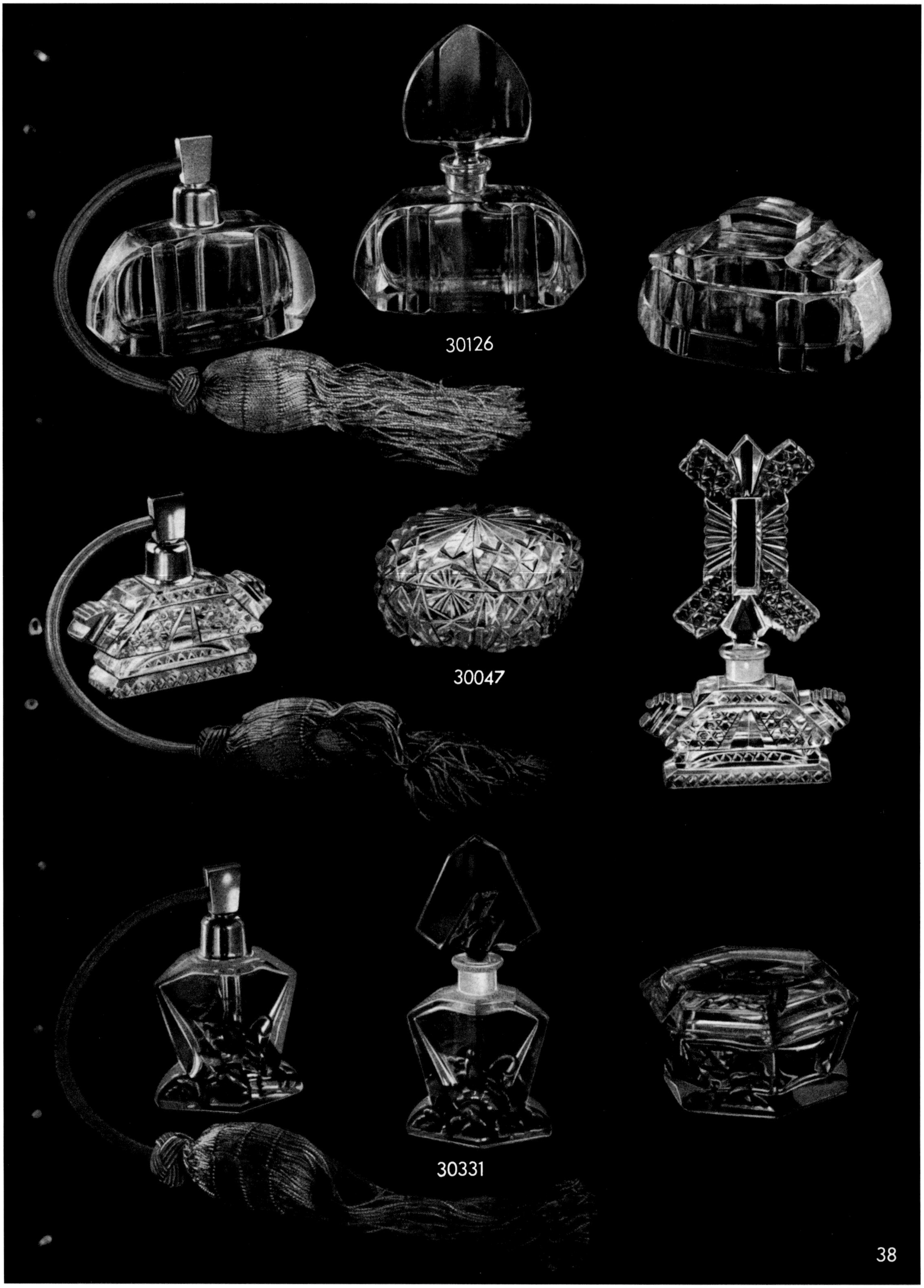
30126
30047
30331
38

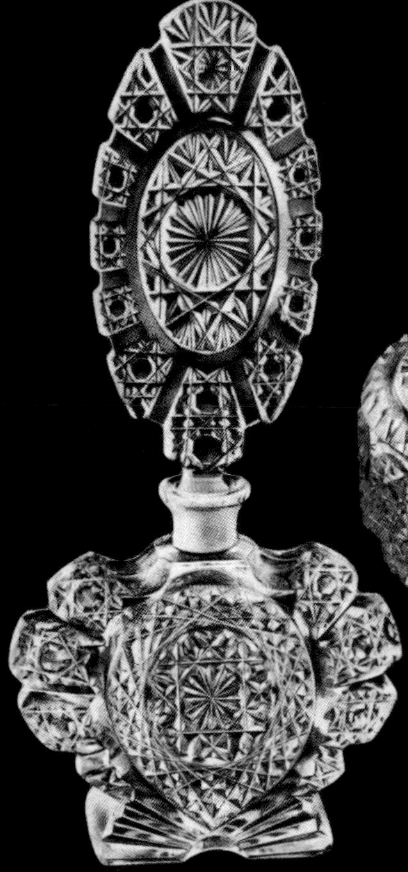

30300
105×45×230 mm

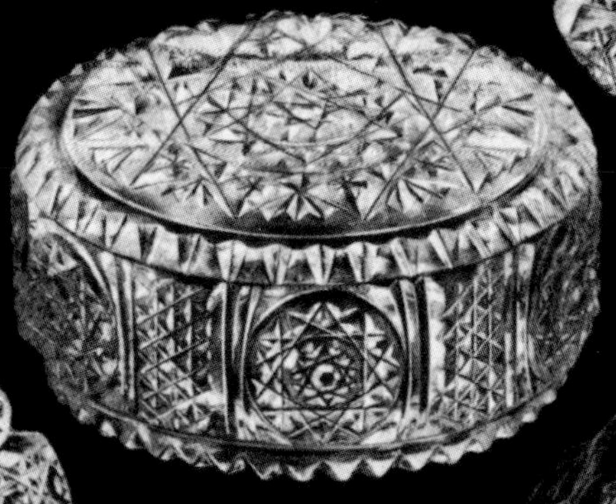

30300
105×105×47 mm

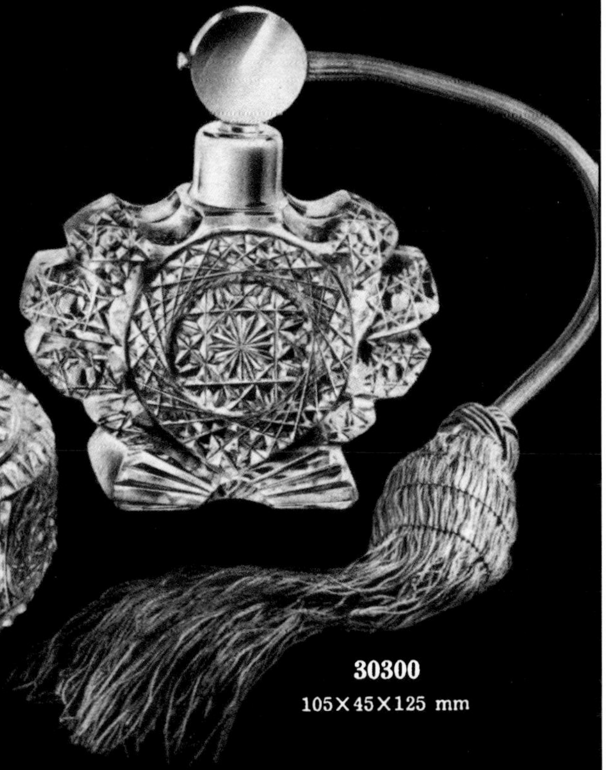

30300
105×45×125 mm

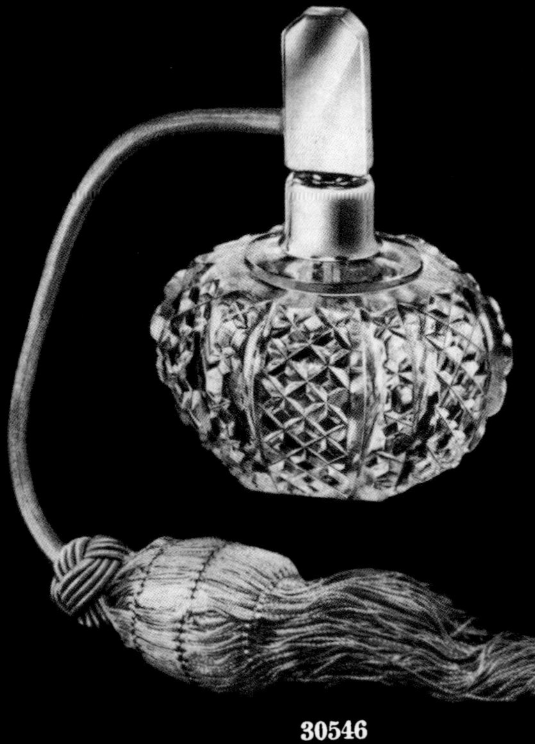

30546
80×80×75 mm

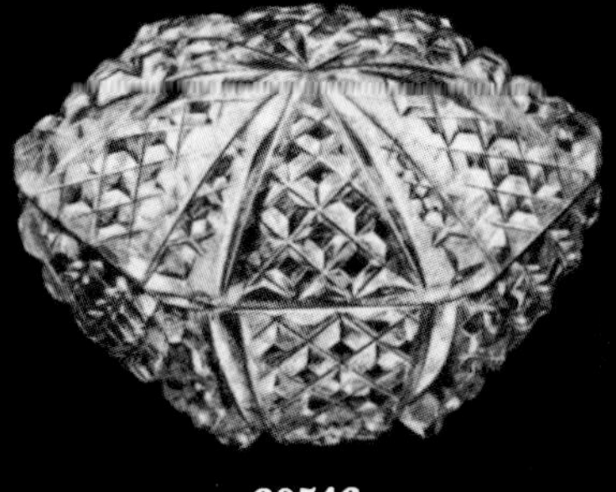

30546
90×90×45 mm

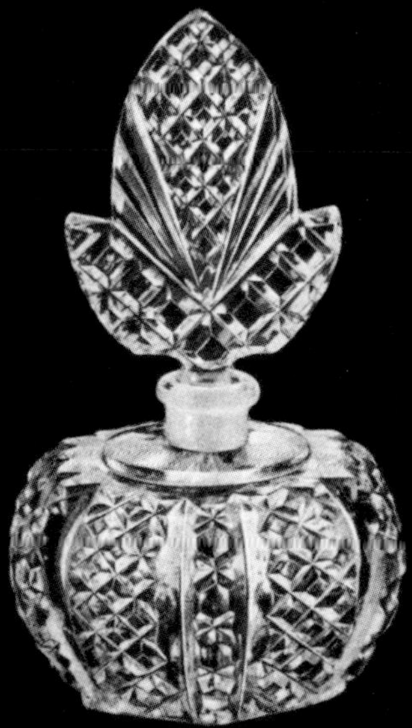

30546
80×80×130 mm

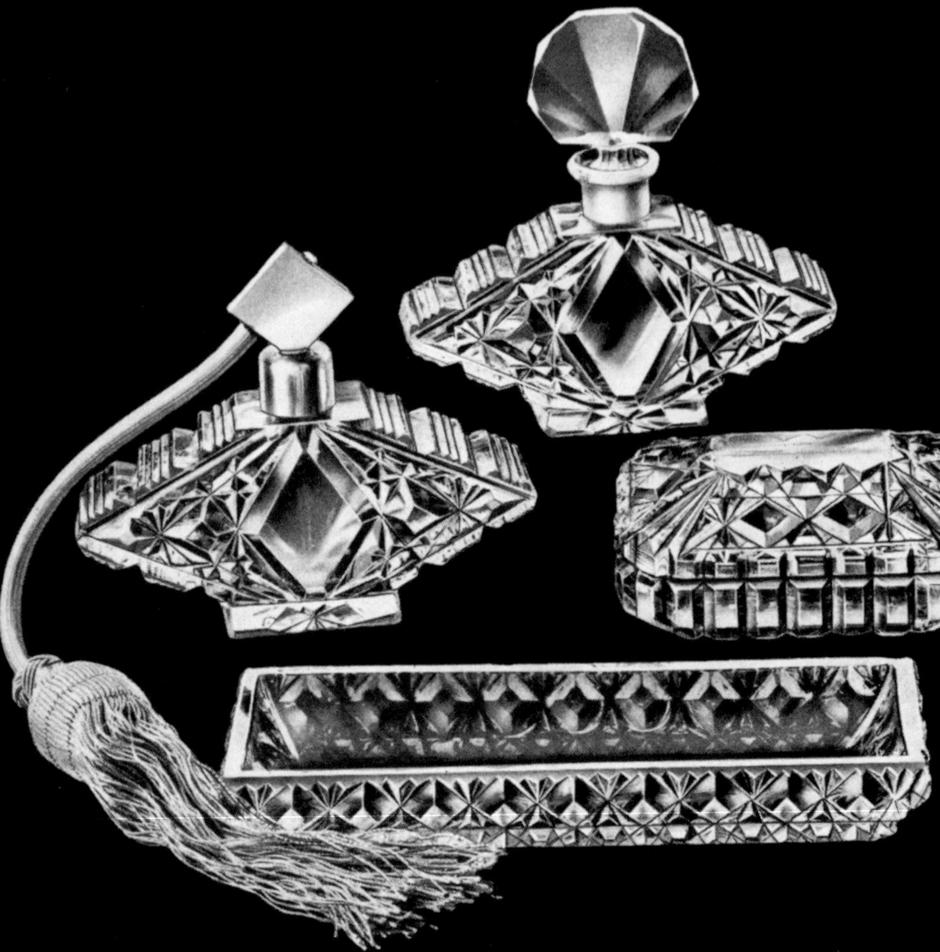

30026

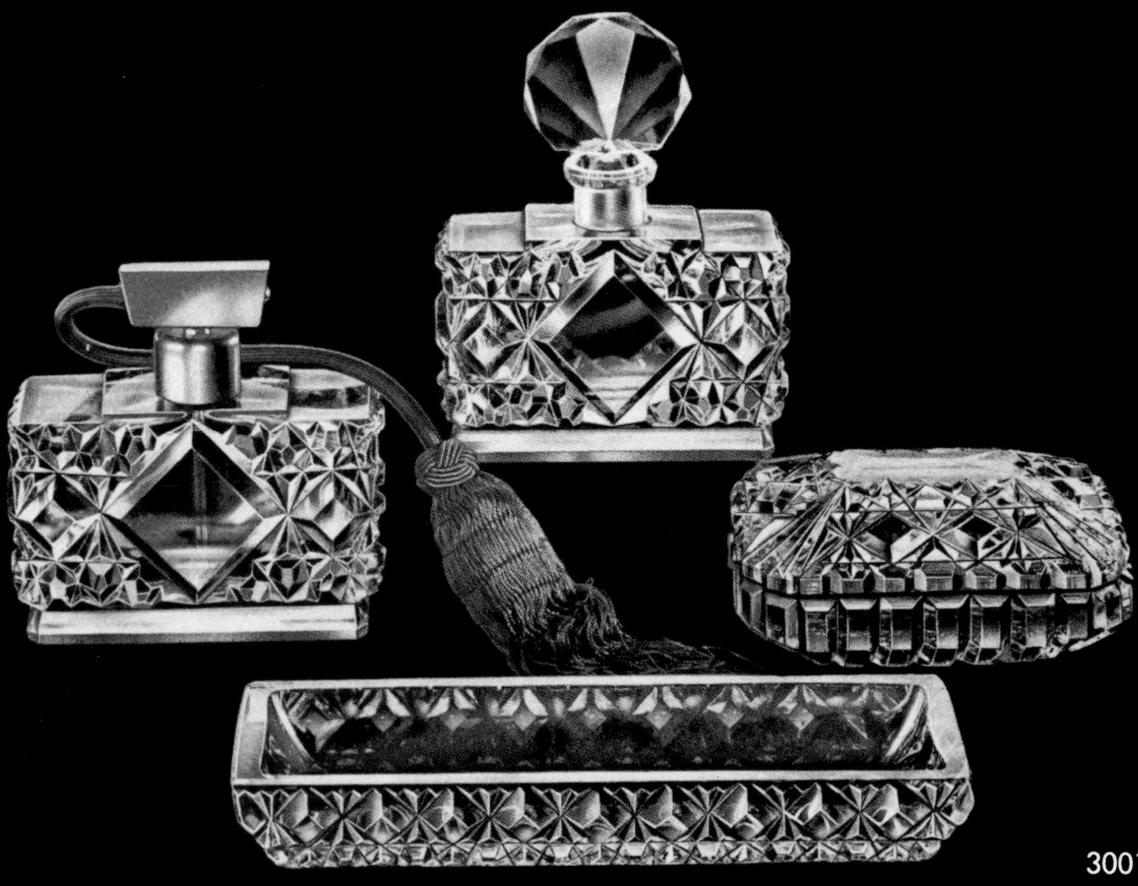

30012

47

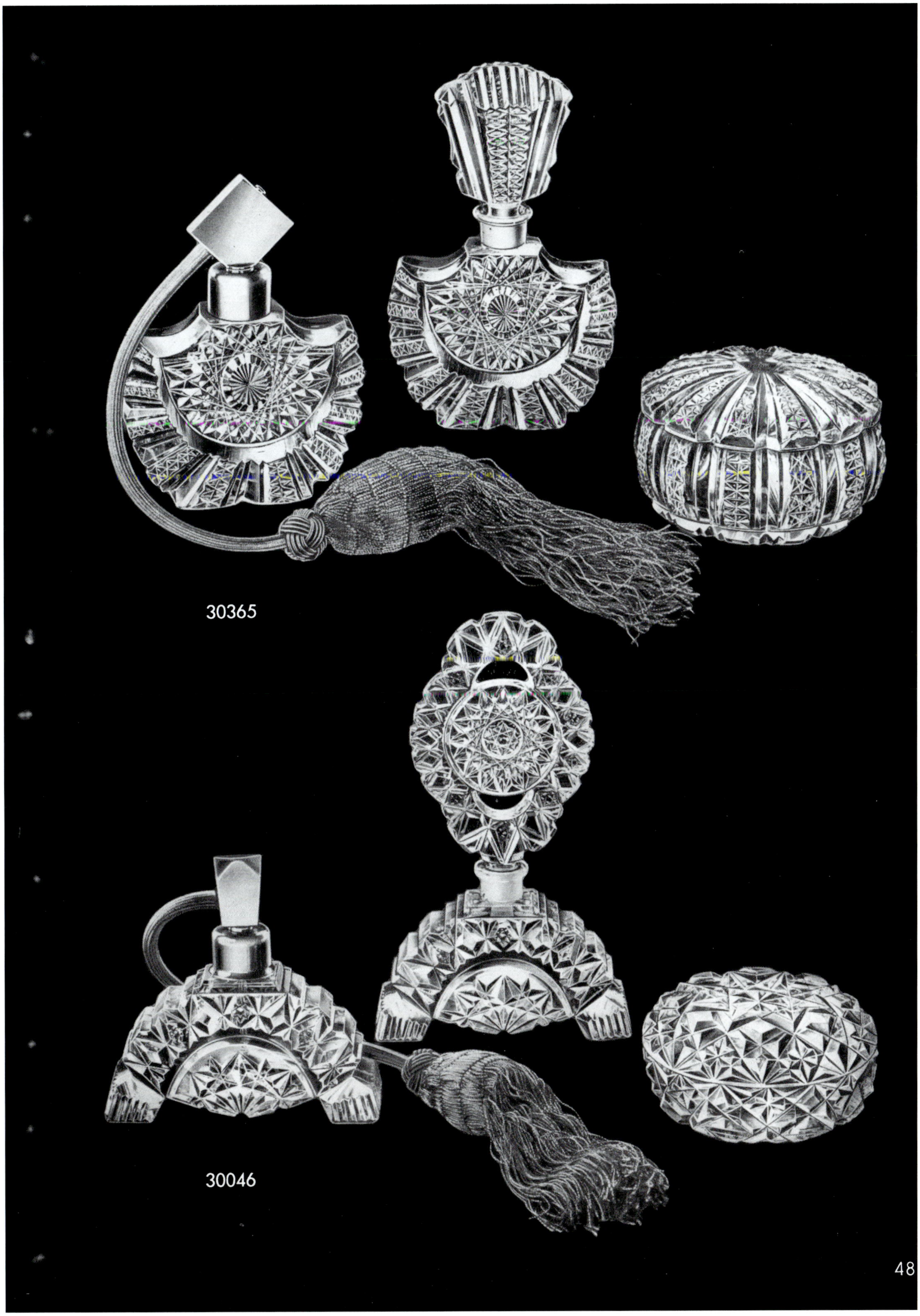
30365
30046
48

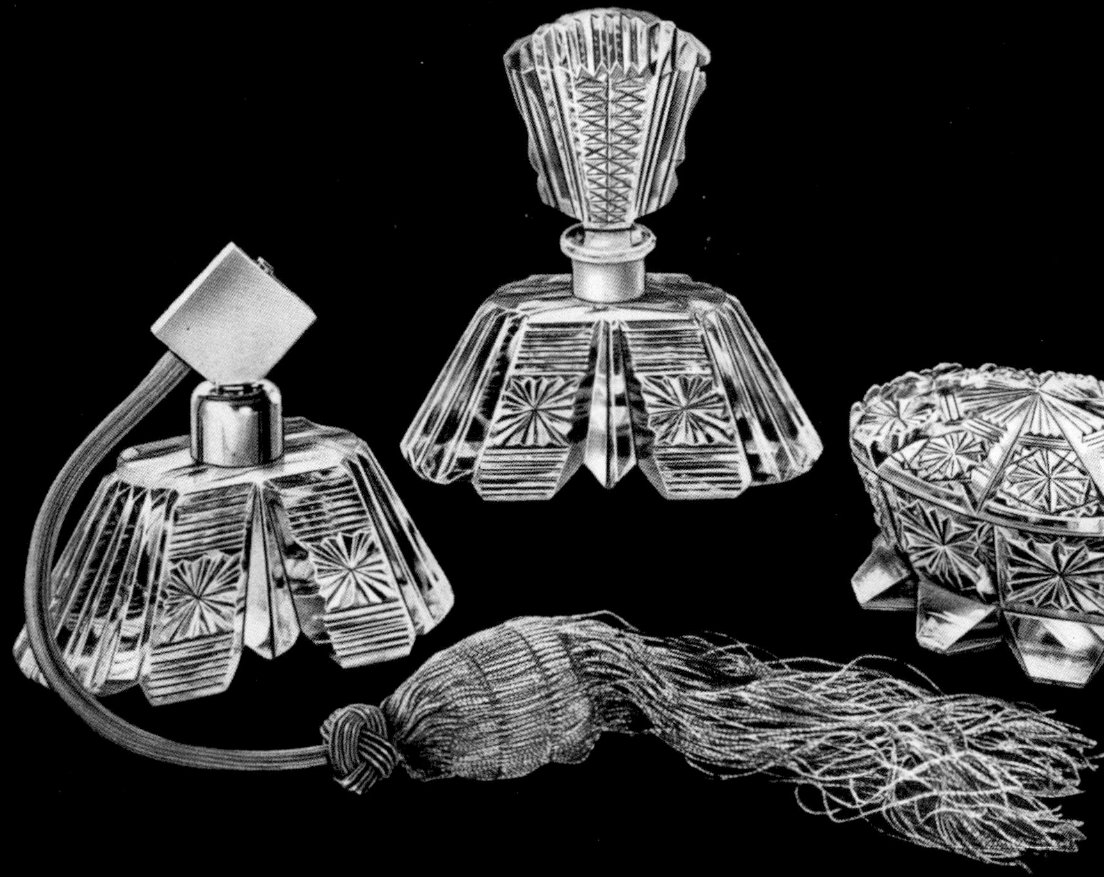

30366

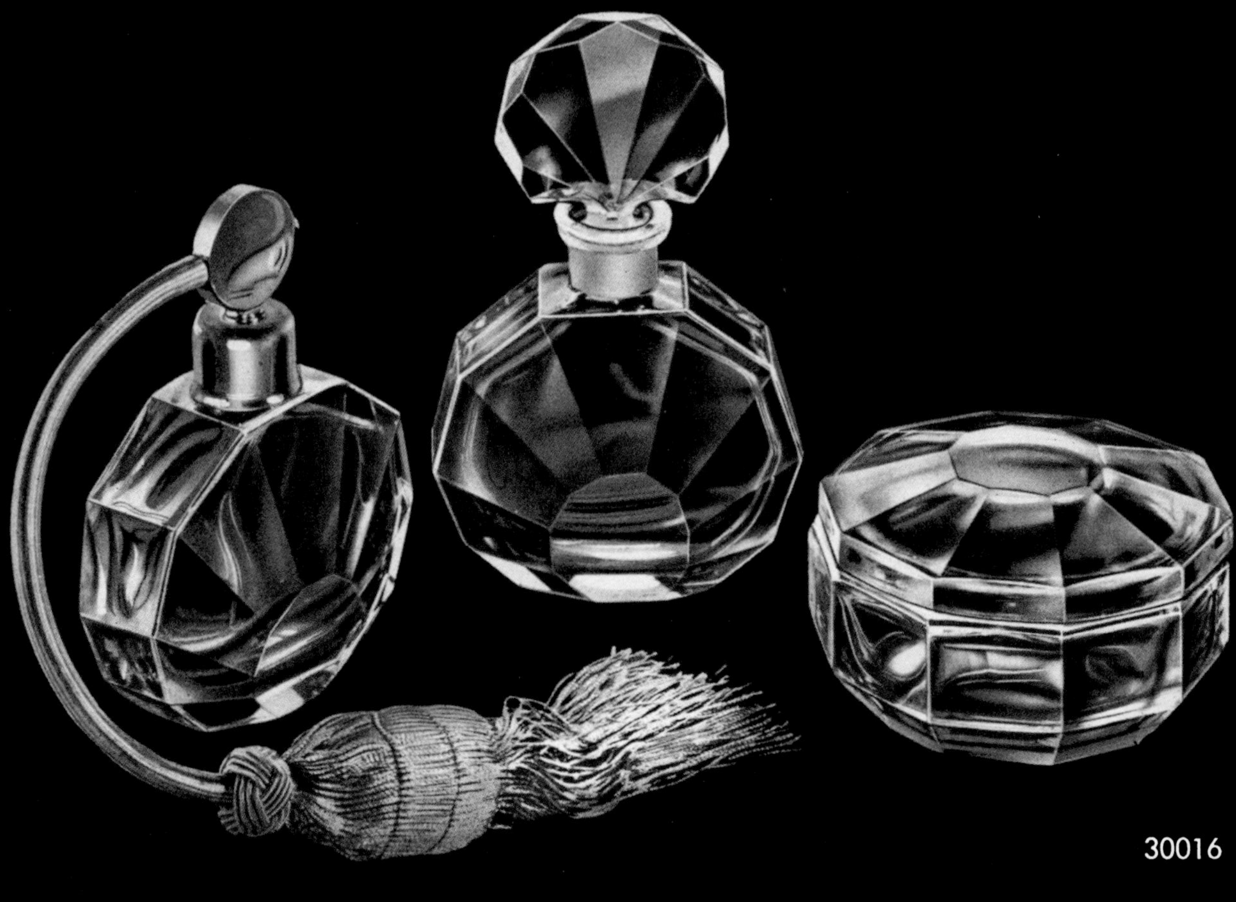

30016

49

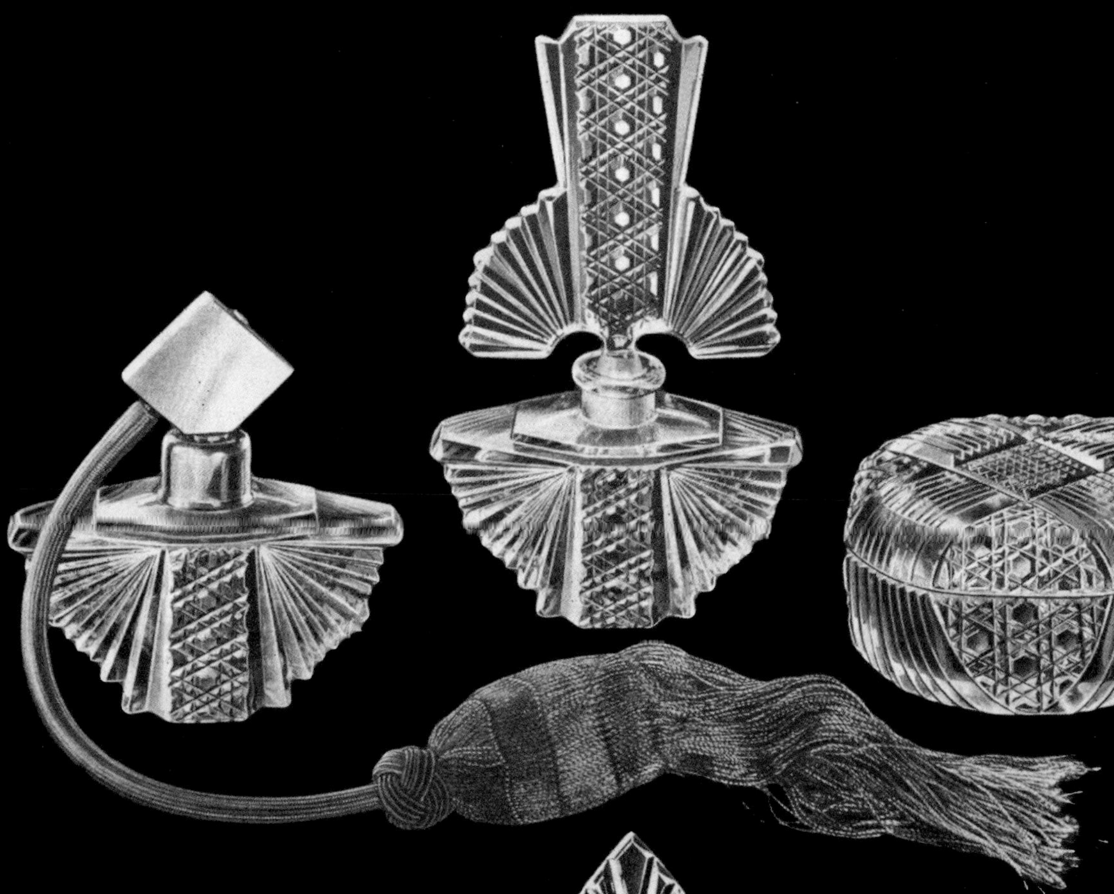

30051

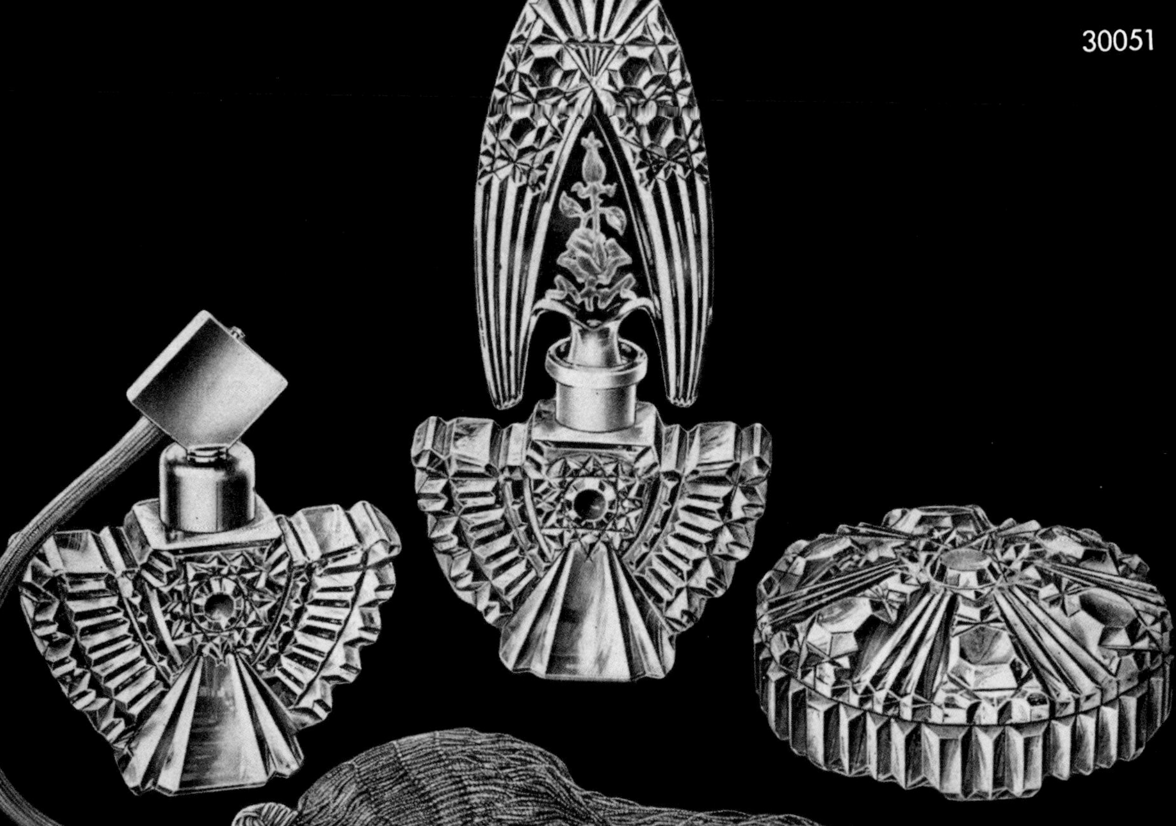

30443

50

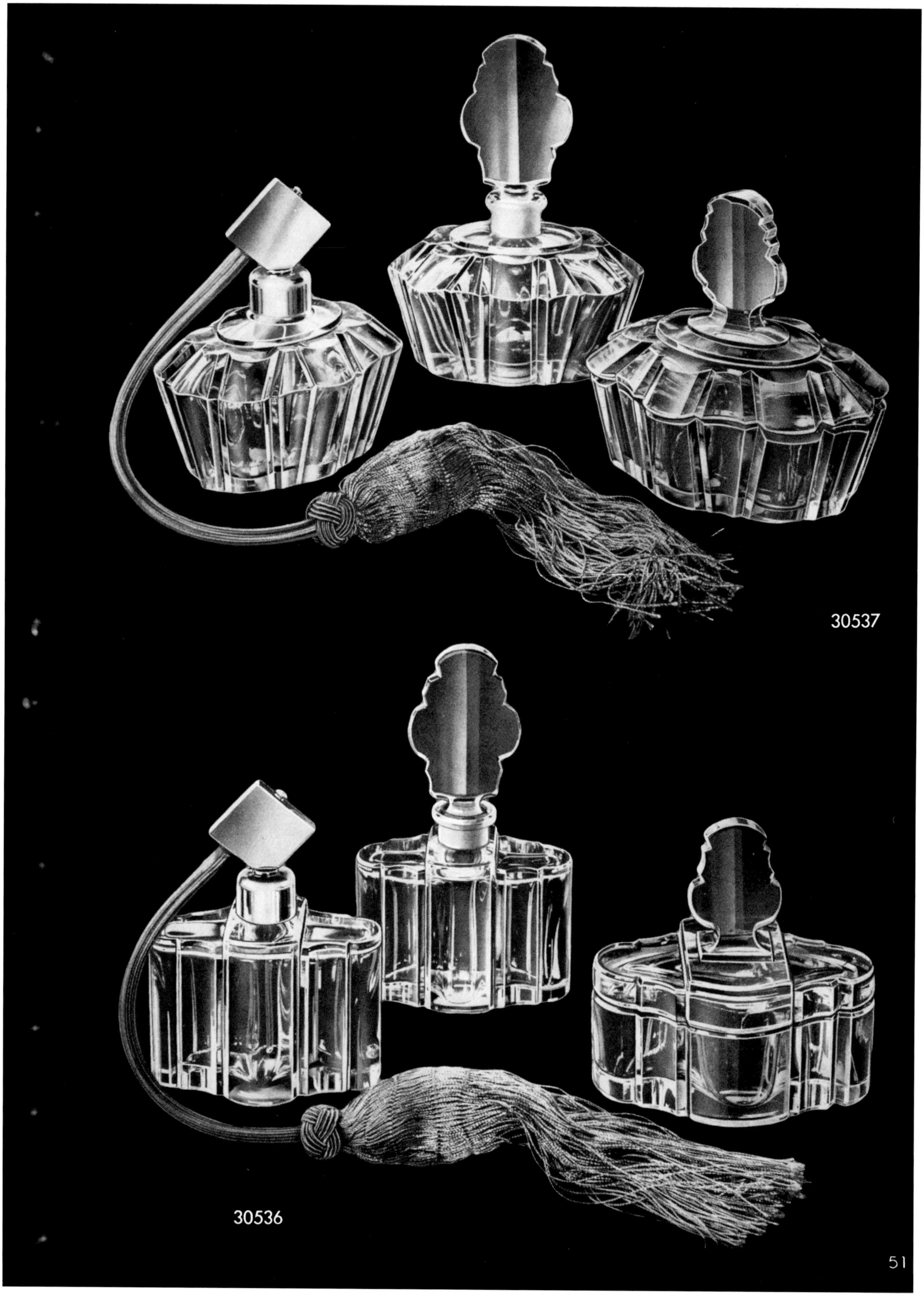
30537
30536
51

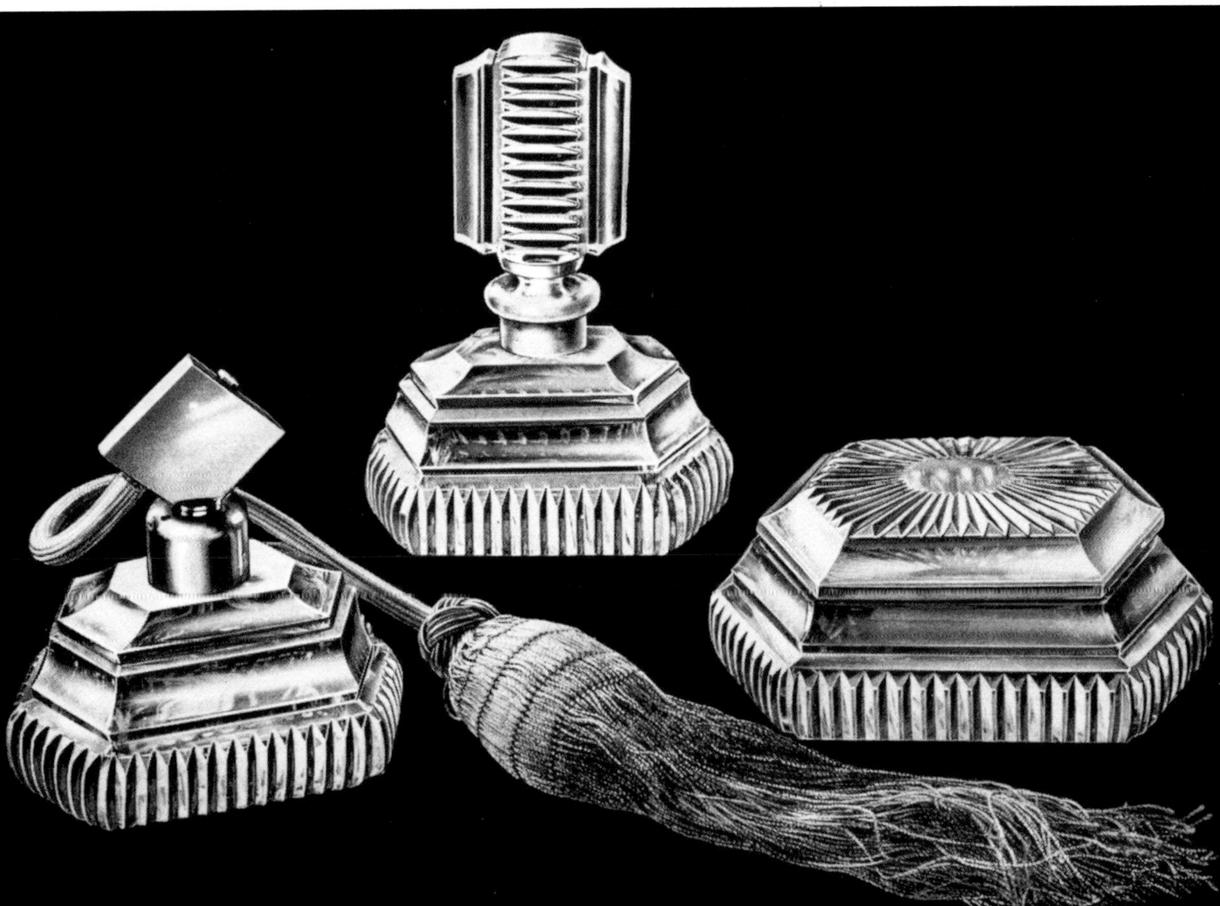

30524

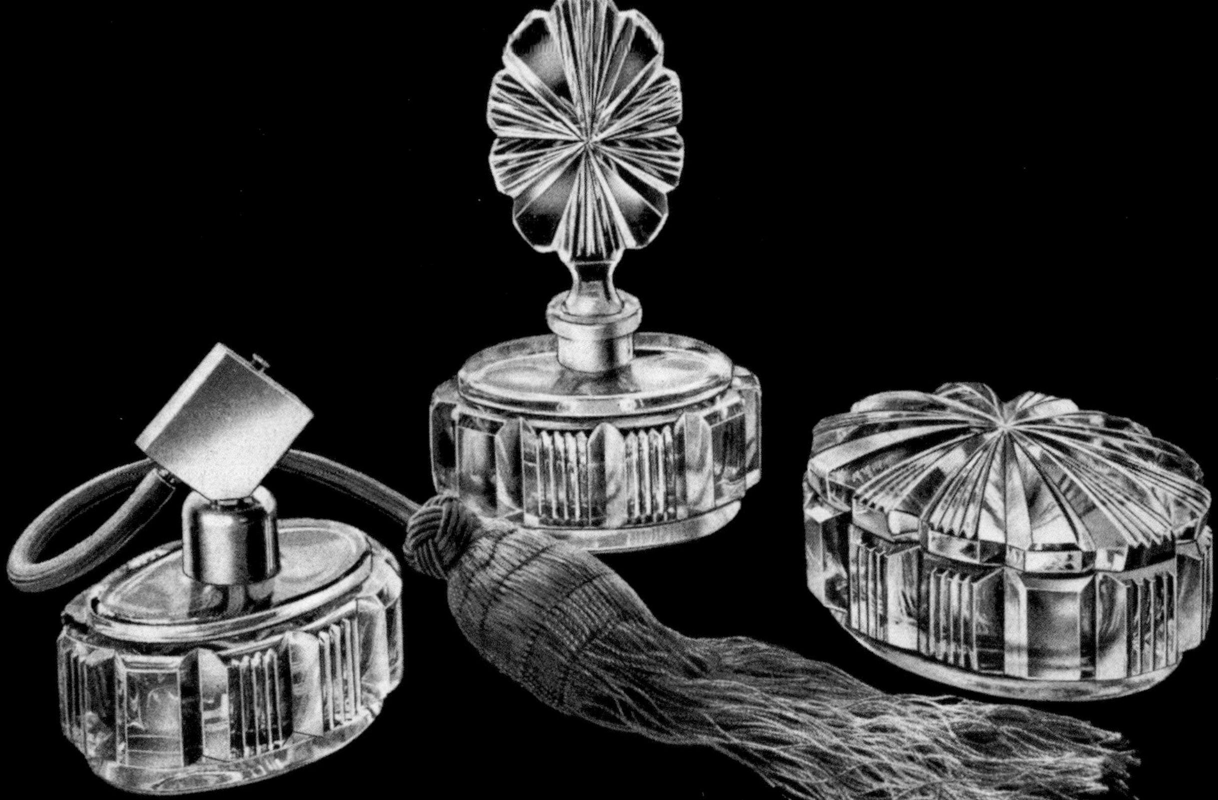

30523

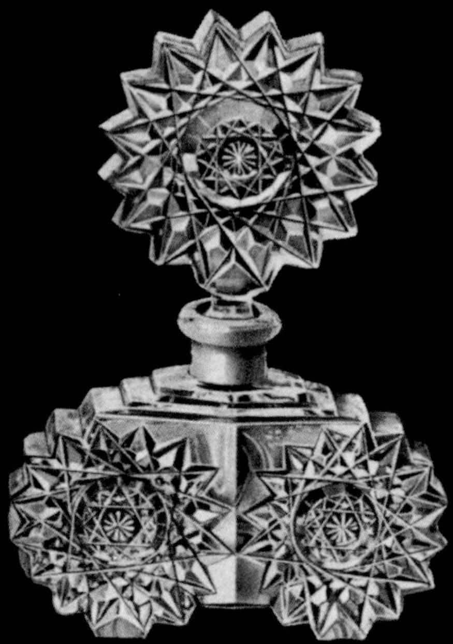

10027

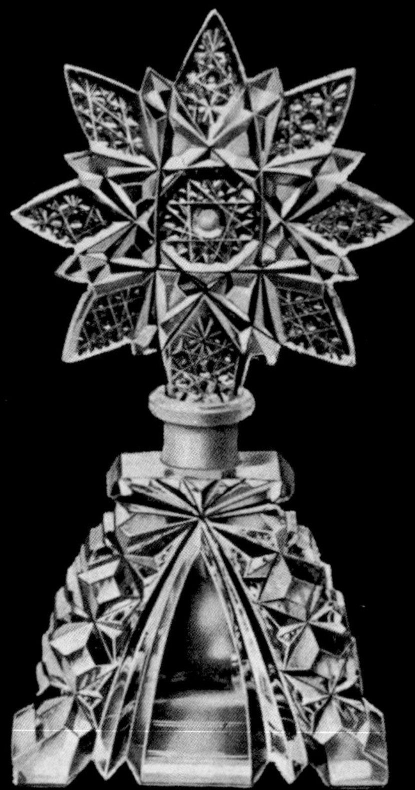

13440

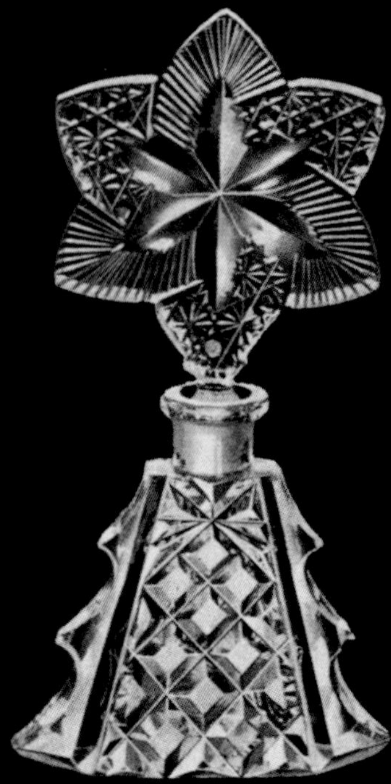

11964

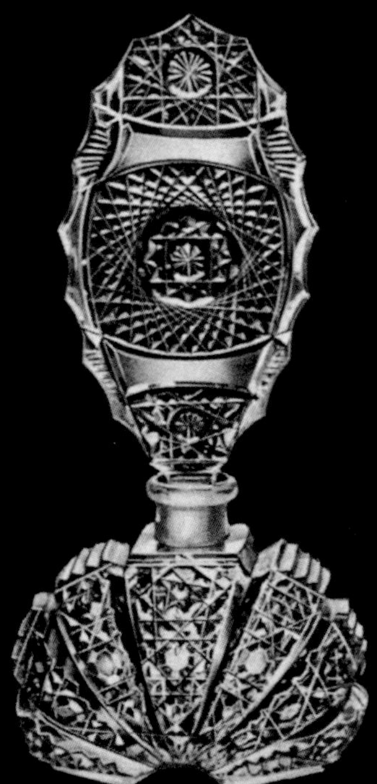

13466

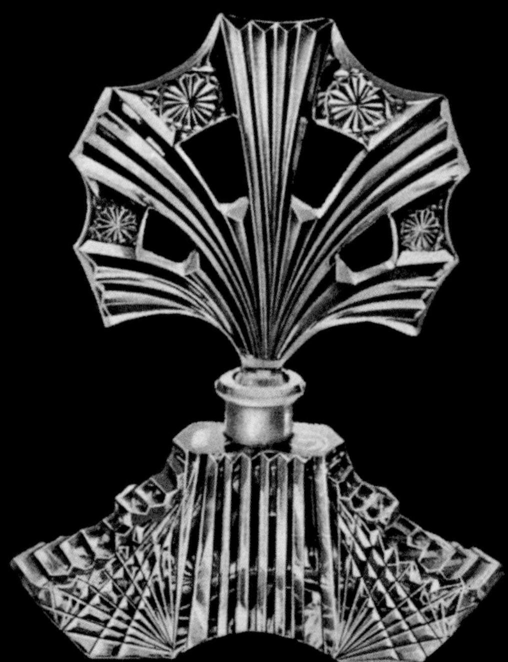

13465

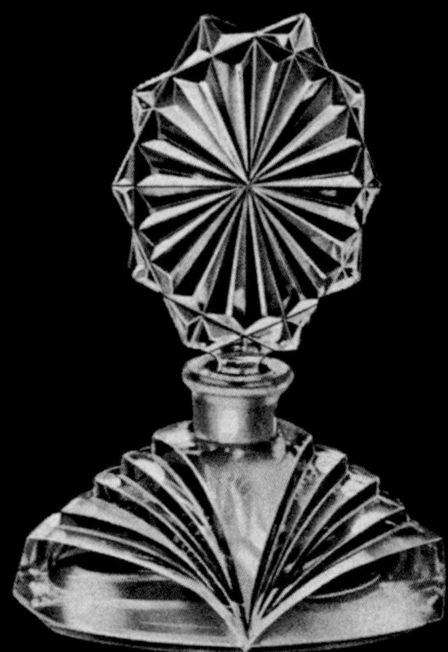

13462

64

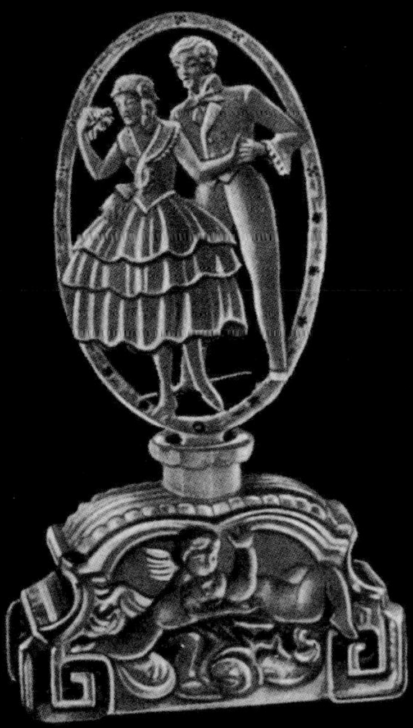

13437

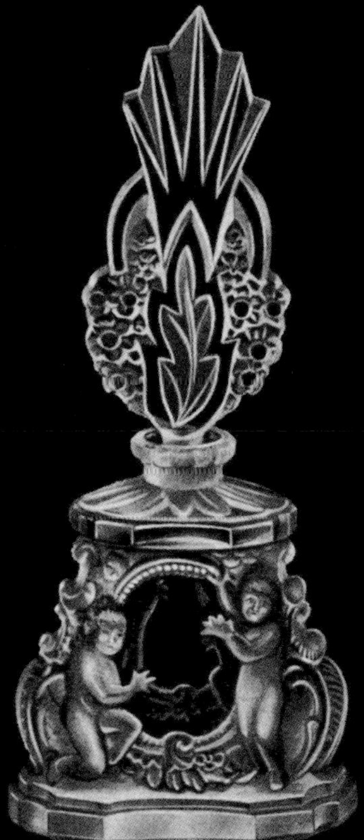

13461

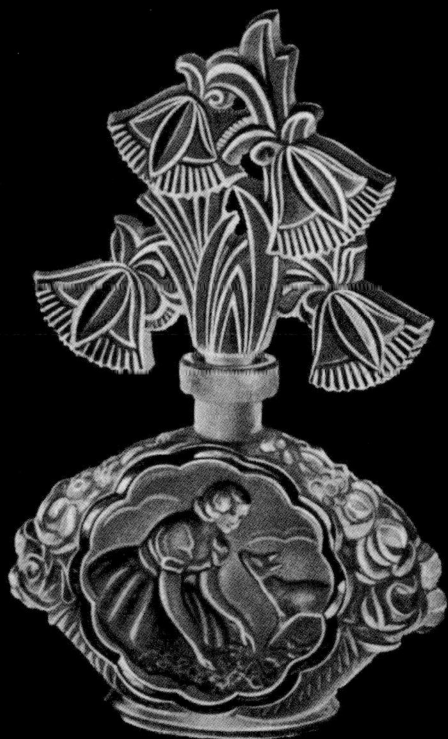

13458

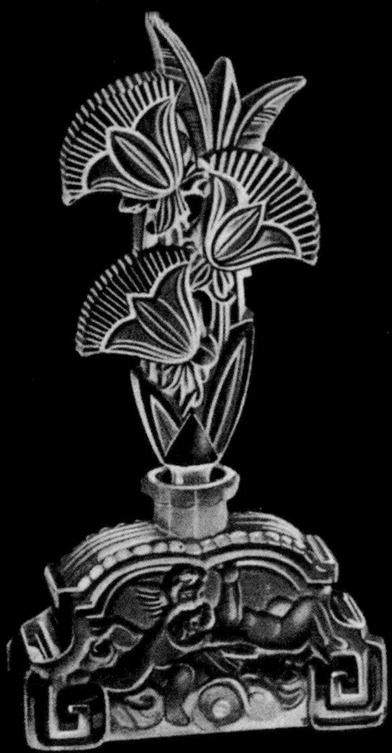

13459

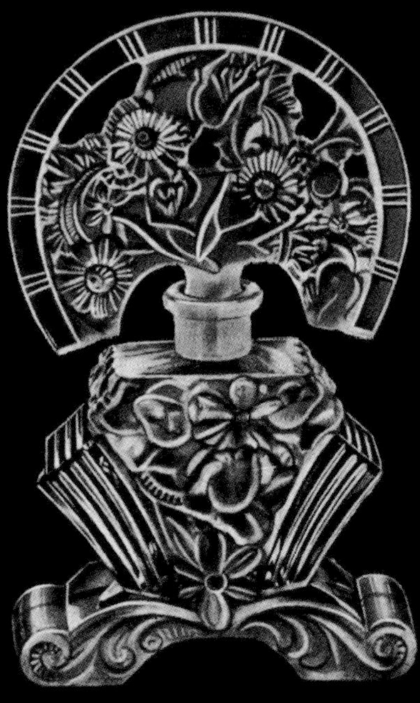

13457

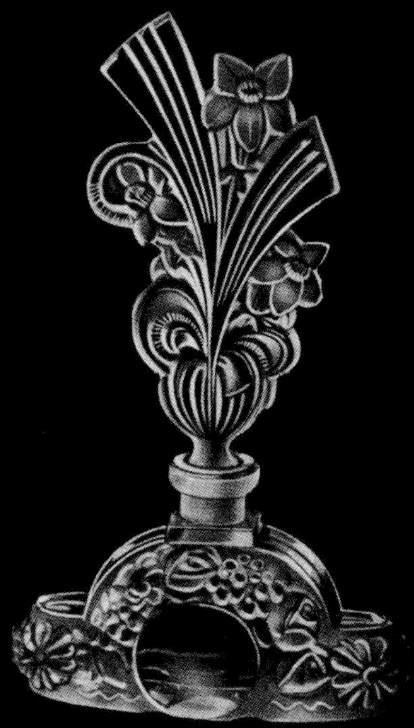

13460

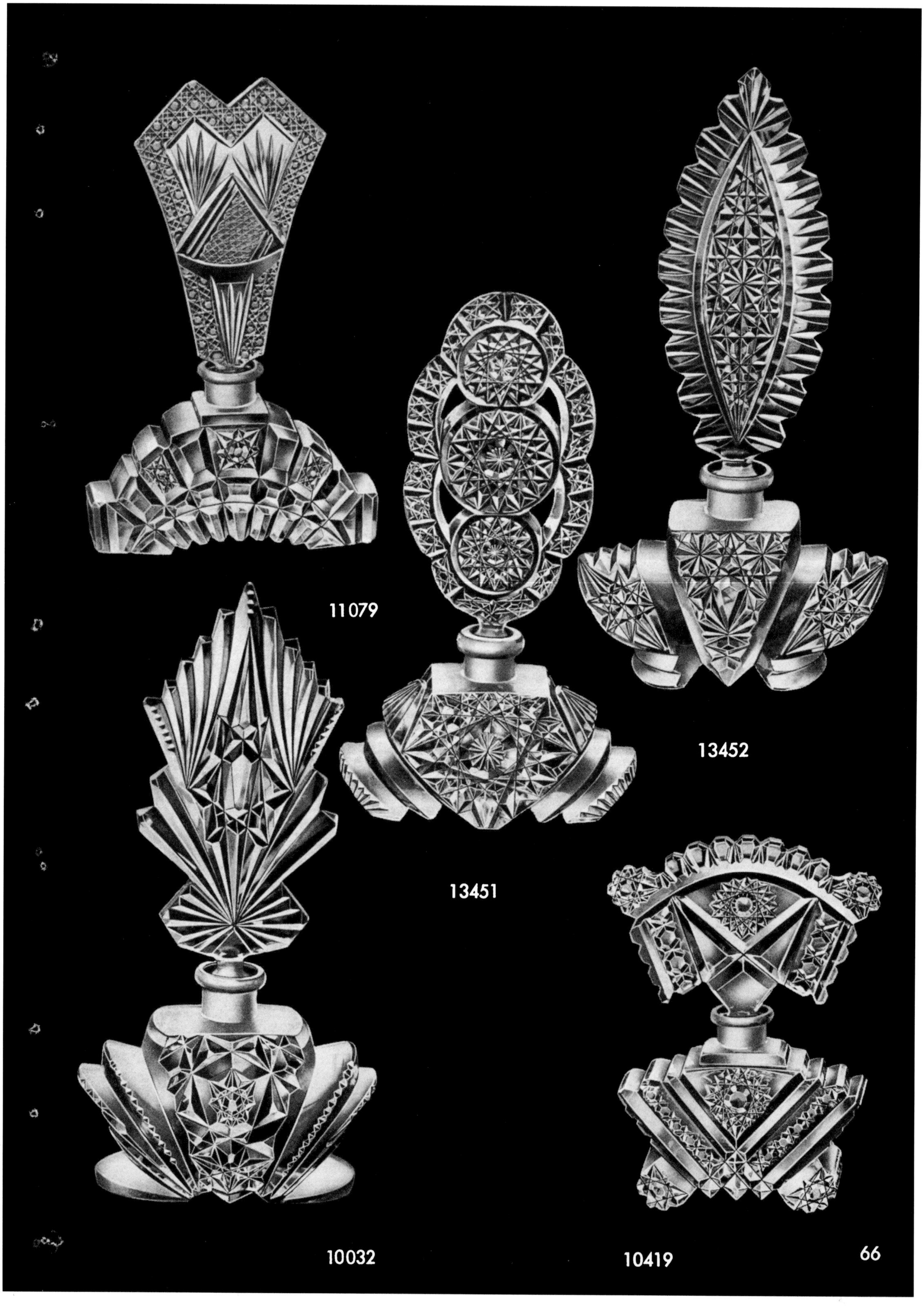
11079
13452
13451
10032
10419
66

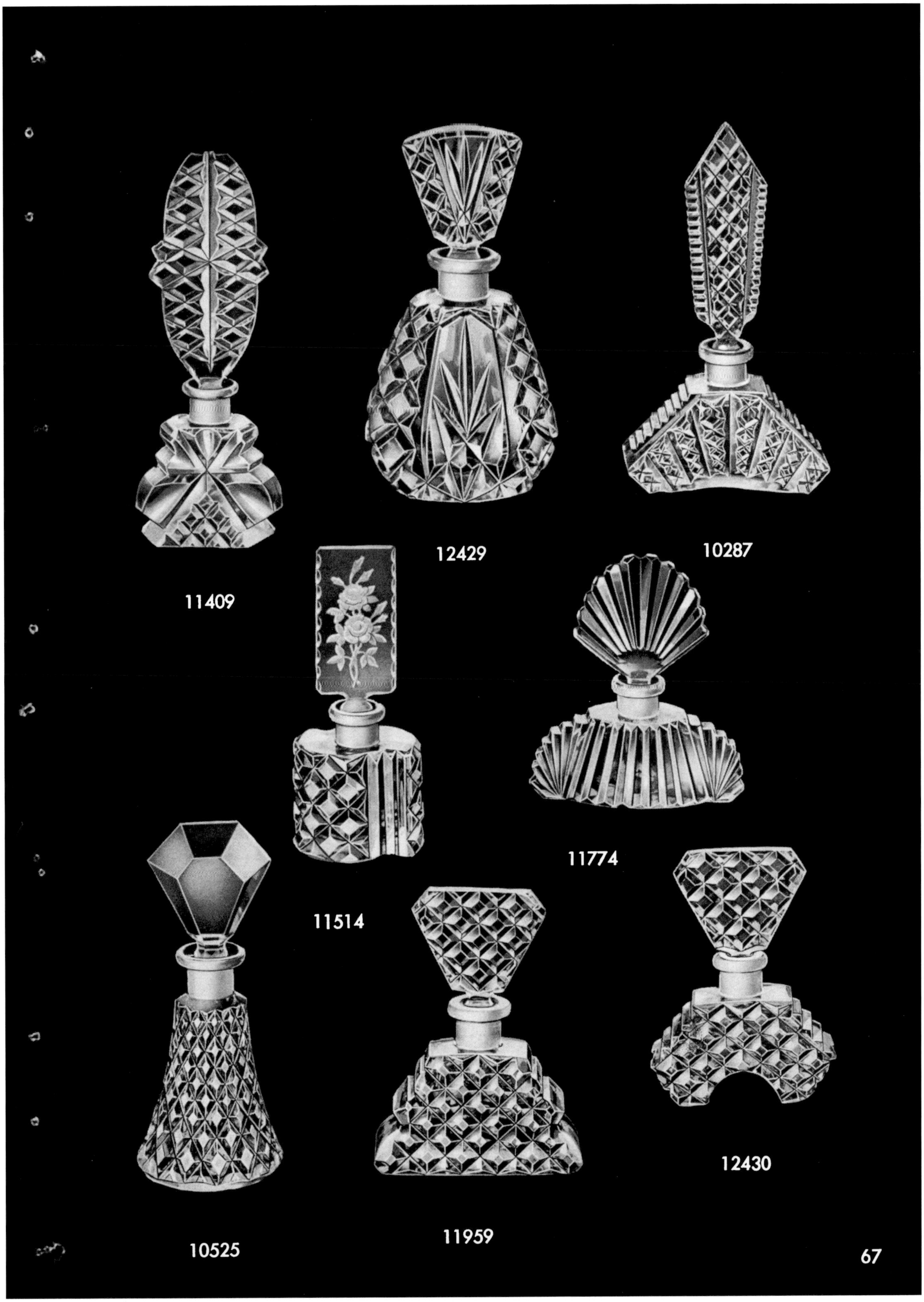
11409
12429
10287
11514
11774
10525
11959
12430
67

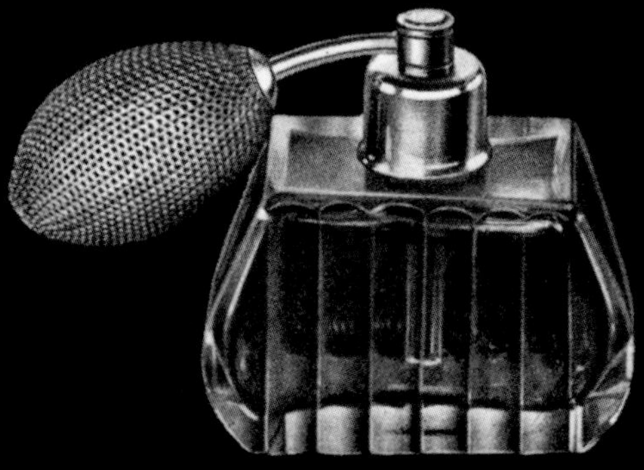

11931

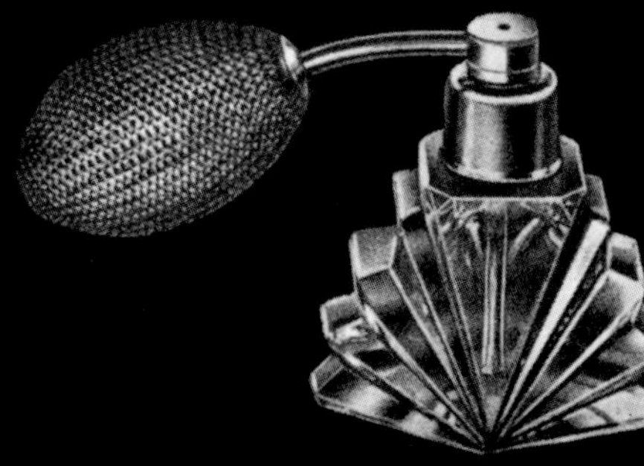

11667

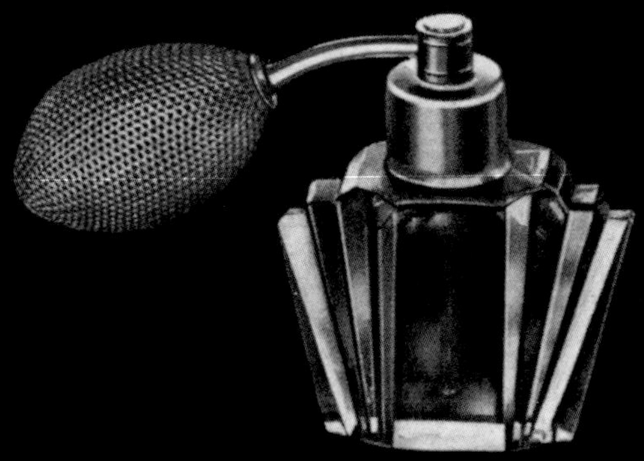

12459

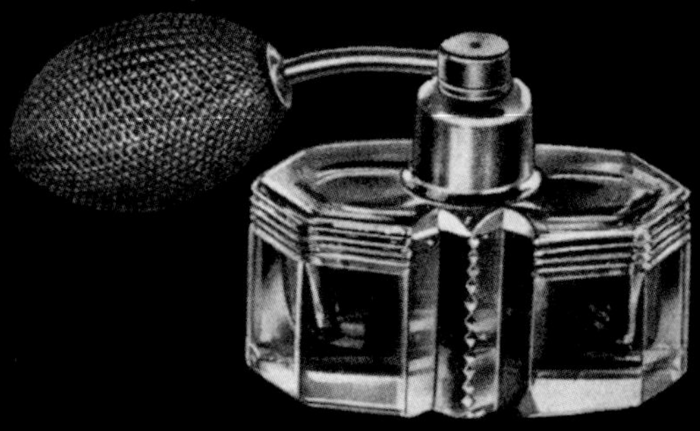

11674

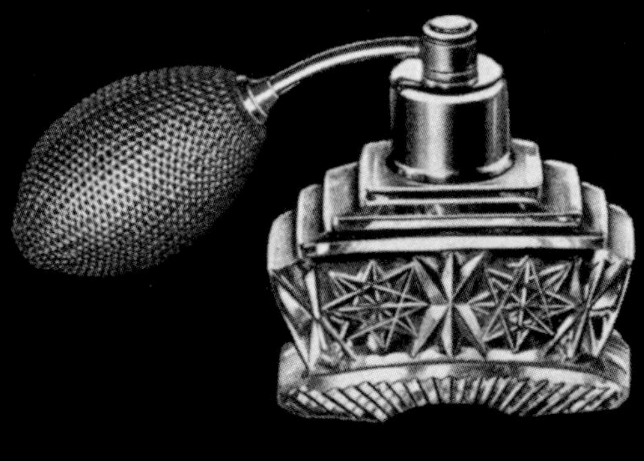

10463

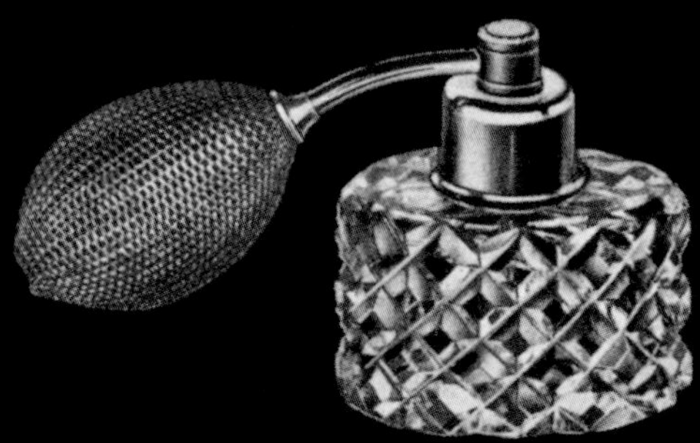

12728

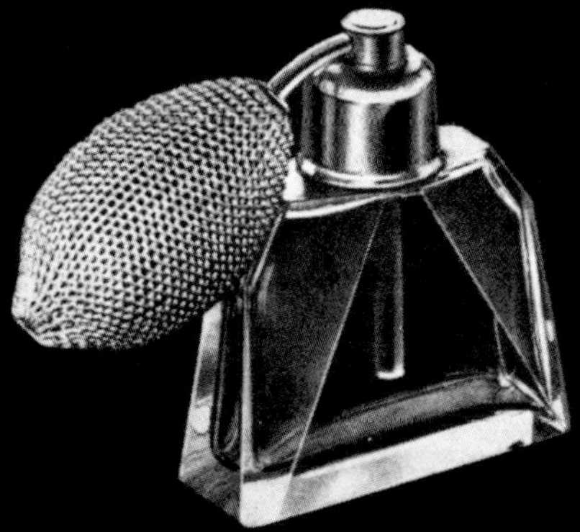

11634

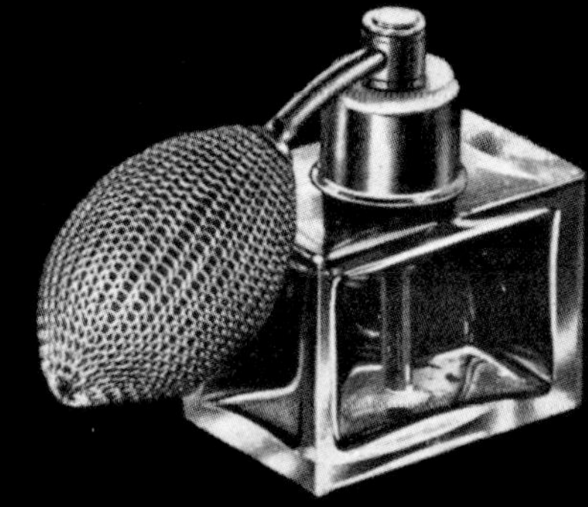

11610

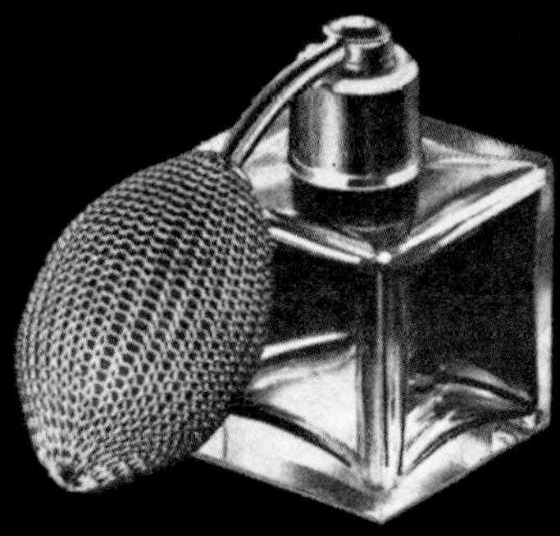

11607

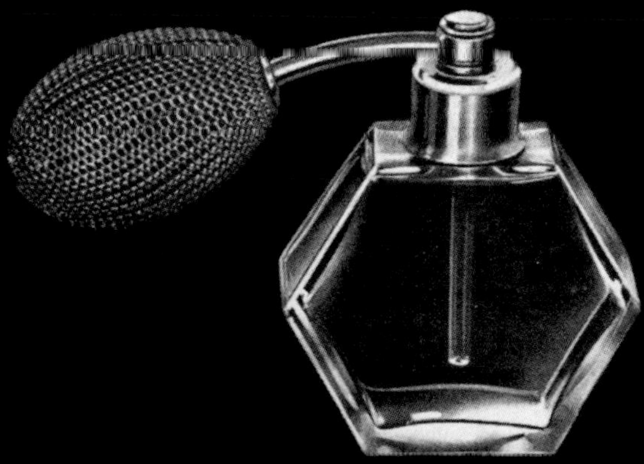

10410

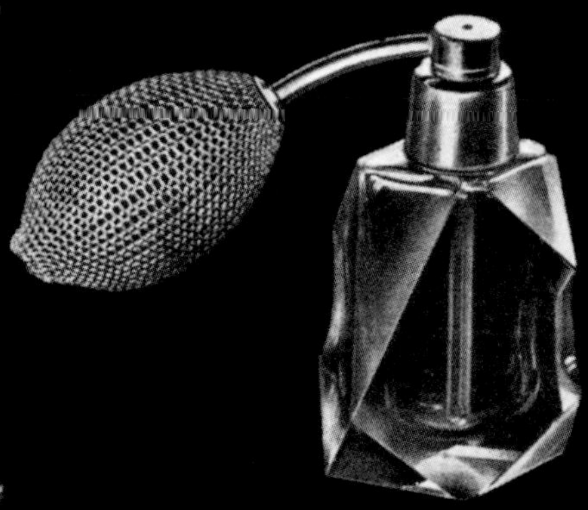

11695

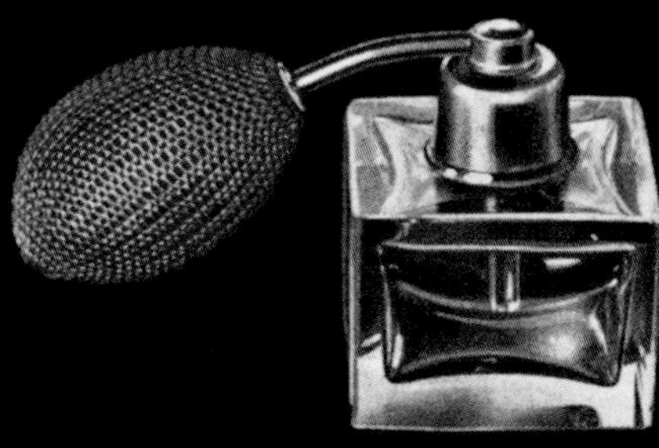

11615

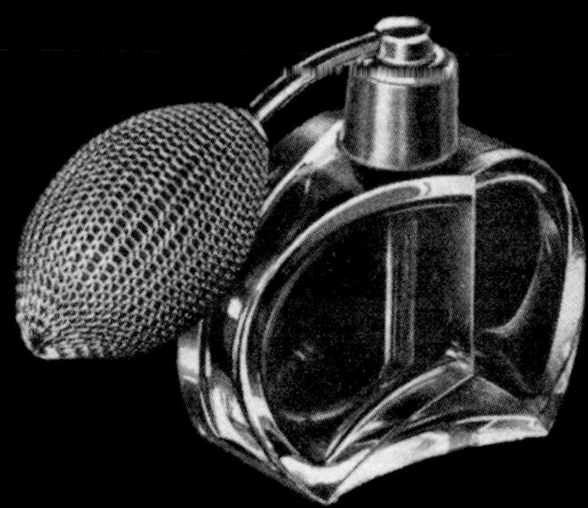

11703

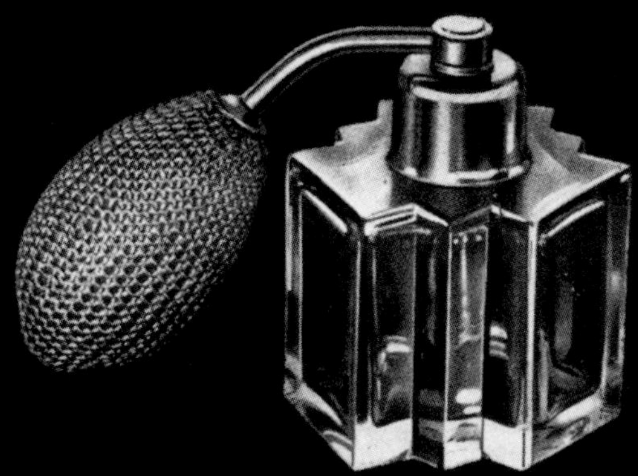

11635

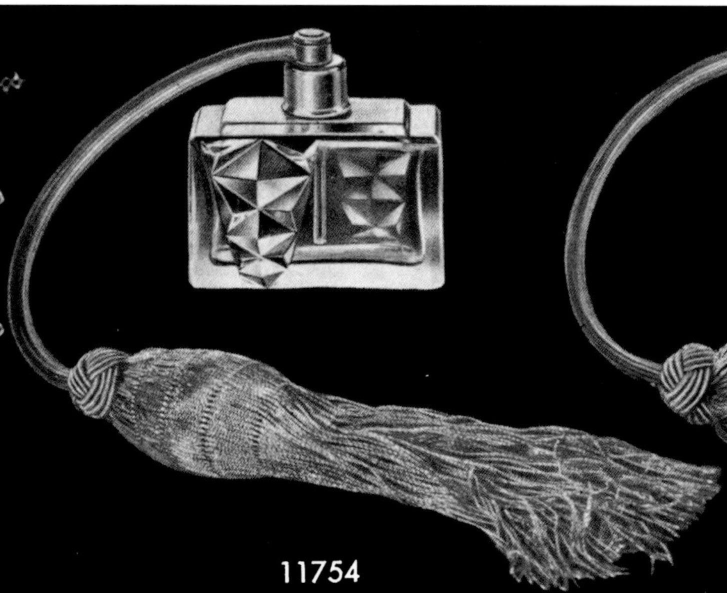

11754

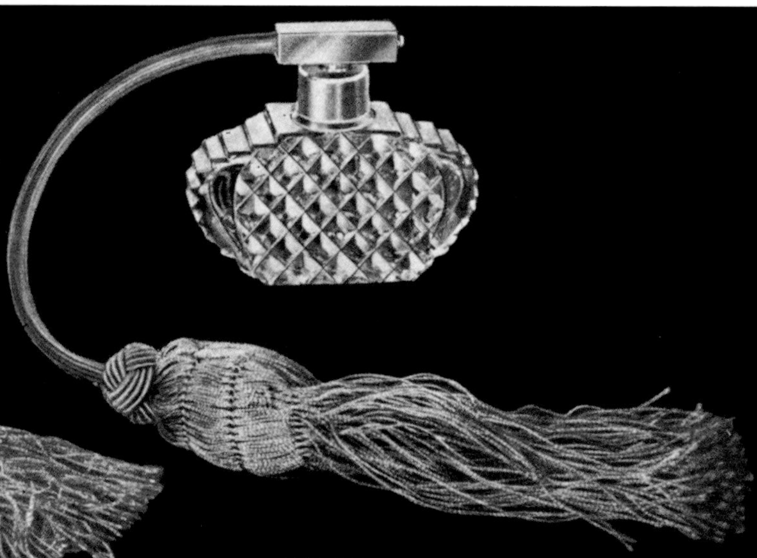

11910

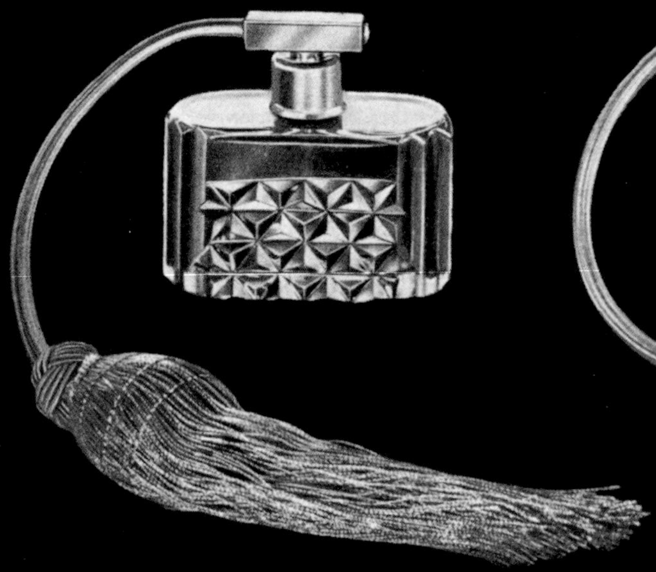

11539

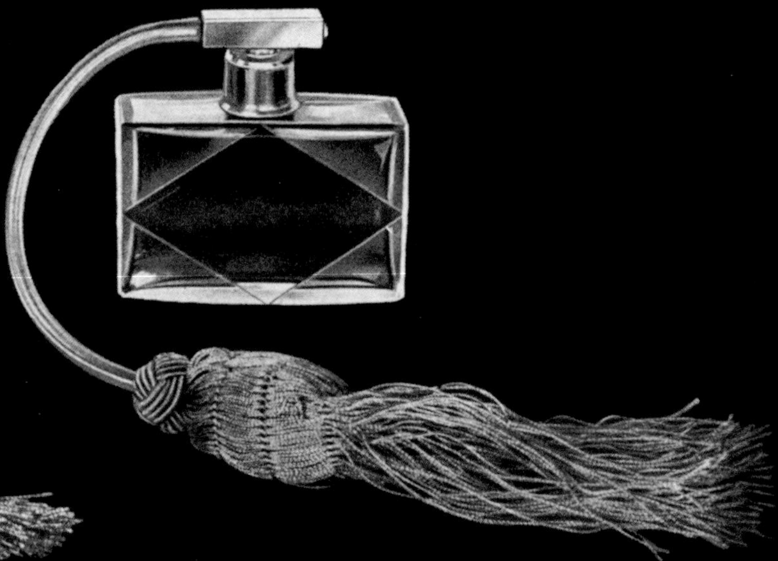

11537

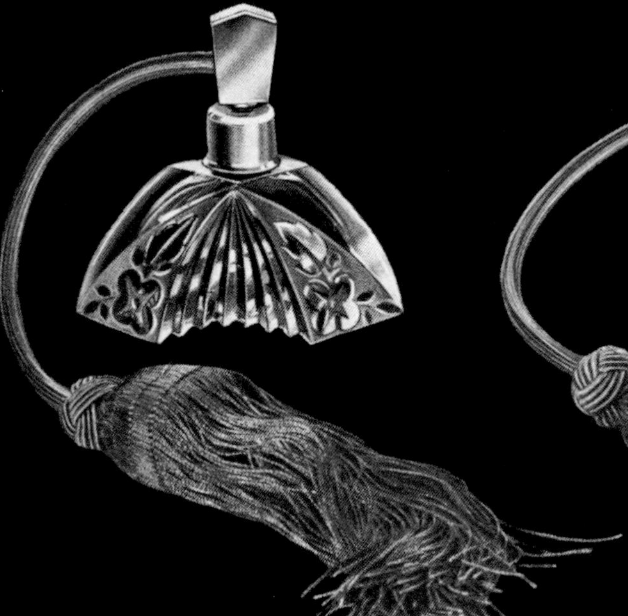

11040

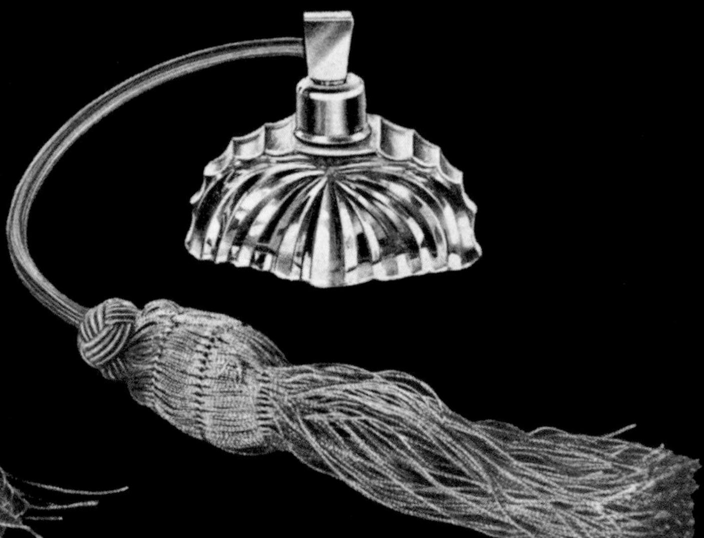

11504

74

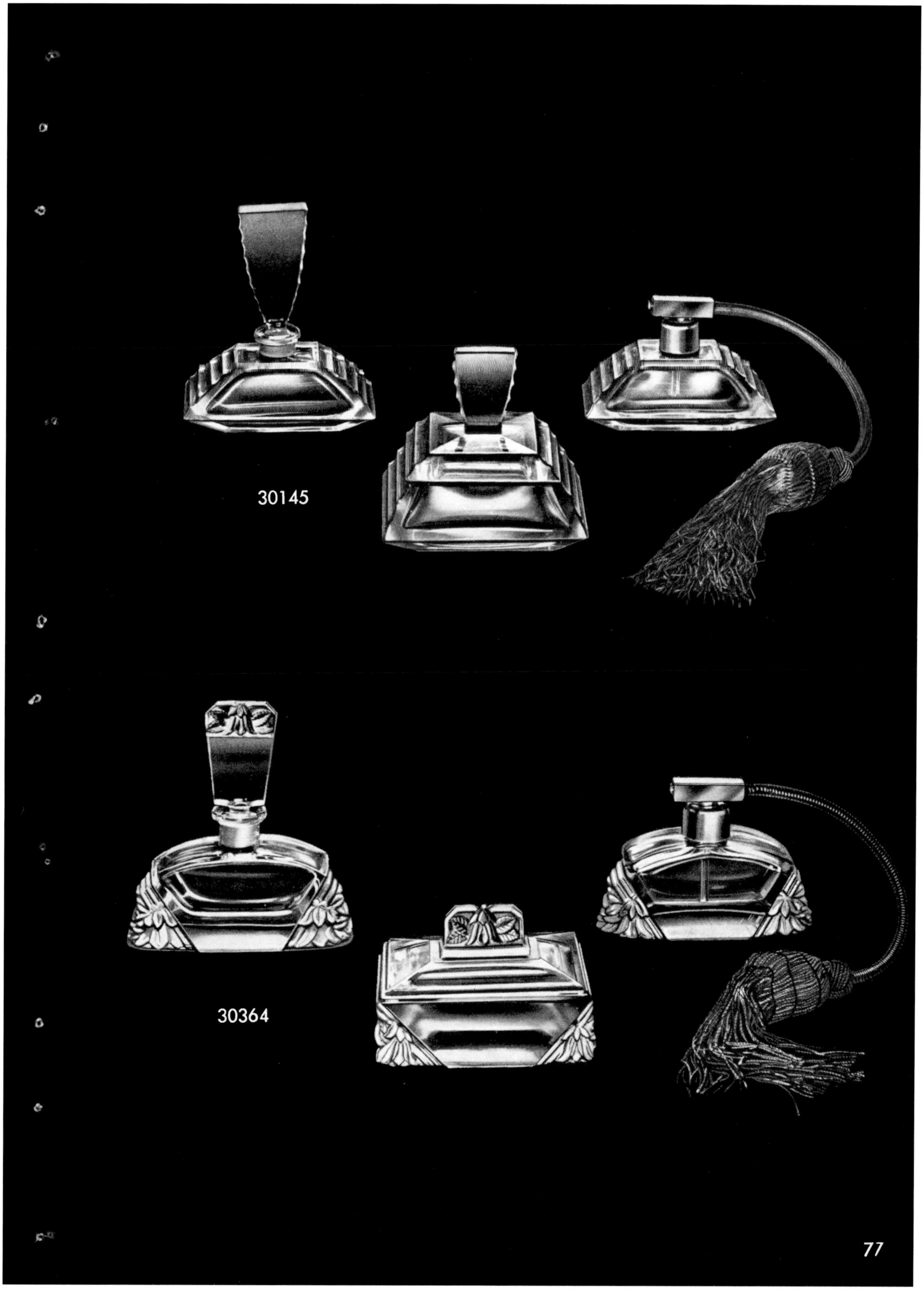
30145
30364
77

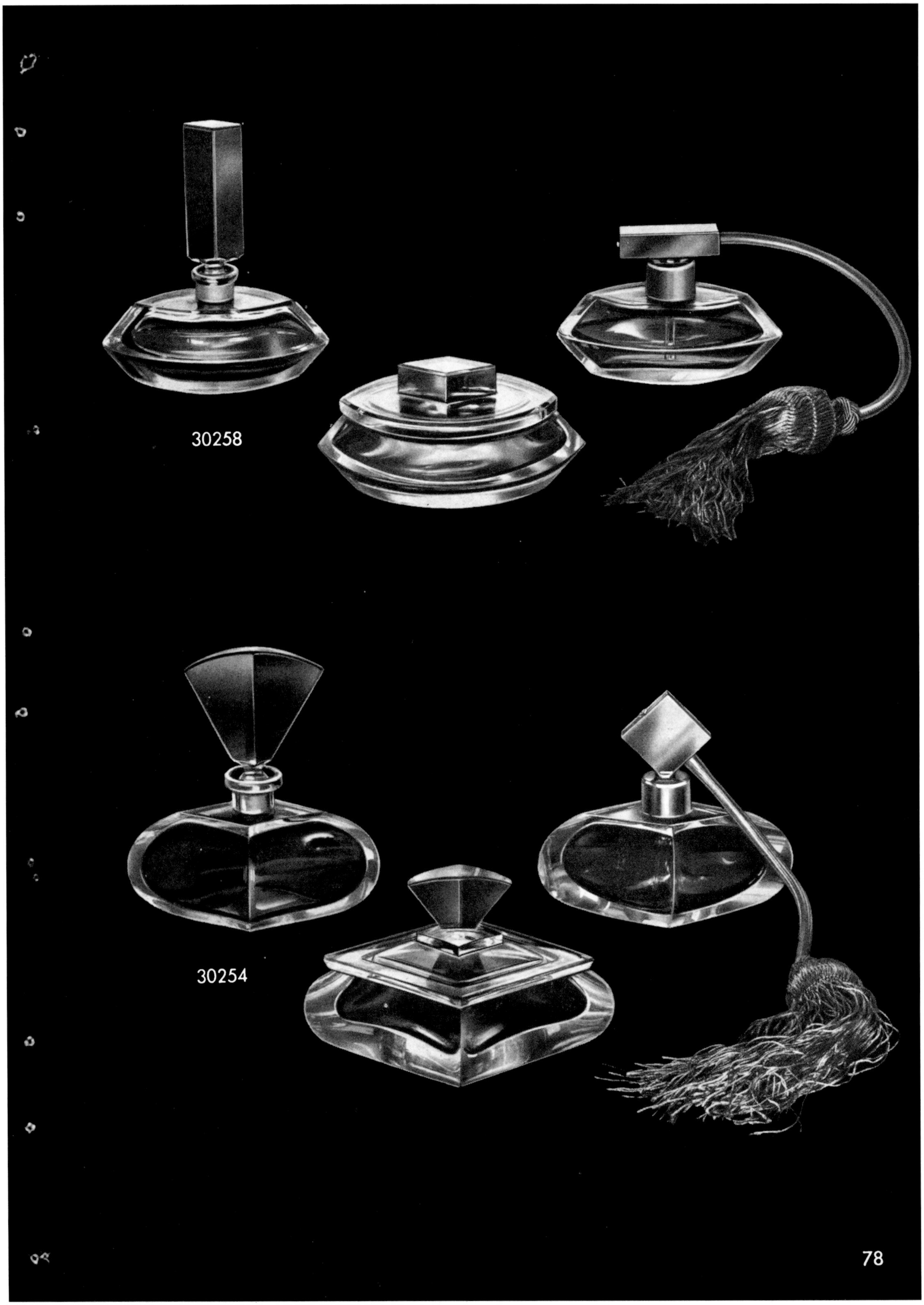
30258
30254
78

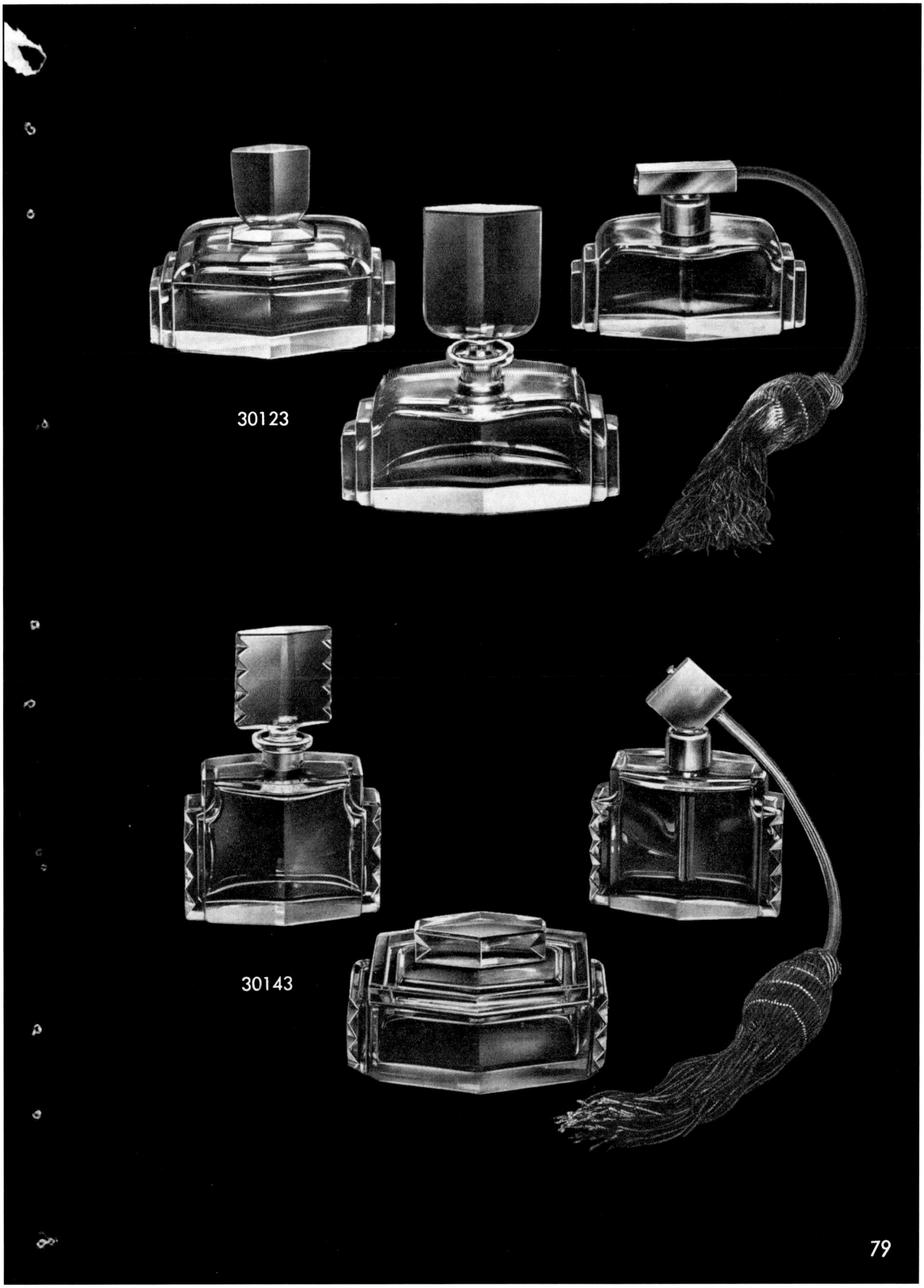
30123
30143
79

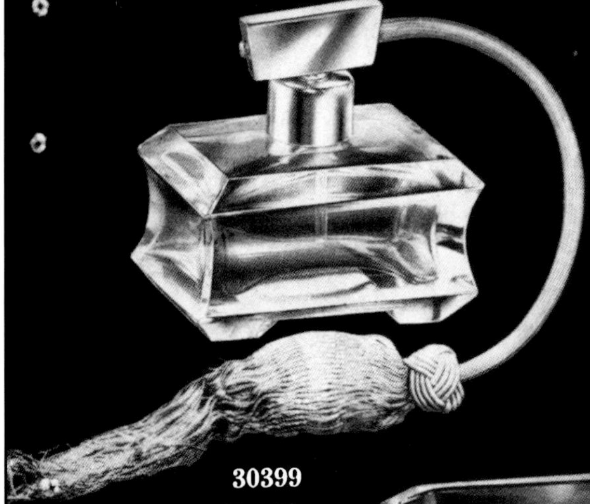

30399
95×60×100 mm

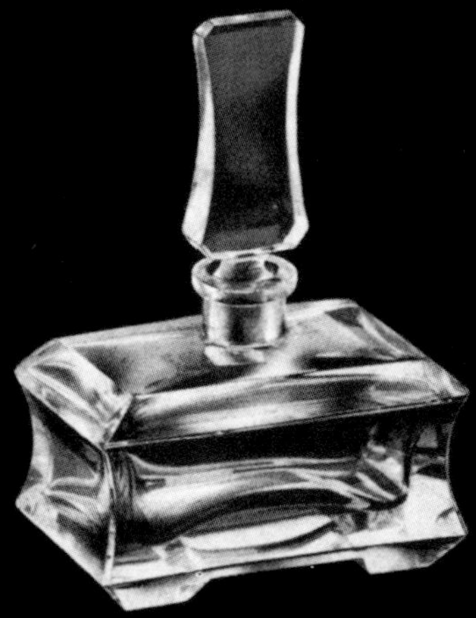

30399
95×60×135 mm

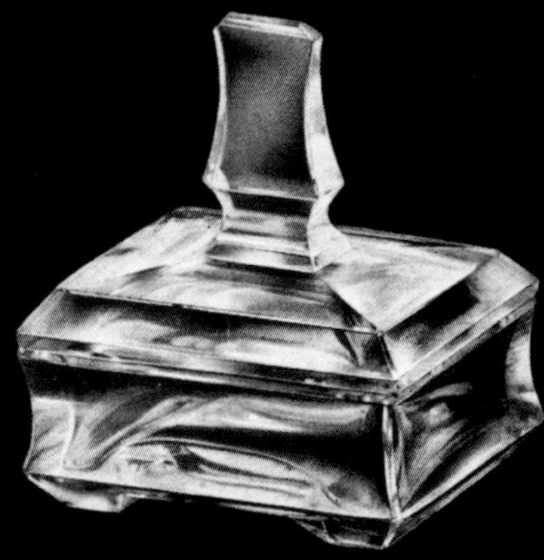

30399
105×85×110 mm

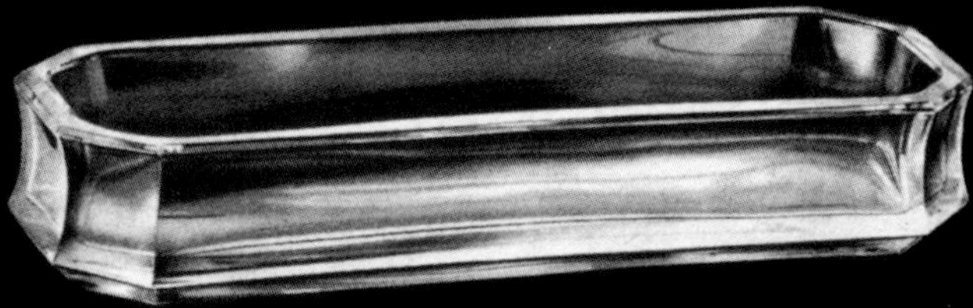

30399
220×70×35 mm

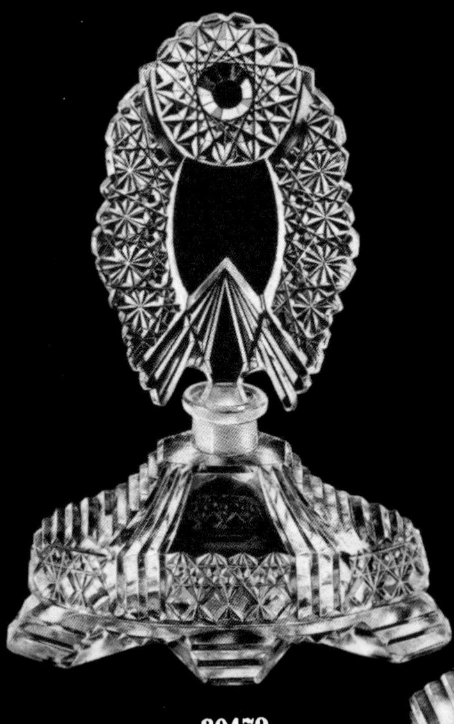

30479
150×78×215 mm

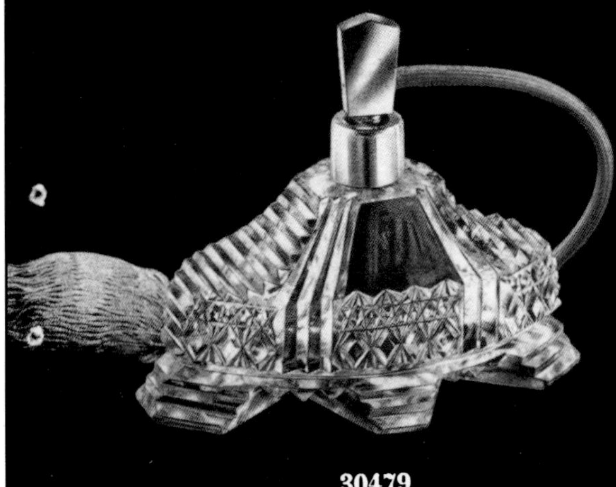

30479
150×78×110 mm

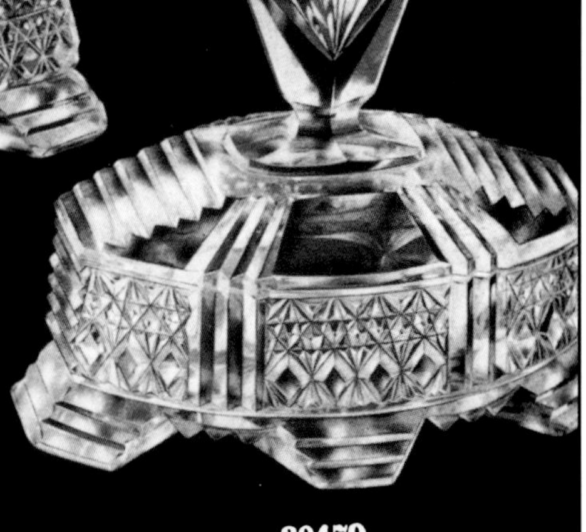

30479
162×100×130 mm

98

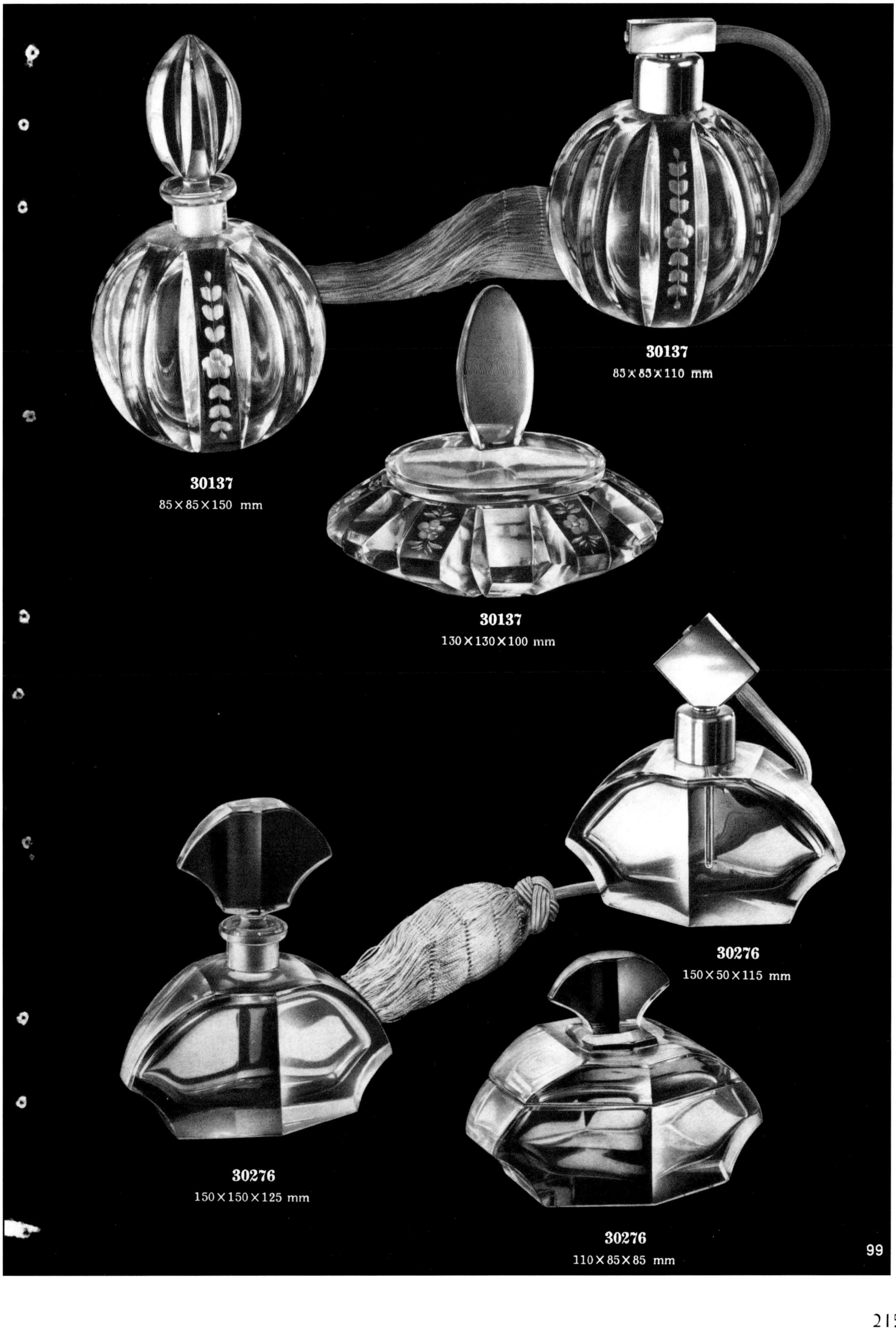

30137
85 X 85 X 110 mm

30137
85 X 85 X 150 mm

30137
130 X 130 X 100 mm

30276
150 X 50 X 115 mm

30276
150 X 150 X 125 mm

30276
110 X 85 X 85 mm

99

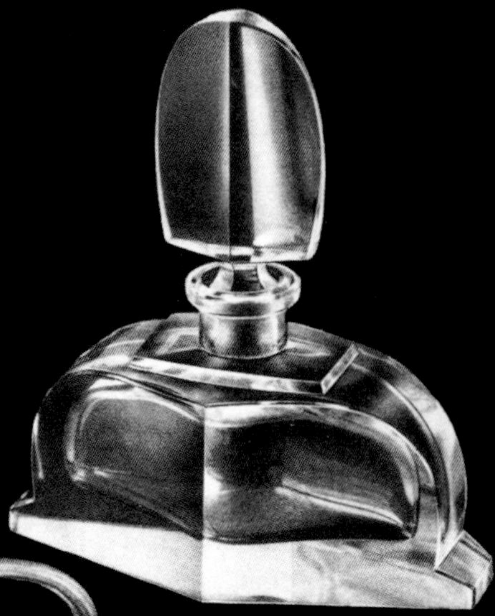

30039
120×60×135 mm

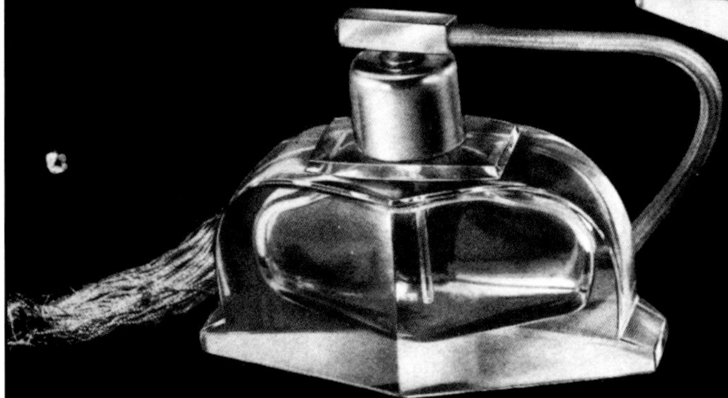

30039
120×60×85 mm

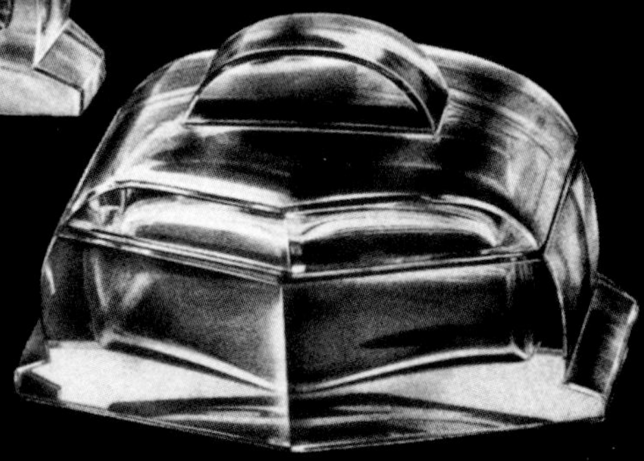

30039
120×80×65 mm

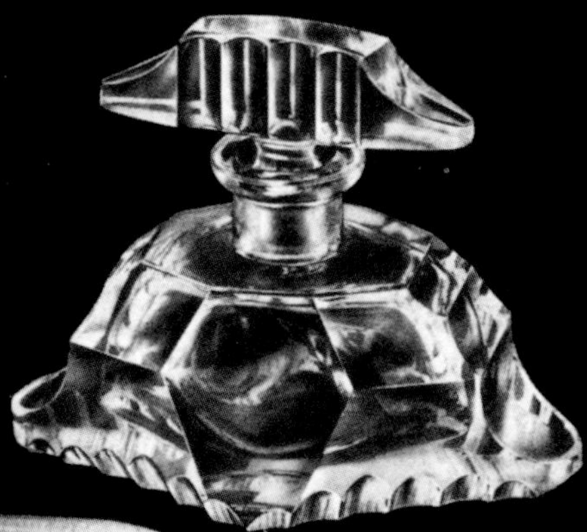

30327
120×75×90 mm

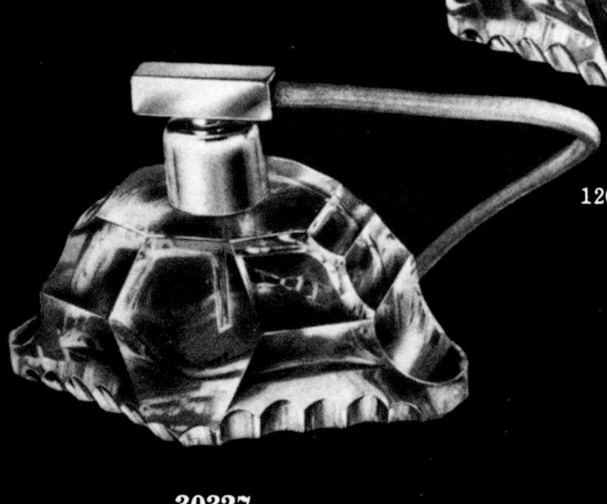

30327
120×75×75 mm

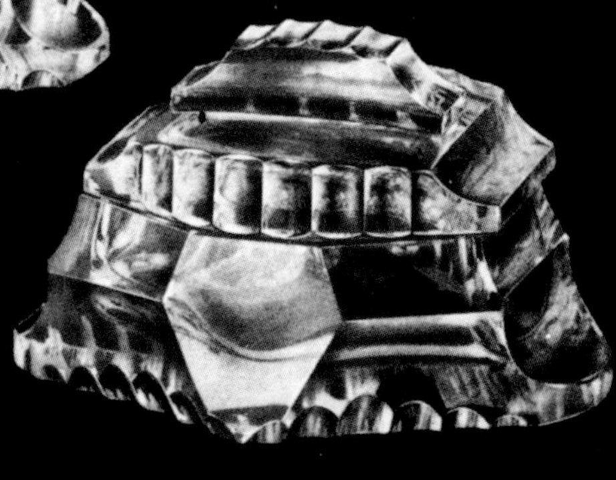

30327
120×95×70 mm

100

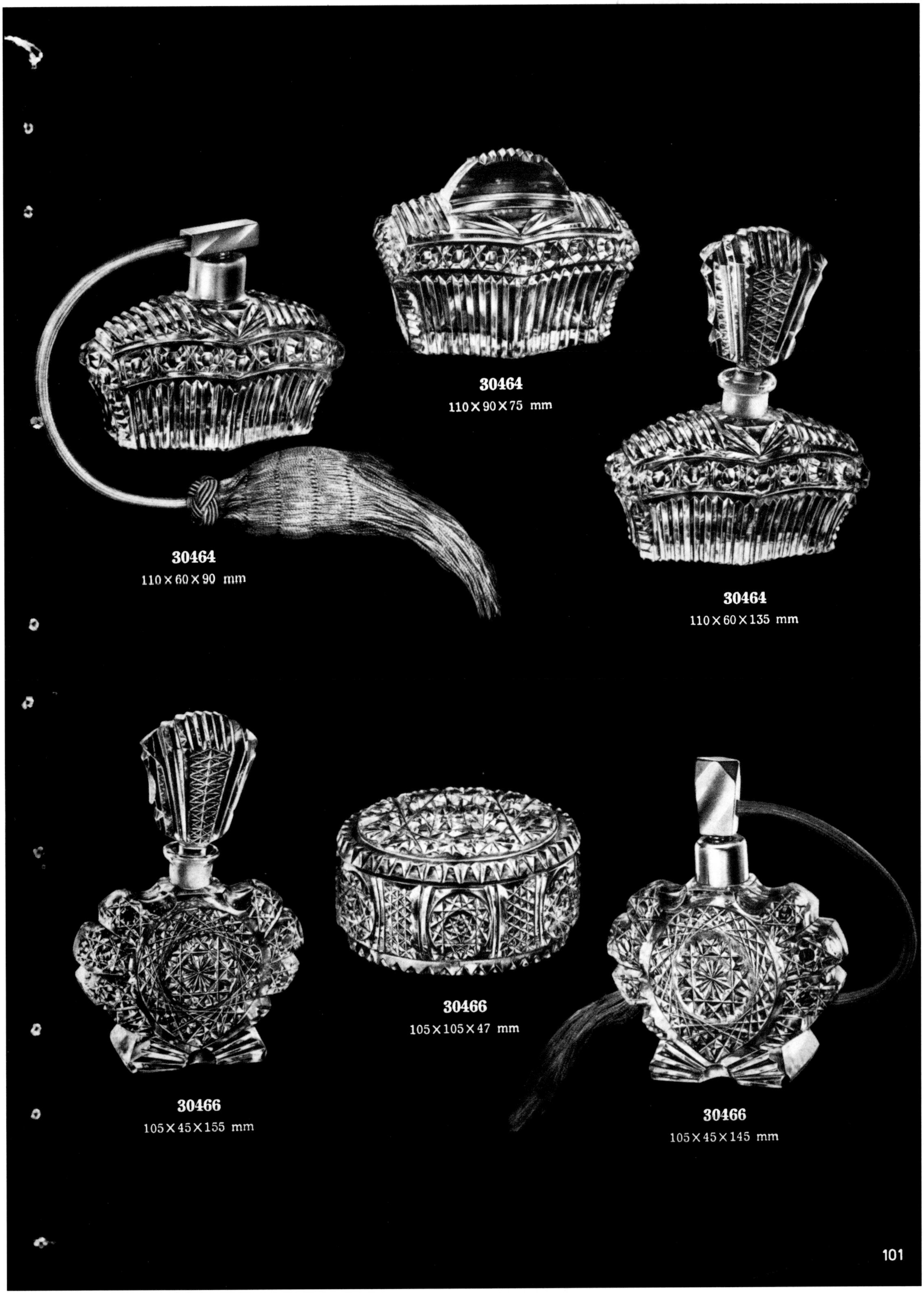
30464
110×90×75 mm
30464
110×60×90 mm
30464
110×60×135 mm
30466
105×105×47 mm
30466
105×45×155 mm
30466
105×45×145 mm
101

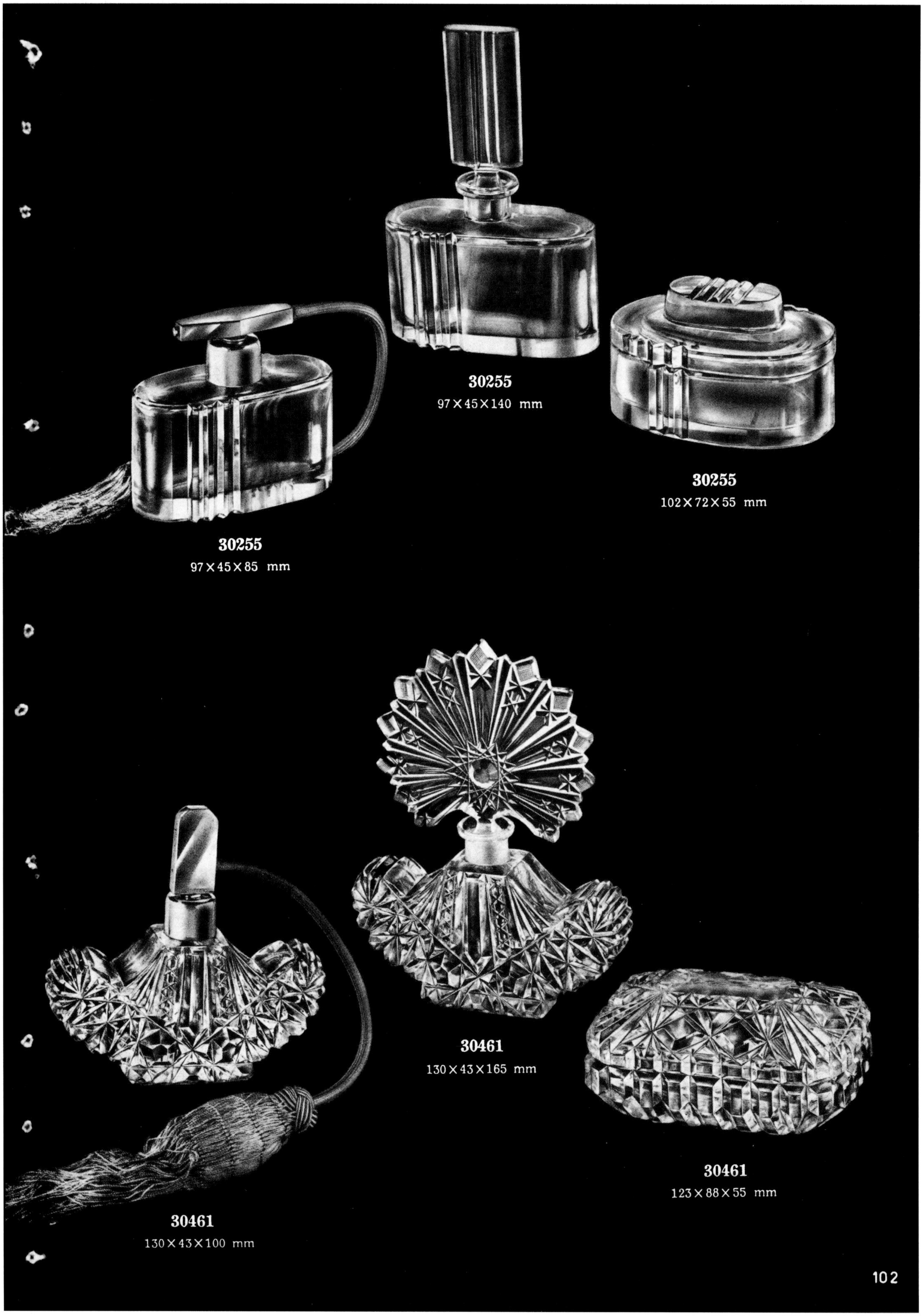

30255
97×45×140 mm

30255
102×72×55 mm

30255
97×45×85 mm

30461
130×43×165 mm

30461
123×88×55 mm

30461
130×43×100 mm

102

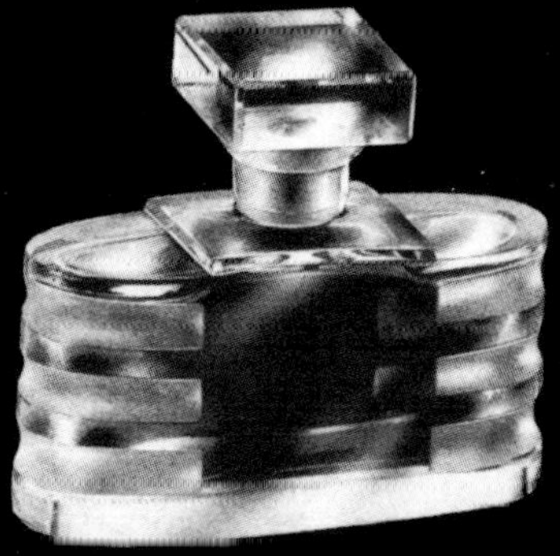

30013
95×36×82 mm

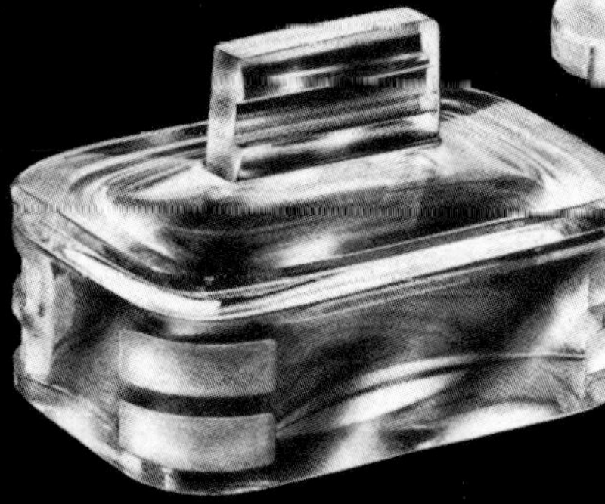

30013
113×75×65 mm

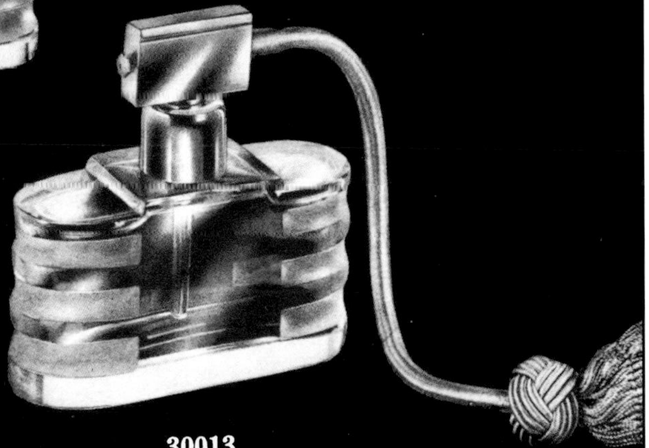

30013
95×36×90 mm

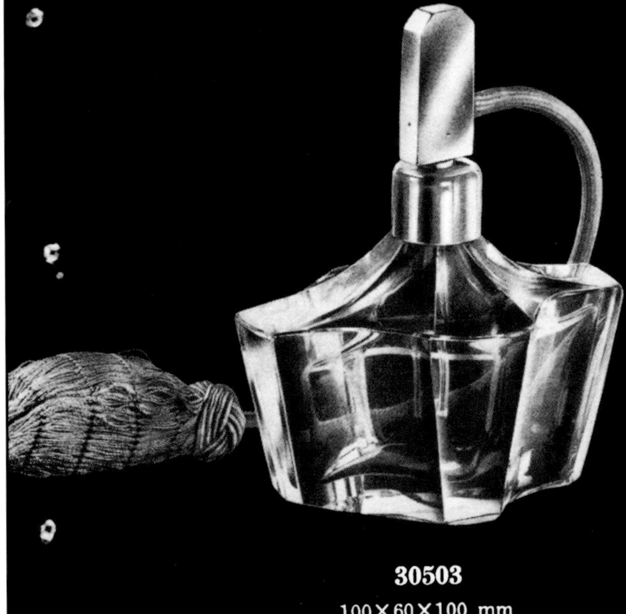

30503
100×60×100 mm

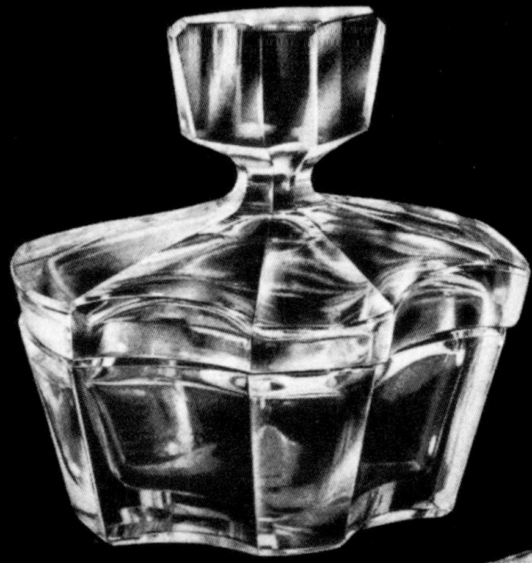

30503
110×80×100 mm

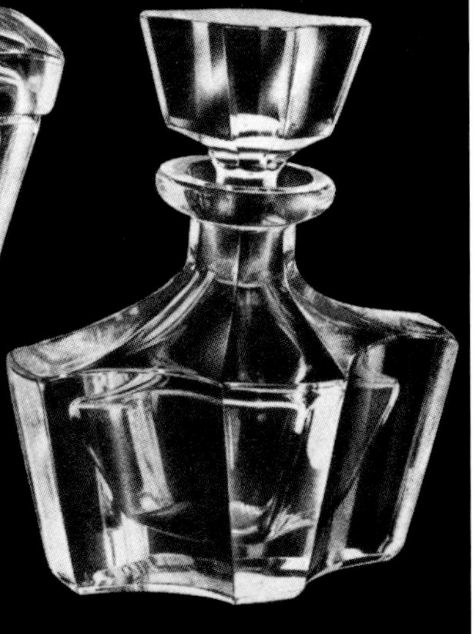

30503
100×60×125 mm

103

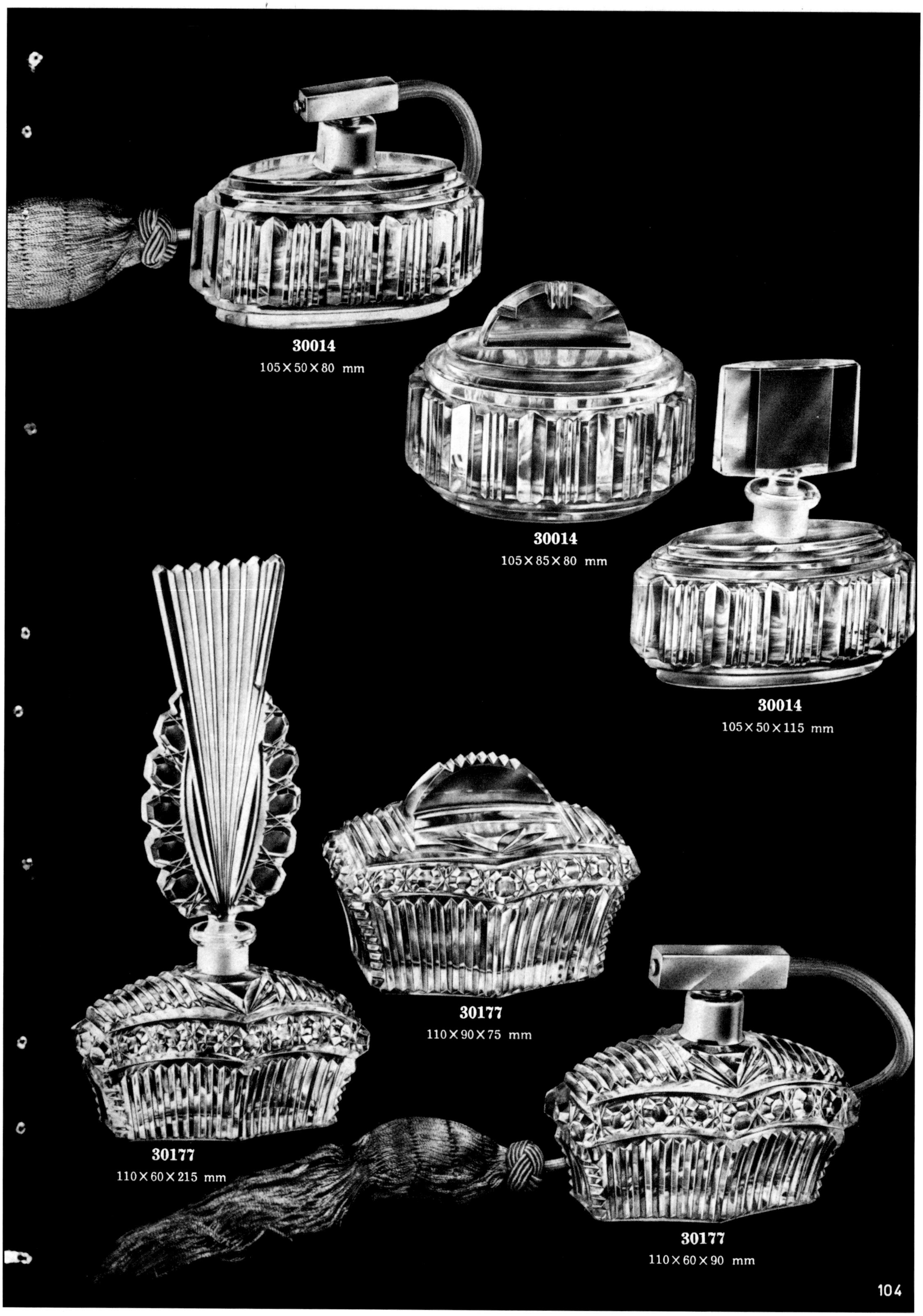

30014
105 X 50 X 80 mm

30014
105 X 85 X 80 mm

30014
105 X 50 X 115 mm

30177
110 X 90 X 75 mm

30177
110 X 60 X 215 mm

30177
110 X 60 X 90 mm

104

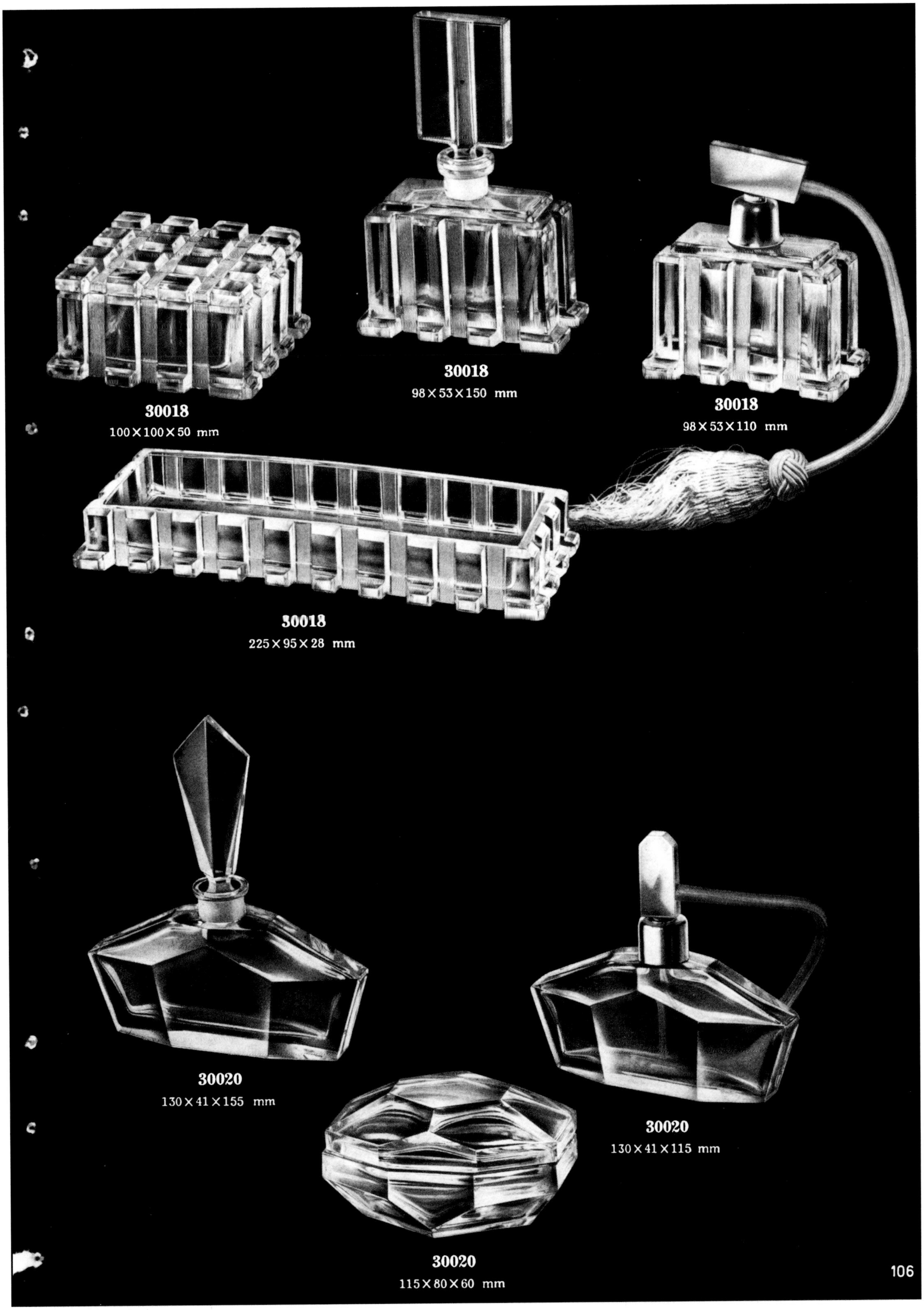

30018
100×100×50 mm

30018
98×53×150 mm

30018
98×53×110 mm

30018
225×95×28 mm

30020
130×41×155 mm

30020
130×41×115 mm

30020
115×80×60 mm

106

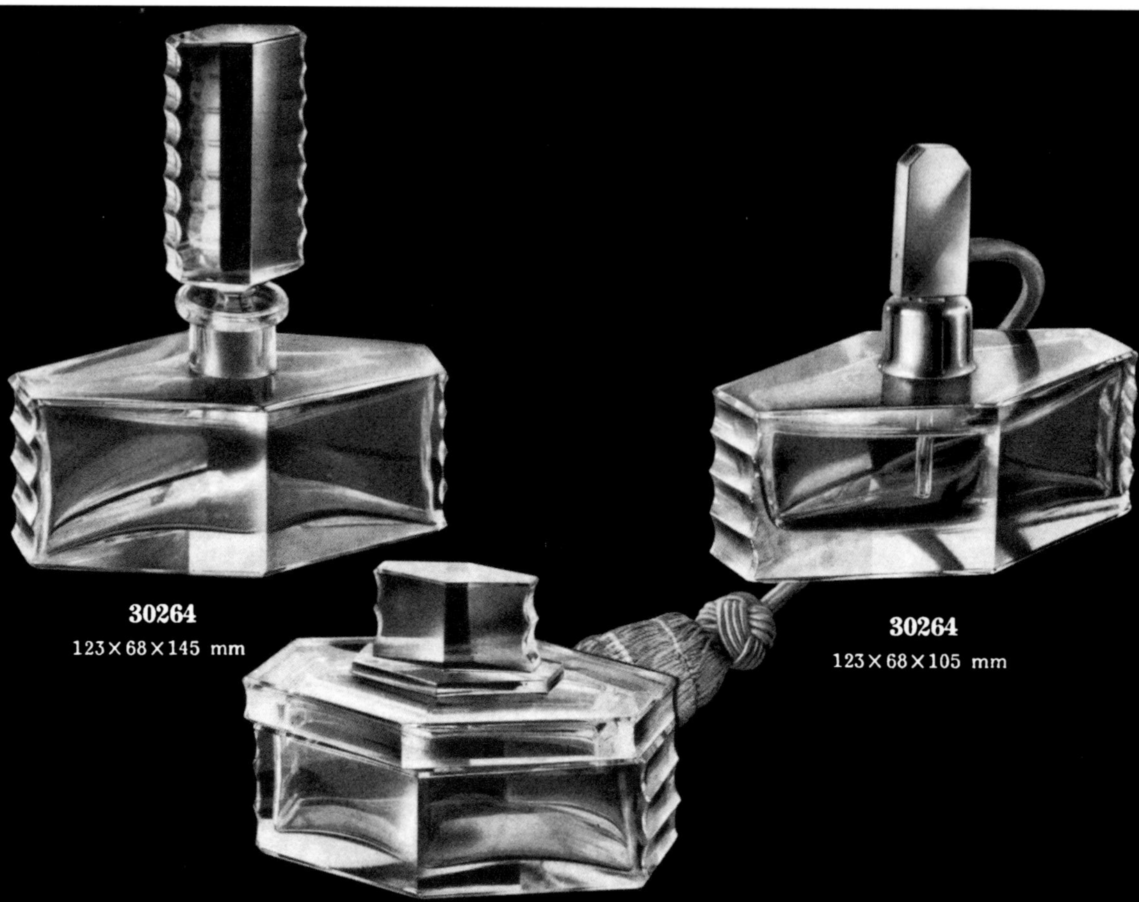

30264
123×68×145 mm

30264
123×68×105 mm

30264
110×83×75 mm

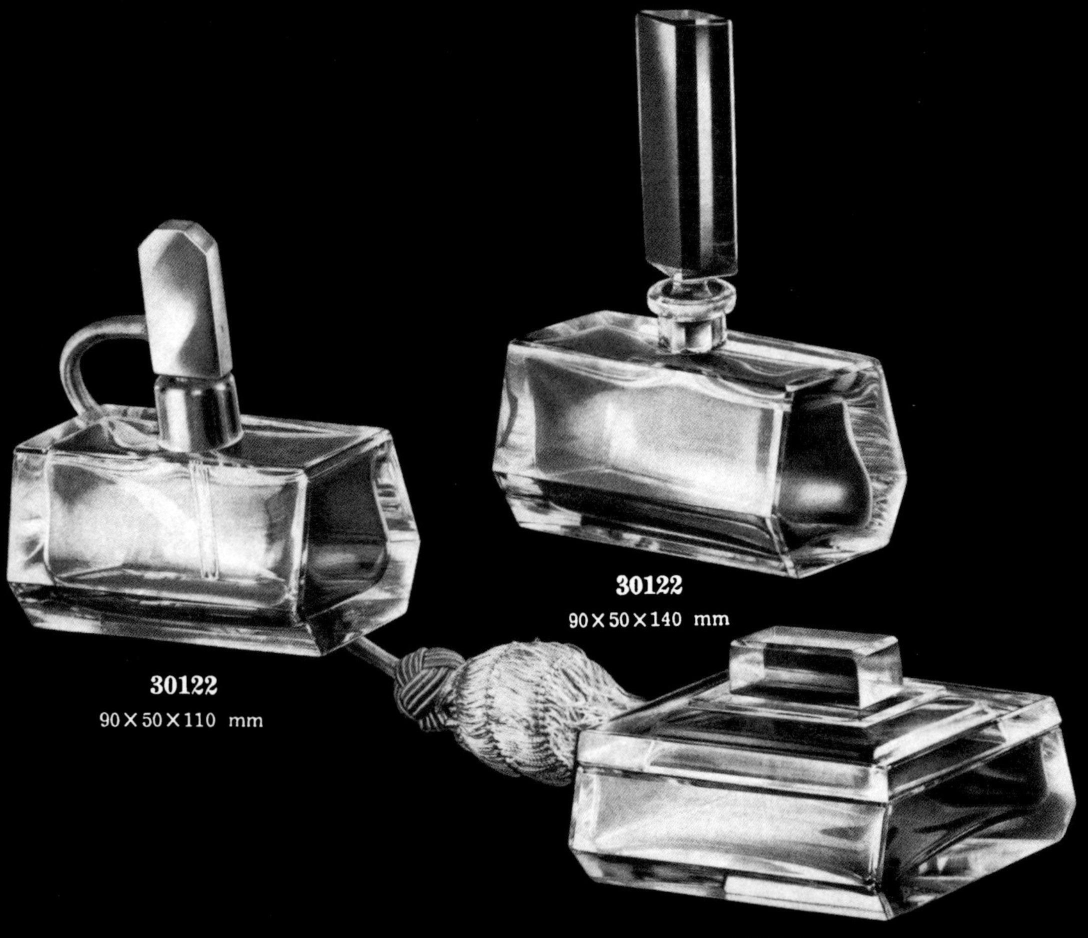

30122
90×50×140 mm

30122
90×50×110 mm

30122
135×95×60 mm

107

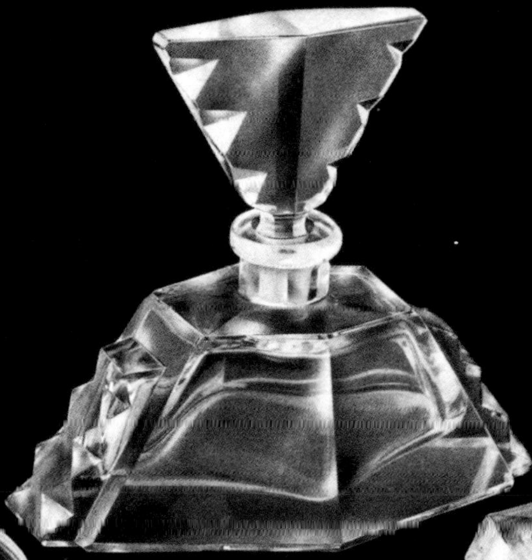

30146
138×78×125 mm

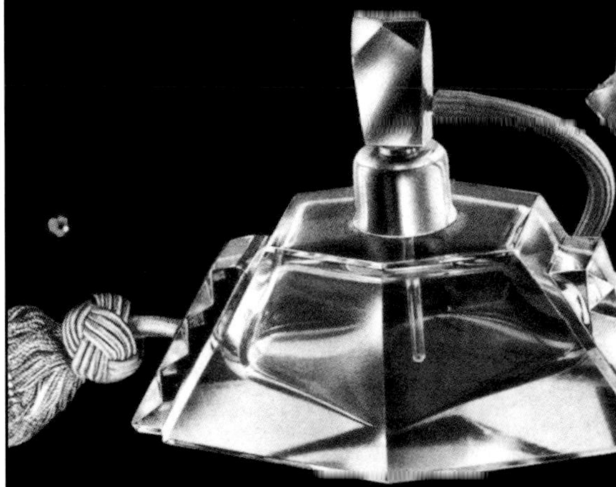

30140
138×78×105 mm

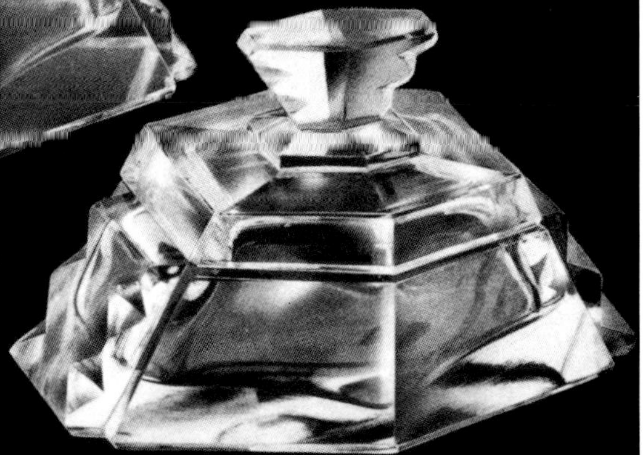

30146
138×103×78 mm

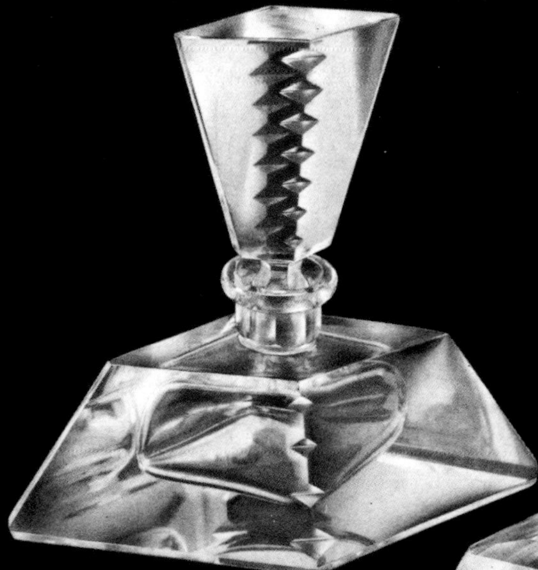

30124
155×80×140 mm

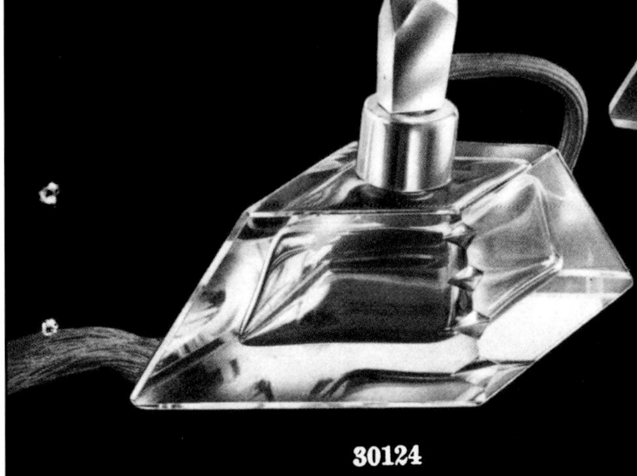

30124
155×80×100 mm

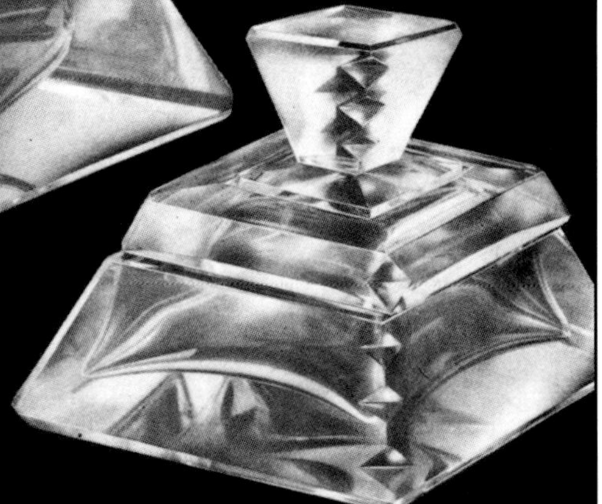

30124
150×110×85 mm

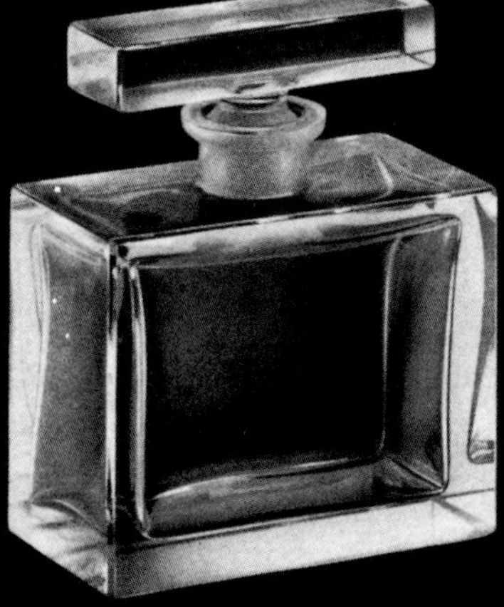

10916
92×49×110 mm

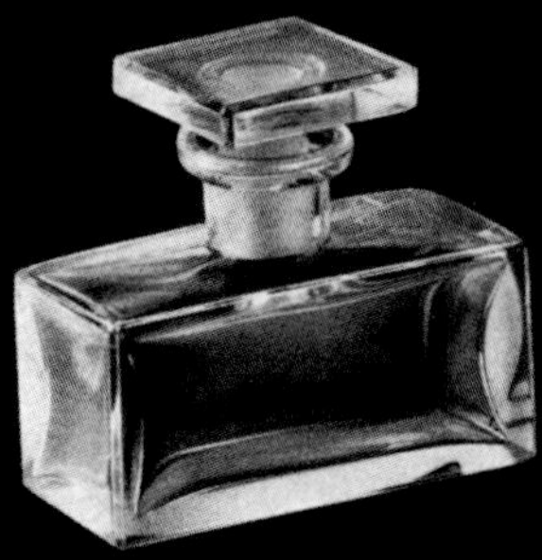

11741
75×35×70 mm

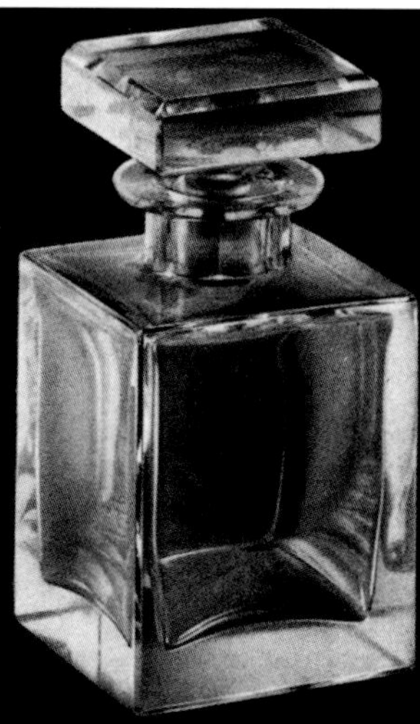

12867
60×60×120 mm

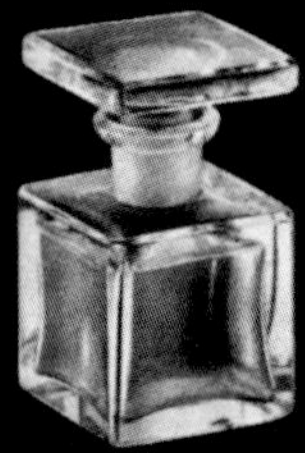

12254
30×30×55 mm

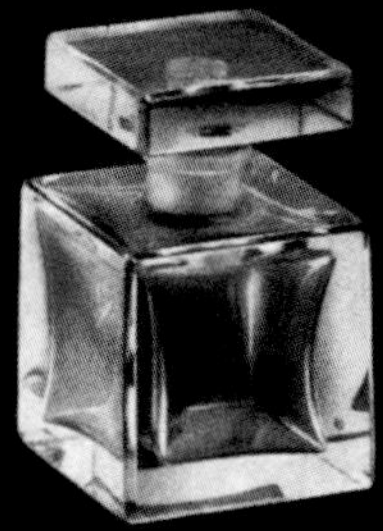

13183
40×40×65 mm

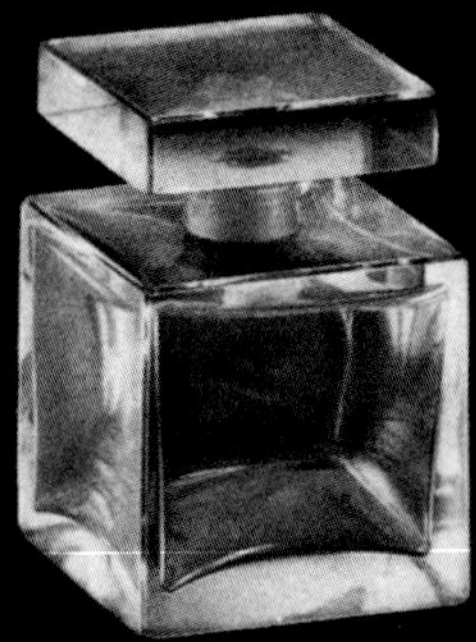

13427
50×50×75 mm

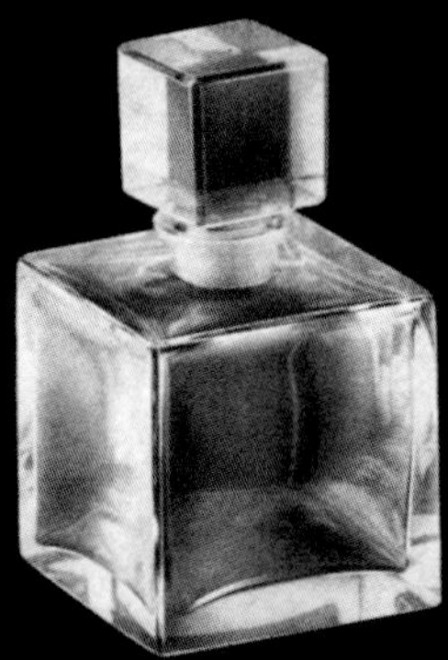

11378
50×50×90 mm

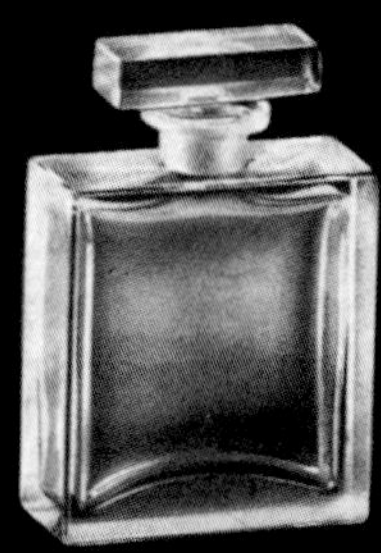

10497
48×19×73 mm

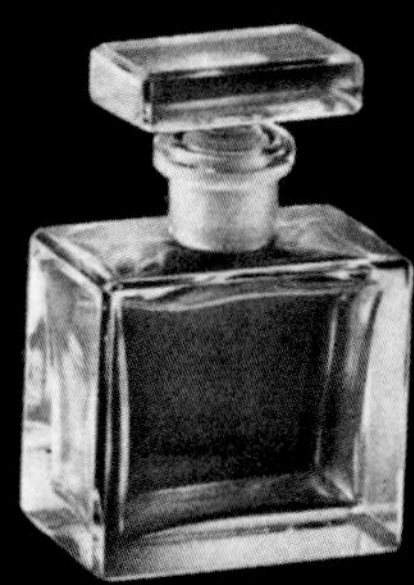

11197
50×31×74 mm

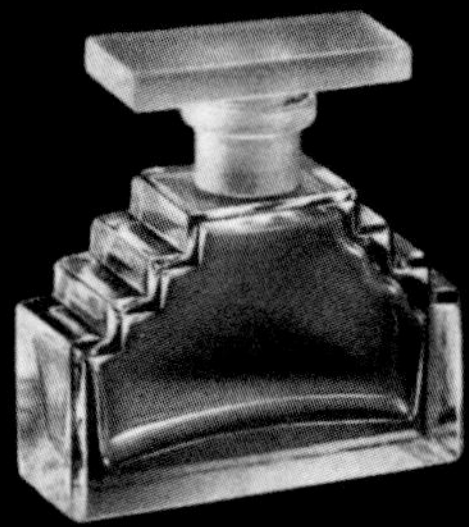

10209
65×24×65 mm

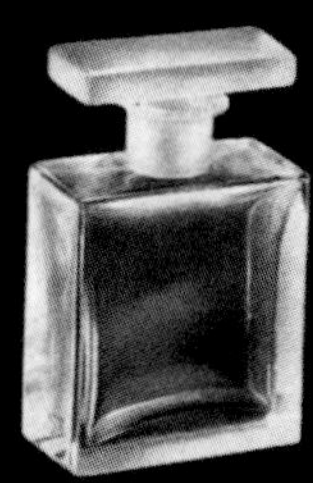

13432
39×19×60 mm

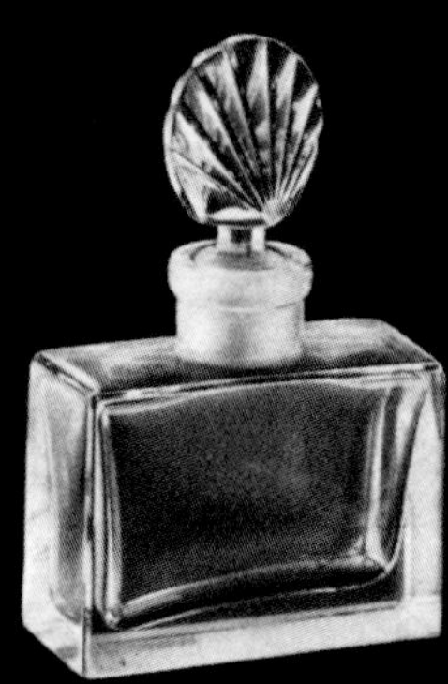

13179
60×27×95 mm

Part IV

Collecting Tips

Copies

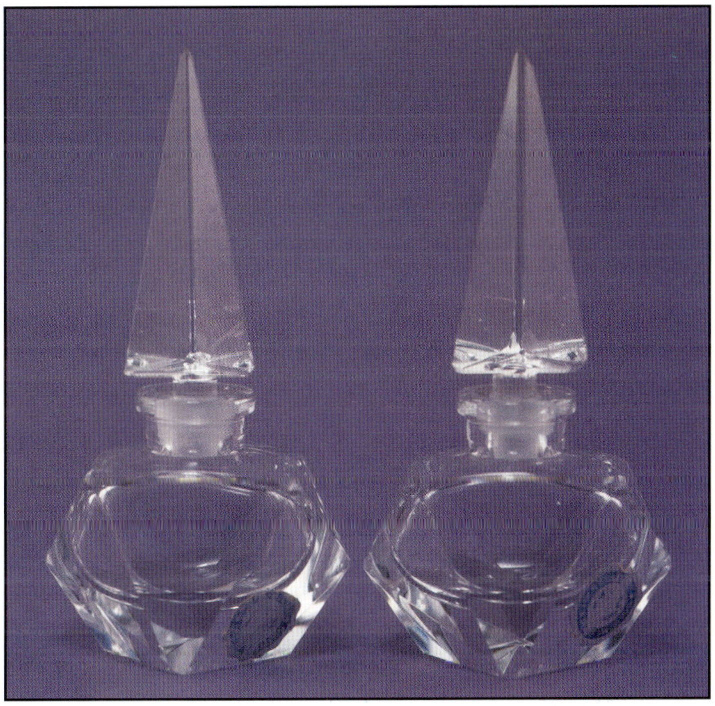

In the quest for Czech perfume bottles, the collector will most likely encounter bottles that have some characteristics of what is sought, but not all. This makes identifying the bottles difficult. With dresser bottles, one looks for the acid mark on the base. It usually appears in a circle, an oval, or a line. If metal work is present, the mark is sometimes there and can be well hidden in a straight line on filigree.

The absence of any identifier could mean a number of things: the item may predate the requirement to note the country of origin; the bottle may not have been sold or shipped to a country, like the US, where the mark is required; it might have been part of a set, the marking having been placed on another part of the set; it might have been marked with a paper label or sticker that has been removed; or, lastly, it might not be Czech.

Japan also produced perfume bottles and was willing to adjust to the specifications of the importer, like Irice. It is not surprising that bottles made in Japan looked so similar to Czech bottles, if that is what the importer had been buying and expected to find. The clear glass pair shown here bear the Irice sticker, by now printed in blue on silver and naming Japan as the country of origin.

Many of the Japanese bottles, though similar in shape or style to their Czech counterparts, were not of good quality. Some twin and triplet sets on trays are similar to Czech designs, but the glass is obviously pressed and cloudy. With some bottles, however, the copies are good enough to cause the collector to examine them very carefully.

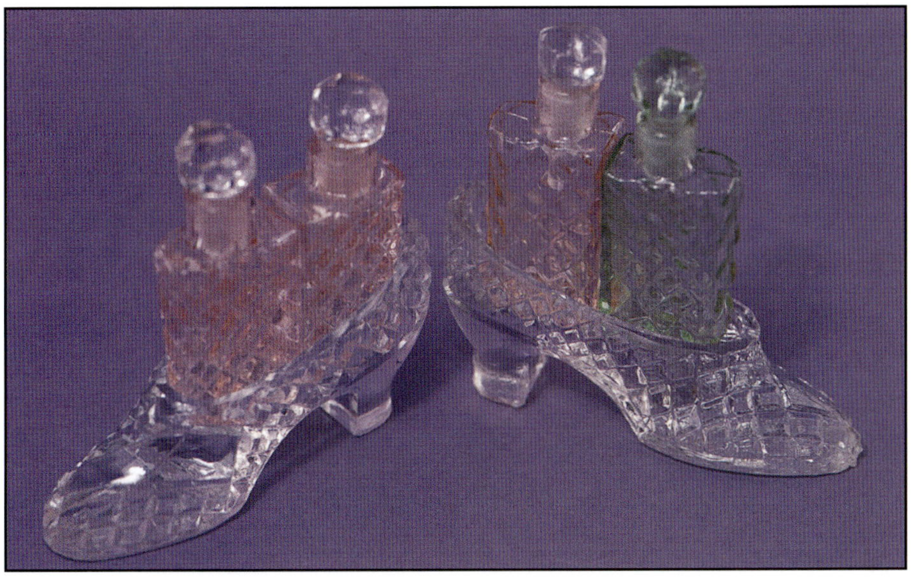

These Cinderella slippers look the same at first glance. The stopper balls show the difference in quality and detailing, however. The pair on the left, with both pink bottles, is marked "Czechoslovakia," while the one on the right is marked "Japan." Left: 2.75". $300-400. Right: 3". $175-225.

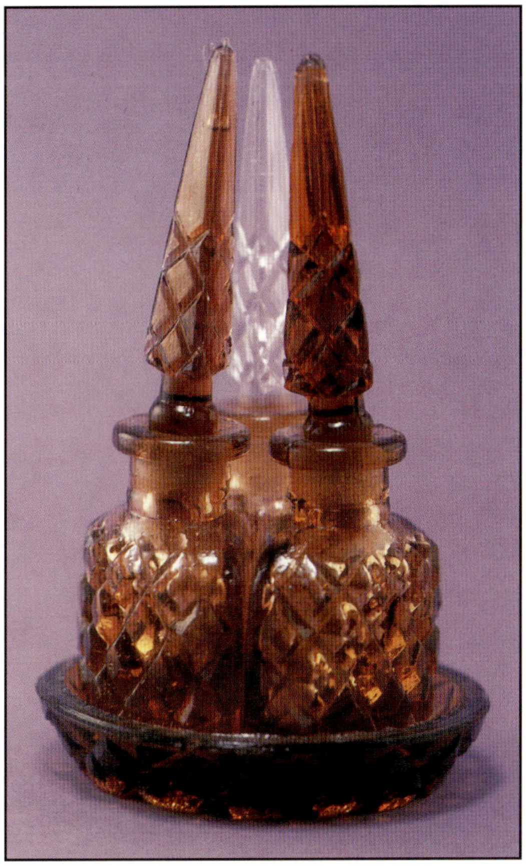

The unmarked green bottle in this photograph is probably Japanese. The color is different—bluer than the Czech greens. The base is thicker and the stopper has a very simple design with only simple edge cuts. The dauber has mold seams and is all one piece, rather than having been applied later.

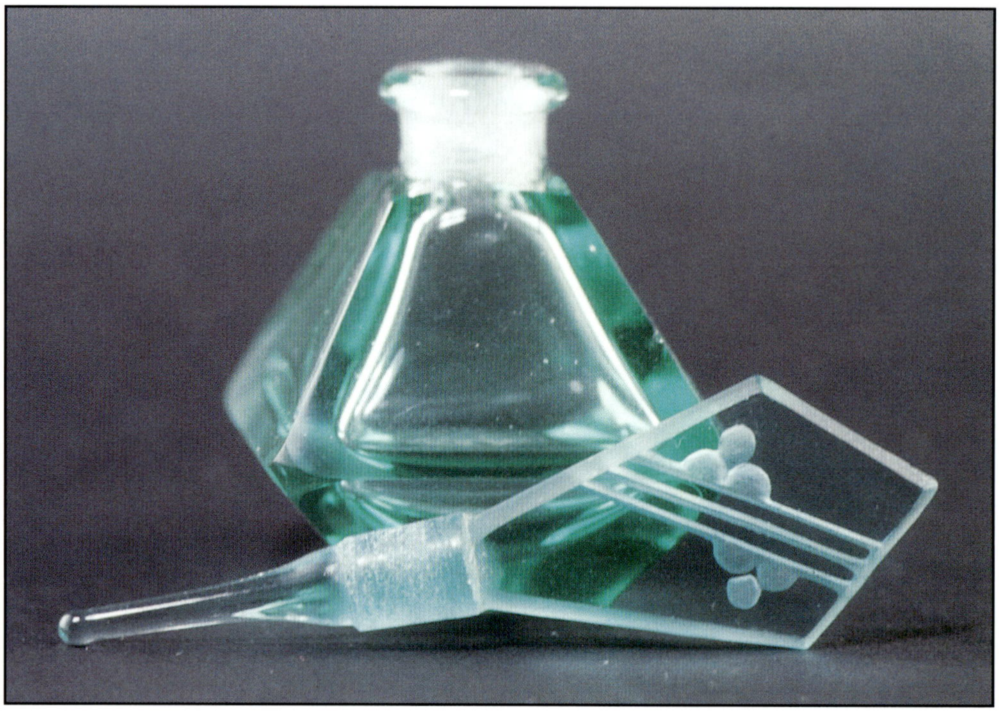

The next two bottles could easily be mistaken for Czech. The color is right and the dauber is a clear glass rod affixed to the plug. However, both are acid marked "Japan."

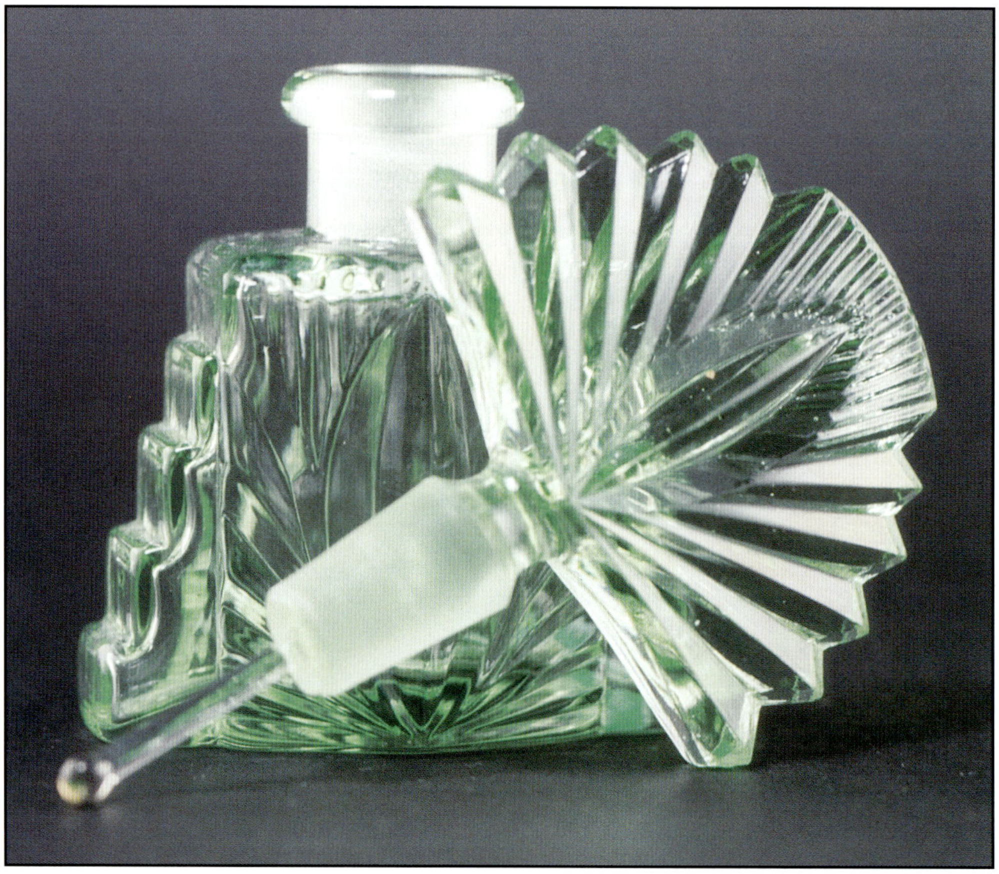

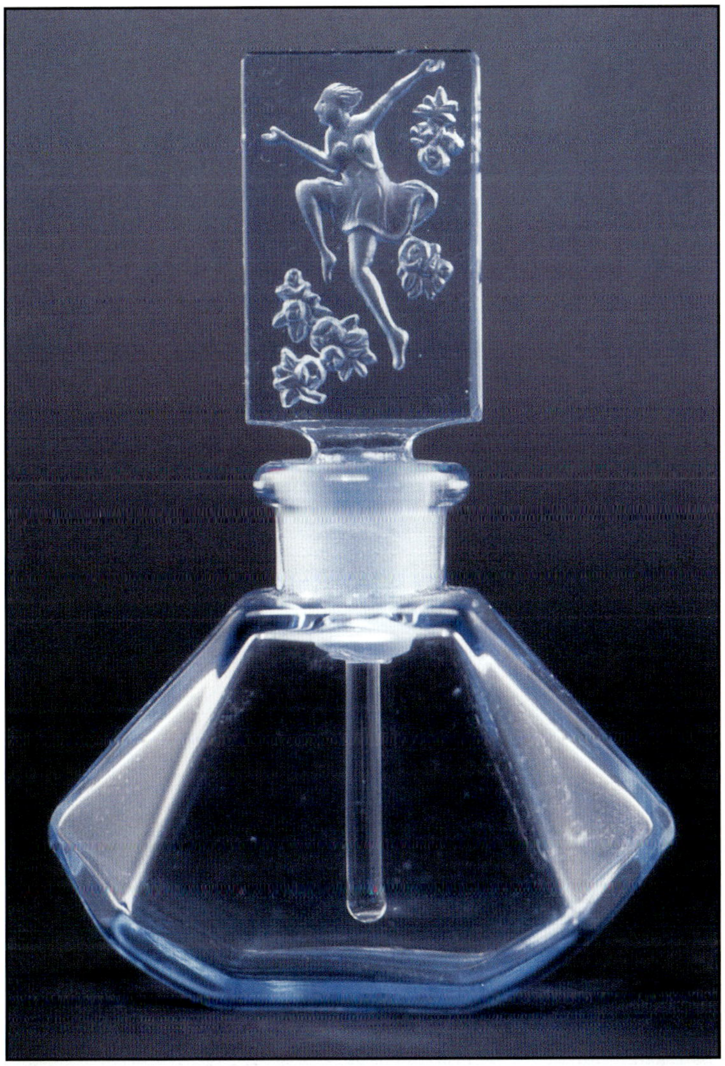

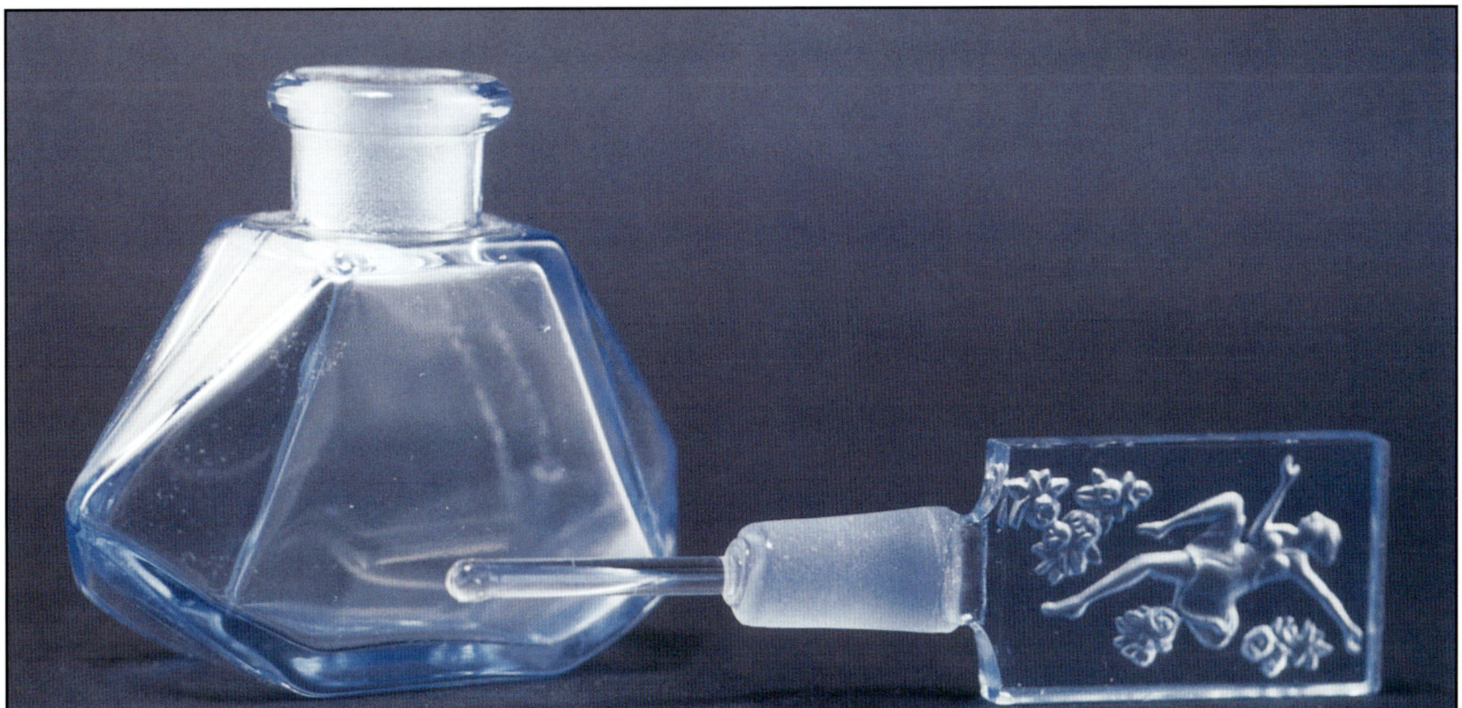

The last two pictures show a novelty bottle by Lander. The "fine" stopper fan is plastic over a screw cap. Other companies also produced "faux" stoppers mimicking the finer Czech glass and showing how popular and luxurious the style was thought to be. The second picture here shows the interesting floral shaping of the bottom of the bottle.

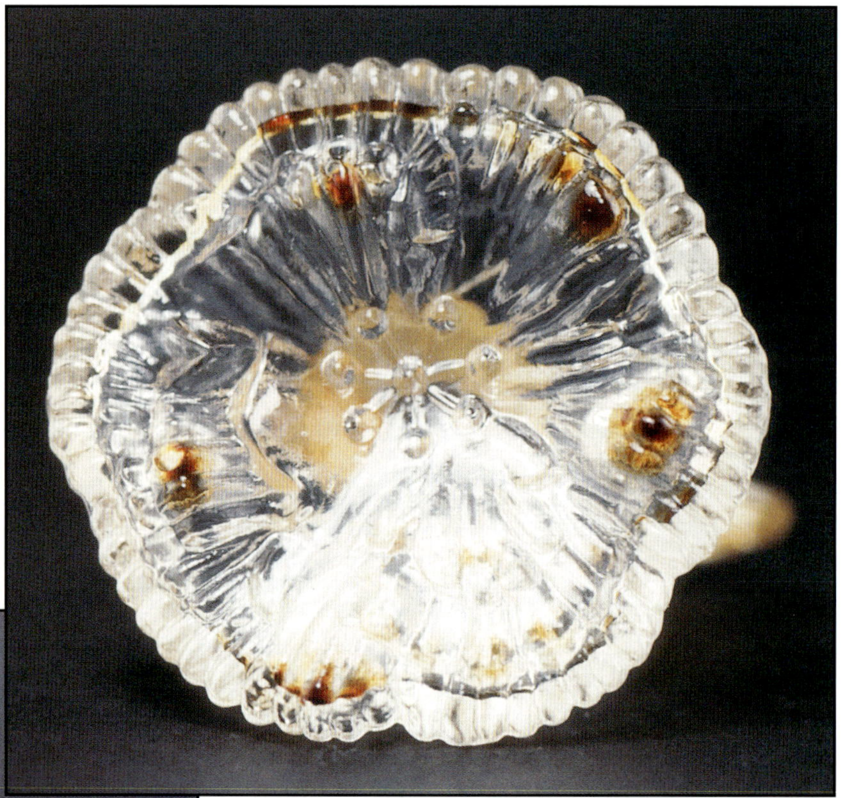

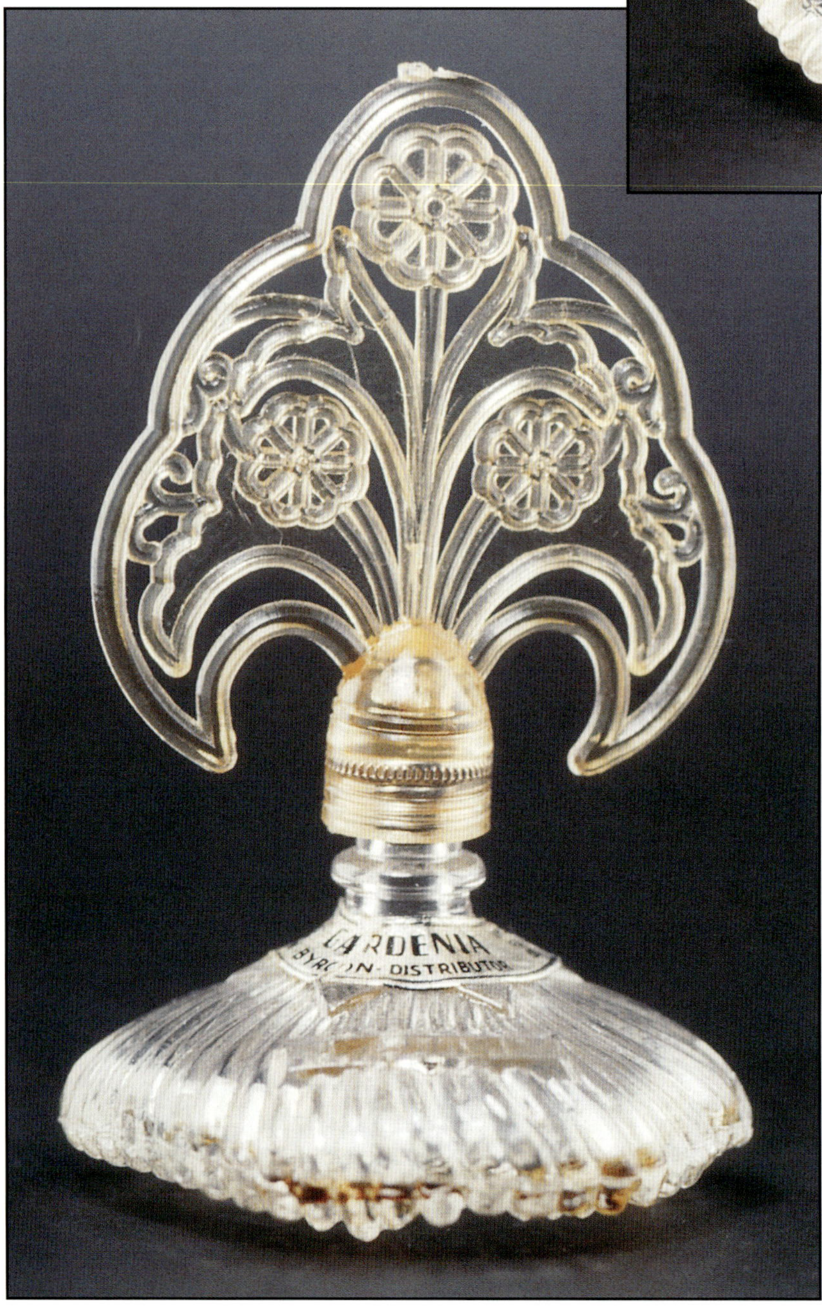

Reproductions

Czech art glass has been back on the market since the early 1990s. Many of the classic molds for perfume bottles and stoppers have been restored and placed in production. As one might imagine, the arrival of reproduction pieces brought a degree of alarm to many collectors who had literally thousands of dollars invested in originals. The concern was that new pieces would flood the market passing for old and that buyers would not be able to tell the difference.

The reality has been that while pieces emerge from the same molds, there are differences in color and in finishing that set them apart. Close inspection should allow the careful collector to be reasonably certain of what he or she is buying.

That being said, it should be also noted that the emerging Czech Republic glass industry produces some lovely, quality pieces, many of which are signed by the contemporary artist or marked by the production company. There is no intent or need to misrepresent product that is art in its own right. Also, current producers are not responsible for the few who misrepresent new pieces with intent to defraud buyers.

It is the responsibility of each buyer to buy intelligently. And, experience is a thorough teacher. I once bought a teal-colored "lady and the peacock" piece from an antique mall in Seattle. The color was unusual, while the price of $175 made it a real bargain if it was old—and quite expensive, if new. I was rushed, as the mall was closing and I would be leaving town, so my examination of the bottle was hurried. I took the card for the mall and noted the dealer's booth number. I called back from home to make further inquiries about the history of the bottle, but the dealer had purchased it from an estate sale and could not tell me more. I bought the bottle and it is a new production. But it is lovely and sits in my bathroom window, set apart from my antique bottles, but enjoyed for its own sake.

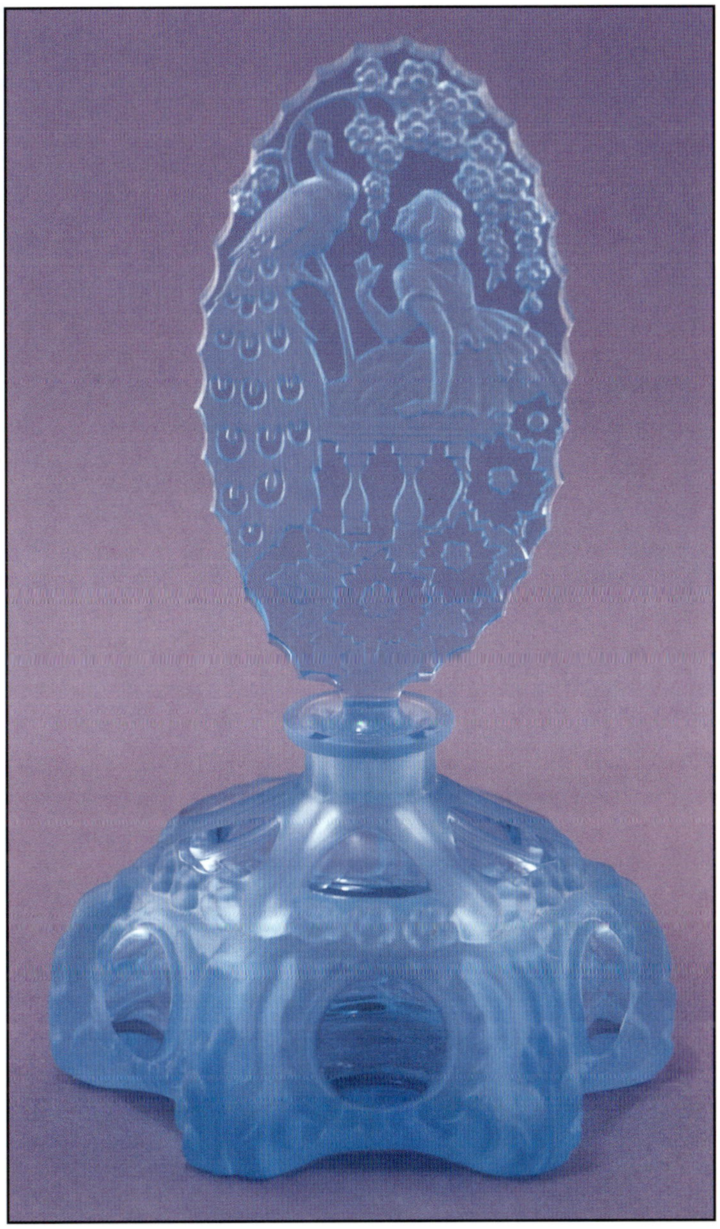

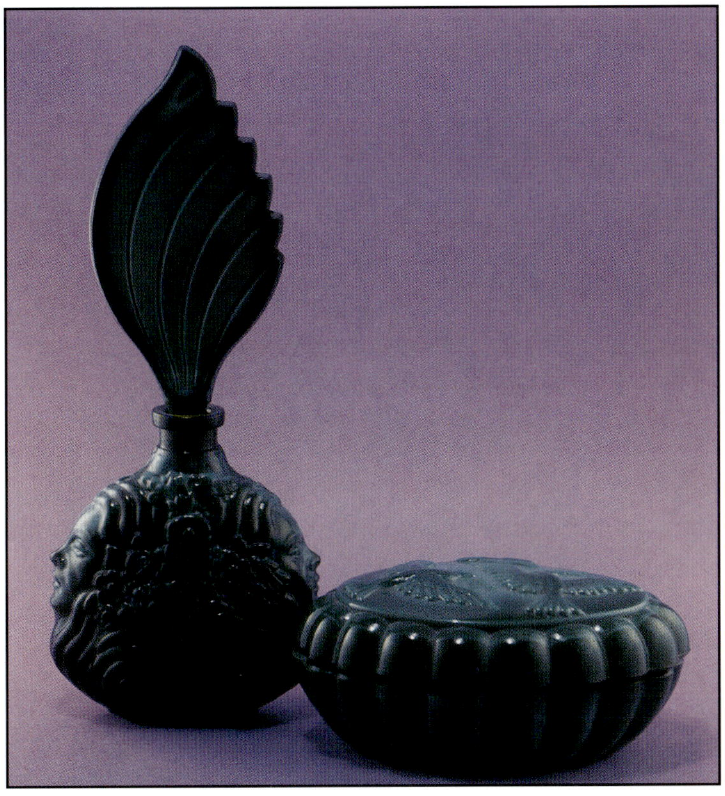

The lesson is, "do not be rushed." Take the time to inspect the bottle—handling it, looking at the finish detailing, and checking for signs of use and normal wear. Be skeptical of any bottle that looks new and does not have a verified history. Consider carefully what the bottle is worth to you, and if it does not look and feel right, remember, a better investment is somewhere in your future.

Malachite glass is popular in reproduction. The bottle and box shown here have the bright, high gloss of new pieces.

Michael Genger, an American who resides in Prague, deals with integrity in both the old and the new Czech pieces. He sent a list of bottles and stoppers that are in current production. His numbers correspond with item numbers in Jones-North's 1990, 1999 revision edition. He asked me to publish his list to inform and assist collectors. Genger notes, "this information is vital, as few collectors are aware of the vast array of articles which are in current production as well as which molds do exist, but are not currently being made." His list is as follows:

> #132, 134, 154, 164, 177, 183, 203 (in Malachite/Lapis/Crystal, and Black), 205 bottle exists (not currently being made, was made in the mid 1990s...) 220, 222, 230, 301 (both bottle and stopper), 303, 304 and 305 (bottle only) 306, 307, 308, 309, 311, 312, 313, 339 (bottle only), 340, 362 (both stopper and bottle), 365, 366, 367, 369, 370, 382 (stopper), 390 (bottle only), 394 (both stopper and bottle were made in the mid 1990s, still exists, not being made today), 397, 398, 399, 400, 401, 403, 406, 409 (both stopper and bottle), 468 (stopper and bottle), 515, 545, 564, 574, 576 (mold still exists and will be made soon), 575, 579, 580, 587, 588, 589, 590 (I own this mold and it is being made by my company), 592, 696, 698, 835 (I own this mold and it is being made by The CIO Collection through a strict limited edition of 750 signed and numbered pieces in each color; has been sold already in Alexandrite, Crystal, Pale blue, Sea Foam, Teal, Citrin, Cobalt, Amber [these colors aside from the crystal and amber are all sold out and now only available on the secondary market]. This year's colors: Ruby, Black, Amethyst, Honey), 771, 800 (this mold I won and is being produced by my company), 799, 806 and 807, 810, 815 (stopper only), 816. On page 102, perfume bottle in the advertisement which appears on the lower right hand side of Art Nouveau Lady, 817, 829 (stopper and bottle), 834 (stopper and bottle) 836, 839, 848 (both stopper and bottle were made in the mid-1990s), in grouping #854, the third bottle from the left, the pierced, clear tiara, the stopper is in current production), 857 (face stopper), 861, 862 (already mentioned), 863, 865, 866, 867, 868 869, 870 (all already mentioned), 873, 874, 875, 883 (already mentioned).

Note: for further information on reproductions, including photos, see Ruth Forsythe's addenda to Jones-North, 1999 edition, pp. 141-144.

Other Fun Stuff

Once a person gets "hooked" on Czechoslovakian perfume bottles, it becomes natural to start noticing other items made in Czechoslovakia as well. For example, the jewelry that accompanies some of the bottles shown in this book seemed too pretty or interesting to pass up. It does not hurt that "retro" is still great to wear. As with perfume bottles, the stones in the settings are usually intact, and if the color combinations are a little different from what we are used to...well, they serve to remind us of how styles and "looks" change.

Salt cellars, dating from a time when salt did not pour easily out of a Morton™ box, are another category of eye-catching Czech items. Those shown here range in size from 2.25" to 3" across. Plain intaglio salts can be found for between $50-100; jeweled ones run as much as $250. The boxed set with the glass spoons would cost between $75-125.

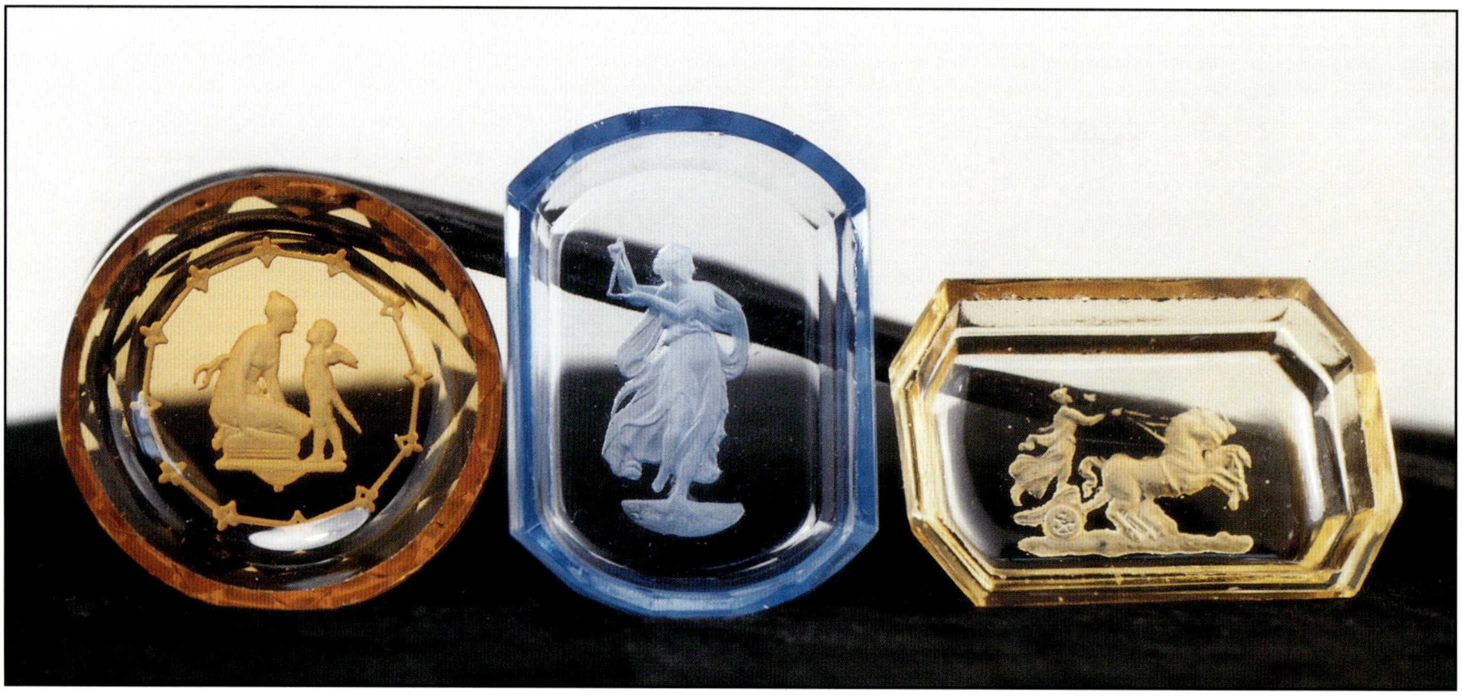

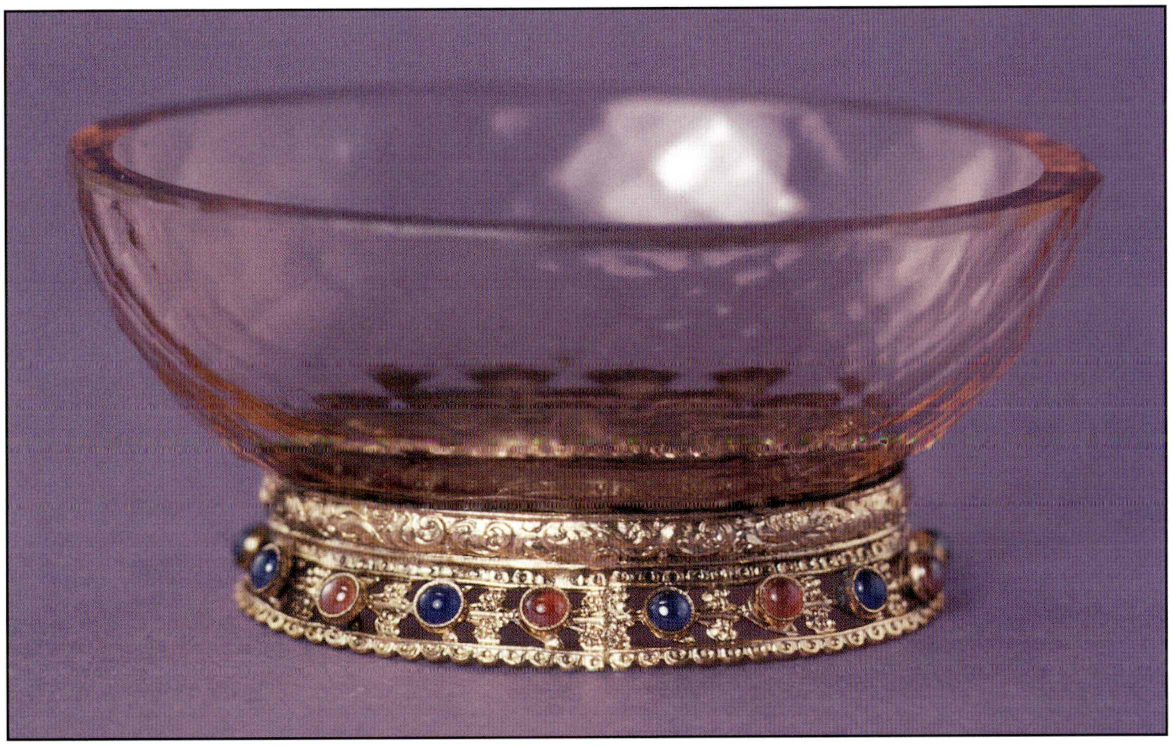

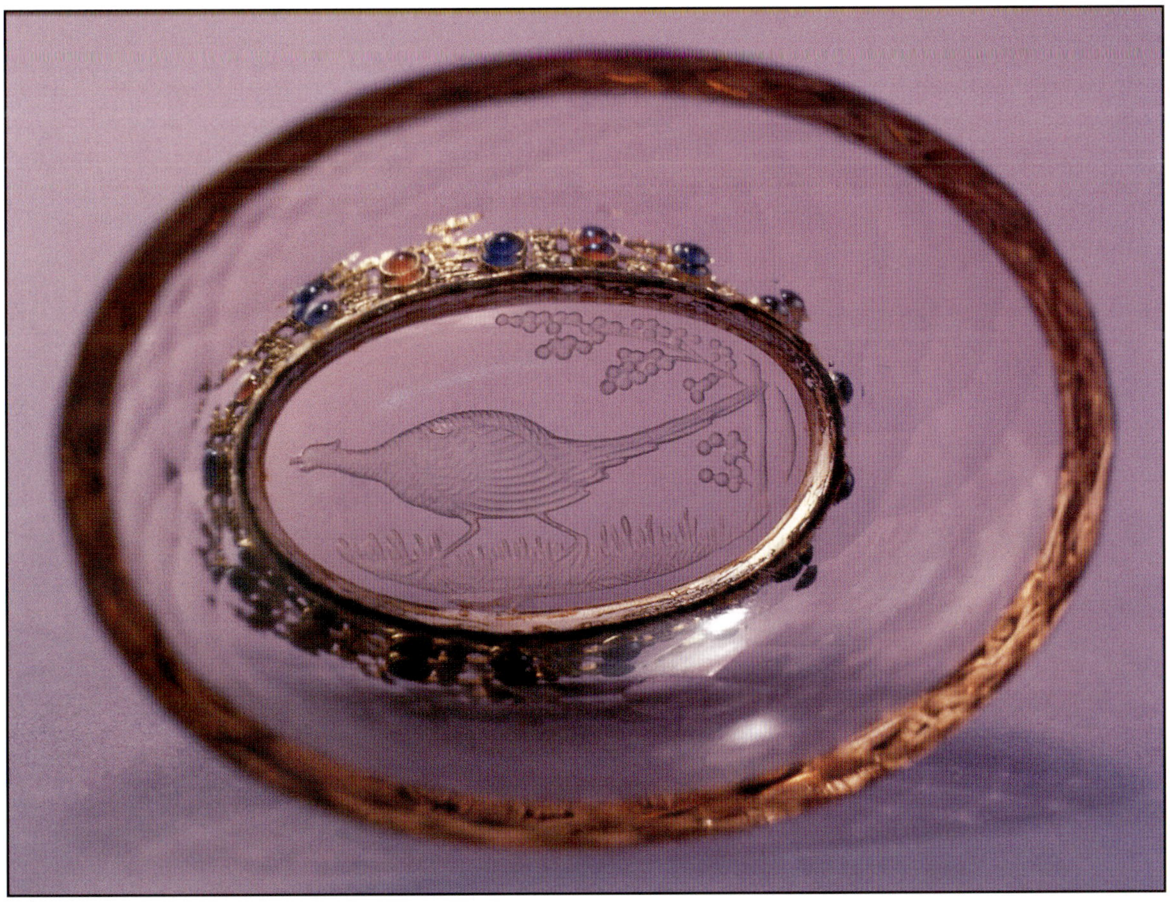

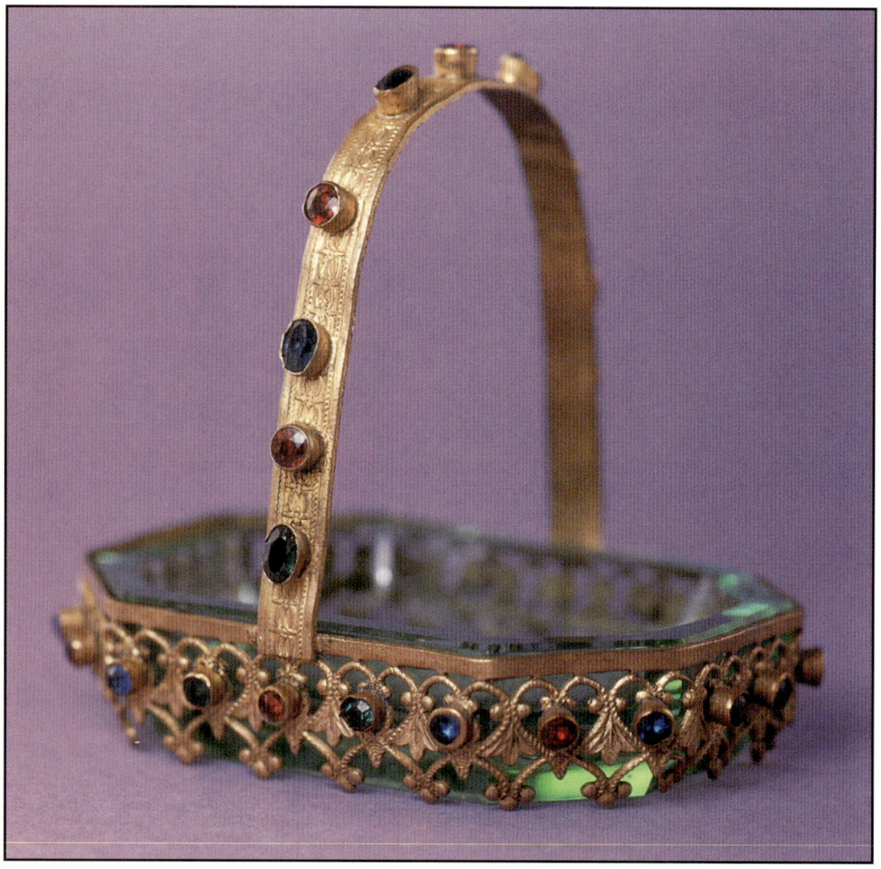

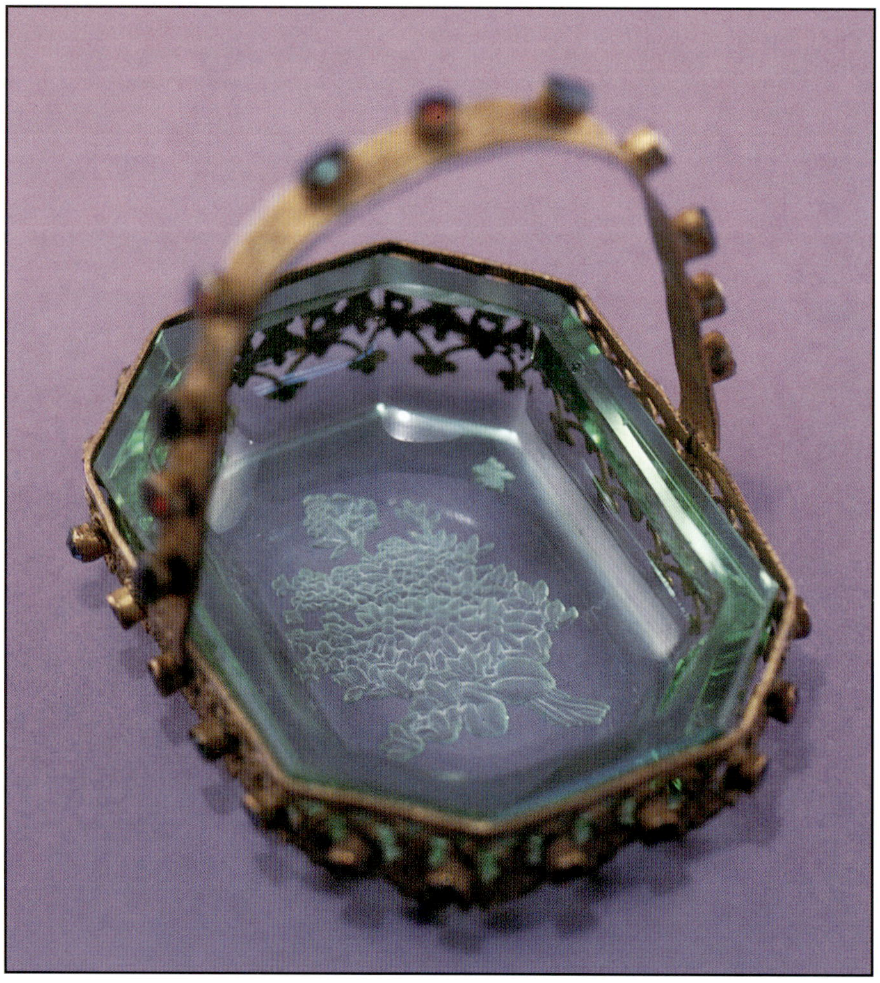

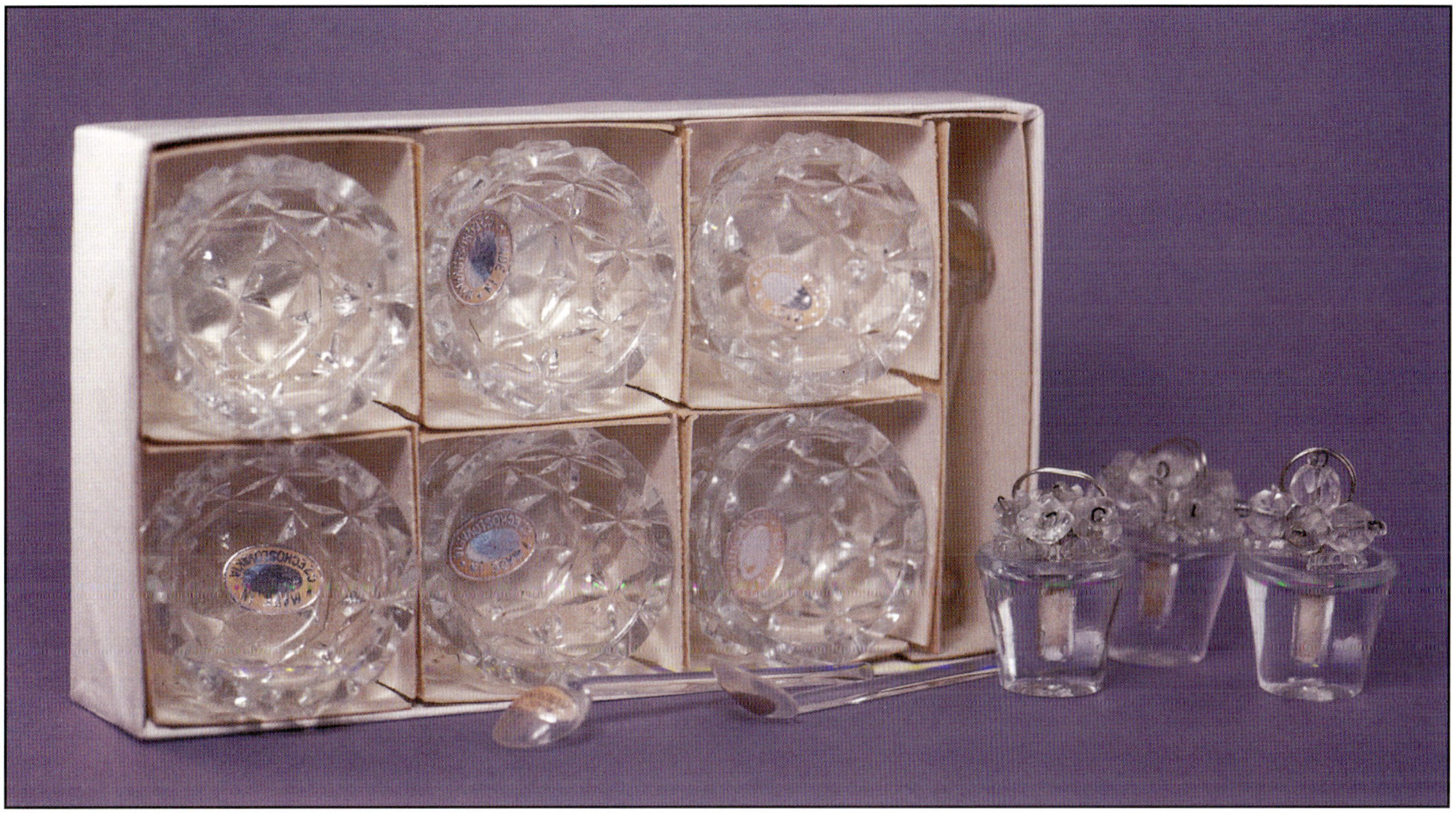

Place card holders are also part of an earlier era, but still add grace to a formal dinner or a party. Those shown were purchased at an average of $10-15 apiece. The clear intaglio one is set onto a silver stand and marked "Austria"; the purchase price was $75.

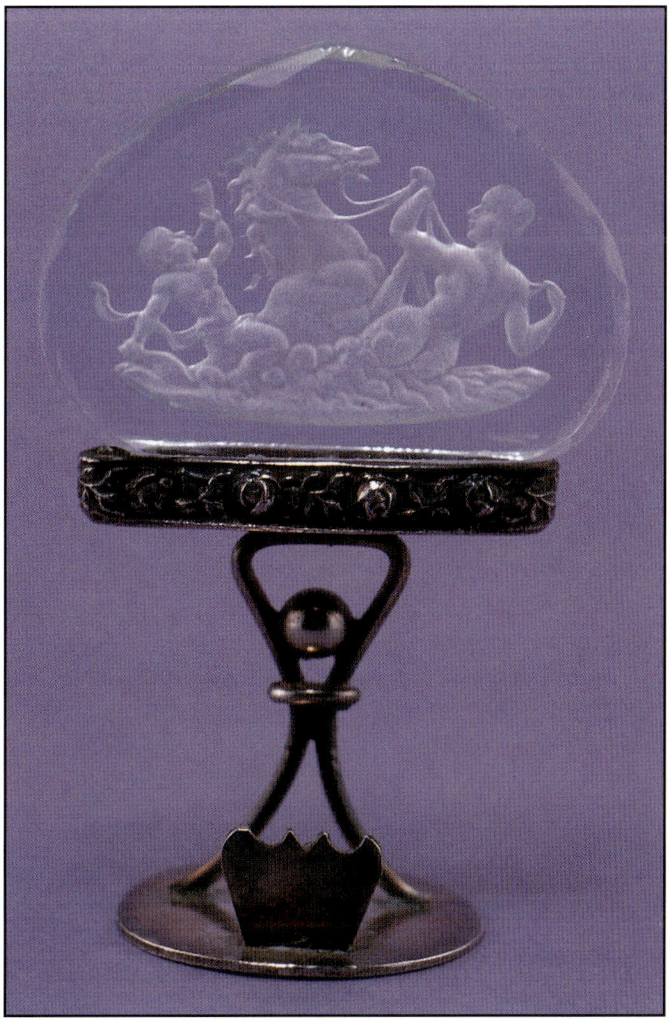

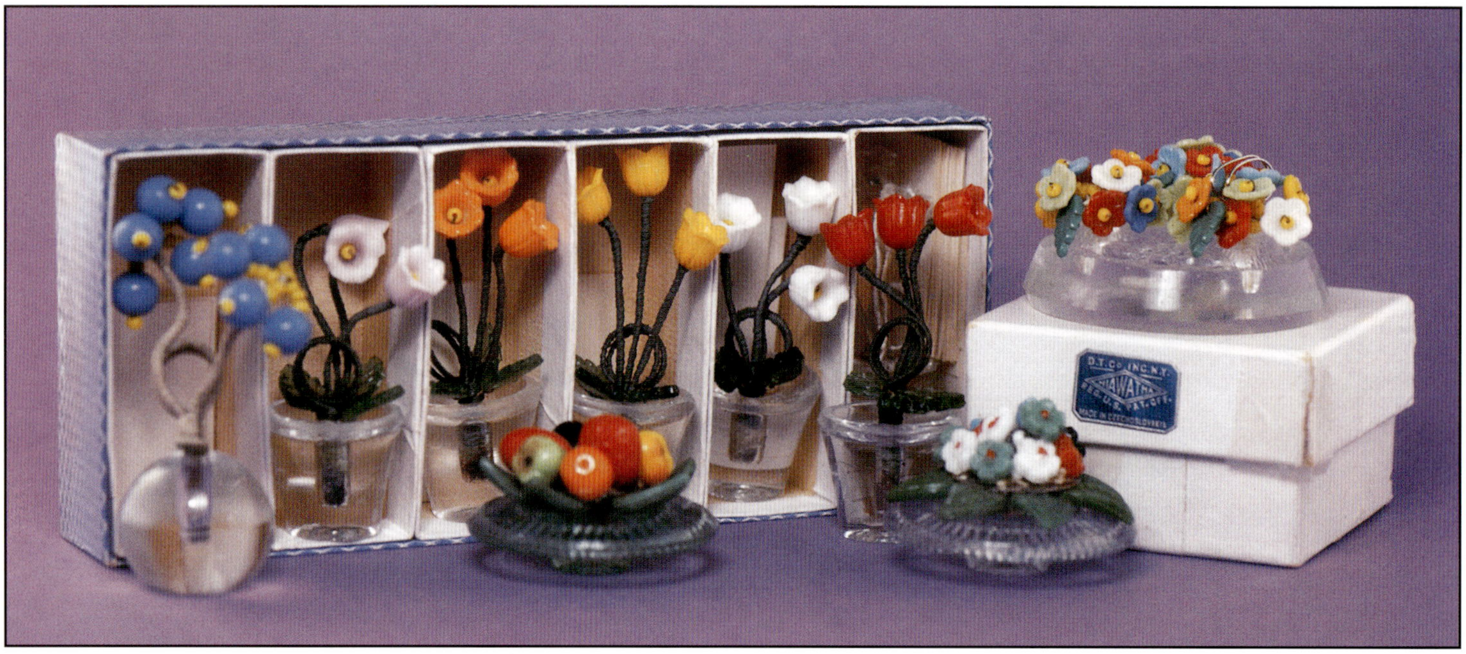
D.T.Co INC. N.Y.
REG. U.S. PAT. OFF.

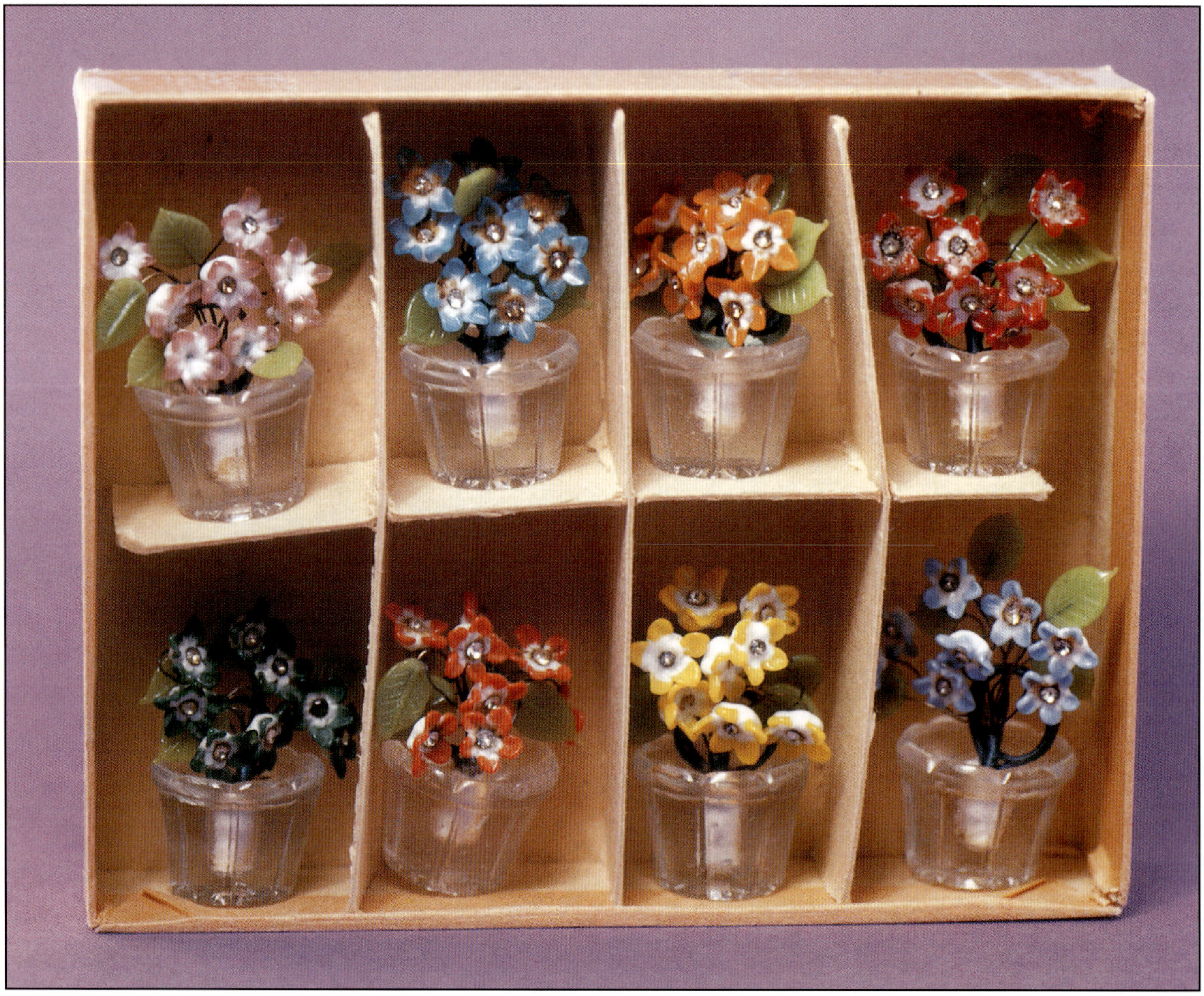

Shown next is a grouping of "Czech pets," small molded glass animals, originally with metal collars and jewel eyes. They are thought to have been used as charms on bracelets and prizes in caramel corn boxes as well as for perfume bottle dangles. The group includes dachshunds, bulldogs, cats, pigs, and a monkey. Other animals were made as well, including camels, bears, rabbits, frogs, and other types of dogs. A St. Nicholas figure was also produced. I purchased my first Czech pet for $15 in the mid 1990s, but the current price is between $35 and $50, with harder-to-find animals sometimes selling for over $100.

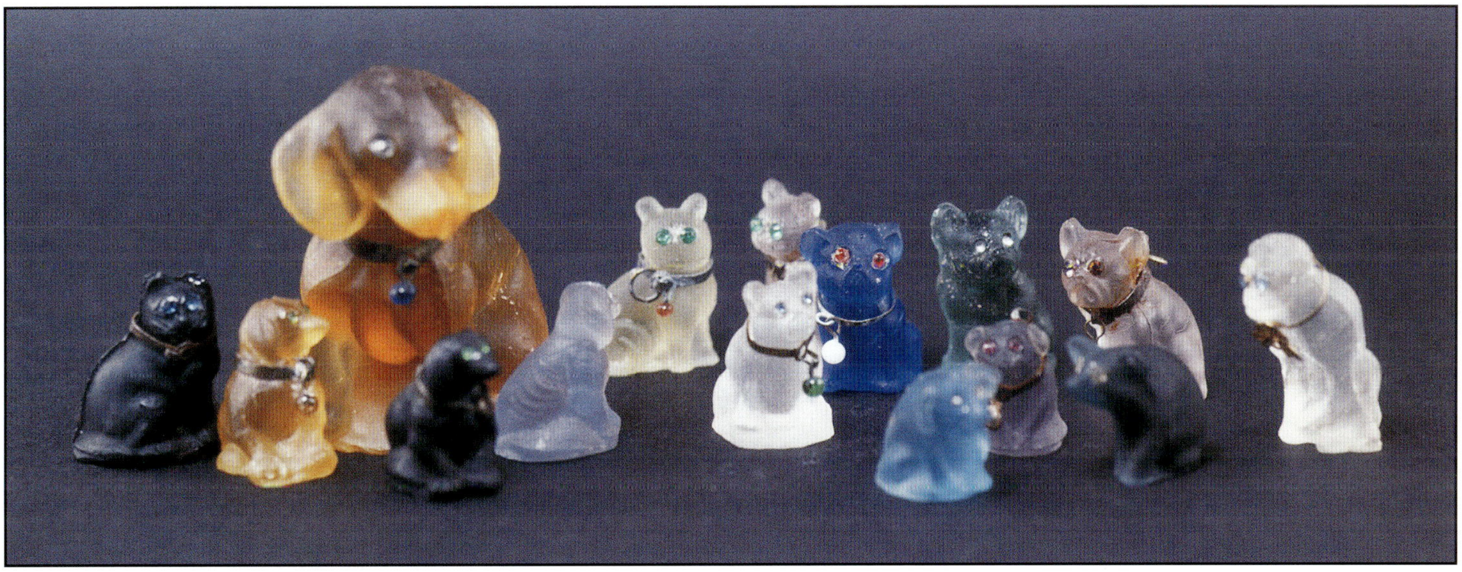

Powder and trinket boxes vary in style and price. The pictured orange box is cased with clear and silhouetted in black enamel. The clear cut glass intaglio box is 3.5" in diameter by 2.625" in height. The pressed green cotton picker is 2.375" tall and 3.25" at the widest point. Expect to pay between $65 and $125 for any of these.

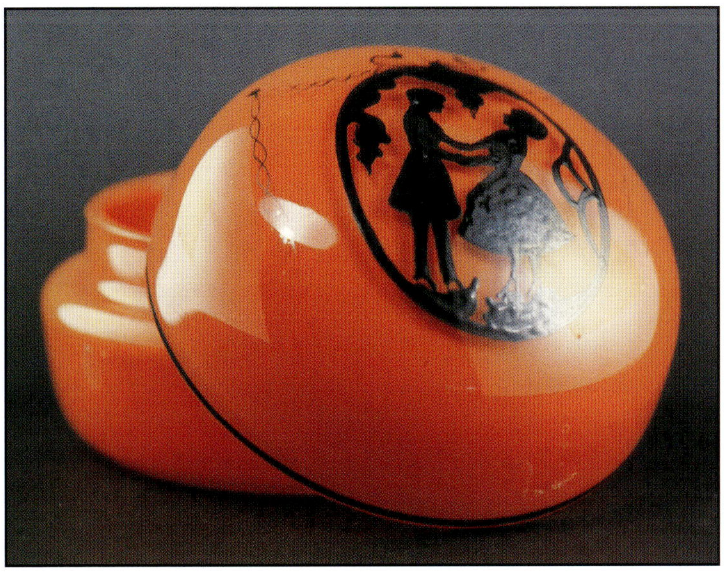

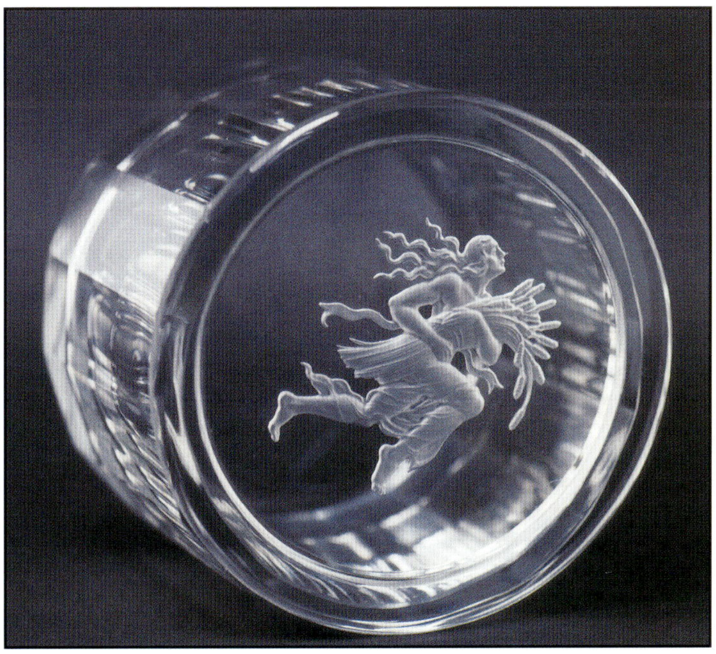

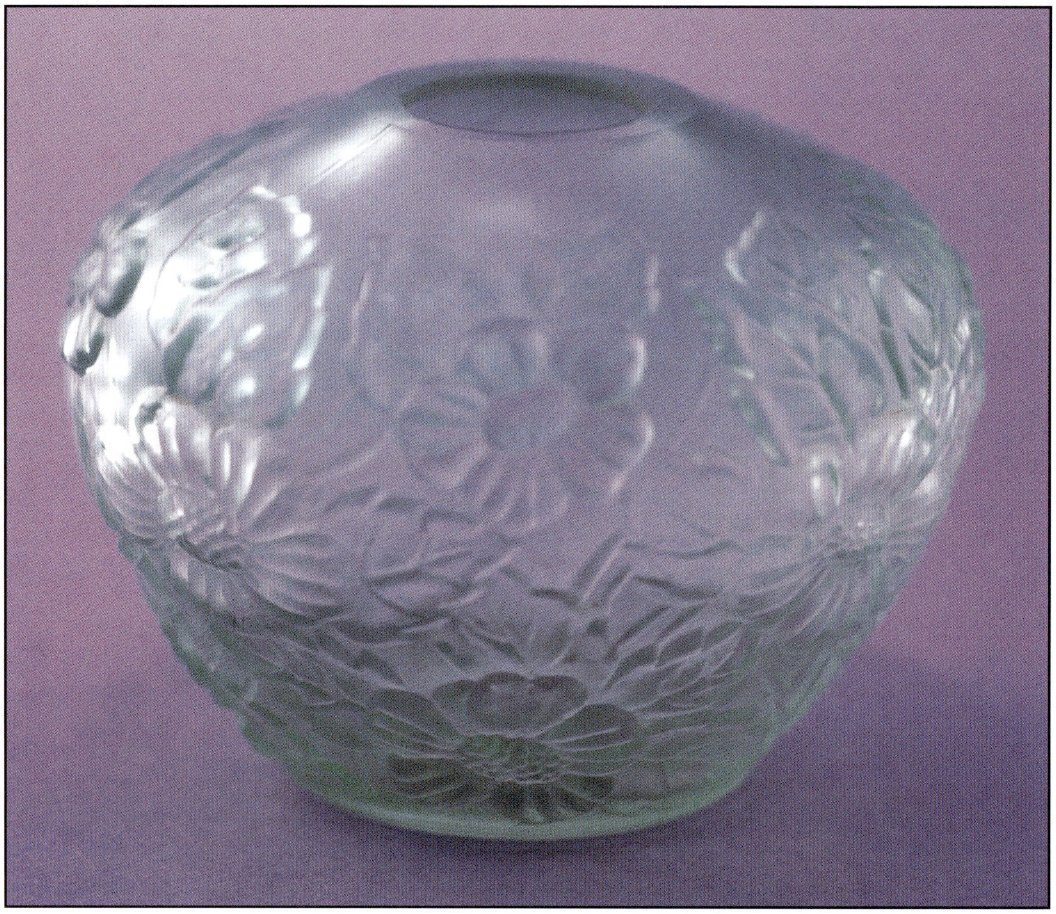

In the next photo, the ash tray shown with a colorful necklace bears a design pictured in the Glassexport catalog. The value would be in the neighborhood of $50. The necklace, however, would be worth between $150-200.

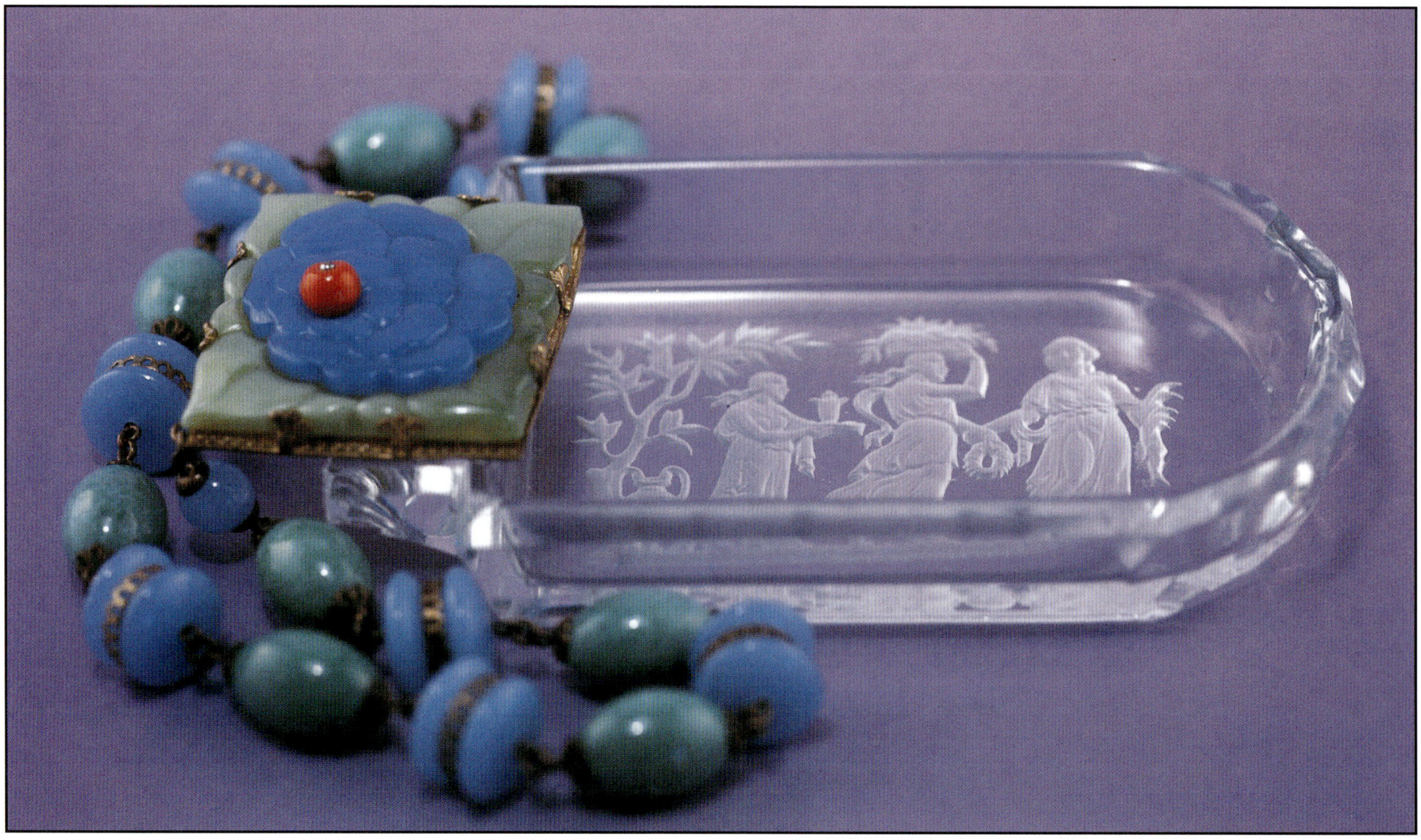

The collector can find many other vanity items, including mirrors, compacts (as shown), puff pats with swans down and a variety of handles, and mirrored trays. Whenever "fun stuff is found, it is always "something to crow about."

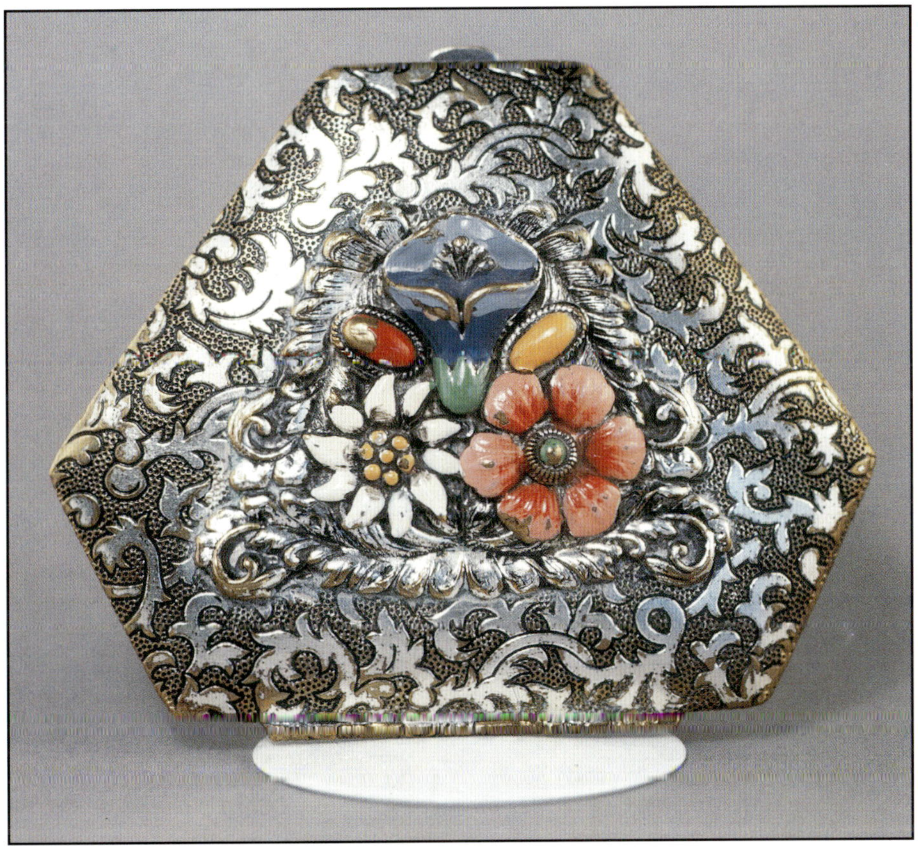

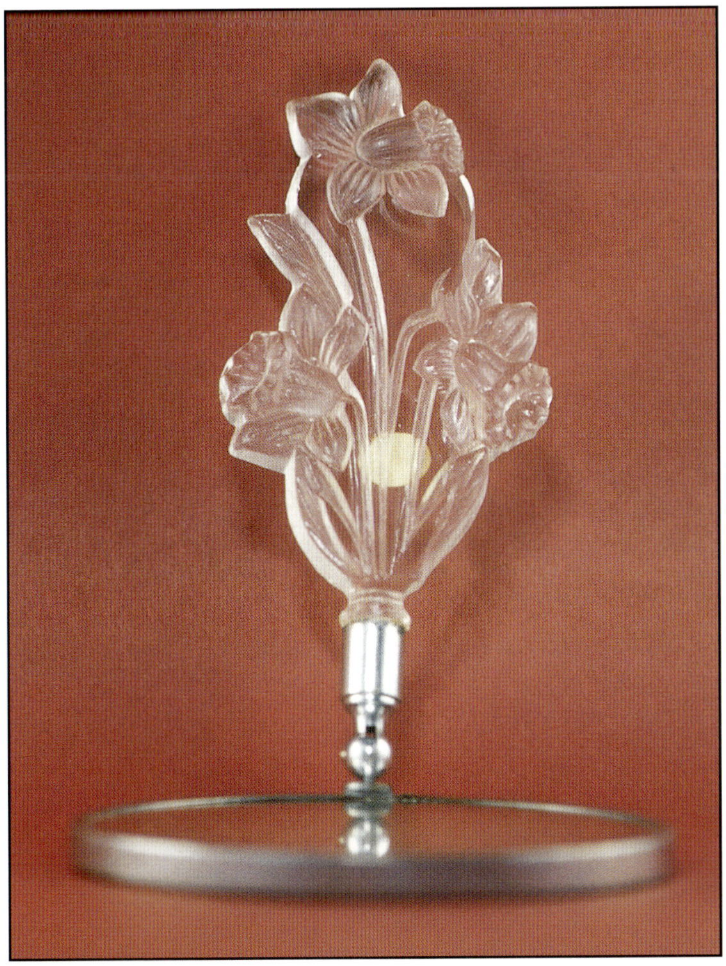

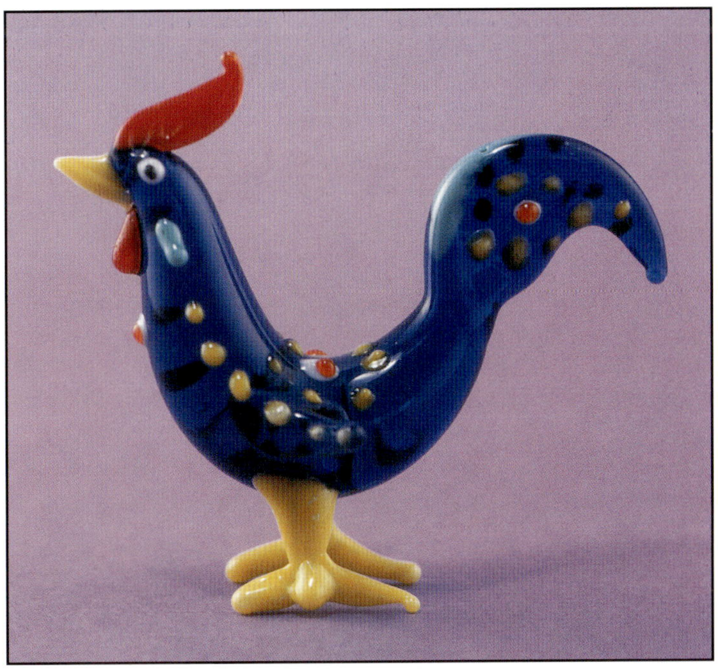

Buying Wisely on the Internet

Buying on the Internet, particularly through eBay auctions, can be both fun and frustrating. If there is any one useful piece of advice, it is to be patient. Discover the resources open to you. Develop a "My eBay" site and move items that interest you to that site where you can examine them on the screen and track the bidding.

Read the item description carefully and examine the pictures. Though most sellers are careful to describe or point out any defect, sometimes the pictures clearly show an unmentioned flaw—which the buyer, it is assumed, will have noticed. Filigree on bottles, for example, is usually symmetrical. What appears to be an asymmetrical design might actually reflect a missing part. Look for missing gems. Look for identifying tags or marks and ask about them if you do not see them. Invest in references and check for the value of similar pieces. Most importantly, do not hesitate to ask questions of the dealer.

Arm yourself with knowledge. An unusual bottle was recently listed on an eBay auction. The art deco stopper was a woman's face in lapis glass; the base was plain, an opaque black cylinder. A similar piece shown in Jones-North (1999, item 589, p. 56) but with the stopper in the more common malachite glass was valued at $2000. This piece, in the more rare blue, sold for about $1250. Probably the seller, who did not seem to know what he had, was delighted, but the buyer got the prize. The more you know, the less likely you are to pay too much for an item or to be fooled by something that is not authentic. Sometimes you get a real bargain.

When you are ready to bid, do it "coolly." Decide how much the item is worth to you and put your bid at that amount. What you have done, then, is to "own" all the prices between the current bidder's top price and your top price. Anyone else bidding will have to go over your top price to get the item—and he or she does not know what that price is. Many people do not want to bid too early in the process because activity calls attention to the item, but there is a bit of an advantage to being the first bidder, especially if you bid the full amount you are willing to pay.

The seller can place a reserve on an item to be sold. That means there is a safety net for the seller, which is usually well above the listed opening amount. If the bidding does not reach that reserve, it does not sell, even if it receives several bids. If your ceiling bid is more than the reserve, the bid raises to the reserve amount and stops. If, however, your highest bid is still below the seller's reserve, the bidding goes to the last active bid and the auction increment is added. You are then the high bidder, but you will not get the item at that bid.

One part of the eBay item screen tells how many bids have been made on this item. Clicking on it will provide a bidding history. This tells you who has bid on the item and the amounts they gave. It will not give you the high bidder's top amount. It is good to track an item even if you have decided that you will not bid on it. At the end of the auction, you can easily see not only the final price, but also the patterns of the bidders.

Unlike a live auction, where bidding is encouraged until the house falls silent under the auctioneer's hammer, an online auction like eBay has a timed item closing. I have made what I consider to be a fair market bid and have "refreshed" my screen to monitor the last minutes of an item only to see that the name on the winning bid is not mine. The person entering an unanswerable bid in the final second has walked away with the item I want for just a dollar or two above my high bid. How did that person "magically" know the exact amount needed to "trump my ace"? In actuality, all he or she needed to do was enter any bid amount with a ceiling higher than mine. The price then advanced to my top bid, the next bidding increment was added, and the item was gone.

I get angry when that happens and end up thinking that the whole thing is stupid and unfair. This kind of disappointing loss is enough to make one wish that on-line auctions could not close until five minutes past the last bid. However, I have also experienced satisfied moments when two people have "cut in" in during the last few seconds and one of them gets stuck paying the other person's inflated ceiling amount.

On the other hand, I have, on occasion, waited until I recovered from my pout and then contacted and congratulated the winner regarding their good taste on the item won. I have ended up with some nice friendships this way, and some good dialogue and picture exchanges. After all, we each share the same passion.

It is good to be philosophical about bidding losses. Few of these bottles were one-of-a-kind, and there are generally other prizes out there if one is patient. Dialogue with other collectors is useful, as sometimes they will sell their duplicates or steer you to a dealer who specializes in what you are looking for. Membership in an organization like the International Perfume Bottle Association also provides collectors with a wonderful support group, great resource information, and opportunities to add to the collection.

Managing the Collection

At some point, the gathering of a number of related items becomes a collection. A growing collection is more than a passion; it is an investment of energy, time, space, and resources. Keeping an item-by-item record, in whatever form it takes, is a needed tool for valuing, insuring, selling, or otherwise disposing of the collection. The objects, in this case perfume bottles, are artifacts—survivors of their time—and thus worthy of thoughtful, careful handling. Their history, too, is important to keep, almost like a genealogy, beginning with the current owner and learning whatever is available including establishing the place and approximate date of origin.

A system for record-keeping, set into place early in the collecting process, saves searching through receipts and check registers later. The easiest method is to record information as each piece enters the collection. Three by five inch index cards are useful, easy to handle, sort, and store. They are available in colors and can be "keyed" to the dominant color of the bottle or to the capstone or focal stone of a purse bottle. For clarity, use one card per item. Information placed on each index card should include, in a consistent format, the general classification of the bottle, its height, identifying marks (or their absence), and a description of the bottle that is accurate enough to differentiate the individual bottle from the group. Other important information includes the name of the seller, date of purchase, and the cost of the item. If a reference to the item is known, that should also be noted specifying the source, publication date, and value, if given. It is also helpful to number the card and place a small removable paper tag with the same number on the bottle. The tag should be placed inconspicuously and should not cover or obscure other original labels, tags, or marks. The back of the card is a good place to store secondary information: a contact number or address of the seller, the original price tag, auction card, or lot number, and perhaps a thumbnail picture of the item.

Besides providing a summary of the collection at one's finger tips, the card is a good location for adding new information; after all, collecting is an ongoing process of discovery. Index cards, especially if they are clearly and consistently organized, will also simplify data entry should one choose to later record onto a database. They also provide a hard copy separate from the computer.

However it is done, keeping a record will save time and frustration in the long run. But if you are not likely to ever construct a formal record, do at least save receipts, storing them in a particular place. Some receipts are pre-printed with the shop or dealer's name, address, and other information, but many are not. Look at the information on the receipt and add a note or two that will help identify the item purchased and supply any other pertinent information.

It is important in gathering artifacts to protect their vulnerable aspects. Labels or packaging can be soiled or damaged by handling or exposure to cleaners or to direct sunlight. Also, since perfume becomes rancid and stale and can even damage bottles, many collectors clean out the residue. Alcohol or inexpensive nail polish remover are effective for cleaning. I recommend putting a small amount into a cap, then pouring from the cap into the bottle by using a funnel. Because any strong solvent or soap has the potential for damaging labels or metal finishes, it is important to control the amount used and the application process. Use the least potent solvent for getting the job done.

Cleaning around filigree should be done with care. Stones, especially those with foil backs, can be damaged, even by water. A set of useful cleaning tools would include a soft-bristled toothbrush, pipe cleaners and cotton swabs. A soft cloth is better than tissue or paper or terry towels for applying cleaner or for drying. Metal filigree that is discolored by contact with perfume can be improved with gentle cleansing, but the metal discoloration overall appears to be permanent.

Placing bottles behind glass allows the collector to control the handling of delicate items by those who are interested in touching them but are not aware of the damage they can do—or, for that matter, the value of what they are holding. Displaying bottles in curio cabinets or other glass fronted cabinets not only shows off the collection nicely and protects it from casual accidents, it also reduces the need to dust—which to some of us is a compelling feature!

Bibliography

Ball, Joanne Dubbs, and Dorothy Hehl Torem. *Commercial Fragrance Bottles*. Atglen, PA: Schiffer Publishing Ltd., 1993.

Ball, Joanne Dubbs, and Dorothy Hehl Torem. *Fragrance Bottle Masterpieces*. Atglen, PA: Schiffer Publishing Ltd., 1996.

Barta, Dale and Diane, and Helen M. Rose. *Czechoslovakian Glass & Collectibles Book II*. Paducah, KY: Collector Books, 1997.

Bowman, Glinda. *Miniature Perfume Bottles*. Atglen, PA: Schiffer Publishing, Ltd., 1994.

Bowman, Glinda. *More Miniature Perfume Bottles*. Atglen, PA: Schiffer Publishing, Ltd., 1996.

Czechoslovak Export Company Ltd. *Jaco Jablonex*. (Product Catalog). Jablonec, Czechoslovakia.

Farnsworth, Helen. *Helen Farnsworth's 30 Year Perfume Library: Perfume Catalogs. Disc I & Disc II*. 2003.

Forsythe, Ruth. *Made in Czechoslovakia*. Galena, OH: Ruth A. Forsythe, 1982.

Forsythe, Ruth. *Made in Czechoslovakia Book 2*. Marietta, OH: Antique Publications, 1993.

Forsythe Auction Book: Czechoslovakian Perfume Bottle Auction: The Ruth Forsythe Collection. Greenville, OH: Jim Wroda Auction Services, Nov. 2, 2002.

Glassexport, No. 1, Section 14. (Product Catalog) Praha, Czechoslovakia.

International Perfume Bottle Quarterly. Volume XIV, Number 3. Spring 2002.

Jargstorf, Sibylle. *Baubles, Buttons and Beads: The Heritage of Bohemia*. Atglen, PA: Schiffer Publishing Ltd., 1993.

Jargstorf, Sibylle. *Glass in Jewelry: Hidden Artistry in Glass*. Atglen, PA: Schiffer Publishing Ltd., 1991.

Leach, Ken. *Perfume Presentation: 100 Years of Artistry*. New York, NY: KRES Publishing Inc., 1997.

Monsen and Baer. *Perfume Bottle Auction Catalogs*. Vienna, VA: Monsen and Baer, 1996, 1997, 2000, 2001, 2002, 2003, 2004, and 2005.

North, Jacquelyne Y. Jones. *Commercial Perfume Bottles*. Atglen, PA: Schiffer Publishing Ltd., 1986.

North, Jacquelyne Y. Jones. *Czechoslovakian Perfume Bottles and Boudoir Accessories Revised Edition*. Marietta, OH: The Glass Press, 1999.

Nový, Petr. *Lisované Sklo a Krystalerie V Jizerských Horách*. Ornela a. s. Desenské sklarny Desná V Jizerských horách a Muzeum skla a bizuterie v Jablonci nad Nisou, 2002.

Rago Arts & Auction Center. *The Fifth Annual Lalique Auction and Perfume Presentations*. Lambertville, NJ: November 6, 2004.

Utt, Marylou and Glen, with Patricia Bayer. *Lalique Perfume Bottles*. New York, NY: Crown Publishers, Inc., 1989.

Revi, Albert Christian. *Nineteenth Century Glass: Its Genesis and Development. Revised Edition*. Atglen, PA: Schiffer Publishing, Ltd., 1959, 1967.

Sloan, Jean. *Perfume & Scent Bottle Collecting*. Radnor, PA: Wallace-Homestead Book Company, 1986.

Truitt, Robert and Deborah. *Collectible Bohemian Glass 1880-1940*. Kensington, MD: B&D Glass, 1995.

Truitt, Robert and Deborah. *Collectible Bohemian Glass Vol. II 1915-1945*. Radnor, PA: Wallace-Homestead Book Company, 1998.

US $69.95

9 780764 324123 56995

ISBN: 0-7643-2412-8